PREVENTION PRACTICE IN PRIMARY CARE

PREVENTION PRACTICE IN PRIMARY CARE

SHERRI N. SHEINFELD GORIN

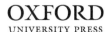
OXFORD
UNIVERSITY PRESS

OXFORD

UNIVERSITY PRESS

Oxford University Press is a department of the University of Oxford.
It furthers the University's objective of excellence in research, scholarship,
and education by publishing worldwide.

Oxford   New York
Auckland   Cape Town   Dar es Salaam   Hong Kong   Karachi
Kuala Lumpur   Madrid   Melbourne   Mexico City   Nairobi
New Delhi   Shanghai   Taipei   Toronto

With offices in
Argentina   Austria   Brazil   Chile   Czech Republic   France   Greece
Guatemala   Hungary   Italy   Japan   Poland   Portugal   Singapore
South Korea   Switzerland   Thailand   Turkey   Ukraine   Vietnam

Oxford is a registered trademark of Oxford University Press
in the UK and certain other countries.

Published in the United States of America by
Oxford University Press
198 Madison Avenue, New York, NY 10016

Library of Congress Cataloging-in-Publication Data
Gorin, Sherri N. Sheinfeld, author, editor of compilation.
Prevention practice in primary care / Sherri N. Sheinfeld Gorin.
p. ; cm.
Includes bibliographical references.
ISBN 978–0–19–537301–1 (alk. paper)
I. Title.
[DNLM: 1. Preventive Health Services.   2. Primary Health Care. WA 108]
RA427.8
362.1—dc23
2013019025

9 8 7 6 5 4 3 2 1
Printed in the United States of America
on acid-free paper

I dedicate this book to my beloved family.

אלמ סלוע סייק וליאכ בותכה וילע הלעמ לארשימ תחא שפנ סייקמה לכו

He [sic] who saves a single… life (is) as if he [sic] has saved the entire world.

—BABYLONIAN TALMUD, *Sanhedrin* 37a

הופטשי אל תורהנו הבהאה תא תובכל ולכוי אל סיבר סימ

Vast floods cannot quench love, no river can sweep it away.

—*Song of Songs* 8:7

Translated by Rabbi Evan (Moshe) Gorin

CONTENTS

FOREWORD

Nearly two decades ago, when my colleagues and I directly observed and carefully analyzed 4,454 patient visits to 138 family physicians, we were shocked at how much prevention work was done, considering how little was paid for. Prevention was the main focus of 12% of visits;[1] a third of illness visits included "opportunistic" preventive service delivery;[2] family information was addressed during half of new patient visits and nearly a quarter of follow up visits;[3] health behavior change was pursued during half of all visits.[4]

Now is a different era. Both prevention[5] and primary care[6] are "in"—driven by widespread recognition of the poor performance, fragmentation, and unsustainability of solely disease-focused health care systems. Primary care still is where most clinical preventive services are delivered, and where prevention is integrated with chronic disease management, family care, and teachable moments for behavior change.

The core attributes of primary care[7, 8] provide a perfect platform for prevention:

- first contact access;
- a comprehensive whole-person focus;
- integration and coordination of care;
- an ongoing relationship with individuals, families, and communities.

Primary care adds a focus on person, family, and community to a health care system that often is driven more by relentlessly delivering commodities of health care than by integrating, personalizing, and prioritizing what is needed to make it possible for people and communities to do what is important to them.

The same needs for effectiveness, integration, and sustainability drive a growing recognition of the vital importance of connecting public health and primary care for prevention—bringing together the complementary strengths of focusing on both the person and the population.[9] The linking of primary care and public health in this new era is supported by new understanding of systems science, by the possibility of previously unavailable information support, and by a sense of necessity amidst shortage.[10]

Prevention Practice in Primary Care brings to the current era a guidebook of prevention science, systems, and sense of possibilities.

Prevention science is made clear in chapters addressing theory and epidemiology that help us to understand, focus our interventions, and continue to learn. The rich discussion of both macro- and micro-level theories in Chapter 3 gives us guiding principles of health behaviors and frameworks for developing effective partnerships to help people improve them.

Prevention systems are addressed at multiple levels that interact to support prevention amidst the competing demands of primary care. A systems perspective is essential as primary care reinvents itself to be able to take both a patient-centered approach that is responsive to patient needs and values, and a proactive approach that is necessary to provide clinical preventive service delivery and integrate it with illness management. The discussion in Chapter 11 of systems to support patient-directed approaches highlights an area of growing importance.

Prevention possibilities are highlighted in multiple chapters that address the current policy and payment environment, information technology platforms, and engagement of patients as partners.

Chapter 8, "Personalizing Prevention," details emerging opportunities for complementing the primary care strength of personalizing care for the whole person, with the possibility of tailoring prevention based on genomic information. The important implications of the emerging patient-centered medical home model for prevention are addressed in Chapter 10.

Prevention Practice in Primary Care dances between the big picture and on-the-ground perspectives that are essential to personalizing the population approach and developing the needed partnerships and systems support to harness the disease prevention potential of primary care and engaged patients. This multilevel focus helps us to identify the most fruitful lever points for effective prevention. Most frequently, these points of maximum effect involve not just a base and a fulcrum, but the complex and emergent interactions that occur at the intersections between the person/patient, family, primary care practice, health care and public health systems, community partners, and public policy. *Prevention Practice in Primary Care* provides a platform to make sense of this complexity and to help people and populations to be healthier.

Kurt C. Stange, MD, PhD
Promoting Health Across Boundaries,
www.PHAB.us
Editor, *Annals of Family Medicine*,
www.AnnFamMed.org
American Cancer Society Clinical
Research Professor
Gertrude Donnelly Hess, MD
Professor of Oncology Research
Professor of Family Medicine
and Community Health,

Epidemiology and Biostatistics,
Sociology and Oncology
Case Western Reserve University

1. Stange KC, Zyzanski SJ, Jaen CR, et al. Illuminating the black box: a description of 4454 patient visits to 138 family doctors. *J Fam Pract.* 1998;46(5):377–389.
2. Stange KC, Flocke SA, Goodwin MA. Opportunistic preventive services delivery: are time limitations and patient satisfaction barriers? *J Fam Pract.* 1998;46(5):419–424.
3. Medalie JH, Zyzanski SJ, Langa D, Stange KC. The family in family practice: is it a reality? *J Fam Pract.* May 1998;46(5):390–396.
4. Stange KC, Gjeltema K, Woolf SH. One minute for prevention: the power of leveraging to fulfill the promise of health behavior counseling. A. *J Prev Med* 2002;22(4):320–323.
5. Woolf SH. A closer look at the economic argument for disease prevention. *JAMA.* Feb 4 2009;301(5):536–538.
6. Okie S. The evolving primary care physician. *N Engl J Med.* May 17 2012;366(20):1849–1853.
7. Donaldson MS, Yordy KD, Lohr KN, Vanselow NA, eds. *Primary Care: America's Health in a New Era.* Washington, DC: National Academy Press; 1996.
8. Stange KC, Nutting PA, Miller WL, et al. Defining and measuring the patient-centered medical home. *J Gen Intern Med.* 2010;25(6):601–612.
9. Institute of Medicine. *Primary Care and Public Health: Exploring Integration to Improve Population Health.* Washington, DC: National Academies Press; 2012.
10. Sweeney SA, Bazemore A, Phillips RL, Jr, Etz RS, Stange KC. A reemerging political space for linking person and community through primary health care. *Am J Public Health.* Jun 2012;102 Suppl 3:S336–341.

ACKNOWLEDGMENTS

It is with deep appreciation that I thank the following individuals for their contributions to this book:

William Lamsbeck, who brought the proposal to Oxford University Press.

Chad Zimmerman, for his support of the book over an extended period of time.

Kurt Roediger for his copy editing of the initial stages of the book.

Newgen Knowledge Works Pvt Ltd for their attentive copy editing.

I thank the outstanding contributors, each of whom greatly shaped this book and to whom I am indebted.

Finally, although this book is dedicated to my family, I wish to again acknowledge the special contributions of my husband, Brian, my father and mother, Albert and Gertrude Sheinfeld, each of whom encouraged me to complete the book despite many delays. I am grateful to my children, Aaron and Evan (Moshe), their spouses, and a growing group of grandchildren, my brother, Stephen, sister-in-law, Jane, and my nephews, all of whose lives I hope to extend and enrich with a focus on prevention.

Sherri N. Sheinfeld Gorin

CONTRIBUTORS

FARUQUE AHMED, PHD, MPH
Senior Scientist, Immunization Services Division
National Center for Immunization and Respiratory
  Diseases
Centers for Disease Control and Prevention
Atlanta, GA

CHARLES BENNETT, MD, PHD, MPP
Professor
Clinical Pharmacy and Outcomes Sciences
University of South Carolina College of Pharmacy
Columbia, SC

SENAIDA FERNANDEZ, PH.D.
California Breast Cancer Research Program
University of California Office of the President
Oakland, CA

AARON P. GORIN, MHA
Director of Research, Juvenile Diabetes Cure
  Alliance
New York, NY

SHERRI N. SHEINFELD GORIN, PHD
Senior Scientific Consultant (SAIC), Division of
  Cancer Control and Population Sciences
National Cancer Institute, National Institutes
  of Health
Bethesda, MD
Director, New York Physicians Against Cancer
  (NYPAC)
New York, NY
Formerly
Associate Professor, Columbia University
Senior Member, Herbert Irving Comprehensive
  Cancer Center
New York, NY

RAMSAY HOGUET, JD, MPH
Massachusetts Center for Health Information
  and Analysis
Boston, MA

KATHLEEN KENNY, MD
Clinical Associate Professor
Stanford School of Medicine
Stanford, CA

ZHIQIANG LU, PHD
University of South Carolina College of Pharmacy
Columbia, SC

ALANNA MURDAY, BS
University of South Carolina College of Pharmacy
Columbia, SC

GBENGA OGEDEGBE, MD, MS, MPH, FACP
Professor of Population Health and Medicine
Department of Population Health
New York University School of Medicine
New York, NY

JOSEPH RAVENELL, MD, MS
Assistant Professor of Medicine
Division of General Internal Medicine
New York University School of Medicine
New York, NY

FRED RINCON, MD, MSC, FACP
Assistant Professor of Neurology and Neurological
  Surgery
Jefferson Medical College of Thomas Jefferson
  University
Philadelphia, PA

ANTOINETTE SCHOENTHALER, EDD, MA
Assistant Professor of Medicine
Division of General Internal Medicine
New York University School of Medicine
New York, NY

YALINI SENATHIRAJAH, PHD
Assistant Professor
Department of Medical Informatics
SUNY Downstate Medical Center
Brooklyn, NY

STEVEN TEUTSCH, MD, MPH
Chief Science Officer
Los Angeles County Department of Public Health
Los Angeles, CA

SANDRA A TSAI, MD, MPH
Clinical Assistant Professor, Medicine
Stanford School of Medicine
Stanford, CA

MARC S. WILLIAMS, MD, FAAP, FACMG
Director of the Genomic Medicine Institute
Geisinger Health System
Danville, PA

CLINTON WRIGHT, MD, MS
Associate Professor of Neurology, Neuroscience,
    and Epidemiology and Public Health
University of Miami
Miami, FL

BARBARA P. YAWN, MD, MSC, FAAFP
Director of Research, Olmsted Medical Center
Adjunct Professor, Family and Community Health
University of Minnesota
Rochester, MN

ABOUT THE EDITOR

Sherri N. Sheinfeld Gorin, Ph.D., Fellow, Society of Behavioral Medicine, is a Senior Scientific Consultant (Leidos Biomedical Research, Inc.) to the Division of Cancer Control and Population Sciences, National Cancer Institute, U.S. National Institutes of Health. She is also Director of New York Physicians Against Cancer, (NYPAC), a grant-funded research and training group that works with primary care physicians to reduce health disparities in cancer prevention and screening. Most recently, she was Associate Professor, Columbia University, and Member, Herbert Irving Comprehensive Cancer Center. On her recent sabbatical at the Mayo Clinic Arizona, she established and directed their first Office of Cancer Health Disparities Research, a unique entity among comprehensive cancer centers nationwide. A Fellow of the Society of Behavioral Medicine, she has authored over 250 peer reviewed publications, book chapters, and presentations. She has also published two books (*The Health Promotion Handbook* and *Health Promotion in Practice*). She serves as a reviewer and/or editorial board member for more than 30 scientific journals.

Her scholarly interests span the fields of cancer and social epidemiology, health services research, health policy and management, behavioral medicine, social work, health psychology, and implementation science. Her primary interests are in the implications of disparities, particularly among ethnic and racial subgroups,, in cancer prevention, screening, and treatment outcomes for breast, colorectal, prostate, and cervical cancer. She and her team have pioneered the theory and systematic educational approach of "academic detailing," sharing the evidence for cancer prevention, screening, and surveillance using brief, repeated, face-to-face or digital "visits" with primary care physicians who work in under-resourced communities. Their published findings, including a high impact cost-effectiveness analysis, have influenced the adoption of academic detailing approaches by local Departments of Health, the American Cancer Society at the national level, and internationally. Similarly, she has published several high impact systematic reviews and meta-analyses that examine primary care approaches to public health problems of smoking, pain among cancer survivors, and cancer care coordination.

Using US population databases, she has examined race and ethnicity as a predictor of breast cancer diagnosis and treatment delay and survival, and the impact of dementia on cancer treatment. She has examined inter-ethnic variations among Hispanics in genetic testing and screening across the United States. Dr. Sheinfeld Gorin has explored the impact of social context on health related quality of life among Medicare health plan participants. These papers have received repeated national media coverage, have informed national policy debates, led to changes at local health care systems and in clinical practice.

She and her research team have received large, multi-year grant awards from NCI, DOD, CDC, the Robert Wood Johnson Foundation, and other highly competitive funders. In addition, she has received recognition and awards for her scientific contributions and leadership from entities as diverse as the Prostate Cancer Foundation, an African American–led patient prostate cancer prevention advocacy group, the American Society for Clinical Oncology (ASCO), and the international Women against Cervical Cancer (WACC).

Dr. Sheinfeld Gorin has been a leader in the international Cochrane Collaboration, the American Society for Preventive Oncology and the American Association for Cancer Research. In addition to being an elected Fellow, she is Chair, Scientific and Professional Liaison Council, and sits on the Board of the Society for Behavioral Medicine (SBM). Dr. Sheinfeld Gorin is a frequent invited scientific contributor to NIH study sections, having served as a permanent member of the NIH Health Services Organization and Delivery study section (HSOD), the primary review group for health services research at the NIH.

Her career has been devoted to prevention in primary care and to increasing health equity.

1

Challenges and Strengths of Prevention Practice in Primary Care

SHERRI N. SHEINFELD GORIN

Health care in America has experienced an explosion in knowledge, innovation, and capacity to prevent and manage previously fatal conditions. Yet, paradoxically, it falls short on such fundamentals as quality, outcomes, cost, and equity (Institute of Medicine, 2012).

Some 40% of deaths are caused by behavior patterns that could be modified by preventive interventions (McGinnis, Williams-Russo, Knickman, 2002). In particular, tobacco use, poor diet, and physical inactivity have contributed to the largest number of deaths, and deaths related to these behaviors have been increasing (Mokdad et al., 2005). Yet, only about 5% of the $2.7 trillion dollars—a 17.9% share of gross domestic product (GDP)—that we spend as a nation on health goes to population-wide health improvement, while 95% goes to direct medical care services (Centers for Medicare and Medicaid Services, 2000; Brown et al., 1992). And, of late, out-of-pocket personal health care spending for direct medical care services has accelerated, so more of these monies are coming from patients themselves (Hartman et al., 2013). Despite this high cost, the United States health care system often fails to provide high-quality and efficient health care (McGlynn, Asch, Adams, et al., 2003; Jencks, Huff, Cuerdon, 2003; Saaddine, Cadwell, Gregg, et al., 2006; Grant, Buse, Meigs, 2005; Nolte & McKee, 2008).

Each action that could improve quality–developing knowledge, translating new information into medical evidence, applying the new evidence to patient care—is marred by significant shortcomings and inefficiencies that result in missed opportunities, waste, and harm to patients. And clinical preventive services are a small proportion of the influences on personal disease risk.

The World Health Organization defines health as "…a state of complete physical, mental and social well-being and not merely the absence of disease or infirmity" (Preamble to the Constitution of the World Health Organization, 1948). This definition of health—as well as others, including health as a balanced state, health as goodness of fit, health as transcendence, and health as power (Arnold & Breen, 2006)—suggests that prevention includes not only the reduction of preventable deaths but also the promotion of optimal health, by mobilizing multilevel approaches toward change (as will be discussed further in Chapters 2 and 3).

Using the best available estimates, on a population basis, the impacts of various domains on early deaths in the United States distribute roughly as follows: genetic predispositions, about 30%; behavioral patterns, 40%; social circumstances, 15%; environmental exposures, 5%; and better availability or quality of medical care, 10%. Ultimately, the health fate of each of us is determined by the interaction of these multi-level factors within us (McGinnis & Foege, 1993). Looking at clinical services for prevention, overall, Americans receive only about half of the recommended care (McGinnis & Foege, 1993)—a finding that highlights the national need for improved health promotion (McGlynn, Asch, Adams, et al., 2003). A significant underuse of preventive care results not only in lost lives, but in inefficient use of health care dollars. Clinical preventive services are immunizations, disease screenings, and behavioral counseling interventions delivered to individuals in clinical settings for the purpose of preventing disease or initiating early treatment for conditions that are not yet apparent. Their health impact can be considerable (see Table 1-1). In 2007, the use of just five preventive services that are recommended by the US Preventive Services Task Force (USPSTF; described in Chapter 2) or the national Advisory Committee on Immunization Practices

TABLE 1-1. MOST COST-EFFECFIVE CLINICAL PREVENTIVE SERVICES*

Cost saving

Advising at-risk adults to consider taking aspirin daily

Childhood immunizations

Pneumococcal immunization (adults 65+)

Smoking cessation advice and help to quit

Screening adults for alcohol misuse and brief counseling

Vision screening (adults 65+)

$0 to $15,000/QALY

Chlamydia screening (sexually active adolescents and young women)

Colorectal cancer screening (adults 50+)

Influenza immunization (adults 50+)

Pneumococcal immunization (adults 65+)

Vision screening in preschool age children

$15,000 to $50,000/QALY

Breast cancer screening (women 40+)

Cervical cancer screening (all women)

Cholesterol screening (men 35+ and women 45+)

Counseling women of childbearing age to take folic acid supplements

Counseling women to use calcium supplements

Injury prevention counseling for parents of young children

Hypertension screening (all adults)

QALYs, Quality Adjusted Life-Years, are metrics in which the harms (of worsening health states) are subtracted from the benefits (of improved health states) over a specific period of time.
*Most cost-effective preventive services among the 25 preventive services recommended by the USPSTF and ACIP that were evaluated by the National Commission on Prevention Priorities.
Source: Partnership for Prevention. A National Profile on Use, Disparities, and Health Benefits (2007). Retrieved December 14, 2012, from: www.prevent.org/NCPP. Maciosck MV, Coftfield AB, Edwards NM, Goodman MJ, Flottemesch TJ, Solberg LI, Priorities among effective clinical preventive services: result of a systematic review and analysis. *Am J Prev Med.* 2006;31(1):52–61.

(ACIP), which evaluates the clinical appropriateness of immunizations, would have saved more than 100,000 lives each year in the United States.

Further, using national data sources, the *Partnership for Prevention* found that:

- 45,000 additional lives would be saved each year if we increased to 90% the portion of adults who take aspirin daily to prevent heart disease. In 2013, fewer than half of American adults took aspirin as a preventive measure.

- 42,000 additional lives would be saved each year if we increased to 90% the portion of smokers who are advised by a health professional to quit and are offered medication or other assistance. In 2013, only 28% of smokers received such services.

- 14,000 additional lives would be saved each year if we increased to 90% the portion of adults aged 50 and older who are up to date with any recommended screening for colorectal cancer. In 2013, fewer than 50% of adults were up to date with screening.

- 12,000 additional lives would be saved each year if we increased to 90% the portion of adults aged 50 and older immunized against influenza annually. In 2013, 37% of adults had an annual flu vaccination.

- 3,700 additional lives would be saved each year if we increased to 90% the portion of women aged 40 and older who have been screened for breast cancer in the past 2 years. In 2013, 67% of women had been screened in the past 2 years.

- Breast and cervical cancer screening rates were lower in 2005 compared to five years earlier for every major racial and ethnic group: White, Hispanic, African American and Asian women all experienced declines.

- 30,000 cases of pelvic inflammatory disease would be prevented annually if we increased to 90% the portion of sexually active young women who have been screened in the past year for chlamydial infection. In 2013, 40% of young women were being screened annually.

The underuse of preventive services is even more pronounced among racial and ethnic subgroups, as well as among low-income Americans. For example, Hispanic Americans have lower utilization compared to non-Hispanic whites and African Americans for 10 preventive services:

- Hispanic smokers are 55% less likely to get assistance to quit smoking from a health professional than white smokers.

- Hispanic adults aged 50 and older are 39% less likely to be up to date on colorectal cancer screening than white adults.

- Hispanic adults aged 65 and older are 55% less likely to have been vaccinated against pneumococcal disease than white adults.

- Asian Americans have the lowest utilization of any group for aspirin use as well as breast, cervical, and colorectal cancer screening.
- Asian men aged 40 and older and women aged 50 and older are 40% less likely to use aspirin to prevent heart disease than white adults.
- Asian adults aged 50 and older are 40% less likely to be up to date on colorectal screening than white adults.
- Asian women aged 18 to 64 are 25% less likely to have been screened for cervical cancer in the past 3 years than white women.
- Asian women aged 40 and older are 21% less likely to have been screened for breast cancer in the past two years than white women.
- Despite higher screening rates among African Americans for colorectal and breast cancer compared to Hispanic and Asian Americans, increasing screening in African Americans would have a bigger impact on their health because they have higher mortality for these conditions.
- If the percentage of African Americans aged 50 and older who are up to date with recommended screening for colorectal cancer increased from the current rate of 42% to 90%, 1,800 additional lives would be saved annually. This is a rate of 26 per 100,000 African Americans aged 50 and older, substantially more than the corresponding rates of 17, 15, and 15 per 100,000 additional lives saved for whites, Hispanics, and Asians, respectively.

Low utilization rates for cost-effective preventive services reflect the lack of emphasis that our health care system currently gives to providing these services. Racial and ethnic minorities are receiving even less preventive care than the general US population. Expanding the delivery of this care of proven value would enable millions of Americans to live longer, healthier, and more fulfilling lives. And the United States would get more value—in terms of premature death and illness avoided—for the dollars it spends on health care services.

Since the great majority of patients prefer to seek initial care from a primary care physician rather than a specialist (Grumbach, Selby, Damberg, et al., 1999), the primary care physician is generally the first to deliver clinical services for the prevention of disease and the promotion of health. Specifically, of the nearly 956 million visits that Americans made to

office-based physicians in 2008, 51.3% were to primary care physicians (National Center for Health Statistics, 2011; AHRQ, 2011). *Most important, the primary care physician has the potential to influence the health trajectory for all in this country.*

In 2010, there were approximately 209,000 practicing primary care physicians in the United States (using the American Medical Association Physician Masterfile). Of the 624,434 physicians in the United States who spend the majority of their time in direct patient care, slightly less than one-third are specialists in primary care (National Center for Health Statistics, 2011; AHRQ, 2011). Primary care physicians consist of family physicians and general practitioners, general internists, general pediatricians, and geriatricians.

As US health care has traditionally been based on a solid foundation of primary care to meet the majority of preventive, acute, and chronic health care needs of its population, the recent challenges facing health care in the United States have been particularly magnified within the primary care setting (see Figures 1-1 through 1-4).

Fewer US physicians are choosing primary care as a profession (Bodenheimer, 2006), as a result, the per capita supply of primary care physicians is lower than that of specialty providers (National Ambulatory Medical Care Survey, NAMCS, 2009–2010). At the same time, based on 2009–2010 data, the annual volume of visits per primary care physician exceeded the corresponding volume per specialty physician by 30%. Although primary care physicians' annual visit loads were higher compared with specialty physicians, access to primary care in 2009–2010 was more available than access to specialty care by several measures. Primary care physicians were more likely than specialty physicians to spend more hours per week providing direct patient care, to treat patients in their offices during evening and weekend hours, to report shorter waiting periods for patients to get an appointment for a routine medical examination, and to have practices that set aside time for same-day appointments.

Nonetheless, a growing proportion of patients report that they cannot schedule timely appointments with their physicians. Emergency departments are overflowing with patients who do not have access to primary care. Access is a particularly acute problem for those without private insurance (Decker, 2009; Medicare Payment Advisory Commission. Report to the Congress: Medicare Payment Policy, 2013), and for those who live in rural areas where primary care physicians are particularly scarce and distances

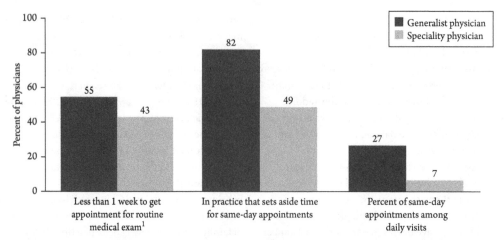

FIGURE 1-1: Percentage of Physicians by Time to Get an Appointment, Whether Practice Sets Aside Time for Same-Day Appointments, and Percentage of Same-Day Appointments, and by Specialty: United States, 2009–2010.

[1]Excludes physicians who did not provide routine medical examinations (14% of specialty physicians).

Note: All differences between generalist and specialty physicians are statistically significant (p <0.05). Generalist physicians include family and general practitioners, internists, and pediatricians; specialty physicians include all other specialties.

Source: CDC/NCHS, National Ambulatory Medical Care Survey.

Note: The health benefits of preventive services were defined as clinically preventable burden (CPB), or the disease, injury or premature death that would be prevented if the service were delivered to all people in the target population. The economic value of preventive services was measured as cost-effectiveness (CE), which compares the net cost of a service to its health benefits. CE provided a standard measure for comparing services' return on investment. Services that produce the most health benefits received the highest CPB score of 5. Services that were most cost-effective received the highest CE score of 5. Scores for CPB and CE were then added to give each service a possible total score between 10 and 2.

Note: Cost-effectiveness (CE) measures economic value, or the cost of producing a unit of health, such as a quality-adjusted life year, or QALY. A QALY is a measure that accounts for both mortality (years of life lost) and morbidity (quality of life lost due to days lived with sickness): CE = $ spent - $ saved = QALYs saved. The fewer dollars spent per QALY, the more cost effective the service. If the dollars saved are greater than the dollars spent, the service is cost saving. By itself, a service's CE ratio does not indicate whether or not the service is cost effective because there is no specific figure that separates services that are sufficiently cost effective from those that are not. CE ratios must be compared to one another to see which services require the fewest dollars to produce the same unit of health. However, as a general rule of thumb, health care services are considered "costeffective" at less than $50,000 per QALY.

A quality-adjusted life year (QALY) is a year of life adjusted for its quality. Saving one QALY through prevention is equivalent to extending a life for 1 year in perfect health.

Source: Partnership for Prevention. A National Profile on Use, Disparities, and Health Benefits (2007). Retrieved December 14, 2012, from: www.prevent.org/NCPP.

are lengthy (see Figure 1-5 for a state-by-state map of the distribution of primary care physicians).

Within the standard 15-minute primary care visit, there is insufficient time to spend on prevention (National Center for Health Statistics, 1997). An oft-cited paper by Yarnall et al. (2003) examined the amount of time required for a primary care physician to provide USPSTF-recommended preventive services to a patient panel of 2500 with an age and sex distribution similar to that of the US population. Their findings revealed that, to fully satisfy the USPSTF recommendations, 1,773 hours of a physician's annual time, or 7.4 hours per working day, are needed for the provision of preventive services. For patients with chronic conditions, it has been estimated that it would take an additional 3.2 hours per day to deliver the USPSTF-recommended services (Bodenheimer, 2006). Therefore, they concluded that time constraints limit the ability of physicians to comply with preventive services recommendations (Yarnall et al., 2003).

Not only has the number of primary care tasks grown exponentially, but physician performance is being measured more comprehensively, and they are often being paid according to their ability to perform these tasks reliably and consistently. These demands invariably result in increased paperwork for data collection and for monitoring adherence

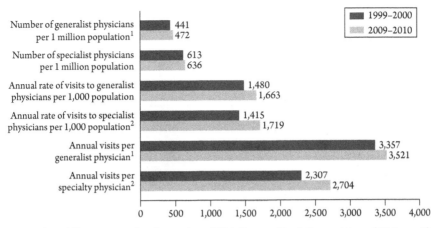

FIGURE 1-2: Number of Physicians per Population, Annual Visit Rate per Population, and Annual Visits per Physician, by Specialty: United States, 1999–2000 and 2009–2010.

[1]*Difference between generalist and specialist rates is statistically significant (p <0.05) in each 2-year time period.*

[2]*Trend is statistically significant (p < 0.05).*

Note: Generalist (primary care) physicians include family and general practitioners, internists, and pediatricians; specialty physicians include all other specialties.

Source: CDC/NCHS, National Ambulatory Medical Care Survey.

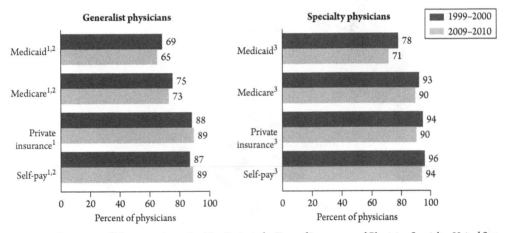

FIGURE 1-3: Percentage of Physicians Accepting New Patients, by Type of Insurance and Physician Specialty: United States, 1999–2000 and 2009–2010.

[1]*1999–2000 difference between generalist and specialty physicians is statistically significant (p <0.05).*

[2]*2009–2010 difference between generalist and specialty physicians is statistically significant (p <0.05).*

[3]*Trend is statistically significant (p <0.05).*

Note: Generalist physicians include family and general practitioners, internists, and pediatricians; specialty physicians include all other specialties.

Source: CDC/NCHS, National Ambulatory Medical Care Survey.

to practice guidelines (Schwartz, Woloshin, and Welch, 1999), leaving many primary care providers feeling burdened. Reimbursement based primarily on the quantity of services delivered through fragmented payment systems (e.g., CMS's Hospital Inpatient Prospective Payment Systems [IPPS], Hospital Outpatient Prospective Payment System [OPPS], and Relative Value Scale [RBRVS] for physicians,), in a fee-for-service model—rather than on quality—forces primary care physicians onto

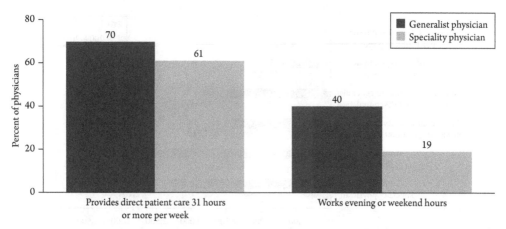

FIGURE 1-4: Percentage of Physicians Providing Direct Patient Care 31 Hours or More per Week, and Percentage Working Evening and Weekend Hours, by Specialty: United States, 2009–2010.

Note: All differences between generalist and specialty physicians are statistically significant ($p < 0.05$). Generalist physicians include family and general practitioners, internists, and pediatricians; specialty physicians include all other specialties.

Source: CDC/NCHS, National Ambulatory Medical Care Survey.

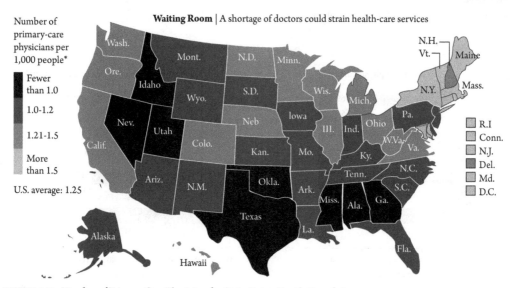

FIGURE 1-5: Number of Primary Care Physicians by State, Kaiser Family Foundation.

a treadmill, devaluing their professional work life (Bodenheimer, 2006).

Satisfaction among primary care physicians has thus waned amid the growing demands of office-based practice (Nolte & McKee, 2008; Bodenheimer, 2006). (Even patients have shared this growing unhappiness, and are often passive and unengaged in their own care [Safran, 2003].) Similarly, primary care physicians are expressing frustration that the knowledge and skills they are expected to master exceed the limits of human capability, making it impossible to provide the best care to every patient (Yarnall et al., 2003). In practice, the clinician must first address the patient's chief complaint, the concerns and symptoms that brought the patient to the office, perhaps expressed by someone with limited English proficiency (Emanuel & Emanuel, 1992; Bodenheimer, 2006). Since most diseases seen in primary care—including diabetes, coronary heart disease, arthritis, and depression—are preventable, their attention must quickly turn to prevention or risk reduction. In this, their tasks range from patient assessment to motivating change in behavior (such as recommending smoking cessation) to referral or provision of behavioral counseling to follow-up. For each of these behaviors, there are challenges, including uncertain evidence or professional guidelines (for example, in obesity prevention); unavailable or inaccessible professional guidelines at the time of the office visit; difficult communication with patients who often have limited health literacy (Koh, Brach, Harris, & Parchment, 2013); and uncoordinated (and often limited) services for referral and follow-up. All of these tasks require effective communication with patients (as well as family members and other clinicians); few primary care providers receive such training (Schwartz, Woloshin, & Welch, 1999). As a result, the majority of patients with diabetes, hypertension, and other chronic conditions do not receive adequate clinical care (Roux et al., 2012), partly because half of all patients leave their office visits without having understood what the physician said (Pagoto, Pbert, Emmons, 2012).

Given the foregoing, it is not surprising that there has been growing concern that current models of primary care will not be sustainable for meeting the health care needs of the population (Jackson et al., 2013; Kalet, Roberts, Fletcher, 1994; Schwartz, Woloshin, & Welch, 1999; http://effectivehealthcare.ahrq.gov). In particular, as the overall population ages, educators and policy makers are focusing on this unbalanced distribution of primary care physicians and an overall shortage in the primary care workforce, particularly as provisions of the Patient Protection and Affordable Care Act, (P.L. 111-148, March 23, 2010; the Affordable Care Act, or ACA) expand health insurance coverage (Carrier, Yee, Stark, 2011; Colwill, Cultice, Kruse, 2008; Staiger, Auerbach, Buerhaus, 2009).

Some solutions to this crisis in primary care have been proposed, and some are in the process of implementation, notably under the ACA. Several are discussed in this Chapter, and others are explored throughout this book, particularly in Chapters 10, 11, and 12.

A SUSTAINED PARTNERSHIP

In its interim report on primary care, the Institute of Medicine stressed the importance of the relationship between patients and their primary care providers, which it defined as a "sustained partnership" (Institute

of Medicine, 1996.) For this sustained partnership to become actualized, practices need to recognize that there are limits to the number of services that each provider can deliver and the number of patients for whom each provider can be accountable (commonly referred to as "panel size"), and these limits must be defined (Hall, 2007). Defining (and limiting) panel size has been a more common focus of primary care practices of late. Its advantages include providing patients with the opportunity to choose, and have access to that primary care provider; defining the workload to predict patient demand and ensure that providers are each carrying his or her "fair share" and improving provider practice patterns (as discussed further in Chapter 10). Identifying individual panels enables providers to make a commitment to continuity (e.g., to taking care of their own patients for all of their visits). There is some evidence for improved clinical outcomes from panels (Ettner, 1999; Dietrich & Marton, 1982; Davis, McBride, & Bobula, 1992; Taplin, Galvin, Payne, Coole, & Wagner, 1998; Carney, Dietrich, Keller, Landgraf, & O'Connor, 1992), in reduced costs and enhanced revenue per visit (Christakis, Mell, Koepsell, Zimmerman, & Connell, 2001; Raddish, Horn, Sharkey, 1999; O'Hare & Corlett, 2004; Lewandowski, O'Connor, Solberg, et al., 2006). The most recent work on provider teams, however, suggests that, in addition to identifying provider panels, effective care must be delivered by collaborative teams of clinicians, with each member playing a vital role (Institute of Medicine, 2012). Collaborative primary care teams, or "pods," (Green, Savin, & Lu, 2013) alongside better information technology, the sharing of data, and the use of other medical team members are effective means for patient engagement, as well as for ensuring more care coordination, better access, and more effective primary care prevention with a limited and burdened physician workforce.

Engaging patients in prevention (and other aspects of their care) remains a challenge, even under the new models of health care. A recent survey of 112 Patient-Centered Medical Home (PCMH) practices in 22 states found that, while nearly all sought patient feedback—a hallmark of the PCMH—only about one-third (29%) involved patients and families as advisers and sought feedback through surveys. Only about as many (32%) involved patients in a continuing role in quality improvement (Han, Scholle, Morton, Bechtel, Kessler, 2013). The importance of patients' engagement in their care (including quality improvement and governance) is discussed further within the chronic care model in Chapters 3, 10, and 12; approaches for increasing patient engagement are discussed in Chapters 11 and 12.

THE PROMISE OF THE ACA

The ACA is a landmark for prevention and, when fully implemented, promises to address many of the structural impediments to effective primary care practice. While the ACA is discussed in detail in Chapter 2, an introduction follows (adapted from Koh & Sibelius, 2010; a summary of the impact of the ACA on prevention is found in Table 1-2).

The ACA provides individuals with improved access to clinical preventive services by removing cost as a barrier to access. For example, new private health plans and insurance policies (for plans or policy years beginning on or after September 23, 2010) are required to cover a range of recommended preventive services with no cost sharing by the beneficiary. These services include those rated as "A" (strongly recommended) or "B" (recommended) by the USPSTF, vaccinations recommended by the Advisory Committee on Immunization Practices, and preventive care and screening included in both existing health guidelines for children and adolescents and in future guidelines to be developed for women through the US Health Resources and Services Administration (HRSA). Examples of covered services include screening for breast cancer, cervical cancer, and colorectal cancer; screening for human immunodeficiency virus (HIV) for persons at high risk; alcohol-misuse counseling; depression screening (when systems are in place to ensure accurate diagnosis, effective treatment, and follow-up); and immunizations. Cancer screening tests are discussed further in Chapter 4.

The prevention theme in the ACA also affects individuals covered by public insurance programs. A number of policy changes will be phased in over time. For example, starting January 1, 2011, Medicare covered, without cost sharing, an annual wellness visit that includes a health risk assessment and a customized prevention plan. Full coverage of many USPSTF-recommended services will also be available under Medicare with no cost sharing. Similarly, in 2013 and beyond, state Medicaid programs that eliminate cost sharing for preventive services recommended by the USPSTF or the Advisory Committee on Immunization Practices (ACIP) may be eligible for enhanced federal matching funds to provide these services (Koh & Sibelius, 2010).

The ACA authorizes heavy investment in bolstering a primary care workforce that can promote prevention. For example, the law appropriates up to $1.5 billion for the National Health Service Corps between fiscal years 2011 and 2015 to place health care professionals in underserved areas; these monies complement other new investments for community health centers administered through the Health Resources and Services Administration (HRSA). To guide future placement of health care professionals, a new National Health Care Workforce Commission will analyze needs (Koh & Sibelius, 2010).

The law provides new health promotion opportunities in the workplace by, for example, authorizing funds for grants for small businesses to provide comprehensive workplace wellness programs. The law also requires the Secretary of Health and Human Services to assess existing federal health and wellness initiatives and directs the Centers for Disease Control and Prevention (CDC) to survey worksite health policies and programs nationally (Koh & Sibelius, 2010). This effort could assist with obtaining more accurate national rates of program efficacy, as discussed in Chapter 2.

The ACA includes components that could strengthen partnerships between local or state governments and community groups. For example, new Community Transformation Grants promise to improve nutrition, increase physical activity, promote smoking cessation, social and emotional wellness, and prioritize strategies to reduce health care disparities. Also, in further recognition that immunization is a foundation for public health, the Act authorizes states to use their funds to purchase vaccines for adults at federally negotiated prices. Grants for states will also support demonstration projects to improve vaccination rates (Koh & Sibelius, 2010). These community-based approaches are discussed throughout the rest of this book.

The ACA elevates prevention as a national priority in policy making (Koh & Sibelius, 2010). For example, a newly established National Prevention, Health Promotion, and Public Health Council, involving more than a dozen federal agencies, will develop a prevention and health promotion strategy for the country. The council will build on the foundation of preceding prevention initiatives, such as

TABLE 1-2. MAJOR SECTIONS RELATED TO PREVENTION IN THE 2010 AFFORDABLE CARE ACT* (KOH & SIBELIUS, 2010)

Section Number	Section Name	Summary
		For individuals
§2502	*Medicaid and Tobacco Pharmaceutical Coverage*	Prevents states from excluding coverage for tobacco-cessation drugs from their Medicaid programs.
§2713	*Coverage of Preventive Health Services*	Requires new employer-sponsored group health plans and private health insurance policies to provide coverage, without cost sharing, for preventive services rated A or B by the USPSTF; immunizations recommended by ACIP; preventive care and screening for infants, children, and adolescents and additional preventive services for women that are recommended by HRSA.
§4103	*Medicare Coverage of Annual Wellness Visit Providing a Personalized Prevention Program*	Eliminates copayments for Medicare enrollees who receive an annual wellness exam that includes a health risk assessment and personalized prevention plan.
§4104	*Removal of Barriers to Preventive Services in Medicare*	Eliminates copayments for Medicare preventive services that are rated A or B by the USPSTF.
§4106	*Improving Access to Preventive Services for Eligible Adults in Medicaid*	Federal medical assistance percentage increased by 1% for preventive services in states that eliminate cost sharing for services rated A or B by the USPSTF and immunizations recommended by ACIP.
§4107	*Coverage of Comprehensive Tobacco Cessation Services for Pregnant Women in Medicaid*	Provides coverage without cost sharing for evidence-based tobacco-dependence treatments for all pregnant women covered by Medicaid.
§4206	*Demonstration Project Concerning Individualized Wellness Plans*	Creates a pilot program to determine the effectiveness of individualized wellness plans at federally qualified community health centers.
		For businesses and workplaces
§4207	*Reasonable Break Time for Nursing Mothers*	Requires employers to provide sufficient break time and appropriate facilities for nursing mothers.
§4303	*CDC and Employer-Based Wellness Plans*	Requires the CDC to provide technical assistance in evaluating employer-based wellness programs, as well as to conduct a survey of existing programs.
§4402	*Effectiveness of Federal Health and Wellness Initiatives*	Requires the secretary of health and human services to evaluate the effectiveness of existing federal health and wellness initiatives and requires a report to Congress.
§10408	*Grants for Small Businesses to Provide Comprehensive Workplace Wellness Grants*	Authorizes a grant program for small businesses to establish workplace wellness programs.
		For communities and states
§4108	*Incentives for Prevention of Chronic Diseases in Medicaid*	Provides grants to states to provide incentives to Medicaid enrollees who adopt and maintain healthy behaviors. Appropriates up to $100 million that became available in FY 2011.
§4201	*Community Transformation Grants*	Authorizes competitive grants for state and local government agencies and community-based organizations for the implementation, evaluation, and dissemination of evidence-based programs to reduce the rates of chronic conditions, improve prevention, reduce disparities, and decrease rates of disease.

(continued)

TABLE 1-2. (CONTINUED)

Section Number	Section Name	Summary
§5313	*Grants to Promote the Community Health Workforce*	Authorizes grants to improve health care in medically underserved areas through the use of community health workers.

National

Section Number	Section Name	Summary
§3011	*National Strategy to Improve Healthcare Quality*	Requires the secretary of health and human services to establish a national strategy to improve the delivery of health care services, patient health outcomes, and population health.
§4001	*National Prevention, Health Promotion, and Public Health Council*	Creates a council to provide coordination and leadership of prevention and wellness and health promotion practices at the federal level, and directs the council to develop a national strategy on prevention.
§4002	*Prevention and Public Health Fund*	Expands and sustains national investment in prevention and public health programs. Appropriates up to $500 million for FY 2010, $750 million for FY 2011, $1 billion for FY 2012, $1.25 billion for FY 2013, $1.5 billion for FY 2014, and $2 billion for FY 2015 and beyond.
§4003	*Clinical and Community Preventive Services*	Promotes expanded coordination among the USPSTF, Community Preventive Services Task Force, and ACIP.
§4004	*Education and Outreach Campaign Regarding Preventive Benefits*	Requires the planning and implementation of a national public-private partnership for a prevention and health promotion outreach and education campaign to raise public awareness of health improvement across the life span.
§4102	*Oral Healthcare Prevention Activities*	Creates education, surveillance, and research demonstration grants.
§4205	*Nutrition Labeling of Standard Menu Items at Chain Restaurants*	Requires the disclosure of specified nutritional information for food sold in certain chain restaurants and vending machines.
§4301	*Research on Optimizing the Delivery of Public Health Services*	Supports research in the area of public health services and systems.
§4302	*Understanding Health Disparities: Data Collection and Analysis*	Requires any federally conducted and supported public health programs to report appropriate data for analysis.
§5101	*National Health Care Workforce Commission*	Establishes a national commission to provide comprehensive information on workforce needs.
§5207	*Funding for National Health Service Corps*	Expands and reauthorizes the National Health Service Corps.
§ 10413	*Young Women's Breast Health Awareness and Support of Young Women Diagnosed with Breast Cancer*	Authorizes a program to support awareness, knowledge, research, and support for breast cancer in young women.
§ 10501	*National Diabetes Prevention Program*	Authorizes a national program focused on reducing preventable diabetes in at-risk adult populations.
§ 10503	*Community Health Centers and the National Health Service Corps*	Provides for expanded and sustained investment in community health centers. Appropriates up to $9.5 billion for Community Health Center Initiative between FY 2011 and FY 2015. Appropriates up to $1.5 billion for National Health Service Corps between FY 2011 and FY 2015. Appropriates up to $1.5 billion for the construction and renovation of community health centers between FY 2011 and FY 2015.

Healthy People (which has set the country's health promotion and disease prevention agenda for the past 30 years), as well as efforts of expert groups such as the USPSTF, the Community Preventive Services Task Force, and the ACIP. (These are discussed further in Chapter 2.) A new Prevention and Public Health Fund, with an annual appropriation that began at $500 million in fiscal year 2010 and increases to $2 billion in fiscal year 2015 and beyond, will invest in a range of prevention and wellness programs administered by the Department of Health and Human Services. Initial funds have already been invested in strengthening public health infrastructure, prevention research, surveillance, integration of primary care into community-based behavioral health programs, HIV prevention, obesity prevention, and tobacco control. Reinvigorated planning will also involve a national strategy to improve the quality of health care, improved data collection on health disparities (Siegel & Nolan, 2009), and authorization of a host of other new programs. Most newly authorized programs await appropriations and future funding as available through the annual budget process (exceptions are noted in Table 1-2; Koh & Sibelius, 2010).

Since tobacco dependence and obesity continue to represent substantial health threats, the ACA addresses these specific challenges in a number of ways. For example, the directives for the new health plans established after September 23, 2010, also included coverage, with no cost sharing, of tobacco-use counseling and evidence-based tobacco-cessation interventions, as well as obesity screening and counseling for adults and children. Starting in 2010, pregnant women on Medicaid received coverage, without cost sharing, for evidence-based tobacco-dependence treatments; in 2014, states will be forbidden from excluding from Medicaid drug coverage any pharmaceutical agents for smoking cessation, including over-the-counter medications, that have been approved by the Food and Drug Administration. To promote healthy weight for populations, the act appropriates funds for fiscal years 2010 through 2014 for demonstration projects to develop model programs for reducing childhood obesity. Menu-labeling provisions require the disclosure of specified nutrient information for food sold in certain chain restaurants and vending machines.

The Affordable Care Act has been met with considerable political opposition, so some of these potential benefits may be too Panglossian. If fully implemented and funded nationally, however, these complementary actions in the clinic and the community could benefit individuals as well as populations (Koh & Sibelius, 2010).[1]

BEST CARE AT LOWER COST: THE PATH TO CONTINUOUSLY LEARNING HEALTH CARE IN AMERICA

In response to widespread demand for an improved health care system, as described earlier in this Chapter, the Institute of Medicine (IOM) convened a committee whose work was reported in "Best Care at Lower Cost: The Path to Continuously Learning Health Care in America (2012). Their major recommendations fell into four major categories: (1) building an adaptive system; (2) delivering reliable clinical knowledge to patients; (3) improving the policy environment; and (4) adopting a continuously learning health care system. Each can be applied to prevention, and all propose multi-level interventions, so most are addressed throughout this book.

Building an Adaptive System

Because health care is complex and constantly changing, a system that learns—in real time with new tools—to better manage problems is proposed. Opportunities now exist that were not available just a decade ago, including vast, increasingly affordable computational power and connectivity that allows information to be accessed in real time. Data generated in health care delivery—whether clinical, delivery process, or financial—should be collected in digital formats, compiled, and protected as resources for managing care, capturing results, improving

---

1 While the focus of the ACA ("Obamacare") is on health, and particularly prevention, the Act has engendered considerable political controversy, including a series of Congressional bills to defund it entirely. As a result, the President has delayed its implementation (e.g., a one-year delay in enforcing the out-of-pocket caps on medical expenses for employees who are insured at their jobs), and its implementation has been highly variable from state to state. In advance of the October 1, 2013, ACA deadline, some major employers (e.g., Walgreens, Sears, Darden Restaurants, Time Warner, and IBM) offered many current employees and retirees coverage through corporate health benefit exchanges instead of the public health exchanges.

processes, strengthening public health, and generating knowledge, as discussed further in Chapter 12.

Human and organizational capabilities offer expanded ways to improve the reliability and efficiency of health care, as explored in Chapters 10 and 11. The Department of Health and Human Services (HHS) can encourage not only this digital capacity, but also the development of distributed data research networks and expanded access to health data resources to improve care, lower costs, and enhance public health. Payers and medical product companies also should contribute more data to research groups to generate new insights. Patients should participate in developing robust data utility; should use new tools, such as personal portals, to better manage their own care; and should be involved in building new knowledge, for example through patient-reported outcomes.

Delivering Reliable Clinical Knowledge to Patients

Improving the data infrastructure and data utility would require revising and streamlining research regulations to improve care, promote capture of clinical data, and generate knowledge. Regulators can clarify and improve rules governing the collection and use of clinical data to safeguard patient privacy while promoting the seamless use of such data for better care coordination and management, improved care, and enhanced knowledge. Decision support tools and knowledge management systems can be included routinely in health care delivery to ensure that decisions are informed by the best evidence.

Among possible actions, clinicians and health care organizations can adopt tools that deliver reliable clinical knowledge to patients, as discussed in Chapters 10 and 11. Research organizations, advocacy organizations, professional specialty societies, and care delivery organizations can facilitate the development, accessibility, and use of evidence-based and harmonized clinical practice guidelines. Also, education programs—such as academic detailing and practice facilitation, as described in Chapter 11—should evolve so that health professionals learn new methods for accessing, managing, and applying evidence, with an emphasis on engaging in lifelong learning; understanding human behavior and social science; and delivering safe care in an interdisciplinary environment. Agencies and organizations that fund research should support investigations into improving the usefulness and accessibility of patient outcome data and

enhancing the implementation of scientific evidence into clinical practice.

Clinicians should place a higher premium on fully involving patients in their own health care to the extent that patients choose. As described more specifically in Chapter 11, clinicians should employ high-quality, reliable tools and skills for sharing decision making with patients, tailored to clinical needs, patient goals, social circumstances, and the degree of control that patients prefer. Health care delivery organizations should monitor and assess patients' perspectives and use those insights to improve care; should establish patient portals to facilitate data sharing among clinicians, patients, and families; and should make high-quality tools available for shared decision making with patients.

In addition, the federal Agency for Healthcare Research and Quality, partnering with the Centers for Medicare and Medicaid Services (CMS), other payers, and stakeholders, should support developing and testing a reliable set of measures of patient-centeredness for consistent use across the health care system. CMS and other payers should promote and measure patient-centered care through payment models, contracting policies, and public reporting programs. And digital technology developers and health product innovators should develop tools to assist individuals in managing their health and health care, as described in Chapter 11.

Improving the Policy Environment

The culture of health care is central to promoting learning at every level. The prevailing approach to paying for health care, based predominantly on individual services and products, encourages wasteful and ineffective care. Instead, payments should reward desired care outcomes and movement toward providing the best care at lower cost. Payers should adopt outcome- and value-oriented payment models, contracting policies, and benefit design to reward and support high-quality, team-based care focused on patients' needs.

Health care delivery organizations, clinicians, and payers should increase the availability of information about the quality, price, and outcomes of care, and professional specialty societies should encourage transparency in the information provided by their members. Likewise, payers should promote transparency to help their members make better decisions. And consumer and patient organizations should disseminate this information to spur conversations and promote informed decision making.

Adopting a Continuously Learning Health Care System

The adoption of a continuously learning health care system will require broad participation by patients, families, clinicians, care leaders, and those who support their work. Health care delivery organizations should develop organizational cultures that encourage continuous improvement by incorporating best practices, transparency, open communication, staff empowerment, coordination, teamwork, and mutual respect, and that align incentives accordingly (see Chapters 3 and 9 in particular). Also, specialty societies, education programs, specialty boards, licensing boards, and accreditation organizations should incorporate basic concepts and specialized applications of continuous learning and improvement into health professionals' education, licensing, certification, and accreditation requirements (see Chapter 10 for evidence-based approaches).

PREVENTION PRACTICE IN PRIMARY CARE: SUMMARIES OF CHAPTERS 2 THROUGH 12

The next two chapters of the book describe the theoretical frameworks on which the work rests. In Chapter 2, "Multilevel Influences in Prevention," the myriad US political and economic forces influencing health promotion are detailed. This Chapter gives special attention to the Affordable Care Act and its implications for the practice of prevention in primary care. These implications are found in legislation, policy, and economic incentives, from the perspectives of governmental and private programs and insurers.

The multilevel perspective that undergirds Chapter 2 and some of the theoretical models in Chapter 3 is emerging as a dominant approach to understanding prevention, a complex problem, with distal, intermediate, and proximal determinants (Holmes, Lehman, Hade, et al., 2008; Taylor, Repetti, Seeman, 1997; Warnecke, Oh, Breen, et al., 2008; Kelley, Baldyga, Barajas, Rodriguez-Sanchez, 2005). The most distal determinants include policies that affect the availability, receipt of, and quality of health care and shared social norms about health. Intermediate determinants include the social contexts, physical environments, and social relationships,

such as neighborhoods or communities, in which the distal effects are experienced (Warnecke, Oh, Breen, et al., 2008). Finally, proximal determinants are embedded in the individual and include genetic susceptibility, biologic markers of disease, socioeconomic status, race/ethnicity, gender, and cultural beliefs. They also include the capacity to address health care needs, to engage in social networks, and to change risk behaviors. Because multilevel interventions may be able to address multiple determinants within these complex contexts, they may be uniquely suited to reducing health disparities in racial and ethnic minorities (Taylor, Repetti, & Seeman, 1997). (While much of dental care is preventive, it is not covered in this book.)

"Models for Prevention," Chapter 3, explores contemporary theoretical approaches to health promotion. It too applies a multilevel approach, from the macrolevel, such as the social ecology and chronic care models, to the microlevel, including the health belief model. It describes the construct of spirituality, and the cross-cutting constructs of empowerment and community capacity-building. Approaches to the evaluation of health promotion programs founded on these contemporary models, as well as their consequent measures of change, are also discussed.

The following Chapters—4 through 7—address prevention approaches to the major causes of mortality among adults (www.cdc.gov), including cancer prevention and screening, cardiovascular disease prevention, stroke prevention, and risk reduction for other major diseases of adulthood. The introduction to each chapter establishes the importance of the area and provides an evidence-based literature review. Each chapter includes interventions that can be implemented in primary care, as well as relevant resources for engaging with patients in a dialogue about prevention.

Chapter 8, "Personalizing Prevention," examines the emerging evidence for personalizing cancer control in genetics and genomics within a primary care practice. The Human Genome Project's generation of a reference human genome sequence ushered in the field of genomics. Advances in bench science are being catalyzed by revolutionary new DNA sequencing technologies that produce prodigious amounts of DNA sequence data, including data from large numbers of individual patients; especially in the comparison of tumor to normal genomes from the same patient (Green, 2012). Further, whether a gene is expressed can be determined by environmental exposures or behavioral patterns. Our genetic pre-dispositions also affect the health care we need, and our social circumstances affect the health care we receive. The growing knowledge and evidence base in these areas provides important opportunities for targeted action and analysis that could develop tools to prompt and facilitate change (McGinnis, Williams-Russo, & Knickman, 2002). Generally, however, the translation of these approaches and understandings to clinical practice has been minimal; this Chapter examines some current applications.

Chapter 9, "Pay for Performance and Quality and Outcomes Frameworks for Prevention," recognizes the pivotal role that "pay for performance" is playing in the emerging changes in health care. In Pay for performance (P4P), payers and health plans offer financial incentives to primary care physicians, specialists, and hospitals for achieving pre-defined quality targets. A conceptual model to describe the influences on the uptake of P4P systems and a case approach anchor the Chapter.

Chapter 10, "Provider and Office-based Approaches to Prevention in Primary Care," and Chapter 11, "Patient-Directed Approaches to Prevention," explore approaches to patient-centered change as the current healthcare environment is transformed.

In Chapter 10, the following provider and office-based approaches are described: the patient-centered medical home, with its central concept of coordination of care, and two critical models for implementing evidence for change in primary care practices: academic detailing and practice facilitation. New health care delivery organizations, such as Accountable Care Organizations, will offer opportunities for more systematic educational outreach to practitioners—including academic detailing and practice facilitation—services that are more difficult to provide as efficiently to a collection of unrelated stand-alone practices (Jerry Avorn, personal communication, November, 2012). The Chapter concludes with a discussion of the use of medical informatics to improve prevention practice in primary care, particularly through meaningful use principles.

Chapter 11, "Patient-Directed Approaches to Prevention," is key to clinical practice. The selected approaches are those that are most likely to enhance patient-centered practices and to increase patient self-management. The Chapter examines some general models for behavior change and the patient/provider encounter; patient decision-making for prevention; and practical approaches to patient behavior change in primary care. Among these approaches are setting SMART (specific, measureable, attainable, realistic, and timely) goals, and shared decision making (an active, individualized exchange of information between provider and patient that leads to common goals and expectations of the process; IOM, 2001). The 5 As (ask/assess, advise, assess/agree, assist, arrange) and motivational interviewing ("a collaborative, person-centered form of guiding to elicit and strengthen motivation for change"; Miller & Rose, 2009) are examined. The Chapter presents a protocol for tailored telephone counseling, that is, a structured form of counseling, often supported by a counseling script that includes (1) gathering information, (2) selecting messages that relate to the patient's concerns or barriers, and (3) delivering a "tailored" message (Rimer & Glassman, 1999). Risk assessment approaches are explored and are illustrated with examples of office-based tools for use in practice. These patient-centered approaches are described, illustrated, and evaluated. The Chapter concludes with select brief, practical assessment and screening tools with patient self-report items for primary care practices.

The final Chapter, 12, "The Future of Prevention in Primary Care," points to the larger influences on prevention practice in primary care yet to come. It is likely that the opportunities will include addressing the needs of the growing elderly population, implementing prevention in a diverse populace, harnessing the forces of information technology to promote health, measuring prevention in a comparative effectiveness framework, and engaging in an ongoing ethical dialogue. Included in this Chapter is a section dedicated to medical informatics, defined as the study of the proper use of information in health care (http://www.amia.org/about/faqs/f7.html). As emphasized throughout the book, the future of prevention is predicated on actions taken at multiple levels of the health care system.

CONCLUSIONS

This Chapter has defined prevention in health care and has explored the myriad challenges to practicing prevention in primary care, including the importance of patient behavior change in provider-based medical care; the demands of patient-centered care in time, expertise, and communication skills; and the fiscal and staffing barriers to providing optimal primary care. The strengths of a major national health policy initiative, the Affordable Care Act, and the novel proposals of the IOM's *Best Care at Lower Cost: The Path to Continuously Learning Health Care in America* address many of these challenges. The Chapter has concluded with an introduction to the remainder of the book.

REFERENCES

AHRQ. *Primary Care Workforce Facts and Stats No. 1: The Number of Practicing Primary Care Physicians in the United States.* AHRQ Publication No. 12-P001-2-EF, October 2011. Agency for Health Care Policy and Research, Rockville, MD. http://www.ahrq.gov/research/pcwork1.htm.

Arnold J, Breen JL. Images of Health. In: Sheinfeld Gorin S, Arnold J. *Health Promotion in Practice.* (pp. 3–20). San Francisco, CA: Jossey-Bass; 2006.

Bodenheimer T. Primary care—will it survive? *N Engl J Med.* 2006;355(9):861–864.

Brown R. et al. Effectiveness in disease and injury prevention: estimated national spending on prevention—United States, 1988. *MMWR.* (July 24, 1992);41(29): 529–531.

Carney PA, Dietrich AJ, Keller A, Landgraf J, O'Connor GT. Tools, teamwork and tenacity: an office system for cancer prevention. *J Fam Pract.* 1992;388–394.

Carrier E, Yee T, Stark LB. *Matching Supply to Demand: Addressing the U.S. Primary Care Workforce Shortage.* Policy Analysis No. 7. Washington, DC: National Institute for Health Care Reform, Center for Studying Health System Change. 2011.

Centers for Medicare and Medicaid Services, Office of the Actuary. *National Health Expenditures, by Source of Funds and Type of Expenditure: Calendar Years 1994–1998* (December 5, 2000). Retrieved December 14, 2012, from www.hcfa.gov/stats/nhe-oact/tables/t3.htm.

Christakis DA, Mell L, Koepsell TD, Zimmerman FJ, Connell FA. Association of lower continuity of care with greater risk of emergency department use and hospitalization in children. *Pediatrics.* 2001;107:524–529.

Colwill JM, Cultice JM, Kruse RL. Will generalist physician supply meet demands of an increasing and aging population? *Health Affairs* 2008; 27(3):w232–w41.

Davis JE, McBride PE, Bobula JA. Improving prevention in primary care: physicians, patients and process. *J Fam Pract.* 1992;35(4):385–387.

Decker SL. Changes in Medicaid physician fees and patterns of ambulatory care. *Inquiry.* 2009;46(3):291–304.

Dietrich AJ, Marton KI. Does continuous care from a physician make a difference? *J Fam Pract.* 1982;15:929–937.

Emanuel EJ, Emanuel LL. Four models of the physician–patient relationship. *JAMA.* 1992;267:2221–2226.

Ettner SL. The relationship between continuity of care and the health behaviors of patients: does having a usual physician make a difference? *Med Care.* 1999;37:547–555.

Grant RW, Buse JB, Meigs JB. Quality of diabetes care in U.S. academic medical centers: low rates of medical regimen change. *Diabetes Care.* 2005;28(2): 337–442.

Green LV, Savin S, Lu Y. Primary care physician shortages could be eliminated through use of teams, nonphysicians, and electronic communication. *Health Affairs.* 2013;32(1): 11–19.

Grumbach K, Selby JV, Damberg C, et al. Resolving the gatekeeper conundrum: what patients value in primary care and referrals to specialists. *JAMA.* 1999;282:261–266.

Hall R, ed. *Patient Flow: Reducing Delay in Healthcare Delivery.* New York: Springer; 2007.

Hartman M, Martin A, Nuccio O, Catlin A, and the National Health Expenditure Accounts Team Health Spending Growth At A Historic Low In 2008. *Health Aff.* 2010;29:147–155.

Han E, Scholle SH, Morton S, Bechtel C, Kessler R. Survey shows that fewer than a third of patient-centered medical home practices engage patients in quality improvement. *Health Affairs.* 2013;32(2):368–375.

Holmes JH, Lehman A, Hade E, et al. Challenges for multilevel health disparities research in a transdisciplinary environment. *Am J Prev Med.* 2008;35(2 suppl):S182–S192.

Institute of Medicine. *Best Care at Lower Cost: The Path to Continuously Learning Health Care in America.* Retrieved December 14, 2012, from http://www.iom.edu.

Institute of Medicine. *Crossing the Quality Chasm: A New Health System for the 21st Century.* Washington, DC: National Academy Press; 2001.

Institute of Medicine. *Primary Care: America's Health in a New Era.* Washington, DC: National Academy Press; 1996.

Jackson GL, Powers BJ, Chatterjee R, Bettger JP, Kemper AR, Hasselblad V, Dolor RJ, Irvine J, Heidenfelder BL, Kendrick AS, Gray R, Williams JW. The patient-centered medical home: a systematic review. *Ann Intern Med* 2013;158(3):169–178.

Jencks SF, Huff ED, Cuerdon T. Change in the quality of care delivered to Medicare beneficiaries, 1998–1999 to 2000–2001. *JAMA.* 2003;289(3):305–312;

Kalet A, Roberts JC, Fletcher R. How do physicians talk with their patients about risks? *J Gen Intern Med.* 1994;9:402–404.

Kelley MA, Baldyga W, Barajas F, Rodriguez-Sanchez M. Capturing change in a community-university partnership: Si Se Puede! Project. *Prev Chronic Dis.* 2005;2(2):A22.

Koh HK, Brach C, Harris LM, Parchment MI. A proposed 'health literate care model' would constitute a systems approach to improving patients' engagement in care. *Health Affairs.* 2013;32(2):357–367.

Koh HK, Sebelius KG. Promoting prevention through the Affordable Care Act. *New England J Med.* 2010;363(14):1296.

Lewandowski S, O'Connor PJ, Solberg LI, et al. Increasing primary care physician productivity: a case study. *Am J Manag Care.* 2006;12(10):573–576.

McGinnis JM, Foege WH. Actual causes of death in the United States. *JAMA.* 1993;270(18):2207–2212.

McGinnis JM, Williams-Russo P, Knickman JR. The case for more active policy attention to health promotion. *Health Affairs.* 2002;21(2):78–93.

McGlynn EA, Asch SM, Adams J, et al. The quality of health care delivered to adults in the United States. *N Engl J Med.* 2003;348(26):2635–2645.

Medicare Payment Advisory Commission. *Report to the Congress Medicare and the Health Care Delivery System.* Washington, DC: June, 2013. http://www.medpac.gov/documents/Jun13_EntireReport.pdf

Miller WB, Rose GS. Toward a Theory of Motivational Interviewing. *Am Psychol.* 2009 September; 64(6):527–537.

Mokdad AH, Marks JS, Stroup DF, Gerberding JL. Correction: actual causes of death in the United States, 2000. *JAMA.* 2005;293(3):293.

National Center for Health Statistics. *Health, United States, 2010: With Special Feature on Death and Dying.* Hyattsville, MD: US Department of Health and Human Services; 2011.

National Center for Health Statistics. *National Ambulatory Medical Care Survey: 1996.* Hyattsville, MD: US Department of Health and Human Services; 1997. Available online from: http://www.cdc.gov/nchswwv/data/ ad295.pdf).

Nolte E, McKee CM. Measuring the health of nations: updating an earlier analysis. [Erratum appears in *Health Aff (Millwood).* 2008 Mar-Apr;27(2):593]. *Health Aff (Millwood).* 2008;27(1):58–71.

Nolte E, McKee CM. Measuring the health of nations: updating an earlier analysis. [Erratum appears in *Health Aff (Millwood).* 2008 Mar-Apr;27(2):593]. *Health Aff (Millwood).* 2008;27(1):58–71).

O'Hare CD, Corlett J. The outcomes of open access scheduling. *Fam Pract Manag.* 2004 Feb;11(2):35–38.

Pagoto SL, Pbert L, Emmons K. The Society of Behavioral Medicine position statement on the CMS decision memo on intensive behavior therapy for obesity. *Trans Behav Med.* 2012; 2:4, 381–383.

Partnership for Prevention. *A National Profile on Use, Disparities, and Health Benefits.* Retrieved December 14, 2012, from www.prevent.org/NCPP.

Preamble to the Constitution of the World Health Organization as adopted by the International Health Conference, New York, June 19–22, 1946; signed on July 22, 1946, by the representatives of 61 States (Official Records of the World Health Organization, no. 2, p. 100) and entered into force on April 7, 1948. http://www.who.int/about/definition/en/print.html

Raddish M, Horn SD, Sharkey PD. Continuity of care: is it cost effective? *Am J Manage Care.* 1999;5:727–734.

Rimer BK, Glassman, B. Is there a use for tailored print communications in cancer risk communication? *JNCI Monogr.* 1999;25:140–148.

Roux AM, Herrera P, Wold CM, Dunkle MC, Glascoe FP, Shattuck PT. Developmental and Autism Screening Through 2-1-1. *Am J Prev Med.* 2012;43:6, S457–S463.

Saaddine JB, Cadwell B, Gregg EW, et al. Improvements in diabetes processes of care and intermediate outcomes: United States, 1988–2002. *Ann Intern Med.* 2006;144(7):465–74.

Safran DG. Defining the future of primary care: what can we learn from patients? *Ann Intern Med.* 2003;138:248–255.

Schwartz LM, Woloshin S, and Welch HG. Risk communication in clinical practice: putting cancer in context. *Monogr Natl Cancer Inst.* 1999;25:124–133.

Siegel B, Nolan L. Leveling the field: ensuring equity through national health care reform. *N Engl J Med.* 2009;361:2401–2403.

Staiger DO, Auerbach DI, Buerhaus PI. Comparison of physician workforce estimates and supply projections. *JAMA.* 2009;302(15):1674–1680.

Taplin S, Galvin MS, Payne T, Coole D, Wagner E. Putting population-based care into practice: real option or rhetoric? *J Am Board Fam Pract.* 1998;11(2):116–126.

Taylor SE, Repetti RL, Seeman T. Health psychology: what is an unhealthy environment and how does it get under the skin? *Ann Rev Psychol.* 1997;48(1):411–447.

The Genomic Landscape circa 2012—Eric Green. http://www.genome.gov.

The Patient Protection and Affordable Care Act, P.L. 111-148, March 23, 2010.

Warnecke RB, Oh A, Breen N, et al. Approaching health disparities from a population perspective: the National Institutes of Health Centers for Population Health and Health Disparities. *Am J Public Health.* 2008;98(9):1608–1615.

Yarnall KSH, Pollak KI, Østbye T, Krause KM, Michener JL. Primary care: is there enough time for prevention? *Am J Public Health.* 2003 April;93(4):635–641.

2

Multilevel Influences in Prevention

SHERRI N. SHEINFELD GORIN, RAMSAY HOGUET
AND AARON P. GORIN

Prevention emerges in a multilevel context of policies, influential groups, organizations, and monetary exchanges. This Chapter[1,2,3] details both the political and economic influences on prevention in the United States and the steps that health care providers may take to change these conditions.

---

1 Sections of this Chapter are adapted from Gorin AP & Sheinfeld Gorin S, Contexts for Health Promotion, Sheinfeld Gorin S & Arnold J, *The Health Promotion Handbook*, 67–123 (San Francisco, CA: Jossey-Bass, 2006).

2 Despite the critical role that multilateral organizations, such as the World Health Organization, have continued to play in the promotion of prevention worldwide, the influence of country-specific models of integrating prevention into a nation-wide health care system, as in Sweden, and the impact of Canadian Leadership and the Lalonde Report (1974) on early US health promotion efforts, this Chapter will focus on the United States and its unique health care system.

3 While *Prevention Practice in Primary Care* focuses on adult health, the SCHIP influences the health care resources available to low income families, in particular, so a brief description of the State Children's Health Insurance Program (SCHIP) follows: The SCHIP, enacted under Public Law 105-33 (passed in 1997), and Title XXI of the Social Security Act, allows states to expand Medicaid or to create their own children's health insurance programs and provides an alternative to employer-based health insurance by using schools as the grouping mechanism to negotiate group health insurance policies. The State Children's Health Insurance Program is administered by the Centers for Medicare and Medicaid Services, but each state sets its own guidelines regarding eligibility and services (Langley, 2013). Children may be eligible for SCHIP if their families have incomes too high to qualify for Medicaid but too low to afford private health insurance. While the program also increases health care stability because coverage is not disrupted if a parent changes or loses his or her job, more than 6 million children are not yet covered by Medicaid

THE POLITICAL ECONOMY FRAMEWORK

Conceptually, health promotion may be characterized as a political economy: that is, a political system (a structure of rule) and an economy (a system for producing and exchanging goods and services) (Wamsley & Zald, 1967; Gargiulo, 1993). In the United States, political support for health promotion is defined by the degree to which important actors at the federal, state, and local levels take an interest in health promotion, have the power and resources to influence it, and communicate their expectations and demands about it to concerned communities, organizations, groups, health care professionals, families, and individuals (Longest, 2002).

From the perspective of the health care professional, the major economic actors in the field of health promotion are the varied payers who reimburse or employ providers for services and programs (e.g., commercial insurance companies, or integrated health systems like Kaiser) and the general types of prevention activities they support (e.g., smoking cessation counseling).

The political economy perspective limits both the contexts and targets for health promotion. Further, although one can separate the political and economic contexts conceptually by their major

---

or SCHIP. Enrollment is lengthy and complicated, particularly for low literacy and non-English-speaking families (Langley, 2013). States are allowed to impose premiums, deductibles, or fees, but no copayments can be charged for pediatric preventive preventative care, including immunizations. Through this cost-sharing method, states can match federal funds provided through the SCHIP program to cover children who otherwise would receive no coverage for a variety of services (American Academy of Pediatrics, 2005).

intent or strategy—health improvement or cost reduction—their aims and tactics may overlap. For example, the content of the U.S. surgeon general's Healthy People 2020 plan, although oriented toward health-promotive goals, is embedded in a legislative context that emphasizes cost reductions, and these reductions are implicit in the suggested preventive actions. Another example is managed care systems, which are designed to reduce costs, in part through the use of preventive services.

POLITICAL CONTEXTS FOR HEALTH PROMOTION

The primary political contexts for health promotion are defined by legislation, influential actors, and organizational policy (see Table 2-1).

Legislation

Traditionally, public health law has been concerned with the protection and preservation of the public's health and the processes of administrative regulation and rule making resulting from the implementation of these aims. Although public health legislation may be enacted by the federal, state, and local governments, each level of government has its own structural features and limited powers.

The US Constitution sets up the structure of the federal government and its relationship with the American people and with state and local governments. The Constitution grants the federal government several powers, including the power to collect taxes, spend money for the general welfare, and provide for national defense. Because American states

TABLE 2-1. SELECTED POLITICAL INFLUENCES ON PREVENTION

Influence	Focus	Example
Federal legislation for health promotion		
Health care and health insurance reform	Provides mechanism for universal health insurance, requires insurers to cover preventive services, reforms health insurance market.	Patient Protection and Affordable Care Act [2010], PL 111-148
Food and Drug Administration	Safety and efficacy of pharmaceuticals, food safety, tobacco regulation, safety of medical devices.	Family Smoking Prevention and Tobacco Control Act [2009, PL 111-31]; FDA Food Safety Modernization Act [2011, PL 111-353]
Nonprofit, religious, or government-funded hospitals and other safety net medical providers	Provide free medical care to indigent people or people on public insurance programs (Medicaid, SCHIP).	Cleveland MetroHealth System.
Environmental Protection Agency	Regulates environmental pollution, pesticides and other toxic substances, monitors pollution and its costs in terms of dollars, morbidity and mortality.	Clean Air Act (42 USC Ch. 85), Clean Water Act [1972, 32 USC 1251 et seq.), Safe Drinking Water Act [1974, 42 USC 300f et seq.]
Occupational Safety and Health Administration	Regulates workplace safety and health, develops and enforces safety standards for workplaces.	Occupational Safety and Health Act of 1970 [29 USC 651 et seq.]
State legislation	Creates and funds state-wide public health authorities and programs. Wide power to legislate for health and safety. Can serve as inspiration for federal programs.	California's Latino Childhood Obesity Prevention Initiative, Massachusettes health insurance mandate and reform, Vermont single-payer system, Maryland health care cost control.
County and municipal legislation	Deals with local public health issues, creates and funds programs for addressing public health at local level. Can serve as experiments and inspiration for state or federal initiatives.	New York City's food safety system, Baltimore's tobacco control legislation, Cleveland's urban gardening program, local sewage regulation, local restaurant food safety, clean indoor air regulation.

now trade heavily with each other in the national economy, one of the most extensive and important powers granted to the federal government is its power to regulate interstate commerce. Another important power granted by the Constitution to the federal government is the power of preemption, which allows the federal government to limit or prevent (i.e., to preempt) states from regulating in a particular area. For example, a federal statute called ERISA prevents states from regulating certain types of employer-sponsored health insurance and pension plans.

Although the power of the federal government may at first blush appear vast, the Constitution is clear that the federal government may not act beyond the powers granted to it. Additionally, the government may not infringe upon any of the Constitutional rights granted to the American people in the Bill of Rights. These rights include freedom of speech, freedom of religion, freedom from unreasonable searches and seizures, and freedom from deprivation of life, liberty, or property without due process of law. However, these rights are not always absolute: the government may limit them in some circumstances, for example, when it criminalizes the publication of state secrets or prohibits the ownership of dangerous animals or substances that may be used in religious ceremonies.

Each state also has its own constitution, which describes the structure and powers of the state government. States generally have broader power to enact public health legislation than the federal government, but like the federal government they may not abridge any of the rights or freedoms described in the Bill of Rights. However, a state's constitution may grant broader rights to the people of that state than the rights described in the federal Constitution, and may also limit the power of the state to act in various ways.

The structure and powers of an American municipality are generally governed by the constitution and statutes of the state in which the city is located. Like the federal and state governments, city governments may not abridge any of the rights described in the federal Constitution, but city governments may also face limitations on their power imposed by the state's constitution or legislation. Many cities, however, have "home-rule" authority, under which they have extensive power to legislate for the health, safety, and morals of the public. In a legislative home-rule system, the state delegates the entirety of police power—or something close

to it—to municipalities, but reserves the right to trump, or "preempt," local authority as it sees fit (Diller, 2007; Diller & Graff, 2011).

The final source of governmental rules concerning public health is administrative agencies, such as the Department of Health and Human Services (HHS), the Environmental Protection Agency (EPA), the Food and Drug Administration (FDA), and their state equivalents. The federal constitutions and many state constitutions allow the legislature to delegate some of their law-making power to administrative agencies, which have greater expertise in the subject matter of the regulation than do members of the legislature. The Constitution also allows administrative agencies to engage in fact-finding and adjudication, as when the Social Security Administration decides whether an applicant is disabled and eligible to receive disability benefits or when the Food and Drug Administration decides that a new prescription drug is safe and effective for its intended use.

Administratively issued regulations and decisions have the force of law, although they must often go through a long and complex process of public comment and revision before they become enforceable. Additionally, administrative rules or decisions, whether at the federal or state level, may not abridge any of the Constitutional rights. The exercise of these public health powers requires a delicate balancing of the state's power to act for the community's common good and the individual's rights to liberty, autonomy, and privacy (Gostin, 1986).

Federal Legislation

Because of its broad statutory authority, the federal government possesses several powers regarding health care: individuals may be denied the right to decide whether or not to submit to a medical examination or treatment; the state may collect sensitive health care information about a person or his or her sexual associates; and if a disease is contagious, compulsory hospitalization or segregation from the community may be imposed. Further, legislation at any level of government may either: (1) require or prohibit certain actions by members of the public (e.g., require the isolation of those infected with active tuberculosis); or (2) create, fund, and govern government benefit programs such as Medicare and Medicaid.

The federal government first began to address health promotion when the Nixon administration created the President's Committee on Health Education in response to decades-long struggles with "the fact [that] the nation does not have the resources, no matter how great a portion of the GNP is allocated to health, to provide sufficient services after the patient becomes ill" (Guinta & Allegrante, 1992). The committee's report recommended the creation of public and private organizations to stimulate, coordinate, and evaluate health education programs. The administration believed it could preserve the health of Americans, control escalating health care costs, and present a less costly alternative to the national health insurance plan that was being proposed at the time (Guinta & Allegrante, 1992).

As a result of this initial interest, the National Consumer Health Information and Health Promotion Act of 1976 was passed during the Ford administration; it was the first legislation to address health promotion comprehensively. The Act defined health education and promotion as "[a] process that favorably influences understandings, attitudes and conduct, including cultural awareness and sensitivity, in regard to individual and community health." Specifically, health promotion affects and influences individual and community health behavior and attitudes in order to moderate self-imposed risks, maintain and promote physical and mental health and efficiency, and reduce preventable illness, disability, and death (National Consumer Health Information and Health Promotion Act of 1976, p. 15). In pursuing the goal of health promotion, the Act established the Office of Consumer Health Education and Promotion and the Center for Health Education and Promotion, set forth national goals for health information and promotion, and developed a systematic strategy for goal achievement. It also established the federal Office of Disease Prevention and Health Promotion to coordinate federal prevention-related activities, to serve as a liaison with the private sector, and to operate a national health information clearinghouse.

A Report of the Senate Committee on Labor and Public Welfare that addressed this Act stressed the influence of "activated patients," who were more involved in decision making; community programs, specifically in schools; and (in conjunction with the Occupational Safety and Health Administration [OSHA]) union and industry initiatives for worksites. Nutrition to educate the "misnourished"—those who lack the knowledge

to choose which foods are best for them—was of particular import to the committee, as were the role of the media and the federal programs to monitor these efforts. The report addressed health education "manpower" and asserted the importance of specialists in this area and the critical role that nurses, in particular, should continue to play. The report also stressed the need to evaluate the effectiveness of community programs. Many of these ideas, for example, of "activated" patients (those equipped with the skills and confidence to engage in their health care) are still on the forefront of prevention; in fact, they have been associated with cost reductions across large health care delivery systems (Hibbard, Greene, Overton, 2013).

This Act was amended by a number of subsequent Acts, including the Preventive Health Amendments of 1993, which addressed breast and cervical cancer screening, injury prevention, prevention and control of sexually transmitted diseases, and production of biennial reports on nutrition and health. This legislation reflects the enormous influence that advocates for women's health—particularly in the area of breast cancer screening and treatment—and advocates focused on AIDS (acquired immune deficiency syndrome) have had on the legislative process. More current legislation reflects continued congressional legislative interest in nutrition (see Table 2-1).

State Legislation

Generally, however, it is state governments, not the federal government that have the most extensive powers in public health. For example, while federal administrative agencies (CDC) provide funding for human papillomavirus vaccines at cost to poor children under the Vaccines for Children Program (VFC), the legislation that requires (or does not require) human papillomavirus immunizations by statute varies state by state (http: www.ncsl. org). Other federal statutes do not preempt stricter state legislation, for example, the federal Healthy, Hunger-Free Kids Act of 2010 (P.L. 111-296) reauthorized the national School Lunch and School Breakfast program, increased per-meal reimbursement, and authorized the secretary of agriculture to set nutrition standards for all products sold on school grounds during the day. Among preschool children, California has enacted even stricter legislation, disallowing sugar-sweetened beverages, either natural or artificial, except for infant formula or complete balanced nutritional products designed for children in licensed day care facilities (CA AB 2084, enacted in 2010; http: www.ncsl.org).

States vary in how actively they use their powers to regulate and provide services, whether concerning public health or other areas: some states adopt strict laws, whereas others adopt more lenient ones (Shipan & Volden, 2005). And, public health is a very common subject of state regulation and programs; for example, all states have legislation designed to impede the spread of infectious and venereal diseases (Gostin, 1986).

While resources to implement prevention programs differ between the federal and state governments, legislation that addresses specific aspects of health promotion, from tobacco control and safety (e.g., the use of motor vehicle seat belts and bicycle helmets) to minority disparity reduction and nutrition and obesity counseling, has passed in numerous states. Smoking control has emerged as important in both state and local legislation, with legislation having increased considerably from 1975 to the present; as of 2010, 35 states have adopted 100% smokefree laws

in workplaces, restaurants, and/or bars, with 79% of their populations covered by these laws (at either the state or the municipal level (see Figure 2-1 for a map of state-by-state regulations on smokefree indoor air; http: www.no.smoke.org). In addition, nutrition and obesity counseling is addressed in numerous state statutes. In 2011 alone, ten states enacted some type of school nutrition legislation or authorized funding for school nutrition grants to ensure that students have access to healthier food and beverage options at school or to encourage other community supports for child nutrition (http: www. ncsl.org).

Local Legislation

Numerous city governments, including those of New York City, Los Angeles, San Francisco, and Houston, have historically instituted legislation concerning the protection of public health, particularly laws dealing with infectious and venereal diseases (Gostin, 1986). As of 2013, 558 municipalities have enacted 100% smokefree workplaces, restaurants, and freestanding bars (http://www. no-smoke.org), an exponential growth over

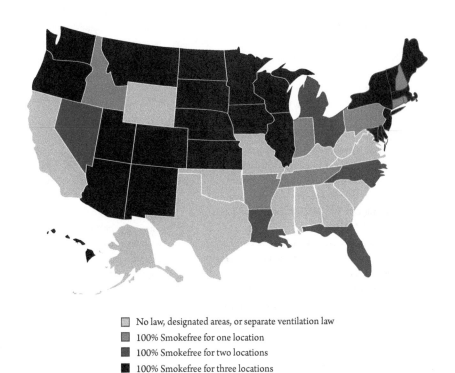

No law, designated areas, or separate ventilation law
100% Smokefree for one location
100% Smokefree for two locations
100% Smokefree for three locations

FIGURE 2-1: State Legislation for Smokefree Indoor Air in Private Worksites, Restaurants, and Bars (2013).

Source: Centers for Disease Control and Prevention State Tobacco Activities Tracking and Evaluation (STATE) System, available at http: www. cdc.govtobacco/statesystem.

the past quarter century (Schroeder, 2004). Nutrition, too, has been a focus of local municipalities. Several examples of municipal regulatory strategies to promote healthy food options and to restrict unhealthy choices are listed on Tables 2-2 and 2-3.

TABLE 2-2. REGULATORY STRATEGIES PROMOTING HEALTHY FOOD OPTIONS

Examples	General Ideas	
Business operations	• New York City committed to issuing 1,000 permits over two years to "green cart" vendors who only sell fresh uncut produce. These vendors are required to operate in designated areas otherwise lacking access to fresh produce. New York City, N.Y., Admin. Code § 17-307(b)(4). • Baldwin Park passed a resolution requiring all city vending machines to carry products that meet certain nutrition standards pertaining to fat, saturated fat, sugar, and calories. Baldwin Park, Cal., Res. No. 2008-014. • Minneapolis requires "grocery stores" to carry certain categories of staple foods, including fresh produce, in order to obtain and retain a business license. Minneapolis, Minn., Mun. Code § 203.10. • Watsonville has a two-tiered award system for restaurants that garner a threshold number of points based on a list of healthy eating options. Watsonville, Cal., Mun. Code § 14-29.	• Enact a streamlined permit program for mobile vendors who sell fresh produce in designated "food deserts." • Set procurement standards for government-run food facilities. • Require food retailers to obtain a license that promotes in some way the sale of healthy food and beverages. • Establish a healthy restaurant certification program that rewards restaurants for reducing the sale and advertising of obesogenic foods and beverages. • Set maximum prices for specified healthy food and beverages. • Enact a menu labeling law that is identical to the federal law (thus enabling local enforcement) and/or that applies to food service establishments that are not covered under the federal law.
Taxes and fees	• New York City provides financial incentives—including real estate tax deductions and a sales tax exemption to developers and store operators—to encourage new full-service grocery stores. New York City Indus. Dev. Agency, FRESH Financial Incentives, available at <http://www.nycedc.com/FinancingIncentives/TaxExemptions/fresh/Pages/fresh.aspx>.	• Offer tax incentives and subsidies to attract healthy food purveyors.
Zoning	• Des Moines allows the establishment of community gardens on city rights-of-way and city property. Des Moines, Iowa, Mun. Code §§ 74-201, 74-202. • Fresno deems farmers' markets an accepted use in residential districts in its zoning code. Fresno, Cal., Mun. Code § 12-105(F)(4.5). • New York City provides incentives to developers of full-service grocery stores, exempting them from zoning requirements regarding the allowable size of stores and the provision of parking spaces. New York, N.Y., Zoning Res. §§ 62-00–63-60.	• Establish comprehensive land-use protections for farmers' markets and community gardens. • Encourage healthier stores and restaurants to move into an area by exempting them from certain zoning requirements. • Establish "conditional uses" that promote healthy food access. For instance, make selling fresh produce a "conditional use" for corner stores or make accepting Supplemental Nutrition Assistance Program benefits (formerly food stamps) a "conditional use" for farmers' markets.

Source: Diller P, Graff S. Regulating food retail for obesity prevention: how far can cities go? *Using Law, Policy, And Research to Improve the Public's Health*; 2011: 89–93.

TABLE 2-3. REGULATORY STRATEGIES RESTRICTING UNHEALTHY FOOD OPTIONS

Examples		General Ideas
Business operations	• Philadelphia prohibits the use of artificial trans fat in restaurant food. Phila., Pa., Heath Code § 6-307. • Santa Clara County enacted an ordinance setting nutrition standards for restaurant meals that include a toy or other incentive item. Santa Clara County, Cal., Health & Welfare Code § A-18. • Phoenix bans mobile street vendors within 600 feet of schools between 7:00 a.m. and 4:30 p.m. Phoenix, Ariz., Mun. Code § 131-24.	• Regulate the ingredients in restaurant food. • Limit toy giveaways with unhealthy food. • Restrict the sale of certain foods near schools. • Require grocery stores to have "healthy check-out aisles," free of obesogenic food and beverages. • Prohibit food sales in non-retail food outlets such as toy and electronic stores. • Set minimum prices for specified obesogenic food or beverages. • Require food retailers to obtain a license that limits in some way the sale of obesogenic food and beverages.
Taxes and fees	• Chicago imposes a tax on soft drink sellers at the rate of 3% of the gross receipts from sales of bottled and canned soft drinks, and 9% of the cost price of fountain soft drinks. Chicago, Ill., Mun. Code § 3-45.	• Impose excise taxes or regulatory fees of at least one penny per ounce on sugar-sweetened beverages and earmark the revenues to fund obesity prevention programs.
Zoning	• Detroit bans fast food restaurants within 500 feet of schools. Detroit, Mich., Mun. Code §16-12-91. • Westwood Village regulates the density of fast food restaurants to at most one per every 400 feet. Westwood Village, Cal., Specific Plan § 5B.	• Prohibit new fast food restaurants from opening near child-oriented locations or in already saturated neighborhoods. • Regulate the density of fast food restaurants or liquor stores. • Ban drive-through windows.

Source: Diller P, Graff S. Regulating food retail for obesity prevention: how far can cities go? *Using Law, Policy, and Research to Improve the Public's Health*; 2011: 89–93.

Influential Actors

The most influential actors in the health promotion field include the US Preventive Services Task Force and selected federal agencies, world health agencies (which are not discussed in this Chapter), voluntary and professional organizations, accreditors, media, and community advocacy groups and coalitions.

US Preventive Services Task Force

Evidence-based medicine—that is, clinical practice based on accepted scientific findings, which are generally reviewed by a professional or scientific body—has become a critical influence on health care providers. One of the key actors in this arena is the US Preventive Services Task Force (USPSTF), established by the US Public Health Service in 1984. It is an independent panel of mostly non-federal experts in primary care and prevention that uses a systematic methodology to review the evidence for the effectiveness of clinical preventive services (e.g., screening tests, counseling interventions, immunizations, and chemoprevention); assigns ratings to the quality of the data; and issues clinical practice recommendations reflecting the strength of the supporting evidence (Woolf, Jonas, & Lawrence, 1996). The USPSTF has collaborated with medical subspecialties committed to evidence-based policy, such as the American College of Physicians and the American Academy of Family Physicians, as well as with its Canadian counterparts. Task force findings have often varied from those of advocacy groups that have relied on older, opinion-based methods of review.

The first USPSTF assessed 60 topic areas in its Guide to Clinical Preventive Services, published in 1989. In 1996, it published a second edition of the

FIGURE 2-2: USPSTF RECOMMENDATIONS FOR PREVENTIVE SERVICES

The U.S. Preventive Services Task Force (USPSTF) recommends that clinicians discuss these preventive services with eligible patients and offer them as a priority. All these services have received an "A" or a "B" (recommended) grade from the Task Force. For definitions of the grades used by the USPSTF, see this Chapter.

| | Adults | | Special Populations | |
Recommendation	Men	Women	Pregnant Women	Children
Abdominal Aortic Aneurysm, Screening[1]	√			
Alcohol Misuse Screening and Behavioral Counseling Interventions	√	√	√	
Aspirin for Prevention of Cardiovascular Disease[2]	√	√		
Asymptomatic Bacteriuria in Adults, Screening[3]			√	
Breast and Ovarian Cancer Susceptibility, Genetic Risk Assessment and BRCA Mutation Testing[4]		√		
Breast Cancer, Screening[5]		√		
Breastfeeding, Primary Care Interventions to Promote[6]		√	√	
Cervical Cancer, Screening[7]		√		
Chlamydial Infection, Screening[8]		√	√	
Colorectal Cancer, Screening[9]	√	√		
Congenital Hypothyroidism, Screening[10]				√
Depression in Adults, Screening [11]	√	√		
Diabetes Mellitus (Type 2) in Adults, Screening[12]	√	√		
Folic Acid to Prevent Neural Tube Defects[13]		√	√	
Gonococcal Ophthalmia Neonatorum, Preventive Medication. [14]				√
Gonorrhea, Screening[15]		√		
Hearing Loss in Newborns, Screening[16]				√
Hepatitis B Virus in Pregnant Women, Screening[17]			√	
High Blood Pressure (Adults), Screening	√	√		
HIV Screenine[18]	√	√	√	√
Iron Deficiency Anemia, Prevention[19]				√
Iron Deficiency Anemia, Screening[20]			√	
Lipid Disorders in Adults, Screening[21]	√	√		
Major Depressive Disorder in Children, Screening[22]				√
Obesity in Children and Adolescents, Screening[23]				√
Osteoporosis, Screening[24]		√		
Phenylketonuria, Screening[25]				√
Rh (D) Incompatibility, Screening[26]			√	
Sexually Transmitted Infections, Counseling[27]	√	√		√
Sickle Cell Disease, Screening[28]				√
Syphilis Infection, Screening[29]	√	√		
Syphilis Infection in Pregnancy, Screening			√	
Tobacco Use in Adults and Pregnant Women, Counseling[30]	√	√	√	
Visual Impairment in Children Ages I to 5, Screening[31]				√

[1]One-time screening by ultrasonography in men aged 65–75 who have ever smoked.
[2]When the potential harm of an increase in gastrointestinal hemorrhage is outweighed by a potential benefit of a reduction in myocardial infarctions (men aged 45–79 years) or in ischemic strokes (women aged 55–79 years).
[3]Pregnant women at 12–16 weeks gestation or at first prenatal visit, if later.
[4]Refer women whose family history is associated with an increased risk for deleterious mutations in BRCA1 or BRCA2 genes for genetic counseling and evaluation for BRCA testing.

FIGURE 2-2. (CONTINUED)

[5]Biennial screening mammography for women aged 50–74 years. Note: The Department of Health and Human Services, in implementing the Affordable Care Act, follows the 2002 USPSTF recommendation for screening mammography, with or without clinical breast examination, every 1–2 years for women aged 40 and older.

[6]Interventions during pregnancy and after birth to promote and support breastfeeding.

[7]Screen with cytology every 3 years (women aged 21–65) or co-test (cytology/HPV testing) every 5 years (women aged 30–65).

[8]Sexually active women 24 and younger and other asymptomatic women at increased risk for infection. Asymptomatic pregnant women 24 and younger and others at increased risk.

[9]Adults aged 50–75 using fecal occult blood testing, sigmoidoscopy, or colonoscopy.

[10]Newborns.

[11]When staff-assisted depression care supports are in place to assure accurate diagnosis, effective treatment, and follow-up.

[12]Asymptomatic adults with sustained blood pressure greater than 135/80 mm Hg.

[13]All women planning or capable of pregnancy take a daily supplement containing 0.4–0.8 mg (400–800 µg) of folic acid.

[14]Newborns.

[15]Sexually active women, including pregnant women 25 and younger, or at increased risk for infection.

[16]Newborns.

[17]Screen at first prenatal visit.

[18]All adolescents and adults and increased risk for HIV infection and all pregnant women.

[19]Routine iron supplementation for asymptomatic children aged 6 to 12 months who are at increased risk for iron deficiency anemia.

[20]Routine screening in asymptomatic pregnant women.

[21]Men aged 20–35 and women over age 20 who are at increased risk for coronary heart disease; all men aged 35 and older.

[22]Adolescents (aged 12–18) when systems are in place to ensure accurate diagnosis, psychotherapy, and followup.

[23]Screen children aged 6 years and older; offer or refer for intensive counseling and behavioral interventions.

[24]Women aged 65 years and older and women under age 65 whose 10-year fracture risk is equal to or greater than that of a 65-year-old white woman without additional risk factors.

[25]Newborns.

[26]Blood typing and antibody testing at first pregnancy-related visit. Repeated antibody testing for unsensitized Rh (D)-negative women at 24–28 weeks gestation unless biological father is known to be Rh (D) negative.

[27]All sexually active adolescents and adults at increased risk for STIs.

[28]Newborns.

[29]Persons at increased risk.

[30]Ask all adults about tobacco use and provide tobacco cessation interventions for those who use tobacco; provide augmented, pregnancy-tailored counseling for those pregnant women who smoke.

[31]Screen children ages 3 to 5 years.

Source: The Guide to Clinical Preventive Services Recommendations of the US Preventive Services Task Force 2012; retrieved January 1, 2013, from www.USPreventiveServicesTaskForce.org.

Guide to Clinical Preventive Services (USPSTF, 1996), comprising evaluations of 200 interventions in 70 areas. This 1996 guide accompanied the Prevention Guidelines of the Centers for Disease Prevention and Control (CDC) (Friede, O'Carroll, Nicola, Oberle, & Teutsch, 1997). In 1998, the Clinicians' Handbook of Preventive Services and the Put Prevention into Practice national implementation program were released.

In late 1998, the Agency for Healthcare Research and Quality (AHRQ) convened the current USPSTF. Its recommendations are based on systematic evidence reviews conducted by two AHRQ-supported Evidence-Based Practice Centers (one at Oregon Health and Science University and the other at Research Triangle Institute–University of North Carolina) and advice from varied government and private panels of reviewers. The final recommendations balance the relative harms and benefits of preventive medicine. The overall net benefits of preventive services are rated from A to D, recommend to not recommend, or I (insufficient). The levels of certainty regarding net benefits range from high to low (U.S. Preventive Services Task Force Ratings. June 2007. http://www.uspreventiveservicestaskforce.org/uspstf07/ratingsv2.htm). The reports do consider the financial costs of preventive services.

The latest *Guide to Clinical Preventive Services* (see Figure 2-2; online updates at: www.USPreventiveServicesTaskForce.org) comprises 64 preventive services, providing the latest available recommendations on preventive interventions, screening tests, counseling, immunizations, and medication regimens for more than 80 conditions. The USPSTF recommendations have created performance measures that are used to judge quality by the National Committee for Quality Assurance (NCQA), peer review organizations (PROs), and the Joint Commission for Accreditation of Healthcare Organizations (JCAHO), holding providers and health care systems accountable for delivering effective health care.

In 1996, the CDC formed the Community Preventive Services Task Force (CPSTF) to address a broad range of interventions, targeting communities and health care systems rather than individual clients, since for some health problems, such as adolescent smoking, community-based interventions are more likely to decrease the problem behavior than are health care provider interventions. The results of the efforts of the CPSTF are published in *The Guide to Community Preventive Services*, which seeks to provide public health decision makers with recommendations on population-based interventions to promote health and to prevent disease, injury, disability, and premature death at the state and local levels, thus complementing the work of the USPSTF (http://www.thecommunityguide.org/index.html; see Figure 2-3).

Barriers to the Dissemination of the USPSTF Guidelines

For a variety of reasons, USPSTF guidelines and other sources of medical evidence or best practices, such as *The Guide to Community Preventive Services*, are not always put into use by health providers, or are put to use only inconsistently. The barriers are multilevel, at the patient, provider, and policy levels.

Patient-related barriers to the uptake of evidence-based prevention practices include; limited or no health insurance; limited literacy; delay in symptom recognition, diagnosis, and treatment; poor cultural matches between patients and providers;

mistrust, low awareness, or limited knowledge of health care services; misunderstanding of provider instructions; low "self-activation," and poor prior interactions with the health care system (reviewed in Institute of Medicine [IOM], 2003; Heck & Sheinfeld Gorin, 2004; Sheinfeld Gorin & NYPAC Study Group, 2004; Sheinfeld Gorin & Albert, 2003; Sheinfeld Gorin, Graff Zivin & NYPAC Study Group, 2003; Sheinfeld Gorin, 2005; Honda & Sheinfeld Gorin, 2005; Sheinfeld Gorin, Heck, Albert & Hershman, 2005; Sheinfeld Gorin & Heck, 2005) as well as limited social support (Berkman & Syme, 1979; Berkman, 1995; Seeman, Kaplan, Knudsen, Cohen, & Guralnik, 1987; Seeman, 2000; example in obesity, Christakis & Fowler, 2007). Provider-level barriers to evidence-based counseling for prevention include limited time, lack of training in prevention, lack of perceived effectiveness of selected preventive services, and practice environments that fail to facilitate prevention (Ashford et al., 2000; Hulscher, Wensing, van der Weijden, & Grol, 2002). Physicians find counseling time-consuming and difficult to track and to charge; in fact, physician time for counseling clients about health promotion is relatively short, under 15 minutes, and often from 2 to 6 minutes (Mullen & Holcomb, 1990; Kushner, 1995; Ockene et al., 1995;

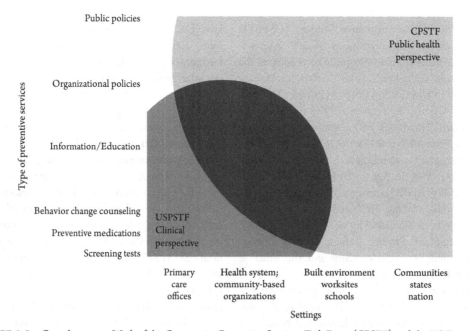

FIGURE 2-3: Complementary Work of the Community Preventive Services Task Force (CPSTF) and the US Preventive Services Task Force (USPSTF).

Source: Community Preventive Services Task Force. 2012 Annual Report to Congress. The Guide to Community Preventive Services; The Community Guide: What Works to Promote Health.

Patton, Kolasa, West, & Irons, 1995; Burton et al., 1995; Price, Clause, & Everett, 1995; Schectman, Stoy, & Elinsky, 1994; Thompson, Schwankovsky, & Pitts, 1993; Ammerman et al., 1993; Cushman, James, & Waclawik, 1991; Logsdon, Lazaro, & Meier, 1989). Further, current methods of reimbursing doctors and hospitals favor testing and procedures over preventive medicine and spending time on patient counseling.

Guides to identifying effective interventions can be difficult in prevention, where randomized, controlled trials are often challenging to conduct. The evidence base is mixed, and there are few effective decision aids for patient use (Sheinfeld Gorin et al., 2006). There is strong evidence for the effectiveness of brief clinician counseling in smoking cessation (Sheinfeld Gorin & Heck, 2004) and in reducing problem drinking. Dietary counseling can lead to increased fruit and vegetable consumption (Pomerleau et al., 2005; Tang et al., 1998; Lin et al., 2010). Primary care–based interventions to increase physical activity demonstrate some short-term effects on cardiovascular health (Lin et al., 2010). For example, the Patient-Centered Assessment and Counseling for Exercise (PACE; Calfas & Hagler, 2006) approach holds promise. Provider counseling of adults and children can increase children's practices of safety behaviors (e.g., the use of seat belts, child safety seats, and bicycle helmets), although the prevalence of this counseling is low, according to a 2007 cross-sectional, list-assisted random-digit-dial telephone survey of randomly selected US children (Chen, Kresnow, Simon, Dellinger, 2007). Brief counseling interventions aimed at high-risk individuals can increase condom use and prevent the spread of sexually transmitted diseases (Noar, 2008). Health provider recommendation is central to compliance with cancer screening tests, such as those for the breast, colon, and cervix (see Mandelblatt & Yabroff, 1999, for a review), but the guidelines differ by patient characteristics, such as age (Journal of the National Cancer Institute, 2013). Often, however, the provider serves as a motivator for, rather than a leader of guideline compliance by patients, as discussed further in Chapter 11.

Similarly, provider-patient process factors, such as poor communication and uncertainty, may limit access to health care and health-promoting counseling, particularly for racial and ethnic subgroups. The time pressures exerted by the demands of modern health care and the beliefs about the likelihood of ameliorating a patient's condition that are inculcated in medical students through their training

can limit counseling; bias and stereotyping may also limit access to health care, particularly among minority patients (IOM, 2003).

Finally, system-level barriers, such as language differences, variations in the geographic availability of health care institutions (including pharmacies) and in the distribution of health-promoting environments (e.g., grocery stores selling healthful foods, Diez-Roux, 2003; parks, bike and walking paths for physical activity), and a lack of coordination among service providers who are treating patients with multiple and complex conditions (IOM, 2003) may influence access to and the provision of quality care.

Further, according to a recent systematic review, evidence-based interventions may vary in their impact on socioeconomic inequalities. Structural workplace interventions, including the provision of resources, and fiscal interventions, such as tobacco pricing, are more likely to reduce socioeconomic inequalities than media campaigns and workplace smoking bans, thus further increasing uncertainty about the relevant intervention choices (Lorenc, Pettigrew, Welch, & Tugwell, 2012). Thus substantial gaps in the delivery of evidence-based preventive health care remain.

Other Influences on Evidence-Based Practice

Internationally (with sites in the US), the Cochrane Collaboration, a voluntary association of academics and clinicians, supports the development and publication of systematic reviews of rigorous studies in health. These reviews are widely available on the Web and through standard bibliographical search engines, such as MedLine. Although, in general, association members' interests align most with treatment evaluations, the Cochrane Public Health Group systematically evaluates public health interventions, and The Cochrane Library publishes the evidence for screening tests. The Campbell Collaboration similarly supports systematic reviews of studies in health, as does the National Institute for Clinical Excellence (NICE) in the United Kingdom, and the Health Evidence Network (HEN) sponsored by the WHO Regional Office for Europe. Generally, the findings of these international collaborations have less influence on health care practice in the United States than do the findings of national groups, such as the USPSTF, although there is burgeoning interest in increasing the US policy-relevance of Cochrane Collaboration reviews, in particular (personal communication with Mark Wilson, CEO, January 24, 2013).

Selected Federal Agencies

Although health promotion policies are housed in several federal agencies, only the actions of the US surgeon general and the CDC are described at any length in this Chapter. In particular the Healthy People documents, presented under the auspices of the surgeon general, have had unprecedented influence on the health promotion field because of the extent of participation that the health care community had in their preparation, their credibility, and the form and content of their texts. They are credited with beginning a "second revolution" in public health.

Centers for Disease Control and Prevention

The Centers for Disease Control and Prevention is unique in the extent of its influence on the health promotion field because it is one of the few (and the oldest) agencies devoted to the singular mission of promoting health and quality of life, by preventing and controlling disease, injury, and disability. Through its 12 centers, institutes, and offices, it stewards a wide range of activities involving chronic disease prevention and health promotion; environmental health; infectious disease (e.g., human immunodeficiency virus [HIV], sexually transmitted disease [STD], and tuberculosis [TB]) prevention; injury prevention and control; occupational safety and health; the national immunization program; epidemiology; and health statistics. Its scope ranges from the international to work with state and local health agencies. Few health promotion efforts fall outside its auspices.

Initiatives Led by Selected Federal Agencies: Healthy People 2020

To place the Healthy People 2020 document in context, a very brief history of public health is offered. The first public health revolution began with the watershed 1848 Public Health Act in Britain; from that point forward, the principle of state intervention in the lives of individuals to promote outcomes of social value was established. In particular, this nineteenth-century revolution sought to improve the social and physical environment to decrease health hazards. This Act, as well as the two that preceded it (the English Towns Improvement Act of 1847 and the Liverpool Sanitary Act of 1846), provided a remedy for particular problems, designated nuisances, and allowed public authorities to order their removal. These nuisances were largely seen as things that smelled offensively, supporting the miasmatic idea that bad smells were a sign of disease. The Act authorized the undertaking of public health works, such as controls over slaughterhouses, common lodging houses, and offensive trades. It contained requirements for all new houses to be built with drains that connected to sewage systems where possible or to a cesspit. It also created a public health structure, the General Board of Health, which functioned as a national public health authority, and local boards of health, which consisted of supervisors of local surveyors and inspectors of nuisances. Responsibility for sewers was vested in the local boards, which had powers to control and cleanse (Reynolds, 1994).

The Second Public Health Revolution

The second public health revolution, reflected in Healthy People: The Surgeon General's Report on Health Promotion and Disease Prevention (US Department of Health, Education and Welfare, Public Health Service, 1979), heralded the importance of lifestyle changes to health promotion and the importance of the reduction of chronic disease and the achievement of a better quality of life for all. Although the report was at first criticized for victim blaming, over time its thesis that lifestyle changes play an important role in health was accepted and led to significant changes in public health practice (Neubauer & Pratt, 1981; Tesh, 1981; Neubauer & Pratt, 1981; Navarro, 1976).

Healthy People 2010

Healthy People 2010 is the most recently completed report; it provided the basis for the planning of the newest national approach to prevention, Healthy People 2020, and thus it will be discussed in some detail. Healthy People 2010 provided a plan of action for the nation's health, with two major goals: to increase quality and years of healthy life and to eliminate health disparities. As did its forerunners, it established a set of specific objectives, 467 in number, organized into 28 focus areas, as a basis for coordinated efforts to improve public health on the national, state, and local levels, and to be used as a teaching tool. Twenty-one of these objectives were found within 10 leading indicators, which involved physical activity, overweight and obesity, tobacco use, substance abuse, responsible sexual behavior, mental health, injury and violence, environmental quality, immunization, and access to health care. The 28 focus areas traversed the three broad categories of public health that were found in *Healthy People 2000*: health promotion, health protection, and preventive services.

An interactive online database, DATA2010, updated quarterly (CDC, 2005b), was available to track the *Healthy People 2010* objectives. Unlike all previous national documents of this type, *Healthy People 2010* placed the reduction of health disparities at its core. It also reflected a more integrated approach to health promotion, from lifestyle to environmental approaches, than previous documents did. In consonance with the *Health 21* document from WHO, and at variance with the individual risk orientation of *Healthy People 2000*, *Healthy People 2010* also reflected goals and objectives related to supportive environments.

Evaluation of Healthy People 2010

Healthy People 2010 Final Review (2011) assessed the overall impact of the Healthy People 2010 initiative on its stated goals, determining that, overall, Americans had met—or were moving toward meeting—71% of the program's 2010 targets, including those associated with reducing deaths from coronary heart disease and stroke. Some of the more promising data released in the assessment revealed that the country met the *Healthy People 2010* objectives of reducing cholesterol levels, while making minor strides toward reducing smoking rates. As a result, according to the National Vital Statistics System, the United States experienced a major drop in deaths from heart disease and strokes over the past decade. In other positive findings, the nation's overall life expectancy continued to rise, and several objectives that tracked mental health status, treatment, and services met their *Healthy People 2010* targets (http://www.hhs.gov/news, October 6, 2011).

While much progress was made with regard to most of the 2010 health objectives, it is clear from the *Healthy People 2010* assessment that the nation still comes up short in a number of critical areas, including efforts to reduce health disparities and the obesity rate. This is particularly telling as eliminating health disparities was one of the two goals of the *Healthy People 2010* initiative.

Over the past decade, health disparities have not changed for approximately 80% of the health objectives and have increased for an additional 13%. And, the report found that obesity rates increased across all age groups. Among children aged 6–11 years, obesity rates rose by 54.5%, and among adolescents aged 12–19 years, the obesity rate rose 63.6%. In addition, the proportion of adults who are obese rose by 48%. These findings are sobering, given the general relationship between obesity and all of the diseases that are discussed in Chapters 4 through 7 of this book.

Healthy People 2020

Healthy People 2020 is informed by the *Healthy People 2010 Final Report*; it is based on the three other Healthy People initiatives that preceded it: the 1979 Surgeon General's Report, *Healthy People: The Surgeon General's Report on Health Promotion and Disease Prevention*; *Healthy People 1990: Promoting Health/Preventing Disease: Objectives for the Nation*; and *Healthy People 2000: National Health Promotion and Disease Prevention Objectives*. *Healthy People 2020*'s goals and objectives are the result of a multi-year process that reflects input from a diverse group of individuals and organizations (www.healthypeople.gov). Under the ACA, the National Prevention, Health Promotion, and Public Health Council, involving more than a dozen federal agencies, will develop a prevention and health promotion strategy that will build on the Healthy People initiatives.

The "Third" Public Health Revolution: The Patient Protection and Affordable Care Act

The most sweeping recent reform in health care is found in the Patient Protection and Affordable Care Act (P.L. 111-148, 124 Stat. 119-1025; ACA; full text: http://www.gpo.gov/fdsys/pkg/PLAW-111publ148/content-detail.html). It will profoundly affect both the way health insurance is purchased and the benefits it will provide. The ACA is designed in part to ensure that all Americans are covered by a health insurance plan that offers adequate coverage of preventive and primary care services, as will be discussed further below. The ACA is a combination of programs (state health exchanges) and requirements for behavior (e.g., the insurance mandate, required benefits coverage), so it has a potential impact on both the politics and economics of health care. It is primarily focused on how insurance is purchased and what benefits it must cover, with cost-containment and quality of care as secondary goals.

The ACA addresses the goal of increased insurance coverage through a requirement that most American citizens and legal aliens purchase health insurance, either with their own pre-tax dollars or, in the case of poor individuals and families, through a subsidy. Individuals who do not purchase health insurance will be subject to a tax penalty. Employers with more that 50 workers must offer health insurance to their employees or face a tax penalty, while small business will be given subsidies and tax advantages when they offer health insurance to their employees. The self-employed, those whose employers do not offer health insurance, or small businesses may purchase it through state-level health insurance exchanges, which create a market for health insurance plans.

To further increase access to adequate health insurance, the ACA imposes a number of requirements on health insurance plans, which must provide a minimum level of benefits, have an adequate network of providers, and place limits on beneficiaries' out-of-pocket expenses, with lower out-of-pocket limits for low-income individuals and families. Health insurance plans may not drop coverage except when it was obtained by fraud, and may not place lifetime limits on the dollar value of coverage provided. Further, insurance plans must spend 85% (80% for plans in the individual and small-group market) of their premium dollars on health services, quality improvements, and other costs, or provide a rebate to customers if they fail to do so.

As discussed in Chapter 1, the ACA affects preventive medicine in several ways. First, it establishes several committees and task forces, such as the National Prevention, Health Promotion and Public Health Council, as well as several funding mechanisms, such as the Prevention and Public Health Fund, to study and pursue prevention and wellness activities. Second, for Medicare and qualified private plans it eliminates cost-sharing (co-pays, co-insurance, or deductibles) on preventive services rated A or B by the USPSTF (i.e., recommended services that should be offered or provided; with either [A] high certainty that the net benefit is substantial; or [B] high certainty that the net benefit is moderate or there is moderate certainty that the net benefit is moderate to substantial; http://www.uspreventive servicestaskforce.org/uspstf/uspsabrecs.htm). It also allows for Medicare to change its coverage of preventive services based on the recommendations of the USPSTF. Additionally, health insurance plans must cover routine immunizations and certain preventive services for children and women without imposing cost-sharing on beneficiaries. Third, it provides a financial reward for states that offer preventive services without cost-sharing requirements as part of their Medicaid benefits (Kaiser Family Foundation, 2011).

The Patient-Centered Outcomes Research Institute (PCORI), which will focus on comparative effectiveness research that evaluates and compares the risks, benefits, health outcomes, and clinical effectiveness of methods to prevent, diagnose, treat, or monitor disease, was also authorized under the ACA. This new institute will seek to apply epidemiologic techniques to provide evidence for patients and medical providers to make informed choices; this process (shared decision making) is discussed further in Chapter 12.

Political opponents of the Act have continued to challenge it, arguing that its individual mandate requirement is beyond the enumerated powers of the federal government, and by claiming that the financial requirements are onerous; they have continued to seek to block its effects through Congressional repeal of the act, and through delaying and defunding implementation activities. The Supreme Court of the United States found the act constitutional, and upheld the individual mandate and the Medicaid expansion; in the latter, by circumscribing the secretary's enforcement authority (in the case, *National Federation of Independent Business v. Sibelius*; June 28, 2012; www. kff.org/healthreform). The Republican presidential candidate in 2012, who had vowed to repeal the act, was defeated. Through the legal and political processes, the debate surrounding the ACA has brought problems in the American health system to the forefront of the political discussion. Significant change is now likely with full implementation of the ACA, although, at present, the process remains both slow and contentious.

Other National Agencies

Several other national agencies are also active in health promotion. The Food and Drug Administration safeguards the nation's food supply (with certain exceptions), prescription and over the counter (OTC) drug supply, medical devices, drugs and devices used for animals, cosmetic products, and biologics, by helping safe and effective products reach the market in a timely way and monitoring them for continued safety after they are in use. Although the FDA has historically been unable to regulate tobacco, the Family Smoking Prevention and Tobacco Control Act gave the FDA expanded powers to regulate the marketing, advertising, and ingredients of some tobacco products. However, the FDA's power with respect to dietary supplements is quite limited. Supplements are not required to be tested for safety and efficacy before they are introduced into the marketplace and may make use of arguably deceptive claims on their labeling. Still, the FDA may impose purity requirements on them and may pull supplements off the market if they are shown to be dangerous, as was the case with ephedra-based supplements.

The Occupational Safety and Health Administration (OSHA) of the US Department of Labor has established guidelines on workplace violence and initiatives in ergonomics that have been important to health promotion. The US Department of Agriculture (USDA) has been particularly influential through the nutritional programs it administers: the food stamps program for low-income Americans; the Special Supplemental Nutrition Program for Women, Infants, and Children (WIC); and child nutrition programs. The Environmental Protection Agency (EPA) enforces the removal of toxic wastes and monitors toxic air pollution and pesticide use, all of which are important to health promotion.

National Voluntary and Professional Organizations

Numerous voluntary organizations such as the American Cancer Society, the American Heart Association, and the American Lung Association, by focusing on a single health issue, have advanced the health promotion agenda nationally and internationally and have educated the public. Similarly, professional groups such as the American Public Health Association and the American College of Preventive Medicine, in pursuing their members' interests, have either directly influenced health promotion legislation concerning a wide array of topics (nutrition, physical activity, pollution, testing and screening, insurance coverage, etc.) or have provided direct service to clients.

The more than 300 professional associations contributing to health promotion in this country have assisted in the development of a national agenda

for health promotion; have influenced legislation; and have engaged in education, screening, and other preventive services for clients. Of course, each organization advocates for the interests of its own members, so their agendas may be rather narrow and may have unintended consequences, like higher fees for specialists than primary care providers—increasing shortages—or over-testing and subsequent over-treatment of their "pet" diseases (like prostate cancer). These associations include the American Public Health Association, Society for Public Health Education, American Nurses Association, American Academy of Family Physicians, American College of Physicians, American College of Preventive Medicine, American College of Nutrition, American Dietetic Association, American Physical Therapy Association, American Dental Association, and National Association of Social Workers. Many of these organizations and groups are represented by some of the more than 18,000 registered lobbyists who incurred roughly $3 billion in 2003 expenses (Mike Scott, director of Government Affairs, American Society of Anesthesiologists, personal communication) to influence legislation and national, state, and local agendas.

Interest in environmental influences (e.g., the "built environment," such as sprawl) on prevention (e.g., on obesity reduction) has grown in recent years. Many of these efforts have been led by national or local voluntary grassroots organizations. For example, California Healthy Cities and Communities has funded community-based nutrition and physical activity programs in several cities, and these programs have included the enactment of policies for land and complementary water use, improved access to produce, elevated public consciousness about health, culturally appropriate educational and training materials, and strengthened community-building skills (Twiss et al., 2003). Active roles for both citizens and communities are central to environmental change approaches.

Accreditors

Accreditation is a self-assessment and external peer review process used by health care organizations to regularly assess their level of performance in relation to established standards and to implement ways to continuously improve the health care system (Tregloan, 2000). According to a recent review, accreditation has an impact on promoting change and professional development (Greenfield

& Braithwaite, 2008). Patient safety is a major stated issue for health care providers, payers, and patients, as reflected in a number of recent quality initiatives. Nonetheless, as noted in a recent IOM report, *Crossing the Quality Chasm* (IOM, 2001) preventable medical errors have remained, with serious health consequences. In fact, of the IOM's six aims of a twenty-first-century delivery system, safety is first (alongside effectiveness, patient-centeredness, timeliness, efficiency, and equity; IOM, 2001).

Two major accrediting groups—the National Commission for Quality Assurance (NCQA) and the Joint Commission on Accreditation of Healthcare Organizations (JCAHO)—maintain standards for the quality of organizations' structured health promotion activities. Other organizations, such as the National Association for Healthcare Quality and the American Society of Health-System Pharmacists, may monitor medication safety, and prestigious scientific groups, such as the Institute of Medicine and the non-profit Institute for Healthcare Improvement, may document the overall quality of health care through their focus on seminal issues, such as health disparities, without issuing certifications. Additionally, rapidly growing groups such as the Utilization Review Accreditation Committee (URAC) serve to promote continuous improvement in the quality and efficiency of health care delivery services by streamlining the processes used to determine whether health care is medically necessary, helping to keep health care costs down for both payers and providers.

Accreditors use a combination of on-site expert surveys of an organization and reviews of written materials to determine whether an organization has met pre-established guidelines for health care. Accreditation indicates that an entity has adopted a set of quality standards and that its performance is continually reviewed. Accreditation is critical to a health care center's continued receipt of insurance funds, competition for employer health care contracts, and licensure for Medicare certification through deemed status (i.e., a status conferred on a hospital or other organization by a professional standards review organization, such as JCAHO, in formal recognition that the organization's review, continued-stay review, and medical care evaluation programs meet certain effectiveness criteria). Often, accreditation by major accreditors serves as an alternative to federal or state inspection of health care facilities. These external accreditations are important adjuncts to the continuous quality improvement (CQI) systems that monitor, correct, and enhance the services of many agencies.

NCQA

NCQA is a private, not-for-profit organization dedicated to improving health care quality and is frequently referred to as a watchdog for the managed care industry. Its Health Plan Employer Data and Information Set (HEDIS) report card requirements guide the managed care industry, as well as many community clinics.

Since 1997, NCQA has produced an annual State of Health Care Quality report that provides an overall assessment of the performance of the health care system. These findings are issued before the annual open enrollment season, when most Americans choose their health plan for the following year. In compiling these data, NCQA requires an organization to evaluate the use of preventive services, including cholesterol measurement; exercise promotion; smoking cessation; and counseling for prevention of motor vehicle injury, sexually transmitted diseases, and alcohol and other drug abuse. The evaluation process includes looking at both the groups at risk and the population as a whole.

Under the guidance of NCQA, consumers, insurance purchasers, and health maintenance organizations (HMOs) developed the HEDIS measures for HMOs to evaluate the quality of services and the care they provide. HEDIS addresses a broad range of important health issues including childhood and adolescent immunization status, high blood pressure control, asthma medication use, antidepressant medication management, breast cancer screening, and smoking cessation counseling. Using the HEDIS findings, NCQA has recently created the Quality Compass,* which allows users to compare health plans side by side and to make health care coverage decisions based on quality and value as well as provider network and price (NCQA).

JCAHO

JCAHO is the predominant standards-setting and accrediting body in the United States, with more than 15,000 health care organizations and programs under its supervision, including ambulatory care centers, home health care centers, behavioral health care organizations, health care networks, corporate health services, long-term care organizations, hospitals, pathology and clinical laboratory services. Since 1994, JCAHO has specified health promotion and disease prevention guidelines for health care networks, including HMOs, preferred provider organizations [PPOs], and other managed care entities that are performance or outcome focused. It addresses each organization's level of performance in areas such as patient rights, patient treatment, and infection control and its performance with respect to health promotion and disease prevention. For behavioral health care organizations, including those that provide mental health and addiction services, JCAHO has developed draft standards for behavioral health promotion and illness prevention (JCAHO, 2005).

JCAHO also awards disease-specific care certification to health plans, hospitals, and other service delivery settings that provide disease management and chronic care services. In 1997, JCAHO launched its ORYX® initiative, which integrates outcomes and other performance measures into the accreditation process, affording a flexible approach that can support quality improvement efforts across all health delivery systems; by 2004, almost all hospitals were expected to comply with new standards and to submit data across several core components (JCAHO, 2005).

Efforts to standardize accreditation procedures were helped when, in 2003, NCQA and JCAHO formed a partnership for the purpose of establishing an accreditation program for efforts to protect human subjects in research. This union also realizes one aim of behavioral health advocates by allaying fears about how informed consent for research participation is obtained from individuals with serious mental illnesses.

Despite all these accreditation bodies, measuring provider performance, developing accurate proxies for performance, and incentivizing providers to meet quality goals remain very difficult. Since performance can rarely be measured directly, it is often the case that compliance with quality proxies is not the same as providing quality care. Some accrediting bodies have conflicts of interest, as in JCAHO's ownership of a for-profit arm that consults with hospitals about how to pass the accreditation process. Some providers may engage in undesirable behavior in order to meet quality goals, like dropping the sickest and most complex cases from their case load. Most hospitals do not have a problem getting accredited, but this does not necessarily mean that they are providing high quality care; for example, the standards for quality may be too low. Further, given the conclusions of *Crossing the Chasm* (IOM, 2001), the accreditation process does not appear to have addressed the high rates of medical errors in the United States.

Medical Licensure

The analogous process for individual physicians, nurses, and other health care providers is medical licensure. Medical licensure is a state-level system designed to ensure that individual practitioners are qualified to practice; however, the system faces problems of conflicts of interest and apparently has not addressed the high rates of medical errors in this country.

The Media

The media provide illumination and a focus of attention that is enormously powerful, particularly when the spotlight can be held in place. Through the agenda-setting process, the mass media may provide the first step in public awareness and change, or by withholding attention, they can leave issues in the dark (Wallack, Dorfman, Jernigan, & Themba, 1993). Even though the media recently have begun to expand their coverage of health-promotive lifestyles, communication challenges remain.

Public education campaigns and commercial advertising have increased interest in low-fat diets, physical exercise, and weight management. Newer screening technologies, such as colonography for the early detection of polyps and newer interventions, such as a vaccine for the human papillomavirus (HPV) to reduce the risk of cervical cancer (Franco & Harper, 2005), are emerging alongside increased public interest. With the growth of social media, health sites and blogs, and other information technologies (as discussed further in Chapters 3, 10, 11, and 12), many individuals have become more knowledgeable about prevention and professional guidelines for screening. The American public depends on the news media for reliable health information. Yet many health care professionals meet with difficulties when sharing science news with the public through the mass media, as discussed further in Chapter 11 (Woloshin, Schwartz, & Welch, 2002). For example, the media may not always report health threats accurately. These inaccuracies may contribute to the public's overestimation of mortality from causes that are actually infrequent (e.g., deaths resulting from illicit drugs) and underestimation of mortality from causes that are frequent (e.g., heart disease) (Adams, 1992–1993; Frost, Frank, & Mailbach, 1997). As discussed further in Chapter 11, there is considerable confusion about how best to discuss health risks in numerical terms, even in clinical settings (Woloshin, Schwartz, & Welch, 2002). Moreover, the media may, at the same time, promote healthful eating through public service announcements while promoting high-fat, high-sugar foods through paid advertising.

Health care providers themselves may enhance their communication with the mass media by using several evidence-based strategies from the CAUSE model (Rowan, Bethea, Pecchioni, & Villagran, 2003). This model involves earning the confidence of respected journalists, creating awareness of health issues, deepening understanding, gaining the satisfaction of news coverage, and motivating enactment or behavioral change. (For a bibliography on health risk communication, see US National Library of Medicine, 2003.) In addition, as discussed in Chapter 11, public training in numeracy and risk assessment would enrich the sophistication of those responding to the media's coverage of health. Mass media interventions can be more cost effective for a large target group relative to individual clinical interventions, supporting the importance of health care professionals engaging in these broader communication approaches (Hastings, 1989; McAlister, 1982; Roberts & Maccoby, 1985; Barker, Pistrang, Shapiro, Davies, & Shaw, 1993; Baylor College of Medicine, 2004; Lorion, 1983). As discussed more fully in Chapter 12, the explosion of the Internet and social media with Web communities and individual Web logs, or blogs, allows for rapid dissemination of information to the consumer seeking quick and easy advice regarding health habits. Blogs (like *Tumblr*) are quickly becoming forums for the rapid exchange of ideas on all topics, alongside social media like *Facebook*, *Twitter*, and *Linked In*; new approaches are emerging regularly. Webinars, video conferences, and podcasts are fast replacing face-to-face training sessions and meetings. These various social media can be used to generate dialogue, but they can also be dominated by those with commercial interests or competing claims, increasing decision conflict. Anonymous Internet portals managed by reputable health care organizations, such as the CDC, may be an effective vehicle for channeling essential messages to consumers who may find it difficult to parse through conflicting information in TV, radio, or print media, however.

Community Advocacy Groups and Coalitions

Community groups, such as Mothers Against Drunk Driving (MADD) and the National Alliance of Breast Cancer Organizations (NABCO), have been effective advocates for change in laws concerning drinking and driving (MADD) and breast cancer (NABCO). In the case of tobacco use, for example, community and professional groups have organized coalitions to lobby successfully for legislation that outlaws smoking in public buildings, workplaces, restaurants, schools, and sporting events across the country, and in conjunction with international partners such as the World Health Organization, in many parts of the developed world. They have influenced schools of medicine to teach smoker counseling, they have provided consultation for clinical trials in community settings (e.g., Community Intervention Trial for Smoking Cessation [COMMIT] and the subsequent American Stop Smoking Intervention Study for Cancer Prevention Trial.[ASSIST]), and they have galvanized community attitudes toward favoring smoking control.

ORGANIZATIONAL POLICY

Organizations such as schools, workplaces, public health departments, and health care facilities are central to the implementation of health promotion legislation, regulations, and policies and are essential to the formation of new initiatives. These organizations wield considerable influence on community, group, and individual behavior.

School Districts and Schools

Lifetime patterns of diet, exercise, smoking, and coping with stress may be established in childhood. Because the roughly 55.3 million children and youth in America spend much of their days in school, the school has become an important context in which to change these patterns, through legislation, policies, and regulation. Children may learn about their bodies and the effects of different lifestyle behaviors in this context. Children may also gain access to necessary preventive services, such as age-appropriate immunizations, nutritious meals, and regular, organized physical activity. The school also may connect families to health insurance programs, potentially through state waiver funding or through Medicaid aid packages, thus enriching a family's ability to continue to receive preventive services.

Worksites and Unions

About 135 million adults go to work every day in the United States (http://www.bls.gov/web/empsit/ceshighlights.pdf, January, 2013); individuals spend more than one-third of their waking hours at work. While labor union membership is declining nationwide, 11.3% of all U.S. workers still belong to a labor union (Bureau of Labor Statistics, (http://www.bls.gov/news.release/union2.nr0.htm, January, 23, 2013); union members generally have access to medical care through their benefit plans. Nonetheless, both worksites and unions are important components of community-wide health promotion efforts. Further, traditional worksite-based health promotion programs are seen as an employee benefit that increases employee morale and attracts and retains good workers at relatively little cost.

Two-thirds of employers with three or more employers who offer health benefits offer at least one wellness program; almost all companies with >1,000 employees offer one. Typical features of wellness programs are health-risk assessments and screenings for high blood pressure and cholesterol; behavior modification programs, such as tobacco cessation, weight management, and exercise; health education, including classes or referrals to online sites for health advice; and changes in the work environment or provision of special benefits to encourage exercise and healthy food choices, such as subsidized health club memberships (http://www.healthaffairs.org/healthpolicybriefs/brief.php?brief_id=69).

Workplaces that are oriented toward promoting good health for employees in order to decrease costs of absenteeism, increase productivity, or create more effective organizations may offer multifaceted supportive programs (e.g., smoking cessation policies and clinics), exercise facilities, employee assistance programs (EAPs) for behavioral health promotion, and health insurance. Since the 1990s, under the Drug-Free Workplace Act of 1988, EAPs have become the linchpin of many workplace-based substance abuse programs, alongside drug-free workplace policies, training and educational programs, and the identification of illegal drug users (Glemigani, 1998; Hoffman, Larison, & Sanderson, 1997; Greenberg & Grunberg, 1995; Delaney & Ames, 1995; Galvin, 2000). In addition, under Occupational Safety and Health Administration (OSHA) regulations, worksites integrate the protection of employee health through setting and enforcing safety standards, training workers, and offering safety education. The Accountable Care Act includes worksite health promotion, as described in Chapter 1; more progressive worksites may see the creation of healthful work as an aim in itself.

Union-based health promotion projects may have access to blue-collar workers who may be otherwise difficult to reach and who have higher rates of smoking and poorer health outcomes than workers in white-collar positions do (Albertsen, Hannerz, Borg, & Burr, 2003; Barbeau, Krieger, & Soobader, 2004; Turrell, Hewitt, Patterson, Oldenburg, & Gould, 2002). There is some evidence to suggest that unions are amenable to worksite risk modification programs, such as smoking cessation interventions that include systematic prevention messages as well as policy changes (Sorensen et al., 2000) and comprehensive programs designed to change dietary behaviors (Heimendinger et al., 1995).

During 2007–2010, a period of economic downturn, the share of Americans under the age of 65 covered by employer-sponsored health insurance (ESI) eroded to 58.6% (marking the 10th year of consecutive declines). As many as 28 million more people under the age of 65 would have had ESI in 2010 if the coverage rate had remained at the 2000 level (http://www.epi.org/publication/bp337-employer-sponsored-health-insurance/). In 2001–2011, the lowest paid workers, those with incomes below 138% of the federal poverty level, had the sharpest decline in ESI, falling from 38% to 29%, while the highest earners saw a much smaller decline, from 92% to 90% (Robert Wood Johnson Foundation; http://ccf.georgetown.edu/ccf-resources/employer-sponsored-insurance-declining-rapidly-low-wage-workers). With the rise in medical and health insurance costs over time, smaller worksites are often unable to offer employee assistance programs and preventive services. Even larger firms are now ceasing to offer health insurance, or are requiring higher employee contributions, reducing access to preventive services.

Evaluation of Worksite Health Promotion Programs

Two meta-analyses of worksite wellness programs have found savings in medical claims due to worksite wellness that have been reported as far more substantial than any other category of health benefit initiative (an average of 24.5% according to one meta-review of 62 studies [Chapman, 2012], resulting in returns-on-investment (ROIs) of 3.27:1 according to another meta-analysis [Baicker, Cutler, & Song, 2010], or roughly $340 per person), which are also far higher than any other voluntary managed care initiative.

Since savings of the magnitude noted in these two meta-analyses (Chapman, 2012; Baicker, Cutler, & Song, 2010) would dramatically multiply the profits for America's roughly 1,000 private health plans, it's unclear why few (if any) of them routinely incentivize wellness programs for fully insured members with their own cash and/or premium discounts. Nor do they routinely require their fully insured members to take Health Risk Assessments (HRAs) or biometric screens, which underlie most corporate wellness programs. Part of the answer lies in the methodologic challenges to the conduct of these workplace studies.

As appropriately noted by the authors of both meta-evaluations (Chapman, 2012; Baicker, Cutler, & Song, 2010), the studies proclaiming wellness program success are subject to methodologic limitations, because by definition there is no "intent to treat" control. Almost invariably, all voluntary participants are in one group and those who didn't want to participate comprise the control, or else the control is a passive matched control, with no indication of whether the control group consists largely of motivated or unmotivated people. In both cases, only motivated participants are included in the study group. This limitation is especially problematic in wellness, because unlike a drug trial, motivation is by far the most important factor in success of an incentivized self-help program. Since the passing of the Health Insurance Portability and Accountability Act (HIPAA) of 1996, individual rights to information privacy have hindered attempts to monitor patients to assess the long-term benefits of wellness promotion programs, thus confounding attempts at achieving accurate cost-benefit analyses of program effectiveness.

Further, encouraging employees to participate in these programs remains a challenge, so the participants are not generally representative of the US working population. Although many worksite-based health promotion programs attempt to maximize participation, some distinguish participation according to employees' health risk profiles (Breslow, 1999). This population health management approach attempts to lower the risks of high-risk employees while maintaining the status of lower-risk employees (Serxner, Anderson, & Gold, 2004), matching the health message and the program component (e.g., newsletters, help lines, workshops, or printed information) to the employee's readiness to change (Prochaska & Velicer, 1997).

The Affordable Care Act of 2010 will, as of 2014, expand employers' ability to reward employees who meet health status goals by participating in wellness programs—and, in effect, to require employees who don't meet these goals to pay more for their employer-sponsored health coverage. Some consumer advocates argue that this ability to differentiate in health coverage costs among employees is unfair and will amount to employers' policing workers' health (http://www.healthaffairs.org/healthpolicybriefs/brief.php?brief_id=69). The implementation of the ACA, in particular, highlights the importance of addressing these methodologic concerns in individual worksite studies so that effective programs are implemented.

Public Health Departments and Health Care Facilities

Public health activities are generally coordinated by a network of municipal, state, and federal agencies and are quite diverse (CDC & the National Association of County Health Officials, 1994). Further, public health departments and other health care facilities are influential institutions in the process of health promotion. Created by state or local statute, public health departments reflect the interests of state and local advocacy groups and government officials (Gebbie, 2000). Public health departments, oriented toward optimizing the health of the entire community, have traditionally been concerned with ensuring health through the control of communicable diseases; health education; environmental sanitation; consumer protection; and the provision of medical and nursing services for the diagnosis, treatment, and prevention of diseases in hard-to-reach populations (McCaig, 1994b). Health departments are, however, changing rapidly under the pressure to improve early detection of disease as part of disaster preparedness (and thus also to improve their rapid, real-time information sharing; Broome & Loonsk, 2004). They are also under pressure to increase access to health care for the culturally and linguistically diverse populations in the communities they serve (Liao, Tucker, Okoro, Giles, Mokdad, & Harris, 2004).

Many Americans receive their clinical services through public health departments (www.cdc.gov, January, 2013). Often, services are offered in a package, including immunizations, health education, tuberculosis screening and treatment, well-child visits, nutritional services for women and children, sexually transmitted disease screening, partner identification and treatment, and HIV testing and counseling. Preventive care is frequently built into the medical protocols that departments must follow; many of these protocols are derived from state or federal statutes.

Hospitals, particularly hospital emergency departments (EDs), provide another context for health promotion. They are the primary sites for clinical care among vulnerable members of the population, such as the homeless, the uninsured, and the working poor. More than 136 million ED visits were provided last year, about 45.1 per 100 persons, generally for the treatment of a presenting illness or injury (www.cdc.gov, January, 2013). Blood pressure measurement, a screening test, is performed in most ED visits (Frew, 1991). Non-urgent problems, often among the more vulnerable in the population, account for many ED visits, thus enabling health care professionals to screen for hypertension, hypercholesterolemia, cervical and other cancers, and syphilis and to conduct other forms of early detection (Chernow & Iserson, 1987; Burns, Stoy, Feied, Nash, & Smith, 1991; Hogness, Engelstad, Linck, & Schorr, 1992; Hibbs, Ceglowski, Goldberg, & Kauffman, 1993). ED staff have an opportunity to counsel patients on injury prevention (McCaig, 1994) and smoking cessation. Although preventive care is provided in this setting and the ED serves as the primary clinical site for many in the population, this usage is not without problems. Ideally, patients would not seek care in the ED unless they were faced with a real emergency, but uninsurance or underinsurance leads some people to delay preventive or other medical care until the problem is acute and they have nowhere to go but the ED. The waits at the ED are often long, and follow-up—critical to prevention of sexually transmitted diseases, for example—is rare (Avner, 1992). Moreover, ED care is costly and inefficient compared to more appropriate settings in which primary and preventive care could occur.

ECONOMIC CONTEXTS FOR HEALTH PROMOTION

In 2011, the United States spent $2.7 trillion dollars on health, or $8,680 per person, up 4% year over year; 95% of these expenditures were for direct medical services (CMS, 2012; https://www.cms.gov/Research-Statistics-Data-and-Systems/Statistics-Trends-and-Reports/NationalHealthExpendData/NHE-Fact-Sheet.html). Approximately 18% of the 2011 gross domestic product (GDP) was earmarked for health expenditures, a figure that has been rising steadily over the past decade. Additionally, according to the Centers for Medicare and Medicaid Services (CMS), per capita expenditure will increase at an annual rate of 5.7% per year from 2011 to 2021 (http://www.cms.gov/, 2012). Despite this generous national expenditure, the United States consistently ranks below many industrialized nations in the effectiveness of their health care system, at 37th (http://thepatientfactor.com/canadian-health-care-information/world-health-organizations-ranking-of-the-worlds-health-systems/, January 2013).

About 85% of Americans are covered by some form of health insurance, according to the US Census (http://www.census.gov/hhes/www/hlthins/data/incpovhlth/2011/highlights.html), whether through employer-provided insurance, policies purchased on the individual market, or government-financed plans like Medicare, Medicaid, and the State Children's Health Program (SCHIP). Importantly, however, 48.6 million were uninsured in 2011—down from 50 million the year before, according to the US Census Bureau (http://www.census.gov/hhes/www/hlthins/data/incpovhlth/2011/highlights.html, 2011). The uninsured are without any health insurance because they are employed by firms that do not offer coverage or because they live below the poverty line and cannot afford it. Uninsured children are more likely than the insured to lack a usual source of health care, to go without needed care, and to experience worse health outcomes (IOM, 2002). In 2011, 9.4% of all children under the age of 18 (7.0 million) were without health insurance; the uninsured rate for children in poverty, 13.8%, was even higher (http://www.census.gov/hhes/www/hlthins/data/incpovhlth/2011/highlights.html, 2011).

Reducing the number of uninsured was the major focus of the ACA, as was providing more access to preventive services, as it seemed difficult for traditional insurers to develop a financially viable business model for providing preventive services. Because health insurance was initially developed to protect individuals from the largely unpredictable and high costs of hospitalization and catastrophic illness, by definition it is generally limited to services that are deemed medically necessary to diagnose and treat illness (Garland & Stull, 2004). The use of health promotion programs such as nutrition counseling is predictable (based on the presence of specific risk factors) and relatively low in cost, so, as preventive services, such programs have never been considered medically necessary (Riedel, 1987). As discussed later in this Chapter, insurance providers have increasingly been criticized for failing to curtail the rapid health care cost increases that are outpacing increases in worker earnings and inflation rates. They have received just as much criticism, if not much more, however, over cost-saving measures like utilization review, coverage limits, dropping coverage, denial of coverage for those with preexisting conditions, and interferences with clinical decision making based on cost.

Generally, the need to cover preventive services must be balanced with the need to have a reasonably affordable health system. Not all preventive medicine is cost-effective, and some preventive screenings are arguably performed too often, leading to unnecessary treatment and high costs. New approaches to

reimbursing preventive and chronic disease care are required (as discussed in Chapter 12).

Through their efforts to bring curative medicines to market, the pharmacological, botanical, and biotechnology industries are briefly discussed in this text as contributors to the economy of prevention (see Table 2-4). In a like vein, the World Bank, another source of funds for government programs, has a significant influence on international economies, so its recent designation of health as an indicator of national development will affect the health promotion field.

Commercial Insurance Companies

Since the 1930s, commercial insurance companies have reimbursed the insured patient, or beneficiary, with stipulated sums of money to be applied against expenditures for the insured risks. Subscribers bear sole responsibility for identifying their need for health care, locating the providers of care, and paying for the care. The insurer reimburses them for their reasonable and customary expenses (Shouldice, 1991). Many large firms bear the financial risk of their employees' health needs because they have in effect set up their own insurance systems and have hired outside insurance firms ("third-party administrators") only to handle the paperwork. As discussed in Chapter 1, in the face of escalating costs, employers have begun to shift costs to employees.

TABLE 2-4. SELECTED ECONOMIC INFLUENCES ON PREVENTION

Program	Focus	Examples of Components
Medicare	Socialized health insurance plan for those over 65. Funded by a combination of general tax revenue and premiums paid by beneficiaries.	Part A) Hospital services, Part B) Outpatient physician services, Part C) Vouchers for private HMO coverage, Part D) Rx drug coverage.
Medicare supplemental insurance	Private plans to reduce out-of-pocket expenses of Medicare beneficiaries, to provide catastrophic coverage and better benefits than Medicare alone.	Reduces or eliminates out-of-pocket expenses associated with some preventive care such as primary care visits.
Health savings accounts and high-deductible health plans	Reduces health insurance premium but increases out-of-pocket expenses.	Beneficiaries may face out-of-pocket expenses for many preventive services, screenings and drugs, but are covered for catastrophic expenses.
Patient Protection and Affordable Care Act (2010)	Increases health insurance coverage, regulates insurance.	Requires individual and some businesses to buy health insurance, subsidizes premiums for the poor, sets up state insurance exchanges, requires preventive coverage, limits ability of insures to deny or drop coverage.

Health insurers plans and policies are driven largely by concerns over rising health care costs. A 2011 survey of national insurance plans conducted by the Kaiser Family Foundation found that health insurance costs increased by an average of 9% in 2011, to $15,073. The overall cost of family coverage has doubled since 2001, when premiums averaged $7,061, while wages have only increased by 34% during the same period of time. The survey represented about 60% of all insured Americans (http://ehbs.kff.org/; Kaiser Family Foundation and Health Research and Educational Trust, 2004).

Among employer groups, any employee demand for preventive services encounters pressures to control costs. Employees, too, may tend to resist raising premiums to pay for additional benefits (Steckler, Dawson, Goodman, & Epstein, 1987). Faced with increasing competition for the business of healthy employer groups, insurers are less likely to add any benefits that increase their costs relative to competitors' costs, unless a clear demand exists. Insurers who elect to cover preventive services, such as smoking cessation programs, may put themselves at risk of adverse selection relative to their competitors— for example, by attracting smokers, who are likely to use proportionately more medical care (Milliman and Robertson Inc., 1987). Adverse selection may be less common in employer-sponsored plans than in the individual market, however, as employees get "locked in" to their employers' plan and have limited choices as far as available plans. Thus, many employees may stay in plans priced above the employee's actuarily fair premium, reducing adverse selection. Although much is known about the impact of health insurance coverage on the outcomes of preventive interventions, such as smoking cessation programs, it remains difficult for insurers to price them and for employers to finance them.

Finally, insurers tend to look at whether any benefits of preventive care will be realized over the time period during which the insurer covers the policyholder. Many of the benefits that accrue after a person quits smoking, for example, may not be realized by the health insurer if the policyholder switches plans, which is likely to occur within 5 years of joining a company. As a result, most insurance companies limit their time frame for realizable benefits from smoking cessation to 3 to 5 years; the reimbursable health care costs for the smoker receiving the benefits must be lower at the end of 2 years than they are for the smoker not receiving these benefits

(USDHHS, 2000b). Health care providers are especially attuned to this time frame and structure health promotion programs to allow insurance companies to realize any short-term benefits; those insurers who have failed to provide preventive care, however, can await their employees' 65th birthdays, when Medicare becomes available, and their obligations to the health care of their employees' cease.

Despite these barriers to health promotion and the economic disincentives to providing insurance for preventive behaviors, as discussed earlier, insurers and employers have recently begun to realize the importance of health promotion in reducing costs (among employees, as discussed previously under workplace wellness), maintaining a healthy, productive workforce, and avoiding customer turnover in the health insurance market. This insurance coverage is a valuable marketing tool for attracting new members, particularly those who may value prevention, and who may be healthier, and thus less and thus less costly over the longer term. Thus, since the 1980s, many insurers have offered rate advantages for non-smokers and individuals who maintain a healthy weight. In addition, some insurers also cover alternative healing methods, such as chiropractic care, massage therapy, or acupuncture (the insertion of hair-thin needles into specific points on the body to prevent or to treat disease), when prescribed by a physician. The components of these programs vary, however, as do their effectiveness. Yet, every US health care plan now offers a covered wellness or health promotion plan.

Health Plans

Health plans, such as Blue Cross and Blue Shield or Group Health Cooperative of Puget Sound, are organizations that insure the health care for a defined population. These plans usually use managed care techniques to pursue the goals of improving the quality of medical care, increasing coordination between medical team members, reducing costs, and reducing unnecessary care. While in many cases these goals are aligned with each other, in some cases they can come into conflict: cost-containment measures may deny beneficial but cost-ineffective care to some patients.

Managed care approaches used by health plans include benefit design, prevention and early treatment programs, provider credentialing and network design, health care quality improvements, coordination of care across multiple providers, disease management programs, utilization review, and restricted formularies and generic drug substitution programs (Manley, Griffin, Foldes, Link, & Sechrist, 2003). According to a 2009 CDC study, 45 of 51 Medicaid programs covered tobacco cessation programs. Notably, if all Medicaid smokers were to quit, the Medicaid program would save $9.7 billion over 5 years. The Centers for Disease Control and Prevention (CDC) reports that the cost of these diseases both to individuals and the nation is substantial, resulting in an estimated $96 billion a year in medical expenses, and an additional $97 billion a year in lost productivity (http://downloads.cms. gov/cmsgov/archived-downloads/SMDL/downloads/smd11-007.pdf).

Blue Cross and Blue Shield

Blue Cross and Blue Shield are nonprofit, independent, community-based health plans that have loosely affiliated with one another (and are known collectively as Blue Cross Blue Shield [BCBS]). BCBS governs a network of nearly 100 million people, one out of every three Americans; offers 38 plans in 50 states, the District of Columbia, and Puerto Rico; processes the majority of Medicare claims, at an estimated $200 billion dollars per year. It contracts with 96% of hospitals and 91% of professional providers, more than any other insurer (Blue Cross Blue Shield, 2013; http://www.bcbs.com/about-the-association/) The BCBS federal health plan is the largest privately underwritten health insurance contract in the world, with 5.2 million federal government employees, retirees, and dependents enrolled (Blue Cross Blue Shield, 2013).

To many, Blue Cross and Blue Shield plans are the insurers of last resort. Blue Cross contracts with local hospitals to cover members at a set reimbursement schedule. To the insured, Blue Cross provides first dollar, first day coverage. Blue Shield plans are nonprofit medical contracts for physician services. Members are reimbursed for those services according to a preset schedule. The two plans complement each other.

Blue Cross Blue Shield has formed HMOs, preferred provider organizations (PPOs), point-of-service (POS) plans, health savings accounts, and government health care plans, including a Medicare managed care network. They offer free health care benefits to eligible uninsured children through the Caring Program for Children, which is financed through matching funds from 40 BCBS plans (Blue Cross Blue Shield, 2013). BCBS has developed integrated delivery systems to partner with hospitals and physicians so that individuals may move more easily from one level of care to another.

BCBS has in some cases developed model benefits for preventive screenings, as well as disease and chronic case management initiatives that promote education to improve consumers' ability to make informed health care decisions. Preventive services covered by BCBS in full (not subject to a deductible) include well-child visits, adult routine physicals, immunizations, mammograms, pap smears, and prostate cancer screening. Health programs may also offer discounts on gym memberships, nutrition and fitness programs, or health fairs and community events promoting wellness as an adjunct to Web-based health assessment tools, as well as personalized support for individuals with chronic conditions such as diabetes, heart conditions, or cancer.

Federal Insurance Programs

The federal government's health insurance programs include Medicare; Medicaid; the Federal Employees Health Benefits Program; TRICARE, for the armed services; Veterans Health Administration medical care; and the Indian Health Service. The Centers for Medicare and Medicaid Services (CMS) is responsible for managing Medicare and Medicaid and the Children's Health Insurance Program (CHIP), spending over $800 billion a year buying health care services for these beneficiaries (CBO, 2012; http://www. beckershospitalreview.com/racs-/-icd-9-/-icd-10/medicare-medicaid-costs-still-expected-to-double-despite-revised-cbo-projections.html).

Medicare

Medicare is a federally administered program that provides hospital and medical insurance protection to 97% of persons 65 years of age and older, disabled persons younger than 65 who receive cash benefits under Social Security or Railroad Retirement programs, persons of all ages with chronic kidney disease, and some aliens and federal civil service employees who pay a monthly premium. The benefit package, administration, and payment methods were modeled on the private sector insurance plans prevalent in the 1960s, such as Blue Cross Blue Shield and Aetna's Plan for Federal Employees (Ball, 1995). In 2011, Medicare financed about 21% of the nation's health care spending (Centers for Medicare and Medicaid Services, 2013). For the portion of the working population covered by Social Security, Medicare provides compulsory hospitalization insurance (Part A) and voluntary supplementary medical insurance (Part B); Part B helps to pay for physicians' services, other medical services, and supplies not covered by the hospitalization plan. Medicare Part D, also called the Medicare prescription drug benefit, is a federal program to subsidize the costs of prescription drugs for Medicare beneficiaries in the United States. It was enacted as part of the Medicare Modernization Act of 2003 (MMA) and went into effect on January 1, 2006.

Managed care plans serve 27% of all Medicare beneficiaries through three types of contracts: risk plans, cost plans, and health care prepayment plans (HCPPs; Gold, Jacobson, Damico, & Neuman, 2013). The largest share (65%) of enrollees are in health maintenance organizations (HMO) plans, followed by local preferred provider organizations (PPOs) and regional PPOs (21% and 7%), and private fee-for-service (PFFS) plans (4%).

Special Needs Plans, a form of Medicare Advantage plans, were authorized in 2003 to provide a managed care option for three groups of beneficiaries with significant or relatively specialized care needs. These include: Medicare Beneficiaries who are dually eligible for Medicare and Medicaid (D-SNPs), beneficiaries requiring a nursing home or institution level of care (I-SNPs), and beneficiaries with severe chronic or disabling conditions (C-SNPs; Gold, Jacobson, Damico, & Neuman, 2013).

Medicare Advantage enrollment tends to be highly concentrated in a small number of firms. About 65% of Medicare Advantage enrollment nationwide is concentrated in six firms or affiliates. These firms include United Healthcare, Humana, Blue Cross Blue Shield (BCBS) affiliates, Kaiser Permanente, Wellpoint, and Aetna. A small number of firms also dominate enrollment in most states, reflecting a mix of national companies, local BCBS affiliates, and in a few states, local independent plan sponsors (Gold, Jacobson, Damico, & Neuman, 2013).

Across all enrollees, plan premiums averaged $35 per month in 2012, down $4 per month from 2011. Medicare Advantage plan enrollees generally must pay Medicare's standard Part B premium, in addition to any premium charged by the plan. More than half of enrollees do not pay any additional premiums to the plan. Premiums for Medicare Advantage plans include supplemental benefits or reduced cost sharing beyond that covered by traditional Medicare, as well as any costs of Part A and Part B benefits that exceed the county benchmark, and any costs for Part D benefits that remain after the plan applies available savings (if any) between what they are paid by the government and what it costs them to deliver benefits. Most (88%) of Medicare Advantage enrollees in individual plans select a Medicare Advantage plan that has a drug benefit (MA-PD) (Gold, Jacobson, Damico, & Neuman, 2013).

The trend toward growing Medicare Advantage enrollment has been persistent over time; it is explained by a combination of historical trends in payment, quality bonuses, the continued erosion of retiree benefits, and other factors affecting beneficiary choice (such as relatively affordable supplemental coverage relative to Medigap; Gold, Jacobson, Damico, & Neuman, 2013). Historically, Medicare Advantage has been most attractive to low- to moderate-income participants who are ineligible for Medicaid or other group plans (AHIP, 2012). Over time, the share of beneficiaries enrolling in Medicare Advantage plans may grow as fewer retirees have access to supplemental coverage from former employers and new Medicare beneficiaries bring more experience with plan choice, particularly with preferred provider plans, as part of their previous employment-based coverage.

Since its inception in 1965, the Medicare program has been reluctant to reimburse for preventive services because they are generally seen as predictable and do not lower reimbursement costs (Schauffler, 1993); however, at present it covers an Annual Wellness Visit (AWV); mammography and colorectal, cervical, and prostate cancer screening; cardiovascular screening (for cholesterol and other blood lipid levels); flu, pneumococcal, and hepatitis B vaccinations; bone mass measurements (for those at risk for osteoporosis) diabetes screening; and glaucoma tests. Some of these services require payment of a deductible, however (www.cms.gov). To fill the gaps in preventive services, 90% of beneficiaries have some sort of supplemental insurance, including 9 million Medicare beneficiaries who have Medigap; in 2010, this represented 20% of all Medicare beneficiaries. In addition, about 3 million beneficiaries of Medigap also have other supplemental insurance policies, primarily through employer-sponsored plans (Kaiser Family Foundation, 2011; http://www.kff.org/medicare/upload/8235-2.pdf).

Among the most common forms of Medicare supplemental insurance (disability income insurance, long-term care insurance, and dental expense insurance), only dental insurance supplies and encourages preventive care (such as X-rays and cleanings). Yet Medicare's involvement in quality assurance for hospitals, nursing homes, and other health care settings allows it to play an important role in setting the agenda for health education as a preventive tool for disease avoidance in at-risk populations (De Lew, 2000).

Medicaid

Medicaid is the nation's largest health program in terms of number of recipients, serving 56 million to Medicare's 48 million. Enacted in 1964 under Title XIX of the Social Security Act, Medicaid provides medical services to low-income people and the disabled, and it is an important source of aid for elderly people in nursing homes (www.cms.gov;http://topics.nytimes.com/top/news/health/diseases conditionsandhealthtopics/medicaid/index.html).

Medicaid is jointly financed and administered by the federal government and the states. For example, the federal government pays 50% of the costs in higher-income states and about 70% in lower-income states like Arkansas. It is a major contributor to all state budgets. Although all states are required to meet certain minimum standards by federal law, they have wide latitude to determine eligibility for Medicaid, set up the specific benefits it will provide, and impose some degree of cost-sharing on recipients. Thus, there is wide variation in how states structure their Medicaid programs (www.cms.gov;http://topics.nytimes.com/top/news/health/diseasesconditionsandhealthtopics/medicaid/index.html).

According to the Congressional Budget Office, in the 2010 fiscal year, 77% of people enrolled in Medicaid were children and families, while 23% were elderly or disabled. But 64% of Medicaid spending was for older Americans and people with disabilities, while 36% went to children and families. Seven of every 10 nursing home residents are on Medicaid, in large part because even middle-class patients often run through their savings while in a nursing home and turn to the entitlement program (www.cms.gov; http://topics.nytimes.com/top/news/health/diseasesconditionsandhealthtopics/medicaid/index.html).

Over its 40-year history, Medicaid has provided medical assistance to persons who are eligible for cash assistance programs, such as Aid to Families with Dependent Children (AFDC) and Supplemental Security Income (SSI). Medicaid benefits may also be available to persons who have enough income for basic living expenses but cannot afford to pay for their medical care. Today it continues to be a safety net for the health and long-term care needs of low-income, elderly, or disabled Americans. It is a source of insurance for more than one in seven Americans, and accounts for approximately 15% of national health care spending (http://www.census.gov/compendia/statab/2012/tables/12s0151.pdf; http://www.kff.org/medicaid/upload/8050-05.pdf).

Under the ACA, with the "Medicaid expansion," the federal government will pay the full cost of covering those newly eligible for Medicaid for 3 years, from 2014 to 2016, and the federal share will then gradually decline to 90% in 2020 and later years. Many state officials worry that Congress will reduce the federal share and shift more costs to the states, however.

When states expand their Medicaid programs and give more poor people health insurance, fewer people die, according to a recent study using county-level data among three states that had expanded their programs during the last decade (Sommers, Baicker, Epstein, 2012). These three states covered a population not normally eligible for Medicaid: adults without children or disabilities. The health care law expands coverage to a similar population nationally.

In this study, Sommers, Baicker, and Epstein (2012) looked at mortality rates in those states—New York, Maine, and Arizona—5 years before and after the Medicaid expansions, and compared them with those in four neighboring states—Pennsylvania, Nevada, New Mexico, and New Hampshire—that did not put such expansions in place.

The number of deaths for people aged 20 to 64—adults too young to be considered elderly by the researchers—decreased in the three states with expanded coverage by about 1,500 combined per year, after adjusting for population growth in those states. In the 5 years before the expansion, there were about 46,400 deaths per year, while in the 5 years after the expansion, there were about 44,900 deaths per year. During the same period, death rates in the four comparison states increased; Medicaid expansions were associated with a reduction in mortality of 2,840 deaths per year, or a relative reduction of 6.1% (Sommers, Baicker, & Epstein, 2012). Clearly, Medicaid spending for enrollees has important ramifications for the health system as a whole. Special payments for rural, inner-city, and teaching hospitals and other safety net providers help to guarantee access to care for all the population groups who live in medically underserved areas.

During the recession, many states had slashed optional benefits, like dental coverage, for millions of poor adults in the program. The ACA requires dental coverage for children only. Many states are also trying to cut the cost of long-term care by profoundly changing Medicaid coverage, through the use of federal waivers. Mandated preventive services only include periodic screening and family planning for children under 21 years of age, as well as cancer screenings (e.g., for breast and cervical cancer), as discussed further in Chapter 1.

The Federal Employees Health Benefits Program (FEHB)

The FEHB provides voluntary health insurance coverage for about 9 million active and retired federal employees and their families (http://www.opm.gov/healthcare-insurance/healthcare/). Depending on the state in which they work, federal employees may enroll in one of the health insurance plans described previously in this Chapter. In addition, federal employees may select Consumer-Driven Plans that offer a wide range of incentives to control the cost of either health benefits or health care under the FEHB Program. With these plans, the employee spends health care dollars up to a designated amount, and receives full coverage for in-network preventive care. In return, employees incur significantly higher cost sharing expenses after using up the designated amount. FEHB is jointly financed by the government, which covers 72–75% of premium costs, and by enrollees, who pay the remaining 25–28%.

TRICARE

TRICARE (formerly CHAMPUS) provides health care for active duty military personnel whose orders do not specify a period of 30 days or less and their dependents, retired and former military personnel entitled to retainer or retirement pay or the equivalent and their dependents, and dependents of deceased members of the US armed forces (http://www.tricare.mil/).

Veterans Health Administration (VHA)

The Veterans Health Administration of the Department of Veterans Affairs (VA) operates over 1,700 facilities (http: //www1.va.gov/health/index.asp) for the care of individuals who served honorably in the armed forces. Under the Veterans' Health Care Eligibility Reform Act of 1996, Veterans Health Administration medical centers may negotiate with managed care entities to provide health services, thus increasing the options for preventive services. Under Public Law 104-262 provisions (US Government Printing Office, 1997), the VA has the authority to furnish health promotion and disease prevention services and primary care and has flexibility to provide outpatient treatment, hospital care, and other means of care in the most efficient way possible.

Indian Health Service

The Indian Health Service, an agency within the Department of Health and Human Services, provides medical care and health services for approximately 1.9 million American Indians, including Alaska Natives, who belong to more than 566 federally recognized tribes in 35 states (http://www.ihs.gov/aboutihs/). The Indian Health Service has adopted a series of quality performance measures, many of which focus on prevention, across behavioral health, cancer screening, cardiovascular disease, dental, diabetes, immunizations, and prenatal HIV screening. Performance across the measures varies by type and year (http://www.ihs.gov/qualityofcare/index.cfm?module=quality). For example, as cardiovascular disease is the leading cause of death for American Indian/Alaska Native people above 45 years of age (Go et al., 2013), health facilities are measured by their provision of a comprehensive CVD Assessment. The comprehensive CVD assessment includes; taking blood pressure at least twice over two years; testing LDL (low density lipid) cholesterol at least once in five years; screening for tobacco use during the year; assessing the patient's weight status (body mass index [BMI]); and counseling patients during the year to encourage changing their nutrition and exercise habits. In 2012, 45.4% of adult patients with ischemic heart disease received a comprehensive assessment; the rate of assessment seems to be increasing over time, although data collection approaches differ (Indian Health Service. Quality of IHS Health Care, 2013).

Managed Care

As discussed previously in this Chapter, managed care is a system that integrates the financing and delivery of appropriate health care services to covered individuals; it has served as an important recent influence on the provision of preventive services. Generally, it includes four elements: (1) arrangements with selected providers to furnish a comprehensive set of health care services to members, (2) explicit standards for the selection of health care providers, (3) formal programs for ongoing quality assurance and utilization review, and (4) significant financial incentives for members to use providers and procedures covered by the plan (American College of Healthcare Executives, 2013). The two broadest arrangements for financing and delivery are fee-for-service indemnity arrangements and prepaid health care. Under fee-for-service indemnity arrangements, the consumer incurs expenses for health care from providers whom she or he selects. The provider is reimbursed for covered services in part by the insurer and in part by the consumer, who is responsible for the amount not paid by the insurer. Under indemnity arrangements, the provider and the insurer have no relationship beyond adjudication of the claim presented for payment, nor is there a mechanism for integrating the care that the consumer may receive from multiple providers (CDC, 2002).

Although the field is changing rapidly, four traditional forms and one emerging type of managed care predominate: (1) health maintenance organizations (HMOs); (2) preferred provider organizations (PPOs); (3) exclusive provider organizations (EPOs); (4) point-of-service (POS) plans; and (5) health savings account, or flexible savings account, plans. Managed care structures are financed under either risk or capitation approaches. A risk contract is generally negotiated between an HMO (or a competitive medical plan, a federal designation for a plan that operates similarly to an HMO) and an entity such as the CMS or an employer. The HMO agrees to provide all services to enrolled members on an at-risk basis for a fixed monthly fee. Capitation is a negotiated amount that an entity such as an HMO pays monthly to a provider whom the enrollee has selected as a primary care physician.

HMOs

The Health Maintenance Organization Act of 1973 committed the federal government to a time-limited demonstration of effort toward and support of HMO development. The Act defines HMOs as entities that provide basic health services to their enrollees, using prepaid enrollment fees that are fixed uniformly under a community-rating system, without regard to the medical history of any individual or family. The HMO provides comprehensive and preventive health care benefits for a defined population, and the consumer of an HMO agrees to use the HMO's providers for all covered health care services. The HMO agrees to provide all covered health care services for a set price—the per person premium fee. The consumer must pay any additional fees (co-payments) for office visits and other services used. The HMO also organizes the delivery of this care through its infrastructure of providers and through the implementation of systems to monitor and influence the cost and quality of care.

HMOs generally are also subject to capitation. The provider is responsible for delivering or arranging for the delivery of health care services required by an enrollee. However, the capitation is paid whether or not the physician has provided services to an enrollee. In this way the health care provider shares with the HMO a portion of the financial risk for the cost of care provided to enrollees (CDC, 1995).

An HMO is generally arranged as one of five kinds of service structures: (1) staff (the HMO contracts with solo salaried physician practices); (2) group (the HMO pays a per capita rate to a physician group); (3) network (the HMO contracts with two or more independent group practices, paying a fixed monthly fee per enrollee); (4) independent practice association (IPA; the HMO contracts with individual physicians or associations of private physicians on a per capita rate, flat retainer system, or negotiated fee-for-service rate); or (5) mixed (the HMO uses a combination of two or more of these models).

In the current US health care system, the HMO is the insurance vehicle best structured to encourage prevention. Over 95% of HMOs cover health-promotive services, including health education about diet, physical activity, and medication use (AHIP, 2002). Persons enrolled in staff-model health maintenance organizations are more likely to be offered health promotion programs—such as cholesterol or blood pressure screening, weight control, stress management, and smoking control—by their plan or physician than are persons enrolled in an independent practice association or indemnity plan (IOM, 2000b).

PPOs

The preferred provider organization (PPO) is a variant of the fee-for-service indemnity arrangement, wherein the PPO contracts with providers in the community to deliver covered services for a discounted fee. Providers under contract are referred to as preferred providers. The PPO gives consumers greater freedom than the HMO does in choosing providers, but like the HMO, it tries to achieve savings by directing clients to providers who are committed to cost-effective delivery of care. PPOs have contracts with networks or panels of providers who agree to provide medical services and to be paid according to a negotiated fee schedule. Enrollees generally experience a financial penalty if they choose to get care from a nonaffiliated provider, but that option is available.

EPOs

The exclusive provider organization, too, is similar to the HMO, but the member must remain within the network to receive benefits. It uses primary physicians as gatekeepers, often capitates providers, has a limited provider panel, and uses an authorization system and other features of the HMO. EPOs are regulated under insurance statutes and are not governed by most state and federal HMO regulations in states where they are allowed to operate (Kongstvedt, 1993). As a result, certain health conditions may not be covered by an EPO.

POS Plans

Point-of-service (POS) plans combine characteristics of both HMOs and PPOs and use a network of contracted participating providers. Enrollees select a primary care physician who controls referrals to medical specialists. If care is received from a plan provider, the plan member pays little or nothing out of pocket; care provided by non-plan providers is reimbursed by fee-for-service or capitation arrangements, and members pay higher copayments and deductibles. Financial incentives are used to avoid provider overuse.

High Deductible Health Plan (HDHP)

High Deductible Health Plans typically feature lower premiums and higher deductibles than traditional insurance plans. As of 2013, HDHPs are plans with a minimum deductible of $1,250 per year

for individual coverage and $2,500 for family coverage. A health savings account (HSA) or a health reimbursement arrangement may be used to pay for qualified out-of-pocket medical costs, reducing federal tax liabilities.

Catastrophic Health Insurance Plan

A catastrophic health insurance plan covers essential health benefits but has a very high deductible, providing a "safety net" coverage in case of an accident or serious illness. Catastrophic plans usually do not provide coverage for services like prescription drugs or immunizations. Premiums for catastrophic plans may be lower than traditional health insurance plans, but deductibles are usually much higher.

Catastrophic plans are available only to people under 30 and to some low-income people who are exempt from paying the fee because other insurance is considered unaffordable or because they have received "hardship exemptions.". Marketplace catastrophic plans cover three annual primary care visits and preventive services at no cost. After the deductible is met, they cover the same set of essential health benefits that other marketplace plans offer. People with catastrophic plans are not eligible for lower costs on their monthly premiums or out-of-pocket costs.

HSAs and FSAs

Health savings accounts (HSAs), or flexible savings accounts (FSAs), are the latest in a continually expanding portfolio of consumer-directed health care products. They are becoming increasingly popular with consumers who demand flexibility to fit their particular health care needs. These plans were created by the 2003 Medicare Modernization Act (CMS, 2003) to allow consumers to save money tax-free and apply withdrawals to health expenses. The accounts may require the purchase of a high-deductible health insurance plan; money in the accounts may be used for health expenses subject to the deductible. Many employers consider these accounts a way of shifting more of the rapidly rising medical costs to workers; generally, younger and healthier workers contribute to these accounts. The ACA act recently modified the contribution levels for 2013 to $2,500 per family, down from $5,000 contribution level in 2012.

Accountable Care Organizations

On March 31, 2011, the Department of Health and Human Services (HHS) released proposed new rules to help doctors, hospitals, and other providers better coordinate care for Medicare patients through Accountable Care Organizations (ACOs). ACOs create incentives for health care providers to work together to treat an individual patient across care settings—including doctor's offices, hospitals, and long-term care facilities. The Medicare Shared Savings Program will reward ACOs that lower growth in health care costs while meeting performance standards on quality of care and putting patients first. Patient and provider participation in an ACO is purely voluntary (http://www.healthcare.gov/news/factsheets/2011/03/accountablecare03312011a.html).

BEHAVIORAL HEALTH CARE

Behavioral health problems encompass a broad range of illnesses, such as anxiety disorder, mood disorder, impulse-control disorder, or substance disorder. Nearly a third of adults and a fifth of children had a behavioral health problem within the past year. These problems range from short-term problems to chronic disorders. Smaller shares—about 5% of adults and 10% of children—have a serious mental illness or behavioral health difficulty. Even people with minor symptoms of mental health problems seem to have a higher risk of death from several major causes, including cardiovascular disease, according to a recent pooled analysis of 10 prospective cohort studies. Those who experience symptoms of anxiety or depression have a lower life expectancy than those without any such symptoms, according to the same study of 68,000 UK adults, perhaps due to biologic changes in the body that increase the risk of other diseases, such as heart (Russ TC, Stamatakis E, Hamer M, Starr JM, Kivimäki M, & Batty GD, 2012).

Treatment for behavioral health problems is most frequently delivered on an outpatient basis. Common treatments for behavioral health problems include psychosocial counseling and pharmacological services; many individuals receive a combination of both types of therapy. People with serious mental illness often require additional non-medical services, such as income support, vocational training, or housing assistance, to help them manage day-to-day activities. Behavioral health services are delivered by both specialty mental health providers and general medical practitioners.

Though utilization of behavioral health services has increased over time, a significant share of people who need services do not receive treatment. Over 60% of adults with a diagnosable disorder and 70% of children in need of treatment do not receive mental health services, and nearly 90% of people over age 12 with a substance use ordependence disorder may not receive specialty treatments for their problems (Kaiser Commission on Medicaid and the Underinsured, 2011).

The 2010 Affordable Care Act (ACA) will lead to a substantial expansion of insurance coverage for behavioral health services, which could replace out-of-pocket or direct government payment for behavioral health services with insurance coverage to finance costs. Medicaid eligibility will be expanded to everyone with incomes up to 133% of the poverty line, and those with incomes up to 400% of poverty will receive subsidies to purchase coverage through newly created Health Insurance Exchanges. These expansions will result in new populations accessing behavioral health services through Medicaid and private insurance. According to the Substance Abuse and Mental Health Services Administration (SAMHSA) 2010 National Survey of Drug Use and Health, there will be an additional 30 million previously uninsured people with behavioral health problems who will be eligible for coverage.

Health reform under the ACA also includes other insurance regulation provisions—such as elimination of preexisting condition exclusions and minimum benefit requirements for participating health plans—that may impact insurance coverage of mental health services. Several specific provisions directly impact mental health, such as the establishment of health homes for individuals with mental illness and new educational training grants for the mental health workforce.

The Affordable Care Act also builds on the Mental Health Parity and Addiction Equity Act of 2008 by requiring coverage of mental health and substance use disorder benefits for millions of Americans in the individual and small group markets who currently lack these benefits, and expanding parity requirements to apply to millions of Americans whose coverage did not previously comply with those requirements. While many operational issues remain to be resolved, it is clear that ACA will impact the financing and delivery of care for individuals with behavioral health needs.

The financing system for behavioral health services differs from that for general medical services. Most notably, public sources play a larger role in financing behavioral health care (representing 61% of expenditures) than they do in overall health services (representing 46% of expenditures). At present, the federal-state Medicaid program is the largest source of financing for behavioral health services in the nation, covering over a quarter of all expenditures. Medicare's role in financing behavioral health care (covering 7% of spending) is much smaller than its overall role in the health system, where it finances nearly a fifth of spending. Many disabled Medicare beneficiaries qualify for coverage on the basis of a mental illness, but other beneficiaries have behavioral health needs as well. Beneficiaries who are dually eligible for Medicare and Medicaid report the highest rates of mental illness (59% and 20% of disabled and aged, respectively). Medicare's behavioral health benefits were initially modeled after private coverage and included many coverage limitations. Some limits on Medicare coverage of behavioral health services have been eased over time, but the program's behavioral health benefits still retain some of their historical limits on psychosocial and support services, inpatient psychiatric hospital care, and certain providers. A large number of other federal, state, and local public programs finance services to support individuals with behavioral health needs. Many of these programs are not targeted to individuals with behavioral health problems, yet they provide key ancillary support services such as housing, income support, and vocational training. The largest federal program dedicated to financing behavioral health services is the Community Mental Health Services Block Grant (MHBG), which allocates grants to states to support and enhance community mental health systems for individuals with serious mental illness. Stemming from a long history of financing and delivering behavioral health services, other state and local funds finance a range of services and account for nearly a quarter of financing for behavioral health services in the nation.

Private insurance finances only about a quarter of spending on behavioral health care. While nearly all (98%) of those with employer-sponsored coverage had mental health benefits included in their health plans in 2008, most had limits on these services, according to the Kaiser Family Foundation. Though they have a long history of funding mental health in the United States, charitable and philanthropic sources account for a small share (4%) of current financing for behavioral health services. Most of these funds are strategically targeted to pilot innovative programs or provide incentives for systems change. Out-of-pocket payments for behavioral health (e.g., co-payments for services covered by insurance; payment for services excluded from insurance plans; or direct payment for all services by individuals with no insurance coverage) account for 11% of spending in this area. Out-of-pocket payment varies by insurance coverage, with the uninsured and those with private coverage paying a higher amount than those with Medicaid coverage.

Managed behavioral health organization (MBHO) is a newer method for providing behavioral care that can be offered by insurance companies. By 2003, 72% of private insurance plans contracted with an MBHO to deliver behavioral health services (Hodgkin, Horgan, Garnick, & Merrick, 2009). Despite these actions, private coverage of behavioral health benefits remain more limited than that for general medical services.

Three core methods are used to manage behavioral health care. In principle these methods are similar to those used to manage medical care; however, because of unique characteristics of the client groups served, their implementation differs. The three methods are (1) managed benefits, which are designed to control care use and expenditures through, for example, gatekeepers who authorize care; (2) managed care, which limits the authorization of benefits for reimbursement to necessary and appropriate care delivered in the least restrictive, least intrusive setting by a qualified provider; and (3) managed health, which offers health advisers, individual health risk assessments, self-help groups, crisis debriefing services, and outreach programs to frequent users of health care services (Freedman & Trabin, 1994).

Between 1970 and 2003, overall health care costs grew faster than GDP, while expenditures for mental health grew in proportion to GDP, due, in part to the growth in MBHOs. These trends in reduced mental health expenditures are due also to budgeting for state and local expenditures, higher cost sharing for behavioral health benefits than for medical care benefits, and lower use of technology in behavioral health treatment compared to overall medical care (Frank, Goldman, & McGuire, 2009).

Some states (e.g., Missouri) and integrated healthcare systems, such as Kaiser Permanente, have integrated behavioral and medical services for individuals with serious mental illness or individuals who co-occurring serious mental illness and substance use disorder. These integrated systems are accompanied by a brief screening for substance abuse, alcohol, depression, and tobacco, alongside early periodic screening for children with the Early and Periodic Screening, Diagnosis and Treatment (EPSDT, a benefit for enrollees under the age of 21; Alliance for Health Reform; May 4, 2012). These integrated programs have yielded considerable cost savings (Alliance for Health Reform; May 4, 2012).

Workers' Compensation

All state legislatures have enacted workers' compensation, or statuary disability benefits—laws that provide health insurance coverage for employees who are injured or become ill during the course of employment (Shouldice, 1991). Benefits are established by state laws and include all reasonable medical care, rehabilitation services necessary to return the injured employee to work, and partial repayment of lost wages. Funds for workers' compensation come from employers and state and local taxes. To promote health and therefore to avoid medical expenses, these programs emphasize the importance of a safe work environment, using education programs, safety inspections, and counseling on safe work practices. Stress prevention and management initiatives that are part of workers' compensation programs represent another emerging area for managed behavioral health care.

PHARMACOLOGICAL, BOTANICAL, AND BIOTECHNOLOGICAL INDUSTRIES

The pharmacological industry is a major force in health care, with a worldwide market of $880 billion in sales (IMS Global, 2009). The United States tops the world in average individual expenditure for medicines, at $806 per person (IMS Health, 2011). Overall, the United States spends 2.1% of its gross domestic product (GDP) on pharmaceuticals, second only to the proportion spent in Japan (IMS, 2011). In 2011, the largest US firms by annual revenues included Pfizer, Novartis, Sanofi, Merck, and GlaxoSmithKline (Roth, 2012). Pharmacologics also include biologic drugs that are proteins made in living cells, like Avastin and Herceptin for cancer and Enbrel and Humira for rheumatoid arthritis

(Pollack, 2011). Biologics are estimated to have reached >$100 billion in 2010, with the top 12 biologics generating $30 billion (IMS global, 2011). The top-selling therapeutic categories globally in 2011 were oncologics ($62.2b), respiratory agents ($39.4b), anti-diabetics ($39.2b), lipid regulators ($38.7b), and anti-psychotics ($28.4b) (IMS Global, 2011) http://www.statista.com/statistics/225118/top-10-therapeutic-classes-by-global-pharmaceutical-sales-2011/). Although mainly oriented toward tertiary prevention, the pharmaceutical industry does contribute to primary prevention through the development of drugs for such conditions such as hypercholesterolemia and osteoporosis and needs such as weight reduction.

The entry of pharmaceuticals into the market is restricted by the Food and Drug Administration (FDA) in the United States and by equivalent agencies in other countries. The FDA's ability to conduct post-marketing surveillance of pharmaceuticals' safety has been a source of considerable contention of late, with the forced removal from the market of several popular drugs after their widespread use resulted in death or injury.

The estimated $240 billion worldwide biotechnology market (IMS Global, 2012) is also growing. Biotechnology is a collection of technologies that focus on the cellular and molecular processes of living organisms. Companies in this industry produce genetic screening tests (e.g., for locating mutations in the breast cancer susceptibility genes BRCA1 and BRCA2), detection and diagnostic products (e.g., for detecting cervical cancer), and pharmaceuticals (often using recombinant DNA technology or developing compounds that act within the cell; Weber, 1997).

The United States continues to dominate the biotechnology market, in terms of both the number of companies in the sector and research and development spending. The latest data (IMS Global, 2011) show that 80% of biopharmaceutical development work is done in the United States, and the pharmaceutical sector employs 272,000 people in the United States (http://selectusa.commerce.gov/industry-snapshots/pharmaceutical-industry-united-states).

Biotechnology companies are also discovering the functions of human genes, as is the Human Genome Project, funded by the National Institutes of Health. The genetic testing products produced by this industry continue to pose ethical quandaries for health care professionals, even with the passage of the Genetic Information Nondiscrimination Act (GINA) in 2009, which provides federal protection from genetic discrimination in health insurance and employment. Questions about the sharing of genetic information with health and life insurance companies and managed care companies continue to challenge these companies. The optimal process a health care professional might use to share genetic information with clients and how that process might encourage behavioral change also remain uncertain, as discussed further in Chapter 8.

COMPLEMENTARY AND ALTERNATIVE MEDICINE

More than one-third (38.3%) of US adults report using some form of complementary and alternative medicine (CAM), according to the 2007 National Health Interview Survey (NHIS), an annual in-person survey of Americans regarding their health- and illness-related experiences (Barnes, Bloom, & Nahin, 2008). According to this same survey, the top ten CAM practices are natural products, deep breathing, meditation, chiropractic and osteopathic, massage, yoga, diet-based therapies, progressive relaxation, guided imagery, and homeopathic treatment (Barnes, Bloom, & Nahin, 2008).

CAM is a group of diverse medical and health care systems, practices, and products. "Complementary" generally refers to using a non-mainstream approach together with conventional medicine. "Alternative" refers to using a non-mainstream approach in place of conventional medicine; true alternative medicine is not common. Most people use non-mainstream approaches along with conventional treatment, although the boundaries between complementary and conventional medicine overlap and change over time. For example, guided imagery and massage, both once considered complementary or alternative, are used regularly in some hospitals to help with pain management. Integrative medicine combines conventional and CAM treatments for which there is evidence of safety and effectiveness (e.g., acupuncture and meditation for symptom management during chemotherapy) (NCCAM, 2013).

The National Center for Complementary and Alternative Medicine (NCCAM), divides CAM into one of two subgroups—natural products or mind and body practices. Natural products include herbs (also known as botanicals), vitamins and minerals, and probiotics. They are widely marketed, readily available to consumers, and often sold as dietary supplements. Interest in and use of natural products have grown considerably in the past few decades. According to the 2007 National Health Interview Survey (NHIS), which included a comprehensive survey on the use of complementary health approaches by Americans, 17.7 percent of American adults had used a non-vitamin/non-mineral natural product in the past year. The most commonly used natural product among adults in the past 30 days was fish oil/omega 3s (reported by 37.4% of all adults who said they used natural products); popular products for children (taken in the past 30 days) included echinacea (37.2%) and fish oil/omega 3s (30.5%). Some of these products have been studied in large, placebo-controlled trials, many of which have failed to show anticipated effects. Research on other natural products to determine whether they are effective and safe is ongoing.

Mind and body practices include a large and diverse group of procedures or techniques administered or taught by a trained practitioner or teacher. According to the 2007 NHIS, the mind and body practices most commonly used included deep breathing, meditation, chiropractic and osteopathic manipulation, massage, yoga, progressive relaxation, and guided imagery. The amount of research on mind and body approaches varies widely depending on the practice. For example, acupuncture, yoga, spinal manipulation, and meditation have had many studies, and some of these practices appear to hold promise in pain management, whereas other practices have had little research to date.

Total visits to CAM providers each year exceed those to primary care physicians, adding up to an annual out-of-pocket cost for CAM exceeding $27 billion in 1997 (Eisenberg et al., 1998). Many hospitals, managed care plans, and conventional practitioners are incorporating CAM therapies into their practices, and schools of medicine, nursing, and pharmacy are beginning to teach about CAM (Institute of Medicine, 2005, p. 1).

Despite the proliferation of CAM among individuals and healthcare organizations, considerable controversy remains about the methodological strength of the evidence supporting the effects of CAM on prevention and their cost effectiveness relative to conventional medical protocols (Joyce, 1994; Ernst, 1994; Sewing, 1994). The Institute of Medicine (IOM) has thus recommended that investigators use and develop as necessary common methods, measures, and standards for the generation and interpretation of evidence necessary for making decisions about the use of CAM. Additional studies are necessary to demonstrate the plausible CAM mechanisms to enhance health.

STRATEGIES FOR HEALTH PROMOTION IN THE POLICY CONTEXT

Health care professionals may adopt a variety of strategies to promote the health of populations. A strategy of policy change, the context of which was explored in this Chapter, may be pursued concomitantly with or subsequent to other strategies discussed throughout this book.

In its most rational form, the policy-making process proceeds from goal determination to needs assessment and the specification of objectives, to the design of alternative courses of action, to the estimation of consequences of alternative actions, to the selection of a course of action, and to implementation and evaluation, with a feedback loop to the goal-setting stage (see Mayer & Greenwood, 1980, for a summary). Concurrently, the policy process may be seen as a "general course of action or inaction rather than specific decisions" (Heclo, 1972, p. 85), ruled by forces that are fluid and unpredictable (Hacker, 1996). The strategies designed to influence policy must therefore consider both its rational and its emergent processes.

The various tactics that the health care professional undertakes are also part of a dynamic process, both directing—in pursuit of a larger aim—and directed—by those affected or potentially affected by the policy change. The first step in this process is building agendas, identifying problems in terms of pressing social issues, and developing a solution that incorporates the interests of affected groups. Second, the problems are defined by their prevalence, location in society, and importance. Their causes are detailed, and appropriate interventions are developed to ameliorate them. In this context, the use of social science methodology is central. Policy options are selected, and proposals advocating particular choices are advanced to an involved policy leader. Methods of policy persuasion, critical to influencing a choice, include determining the objectives of the persuasion (in written or oral form), diagnosing the audience (particularly gauging the

degree of hostility to the idea), and tailoring the objectives to the audience. Concomitantly, health care professionals develop a political strategy grounded in current realities through contact with interest groups, legislators, and others who wield power over the decision-making process and who can assist in the successful development and implementation of policy and its evaluation.

The target of the health care professional's influence determines the role the professional chooses to play in effecting this change. These roles include indirect involvement, such as identifying and communicating information from different sources; consultation through advocacy, such as citizen participation and coalition organization; and direct involvement, such as passing referenda and citizen initiatives and seeking political appointment and public office (Mico, 1978; Simonds, 1978).

CONCLUSIONS

Given the varied contexts, both political and economic, for health promotion, the health care professional has a number of avenues along which to press for change, particularly for policy change. Within these complex contexts, where interests and exchanges are multiple, the health care professional may seek to affect one or several interrelated levels.

A health care professional may seek to advocate for changes in federal, state, local, or international legislation; in a regulation or a policy; or in accreditation standards. He or she may consider organizing coalitions with other voluntary or professional groups to push for change in the definition and practice of prevention or to increase health-promotive practice in underserved community groups. He or she may share information with others about strategies for implementing *Healthy People 2020*, or may organize client groups to advocate for change in Medicare or Medicaid reimbursement policies for health-promotive care. He or she may run for political office on a platform supporting both quality and cost outcomes in managed care or backing provisions to further protect the findings of genetic testing. The contexts for health promotion are rich with possibilities for change.

ACKNOWLEDGMENTS

We thank Jessica Wilen Berg, J.D., M.P.H., Professor of Law and Bioethics, Case Western Reserve University School of Law, Department of

Bioethics, Case Western Reserve University School of Medicine, Cleveland, Ohio for her review and thoughtful guidance on this Chapter.

REFERENCES

Adams WC. The role of media relations in risk communication. *Public Relat Q.* 1992–1993;37:28–32.

Albertsen K, Hannerz H, Borg V, Burr H. The effect of work environment and heavy smoking on the social inequalities in smoking cessation. *Pub Health.* 2003;117(6):383–388.

AHIP Center for Policy and Research. *Low income and minority beneficiaries in Medicare Advantage Plans, 2010.* Washington DC: America's Health Insurance Plans, May 2012.

American Academy of Pediatrics. *Children's health insurance status.* 2005. Retrieved September 2, 2012, from http://www.aap.org.

American College of Healthcare Executives. Accessed January 2013 from http://www.ache.org/CARSVCS/CareerOverviews/managedcare.cfm#intro.

American Health Insurance Plans. *AHIP Survey of Health Insurance Plans: Chart Book of Findings.* 2002. Retrieved September 5, 2012, from http://www.ahip.org/content/default.aspx?docid=2244.

American Managed Behavioral Healthcare Association. Home page. 2005. Retrieved September 2, 2012, from http://www.ambha.org.

Ammerman AS, DeVellis RF, Carey TS, Keyserling TC, Strogatz DS, Haines PS, et al. Physician-based diet counseling for cholesterol reduction: Current practices, determinants and strategies for improvement. *Prev Med.* 1993;22(1):96–109.

Ashford A, et al. Cancer screening and prevention practices of inner city physicians. *Am J Prev Med.* 2000;19:59–62.

Avner JR. The difficulties in providing primary care in the emergency department. *Pediatr Emerg Care.* 1992;8:101–102.

Baicker K, Cutler D, Song Z. Workplace wellness programs can generate savings. *Health Affairs.* 2010;29(2):304–311.

Ball R. What Medicare's architects had in mind. *Health Affairs.* 1995;14(4):62–72.

Barbeau EM, Krieger N, Soobader MJ. Working class matters: Socioeconomic disadvantage, race/ethnicity, gender, and smoking in NHIS 2000. *Am J Public Health.* 2004;94(2):269–278.

Barker C, Pistrang N, Shapiro DA, Davies S, Shaw I. You in mind: A preventive mental health television series. *Br J Clin Psychol.* 1993;32:281–293.

Barnes PM, Bloom B, Nahin RL. *Complementary and Alternative Medicine Use among Adults and Children, United States, 2007.* CDC National Health Statistics Report, #12, 2008. Accessed January 2013 from http://nccam.nih.gov/health/whatiscam.

Barnes PM, Powell-Griner E, McFann K, Nahin RL. *Complementary and Alternative Medicine Use among Adults: United States, 2002* (Advance Data from Vital and Health Statistics; No. 343). 2004. Retrieved September 2, 2012, from http://nccam.nih.gov/news/camstats.htm.

Baylor College of Medicine. *Tobacco Prevention and Control.* 2004. Retrieved September 2, 2012, from http://saludenaccion.org/tobacco/tobacco-mass-media.html.

Berkman LF, Syme SL. Social networks, host resistance, and mortality: A nine-year follow-up study of Alameda County. *Am J Epidemiol.* 1979;109(2):186–204.

Blue Cross Blue Shield, 2013; http://www.bcbs.com/about-the-association/. Retrieved September 3, 2012, from http://www.bcbs.com.

Blue Cross Blue Shield. *Covering America: 75 Years and Counting.* 2005. Retrieved September 2, 2012, from http://www.bcbs.com.

Breslow L. From disease prevention to health promotion. *JAMA.* 1999;281:1030–1033.

Blue Cros and Blue Shield. *About the Blue Cross and Blue Shield Association.* http://www.bcbs.com/about-the-association/, Accessed January 19, 2013.

Broome CV, Loonsk J. Public health information network: improving early detection by using a standards-based approach to connecting public health and clinical medicine. *MMWR.* 2004;53(Suppl.):199–202.

Bureau of Labor Statistics. http://www.bls.gov/news.release/union2.nr0.htm. January 23, 2013.

Burns RB, Stoy DB, Feied CF, Nash E, Smith M. Cholesterol screening in the emergency department. *J Gen Intern Med.* 1991;6(3):210–215.

Burton LC, Paqlia MJ, German PS, Shapiro S, Damiano AM, Medicare Preventive Services Research Team. The effect among older persons of general preventive visits on three health behaviors: smoking, excessive alcohol drinking, and sedentary lifestyle. *Prev Med.* 1995;24(5, Special Issue):492–497.

Calfas KJ, Hagler AS. Physical activity. In: Sheinfeld Gorin S & Arnold J. *Health Promotion in Practice,* pp. 192–221. San Francisco, CA: Jossey-Bass; 2006.

Canadian Task Force on the Periodic Health Examination. *The Canadian Guide to Clinical Preventive Health Care.* Ottawa: Canada Communication Group; 1994.

CBO. Accessed September 2012 from http://www.beckershospitalreview.com/racs-/-icd-9-/-icd-10/medicare-medicaid-costs-still-expected-to-double-despite-revised-cbo-projections.html.

Centers for Disease Control and Prevention. Prevention and managed care: opportunities for managed care organizations, purchasers of health care, and public health agencies. *MMWR.* 1995, November 17;44(RR-14):1–12.

Centers for Disease Control and Prevention. *School Health Profiles.* 2002. Retrieved September 5, 2012, from http://www.cdc.gov/HealthyYouth/profiles.

Centers for Disease Control and Prevention. *CDC Wonder* [Database]. 2005b. Available at http://wonder.cdc.gov.

Centers for Disease Control and Prevention & the National Association of County Health Officials. *Blueprint for a Healthy Community: A Guide for Local Health Departments.* Washington, DC: National Association of County Health Officials; 1994.

Chen J, Kresnow M-J, Simon TR, Dellinger A. Injury-prevention counseling and behavior among US children: results from the Second Injury Control and Risk Survey. *Pediatrics.* 2007;*119*(4): e958–e965.

Christakis NA, Fowler JH. The spread of obesity in a large social network over 32 years. *N Engl J Med.* 2007;357:370–379.

Centers for Medicare and Medicaid Services. *Medicare Modernization Act.* 2003. Retrieved September 5, 2012, from http://www.cms.hhs.gov/medicare.

Centers for Medicare and Medicaid Services, 2013. *About CMS.* Retrieved July 19, 2013, from http://www.cms. gov/About-CMS/About-CMS.html.

Chapman LS. Meta-evaluation of worksite health promotion economic return studies: 2012 update. *Am J Health Promot.* 2012 Mar-Apr;26(4):TAHP1–TAHP12.

Chernow SM, Iserson KV. Use of the emergency department for hypertension screening: A prospective study. *Ann Emerg Med.* 1987;16:180–182.

CMS, 2012; https://www.cms.gov/Research-Statistics-D ata-and-Systems/Statistics-Trends-and-Reports/ NationalHealthExpendData/NHE-Fact-Sheet.html. Retrieved September 5, 2012, from http://www.cms. hhs.gov/medicare.

Cushman R, James W, Waclawik H. Physicians promoting bicycle helmets for children: A randomized trial. *Am J Public Health.* 1991;81(8):1044–1046.

De Lew N. Medicare: 35 years of service. *Health Care Financ Rev.* 2000;22(1):75–103.

Delaney WP, Ames G. Team attitudes, drinking norms and workplace drinking. *Journal of Drug Issues,* 1995;25:275–290.

Description of a Good and Modern Addictions and Mental Health Service System, 2011; http://beta. samhsa.gov/sites/default/files/good_and_mod-ern_4_18_2011_508.pdf

Diez-Roux A. Residential factors and cardiovascular risk. *J Urban Health.* 2003;80:569–589.

Diller P. Intrastate preemption. *Boston Univy Law Rev.* 2007;87:1113–1176, at 1126.

Diller P, Graff S. Regulating food retail for obesity prevention: how far can cities go? *Using Law, Policy, and Research to Improve the Public's Health.* 2011:89–93.

Ernst E. Placebos in medicine: comment. *Lancet.* 1994;345:65.

Franco EL, Harper DM. Vaccination against human papillomavirus infection: a new paradigm in cervical cancer control. *Vaccine.* 2005;23:17–18:2388–2394.

Frank RG, Goldman HH, McGuire T. Trends in Mental Health Cost Growth: An Expanded Role for Management? *Health Affairs.* 2009;28(1):649–659.

Freedman MA, Trabin T. *Managed Behavioral Healthcare: History, Models, Key Issues, and Future Course.* Washington, DC: U.S. Center for Mental Health Services; 1994.

Frew S A. *Patient Transfers: How to Comply with the Law.* Dallas, TX: American College of Emergency Physicians; 1991.

Friede A, O'Carroll PW, Nicola RM, Oberle MW, Teutsch SM. *CDC Prevention Guidelines: A Guide to Action.* Baltimore: Williams & Wilkins; 1997.

Frost K, Frank E, Mailbach E. Relative risk in the news media: a quantification of misrepresentation. *Am J Public Health.* 1997;87:842–845.

Fugh-Berman A. *Alternative Medicine—What Works: A Comprehensive Easy-to-Read Review of the Scientific Evidence, Pro and Con.* Tucson, AZ: Odion Press; 1996.

Galvin DM. Workplace managed care: Collaboration for substance abuse prevention. *J Behav Health Serv R.* 2000;27:125–130.

Gargiulo M. Two-step leverage: managing constraint in organizational politics. *Admin Sci Quart.* 1993;38(1):1–19.

Garland M, Stull J. *Module 9: Public Health and Health System Reform: Access, Priority Setting, and Allocation of Resources.* 2004. Association of Schools of Public Health. Retrieved September 5, 2012, from http:// www.asph.org/UserFiles/Module9.pdf.

Gebbie KM. State public health laws: an expression of constituency expectations. *J Public Health Man.* 2000;6(2):46–54.

Glemigani J. Best practices that boost productivity. *Business and Health* (March 1998), pp. 37–42.

Go AS, Mozaffarian D, Roger VL, et al.; on behalf of the American Heart Association Statistics Committee and Stroke Statistics Subcommittee. Heart disease and stroke statistics—2013 update: a report from the American Heart Association. *Circulation.* 2013;127:e6–e245.

Gold M, Jacobson G, Damico A, Neuman T. *Medicare Advantage 2012 Data Spotlight: Enrollment Market Update.* Accessed January 2013 from http://kaiserfamilyfoundation.files.wordpress.com/2013/01/8323.pdf.

Gostin LO. The future of public health law. *Am J Law Med.* 1986;12(3–4):461–490.

Greenberg ES, Grunberg L. Work alienation and problem alcohol behavior. *J Health Soc Behav.* 1995;36:83–102.

Greenfield D, Braithwaite J. Health sector accreditation research: a systematic review. *International J Quality in Health Care.* 2008;20(3):172–183.

Guinta MA, Allegrante JP. The President's Committee on Health Education: a 20-year retrospective on its politics and policy impact. *Am J Public Health.* 1992;82(7):1033–1041.

Hacker JS. National health care reform: an idea whose time came and went. *J Health Polit Polic.* 1996;21(4):647–696.

Hastings GB. *The Mass Media in Health Promotion: Ten Golden Rules.* Paper presented at the BPS International Conference on Health Psychology, Cardiff, Wales; September 1989.

Health Maintenance Organization Act of 1973, 42 U.S.C. §§ 201 notes et seq. (1994).

Heclo H. Policy analysis. *Br J Policy Sci,* 1972;2:83–108.

Heimendinger J, Feng Z, Emmons K, Stoddard A, Kinne S, Biener L, et al. The Working Well trial: baseline dietary and smoking behaviors of employees and related worksite characteristics. *Prev Med.* 1995;24:180–193.

Hibbard JH, Greene J, Overton V. Patients with lower activation associated with higher costs; delivery systems should know their patients' 'scores.' *Health Affairs.* 2013;32(2):216–222.

Hibbs JR, Ceglowski WS, Goldberg M, Kauffman F. Emergency department–based surveillance for syphilis during an outbreak in Philadelphia. *Ann Emerg Med.* 1993;22(8):1286–1290.

Hodge F. *Center for American Indian Research and Education* (PowerPoint presentation). 1999. Retrieved September 5, 2012, from http://www.cmh.pitt.edu/PPT/Hodge1999.ppt.

Hodgkin D, Horgan CM, Garnick DW, Merrick EL. Benefit Limits for Behavioral Health Care in Private Health Plans. *Admin Policy Ment Health.* 2009;36:15–23.

Hoffman JP, Larison C, Sanderson A. *An Analysis of Worker Drug Use and Workplace Policies and Programs.* Rockville, MD: SAMHSA Office of Applied Studies; 1997.

Honda K, Sheinfeld Gorin S. Modeling pathways to affective barriers on colorectal cancer screening among Japanese Americans. *J Behav Med.* 2005;28:115–124.

Hogness CG, Engelstad LP, Linck LM, Schorr KA. Cervical cancer screening in an urban emergency department. *Ann Emerg Med.* 1992;21:933–939.

Hulscher ME, Wensing M, van der Weijden T, Grol R. Interventions to implement prevention in primary care (Cochrane Review). *Cochrane Library.* 2002;2.

IMS Health. *IMS Health Market Prognosis, March 2009.* Accessed January, 2013 from http://www.abpi.org.uk/industry-info/knowledge-hub/global-industry/Pages/industry-market-.aspx.

IMS Health. OHE. *Figures based on Market Statistics IMS World Review,* 2012 edition. IMS website. Accessed January 2013 from http://www.abpi.org.uk/industry-info/knowledge-hub/global-industry/Pages/industry-market-.aspx.

IMS Health. *IMS Health World Review Analyst 2012.* OECD Health Database. Accessed from http://www.abpi.org.uk/industry-info/knowledge-hub/global-industry/Pages/industry-market-.aspx.

IMS Health. 2011. Accessed January 2013 from http://www.abpi.org.uk/industry-info/knowledge-hub/global-industry/Pages/industry-market-.aspx.

Institute of Medicine. *The Role of Nutrition in Maintaining Health in the Nation's Elderly: Evaluating Coverage of Nutrition Services for the Medicare Population.* 2000b. Retrieved September 5, 2012, from http:/www.nap.edu/openbook/0309068460/html/1.html.

Institute of Medicine. *Health Insurance Is a Family Matter.* Washington, DC: National Academies Press; 2002.

Institute of Medicine. *Unequal Treatment: Confronting Racial and Ethnic Disparities in Health Care.* Washington, DC: National Academies Press; 2003.

Institute of Medicine. *Complementary and Alternative Medicine in the United States.* Washington, DC: National Academies Press; 2005.

Institute of Medicine. *Crossing the Quality Chasm: A New Health System for the 21st Century.* Washington, DC: National Academies Press; 2001.

Joint Commission on Accreditation of Healthcare Organizations. *Facts about Behavioral Health Care Accreditation.* 2005. Retrieved September 5, 2012, from http://www.jcaho.org/htba/behavioral+health+care/facts.htm.

Journal of the National Cancer Institute. Longer span between mammograms okay for older women. February 5, 2013.

Joyce CRB. Placebo and complementary medicine. *Lancet.* 1994;344:1279–1281.

Kaiser Commission on Medicaid and the Underinsured, Mental Health Financing in the United States: a Primer. 2011 Accessed January 2013 from http://kaiserfamily foundation.files.wordpress.com/2013/01/8182.pdf

Kaiser Family Foundation/Health Research & Educational Trust. *Employer Health Benefits Survey,* 2008. Washington, DC: Henry J. Kaiser Family Foundation and Health Research & Educational Trust, p. 141.

Kaiser Family Foundation. *Focus on Health Reform: Summary of the New Health Reform Law.* April 15, 2011. Retrieved from http://www.kff.org/healthreform/upload/8061.pdf.

Kaiser Family Foundation. *Focus on Health Reform: Preventive Services Covered by Private Health Plans under the Affordable Care Act.* September 2011. Retrieved from http://www.kff.org/healthreform/upload/8219.pdf.

Kaiser Family Foundation and Health Research and Educational Trust. *Employer Health Benefits 2011 Annual Survey.* 2011. Retrieved July 19, 2013, from http://www.kff.org.

Koh HK, Sebelius KG. Promoting prevention through the Affordable Care Act. *N Engl J Med.* 2010;363:1296–1299.

Kongstvedt PR. *The Managed Health Care Handbook.* 2nd ed. Gaithersburg, MD: Aspen; 1993.

Kushner RF. Barriers to providing nutrition counseling by physicians: a survey of primary care practitioners. *Prev Med*. 1995;24(6):546–552.

Lalonde M. *A New Perspective on the Health of Canadians*. Ottawa: Information Canada; 1974.

Liao Y, Tucker P, Okoro CA, Giles WH, Mokdad AH, Harris VB. REACH 2010 surveillance for health status in minority communities: United States, 2001–2002. *MMWR*. 2004;53(SS06):1–36.

Lin JS, O'Connor E, Whitlock EP, Beil TL, Zuber SP, Perdue LA, Plaut D, Lutz K. *Behavioral Counseling to Promote Physical Activity and a Healthful Diet to Prevent Cardiovascular Disease in Adults: Update of the Evidence for the U.S. Preventive Services Task Force* [Internet]. Rockville (MD): Agency for Healthcare Research and Quality (US); 2010; Report No.: 11-05149-EF-1. U.S. Preventive Services Task Force Evidence Syntheses, formerly Systematic Evidence Reviews.

Logsdon DN, Lazaro CM, Meier RV. The feasibility of behavioral risk reduction in primary medical care. *Am J Prev Med*. 1989;5(5), 249–256.

Longest BB Jr. *Health Policymaking in the United States*. 3rd ed. Chicago: AUPHA/HAP; 2002.

Lorenc T, Petticrew M, Welch V, Tugwell P. What types of interventions generate inequalities? Evidence from systematic reviews. *J Epidemiol Community Health*. 2012.

Lorion RP. Evaluating preventive interventions: Guidelines for the serious social change agent. *Cancer Epidem, Biomar*. 1983;8:759–767.

Manley MW, Griffin T, Foldes SS, Link CC, Sechrist RAJ. The role of health plans in tobacco control. *Ann Rev Public Health*. 2003;24:247–266.

Mandelblatt JS, Yabroff KR. Effectiveness of interventions designed to increase mammography use: a meta-analysis of provider-targeted strategies. *Cancer Epidemiology, Biomarkers & Prevention*. 1999;8:759–767.

MarketingVOX News. *Blog Stats Redux*. 2004. Retrieved September 5, 2012, from http://www.marketingvox.com/archives/2004/11/23/blog_stats_redux.

Mayer RR, Greenwood E. *The Design of Social Policy*. Upper Saddle River, NJ: Prentice Hall; 1980.

McAlister A. Mass and community organization for prevention programs. In: Jeger AM, Slotnick RS, eds. *Community Mental Health and Behavioral Ecology: A Handbook of Theory, Research and Practice*, pp. 243–256. New York: Plenum; 1982.

McCaig LF. National Ambulatory Medical Care Survey: 1992 emergency department summary. *Advance Data*. 1994a;245:1–12.

McCaig LF. National Ambulatory Medical Care Survey: 1992 outpatient department summary. *Advance Data*. 1994b;248:1–12.

Mico PR. An introduction to policy for health educators. *Health Educ Monog*. 1978;6(Suppl. 1):7–17.

Milliman and Robertson, Inc. *Health Risks and Behavior: The Impact on Medical Costs*. Brookfield, WI: Author; 1987.

Mullen PD, Holcomb JD. Selected predictors of health promotion counseling by three groups of allied health professionals. *Am J Prev Med*. 1990;6(3):153–160.

National Committee for Quality Assurance. *About NCQA*. Retrieved September 5, 2012, from http://www.ncqa.org/about/about.htm.

National Conference of State Legislatures. *Health Promotion: State Legislation and Statutes Database*. 2005b. Retrieved September 5, 2012, from http://www.ncsl.org/programs/health/pp/healthpromo_cfm.

National Conference of State Legislatures (2013). Federal and State Recognized Tribes. Retrieved July 19, 2013 from http://www.ncsl.org/issues-research/tribal/list-of-federal-and-state-recognized-tribes.aspx.

National Consumer Health Information and Health Promotion Act of 1976, 42 U.S.C. §§ 301 et seq. (1994).

Navarro V. *Medicine under Capitalism*. New York: Prodist; 1976.

Neubauer D, Pratt R. The second public health revolution: A critical appraisal. *J Health Polit Polic*. 1981;6(2):205–228.

Noar SM. Behavioral interventions to reduce HIV-related sexual risk behavior: review and synthesis of meta-analytic evidence. *AIDS and Behavior* 2008;12(3):335–353.

Ockene JK, Ockene IS, Quirk ME, Hebert JR, Saperia GM, Luippold RS, et al. Physician training for patient-centered nutrition counseling in a lipid intervention trial. *Prev Med*. 1995;24(6):563–570.

Office of Personnel Management. *Federal Employees Health Benefits Program*. 2005. Retrieved September 5, 2012, from http://www.opm.gov/insure/health/about/fehb.asp.

Patton D, Kolasa K, West S, Irons T. Sexual abstinence counseling of adolescents by physicians. *Adolescence*. 1995;30(120):963–969.

Pollack A. *Obama Pushes More Competition on Biologic Drugs*. September 19, 2011. http://prescriptions.blogs.nytimes.com/2011/09/19/obama-pushes-more-competition-on-biologic-drugs/?_r=0.

Pomerleau J, Lock K, Knai C, McKee M. Interventions designed to increase adult fruit and vegetable intake can be effective: a systematic review of the literature. *J. Nutr*. 2005;135(10):2486–2495.

Preventive Health Amendments of 1993, PL 103-183 (42 U.S.C. §§ 233 et seq).

Price JH, Clause M, Everett SA. Patients' attitudes about the role of physicians in counseling about firearms. *Patient Educ Couns*. 1995;25(2):163–170.

Prochaska JO, Velicer WF. The transtheoretical model of health behavior change. *Am J Health Promot*. 1997;12(1):38–48.

Reynolds C. The promise of public health law. *J Law Med*. 1994;1:212–222.

Riedel JE. Employee health promotion: Blue Cross and Blue Shield plan activities. *Am J Health Promot.* 1987;1(4):28–32.

Roberts DF, Maccoby N. Effects of mass communication. In: Lindzy G, Aronson E, eds. *Handbook of Social Psychology: Vol. 2. Special Fields and Applications*, pp. 539–598. New York: Random House, 1985.

Roth GY. *Top 20 Pharma Report: Our Annual Look at the 20 Biggest Players in the Pharmaceutical Marketplace.* Contract Pharma, 2012. http://www.contract pharma.com/issues/2012-07/view_features/top-20-pharma-report/

Rowan KE, Bethea LS, Pecchioni L, Villagran M. A research-based-guide for physicians communicating cancer risk. *Health Commun.* 2003;15:239–252.

Russ TC, Stamatakis E, Hamer M, Starr JM, Kivimäki M, Batty GD. Association between psychological distress and mortality: individual participant pooled analysis of 10 prospective cohort studies. *MJ.* 2012;345:e4933.

Schauffler HH. Disease prevention policy under Medicare: a historical and political analysis. *Am J Prev Med.* 1993;9(2):71–77.

Schectman JM, Stoy DB, Elinsky EG. Association between physician counseling for hypercholesterolemia and patient dietary knowledge. *Am J Prev Med.* 1994;10(3):136–139.

Schroeder SA. Tobacco control in the wake of the 1998 master settlement agreement. *New Eng J Med.* 2004;350(3): 293–301.

Seeman TE. Health promoting effects of friends and family on health outcomes in older adults. *Am J Health Promot.* 2000;14(6):362–370.

Seeman TE, Kaplan GA, Knudsen L, Cohen R, Guralnik J. Social network ties and mortality among tile elderly in the alameda county study. *Am J Epidemiol.* 1987;126(4):714–723.

Serxner S, Anderson DR, Gold D. Building program participation: strategies for recruitment and retention in worksite health promotion programs. *American Journal of Health Promotion.* 2004;18(4):1–6.

Sewing K-Fr. Placebos in medicine: comment. *Lancet.* 1994;345:65–66.

Sheinfeld Gorin S, Heck J, Albert S, Hershman D. Treatment for breast cancer among patients with Alzheimer's disease. *JAGS.* 2005;53:1897–1904.

Sheinfeld Gorin S, Heck J. Cancer screening among Latino subgroups in the United States. *Prev Med.* 2005;40:515–526.

Sheinfeld Gorin S. Colorectal cancer screening compliance among urban Hispanics. *J Behav Med.* 2005;28:125–137.

Sheinfeld Gorin S, Heck J. Meta-analysis of the efficacy of tobacco cessation counseling: a comparison of physicians, nurses, and dentists. *Cancer Epidem Biomar.* 2004;13:2012–2022.

Heck JE, Sheinfeld Gorin S. Neighborhood-level income inequality and breast cancer stage at diagnosis. *Ann Epidemiol.* 2004;14(8):597.

Sheinfeld Gorin S, NYPAC Study Group. Models of physician colorectal cancer (CRC) genetic counseling referral practices. *Ann Behav Med.* 2004 Supplement;27;S007.

Sheinfeld Gorin S, Albert SM. The meaning of risk to first degree relatives of women with breast cancer. *Women and Health.* 2003;37:97–117.

Sheinfeld Gorin S, Graff Zivin J, NYPAC Study Group. Effects of academic detailing for colorectal cancer screening among primary care physicians: self report and cost effectiveness findings. *Cancer Epidem Biomar.* 2003;12:1276s–1279s.

Sheinfeld Gorin S, Wang C, Raich P, Bowen DJ, Hay J. Decision making in cancer primary prevention and chemoprevention. *Ann Behav Med.* 2006;32(3):179–187.

Sheridan SL, Harris RP, Woolf SH. *Shared Decision-Making about Screening and Chemoprevention: A Suggested Approach from the U.S. Preventive Services Task Force* (AHRQ Publication No. 04-0529). Rockville, MD: Agency for Healthcare Research and Quality; 2003.

Shipan CR, Volden C. *Policy Diffusion from Cities to States: Antismoking Laws in the US.* Presented at the Law, Economics, and Organization Workshop, Yale University; 2005.

Shouldice RG. *Introduction to Managed Care: Health Maintenance Organizations, Preferred Provider Organizations, and Competitive Medical Plans.* Arlington, VA: Information Resources Press; 1991.

Simonds SK. Health education: Facing issues of policy, ethics, and social justice. *Health Educ Monog.* 1978;6(Suppl. 1):17–27.

Sommers BD, Baicker K, Epstein AM. Mortality and access to care among adults after state Medicaid expansions. *New Engl J Med.* 2012;367:1025–1034.

Sorensen G, Stoddard AM, Youngstrom R, Emmons K, Barbeau E, Khoransanizadeh F, et al. Local labor unions' positions on worksite tobacco control. *American Journal of Public Health.* 2000;90:618–620.

Steckler A, Dawson L, Goodman RM, Epstein N. Policy advocacy: three emerging roles for health education. *Adv Health Educ Promot.* 1987;2:5–27.

Tang JL, Armitage JM, Lancaster T, Silagy CA, Fowler GH, Neil HAW. Systematic review of dietary intervention trials to lower blood total cholesterol in free-living subjects. *BMJ.* 1998;316(7139):1213–1220.

Tesh S. Disease causality and politics. *J Health Polit Polic.* 1981;6(3):369–390.

Thompson SC, Schwankovsky L, Pitts J. Counseling patients to make lifestyle changes: the role of physician self-efficacy, training and beliefs about causes. *Family Practice.* 1993;10(1):70–75.

Tregloan ML. Health service quality assessment: defining and assessing health care standards; an international picture. *Healthcare Review* 2000.

Turrell G, Hewitt B, Patterson C, Oldenburg B, Gould T. Socioeconomic differences in food purchasing behaviour and suggested implications for diet-related health promotion. *J Human Nutr Diet.* 2002;15(5):355–364.

Twiss J, Dickinson J, Duma S, Kleinman T, Paulsen H, Rilveria L. Community gardens: Lessons learned from California Healthy Cities and Communities. *Am J Public Health.* 2003;93(9):1435–1438.

U.S. Department of Health and Human Services. A historical review of efforts to reduce smoking in the United States. In *Reducing Tobacco Use: A Report of the Surgeon General* (chap. 2). 2000b. Retrieved September 5, 2012, from http://www.cdc.gov/tobacco/sgr/sgr_2000/Chapter2.pdf.

U.S. Department of Health and Human Services. *Indian Health Service Introduction.* 2005a. Retrieved September 5, 2012, from http://www.ihs.gov/PublicInfo/PublicAffairs/Welcome_Info/IHSintro.asp.

U.S. Department of Health, Education and Welfare. *Healthy People: The Surgeon General's Report on Health Promotion and Disease Prevention* (PHS Publication No. 79-55071). Washington, DC: Author; 1979.

U.S. Government Printing Office. *Public and Private Laws.* 1997. Retrieved September 5, 2012, from http://www.access.gpo.gov/nara/publaw/104publ.html.

U.S. National Library of Medicine. *Current Bibliographies in Medicine 2000–7: Health Risk Communication.* 2003. Retrieved September 5, 2012, from http://www.nlm.nih.gov/pubs/cbm/health_risk_communication.html.

U.S. Preventive Services Task Force. *Guide to Clinical Preventive Services.* 2nd ed. Baltimore: Williams & Wilkins; 1996.

U.S. Preventive Services Task Force. *Guide to Clinical Preventive Services.* 3rd ed. 2004. Retrieved September 5, 2012, from http://www.ahrq.gov/clinic/uspstfix.htm.

Veterans' Health Care Reform Eligibility Act of 1996, PL 104-262, 38 U.S.C.A. §§ 101 note et seq. (1994).

Vernon S, Meissner H, Klabunde C, Rimer B, Ahnen D, Bastain R, Mandelson M, Nadel M, Sheinfeld Gorin S, Zapka J. Measures for ascertaining use of colorectal cancer screening in behavioral, health services, and epidemiologic research. *Cancer Epidem Biomar.* 2004;13:898–905.

Wallack L, Dorfman L, Jernigan D, Themba M. *Media advocacy and Public Health: Power for Prevention.* Thousand Oaks, CA: Sage; 1993.

Wamsley G, Zald M. *The Political Economy of Public Organizations: A Critique and Approach to the Study of Public Administration.* Bloomington: Indiana University Press; 1967.

Weber J. Drugs and biotech. *Business Week,* January 13, 1997, p. 110.

Woloshin S, Schwartz LM, Welch G. Risk charts: putting cancer in context. *J Natl Cancer I.* 2002;94(11):799–804.

Woolf SH, Jonas S, Lawrence RS, eds. *Health Promotion and Disease Prevention in Clinical Practice.* Baltimore: Williams & Wilkins; 1996.

3

Models for Prevention

SHERRI N. SHEINFELD GORIN

This Chapter[1] explains prevention within the constraints of several dominant models in the field of health promotion (global and national policies; the environmental approaches; the life course model; and the health attitude, belief, and behavioral change approaches) and details these models' implicit approaches to health. Using a multilevel approach, the loci of change are at either the rnicrolevel (individual, family, group) or the macrolevel (societal, community, population) (Zaitman, Kotler, Kaufman, 1972).

Models present a simplified picture of part of the phenomenon of prevention in health. Several of the models described in this Chapter could also be characterized as theories of social relations. In general, a theory (1) contains constructs (i.e., mental images, such as health) that it seeks to explain or account for in some way; (2) describes relationships, often causal, among constructs; and (3) incorporates hypothesized relationships between the constructs and observable variables that can be used to measure the constructs (i.e., operationalized constructs; Judd, Smith, & Kidder, 1991). Theory can help to understand and explain the reasons that an evidence-based intervention may work to induce planned change in patients and providers (Sales, Smith, Curran, Kochevar, 2006). Several of these theories, such as that of social cognition, have been empirically verified, and thus strong evidence for their veracity exists. Other models, even as they are guiding research and intervention development, are at the same time undergoing verification and modification, through approaches similar to those outlined in the last part of this Chapter, and in Chapter 12 (e.g., complexity theory; Miller, McDaniel, Crabtree, & Stange, 2001).

---

1 Much of this Chapter is adapted from Sheinfeld Gorin S, Models of Health Promotion. In: Sheinfeld Gorin S. & Arnold J. *The Health Promotion Handbook*, 21–66. San Francisco, CA: Jossey-Bass; 2006.

GLOBAL POLICY

Global health policy sets the context for US health promotion policy, so is discussed in brief. Global health policy is based on the World Health Organization's definition of *health*, as stated in Chapter 1, which is currently the broadest, most inclusive definition and is designed for citizens of the world: "Health is a state of complete physical, mental, and social well-being, and not merely the absence of disease or infirmity."

In 1978, at Alma-Ata, Kazakhstan, representatives of nations throughout the world expressed the need for nations to develop access to primary health care that would enable their citizens to lead socially and economically productive lives. This meeting was followed by one in 1988 in Riga, Latvia, to identify the remaining gaps in health care, particularly for infants, children, and women of childbearing age. Strategies to achieve health for all persons by the year 2000 were drafted. They called for (1) empowering persons by providing information and decision-making opportunities, (2) strengthening local systems of primary health care, (3) improving education and training programs in health promotion and prevention for health care professionals, (4) applying science and technology to critical health problems, (5) using new approaches to health problems that have resisted solution, (6) providing special assistance to the least-developed countries, and (7) establishing a process for examination of the long-term challenges that must be addressed beyond the year 2000 in achieving health for all (World Health Organization [WHO], 1988). To implement the aim of the first conference and to develop the strategies of the second, WHO (1984) adopted the following five principles of health promotion:

1. Health promotion includes the population as a whole in the context of individuals'

everyday lives, rather than focusing on persons at risk for specific diseases.

2. Health promotion is directed toward action on the causes or determinants of health.

3. Health promotion combines diverse but complementary methods or approaches, including communication, education, legislation, fiscal measures, organizational change, community development, and spontaneous local activities against health hazards.

4. Health promotion is particularly aimed at effective and concrete public participation.

5. While health promotion is basically an activity in the health and social fields and not a medical service, health care professionals—particularly in primary health care—have an important role in nurturing and enabling health promotion.

The WHO definition of health promotion offers a multidimensional characterization of health and incorporates a multitude of strategies, including individual and community change and legislation, under its rubric. The WHO definition assumes that a person does not have sole control over his or her health. It does, however, allow people to take responsibility for their choices within a context of concomitant social responsibility for health. Further, on the philosophical level, it implies that health is a means to an end—a *resource*—and an instrumental value, or good, for what it brings. Health, like power, is a resource differentially distributed in society (Gutiérrez, 1990). In the global policy model, health is not a good in and of itself or a value in its own right but a resource for living. Multisectoral cooperation—among public health, transportation, social welfare, and other systems—is necessary for the equitable distribution of health resources.

NATIONAL POLICY

As discussed in Chapter 1, some 40% of deaths are caused by behavior patterns that could be modified by preventive interventions (McGinnis, Williams-Russo, Knickman, 2002). In particular, tobacco use, poor diet, and physical inactivity have contributed to the largest number of deaths, and deaths related to these behaviors have been increasing (Mokdad et al., 2005). Attention to these risks at the population level and federal interest in the

reduction of health care expenses led to the development of *Healthy People 2020*. This monograph is the most recent of several national initiatives to develop health objectives for the country, and it has spawned a number of similar state initiatives. Details of the plan are found in Chapter 2; in general it provides a plan of action for the nation's health; the document mixes both a health promotion and a disease prevention approach. The concept of health promotion developed in these approaches emphasizes the roles of individuals, groups, organizations, and policy makers as active agents in shaping health practices and policies to optimize both individual wellness and collective well-being.

Health Promotion

The health promotion strategies developed in the *Healthy People* documents are related to individual lifestyle—personal choices made in a social context—that can have a powerful influence over one's health prospects. These strategies target issues such as physical activity; nutrition; sexuality; tobacco, alcohol, and other drug use; oral health; mental health and mental disorders; and violent and abusive behavior. Educational and community-based programs can address lifestyle choices in a cross-cutting fashion.

Health Protection

The health protection strategies set out in these documents are related to environmental or regulatory measures that confer protection on large population groups. These strategies address issues such as unintentional injuries, occupational safety and health, environmental health, food and drug safety, and fluoridation of water for oral health. Interventions applied to address these issues generally are not exclusively protective—they may provide a substantial health promotion element as well—and the principal approaches involve a community-wide, rather than individual, focus.

Disease Prevention

The disease prevention model in these documents focuses on the avoidance of illness and the agents of illness, as well as the identification and minimization of risk. This approach is found throughout the health promotion literature, most particularly in the work of the US Preventive Services Task Force (USPSTF), as discussed further in Chapter 2. Epidemiologic data are the foundation for the development of this model. Epidemiology focuses on how diseases originate and spread in populations (Lilienfeld, 1976).

In a preventive approach, the natural history of the disease at issue is examined to identify the interrelationship between the outside etiologic, or causal, agents and the biological response of the host and to determine the effects of environmental, social, and physical factors; community patterns of medical care; and the social and intellectual response of the host (Leavell & Clark, 1953). The target of the preventive intervention is selected based on the prevalence (proportion of the population affected) and the incidence (number of new cases per year) of the condition. In the USPSTF's work, the target conditions selected are relatively common in the United States and are of major clinical significance. The natural history of a disease may depend on environmental conditions, like the prevalence of asthma in areas of high air pollution compared to areas of low air pollution. Similarly, the natural history of a disease may show variations related to sociodemographic characteristics of the affected individuals, such as their race or ethnicity or the health service characteristics of their communities, such as access to care (Hutchison, 1969).

The traditional triad of primary, secondary, and tertiary prevention is often used to distinguish approaches. Primary preventive measures are those provided to individuals to prevent the onset of a targeted condition (e.g., routine immunization of healthy children). Secondary preventive measures identify and treat asymptomatic persons who have already developed risk factors or pre-clinical disease but in whom the condition has not become clinically apparent (e.g., screening for high blood pressure). Tertiary preventive measures are those directed toward persons as part of the treatment and management of their clinical and chronic diseases (e.g., cholesterol reduction in clients with coronary heart disease or insulin therapy to prevent the complications of diabetes mellitus; USPSTF, 2004).

Risk Assessment

In the disease prevention orientation, individuals and groups are characterized by their absolute, relative, or attributable *risk* for various diseases and disorders. According to the Royal Society (1983), "Risk is the probability that a particular adverse event occurs during a stated period of time, or results from a particular challenge." In the field of epidemiology, *absolute risk* measures the magnitude of the incidence of disease in a population, *relative risk* measures the strength of an association between a risk and a disease (e.g., between smoking and lung cancer), and *attributable risk* is a measure of how much of the disease risk (e.g., risk for coronary heart disease) is attributable to a particular exposure (e.g., smoking; Gordis, 2000). The *population attributable fraction* (PAF) refers to the fraction of disease cases (or deaths) in a population that is associated with an exposure (e.g., obesity), generally by age groups. It is not meaningful at the level of the individual (Goodman, 2005).

A critical clinical issue for clinicians is how to portray risk of disease to a client. As posited by the health belief model (to be discussed later in this Chapter), whether individuals respond to a health threat depends in part on how large they perceive their personal risk to be. Even though the definition of the risk denotes that the risk taker's behavior is harmful, the real or perceived benefits of smoking, eating, and drinking may be seen differently by the person engaging in the activity and by an outsider. As discussed more fully in Chapter 11, typical clinical (or media) presentations of health risks may do little to inform these perceptions (Woloshin, Schwartz, & Welch, 2002). Generally, health care professionals and patients are poorly prepared for discussions of health risks (Schwartz, Woloshin, & Welch, 1999; Fong, Rempel, & Hall, 1999; Woloshin, Schwartz, & Welch, 2002; Lipkus & Hollands, 1999).

The discussion of risk should take place in the context of *shared decision making* (SDM); *shared decision making* occurs when the client and the health care professional together discuss the risks and benefits of a proposed decision. Informed decision making occurs when an individual understands the disease or condition being addressed and also comprehends what the clinical service involves, including its benefits, risks, limitations, alternatives, and uncertainties. In SDM the client has considered his or her own preferences, believes that he or she has participated in decision making at a level that he or she desires, and makes a decision consistent with those preferences (Sheridan, Harris, & Woolf, 2004). Numerous decision aids are available to assist with SDM (for a review, see O'Connor et al., 2004; also see Llewellyn-Thomas, 1995; Harvard Center for Cancer Prevention, Harvard School of Public Health, [http://www.diseaseriskindex.harvard.edu/update/]; see Chapter 11 for additional discussions).

Example of a Large Community Risk-Prevention Program

The Framingham Heart Study, begun in 1948 in the town of Framingham, Massachusetts, and funded by the National Heart, Lung, and Blood Institute (NHLBI), is an exemplary epidemiologic study with ramifications for community-based risk modification. The data derived from study of the original cohort of 5,209 healthy residents between 30 and 60 years of age, 5,124 of their children and spouses, and 500 members of the Framingham minority community that have been used to develop approaches to reduce heart disease, stroke, dementia, osteoporosis, arthritis, diabetes, eye disease, and cancer and to understand the genetic patterns of many common diseases (Framingham Heart Study, http://www.framinghamheartstudy.org/biblio/index.html).

DIFFERENCES AMONG THE HEALTH PROMOTION, HEALTH PROTECTION, AND DISEASE PREVENTION CONCEPTS

The critical difference among these concepts lies in the underlying motivation they offer for a particular behavior on the part of individuals and populations (Pender, 1996). Health promotion encourages well-being and is oriented toward the actualizing of human potential and thus is positive in valence, or attractive to the client. Health protection, however, is directed toward a desire to actively avoid illness, to detect it early, or to maintain function within the constraints of illness, and holds a negative valence. Disease prevention is similar to health protection in that one is taking action to thwart the disease process by finding ways to modify the environment, behavior, and bodily defenses so that disease processes are eliminated, slowed, or changed (Parse, 1987).

Environmental Approaches

The ecological model focuses specifically on the components of health-promotive environments. Within this context, some national policies, such as those establishing acceptable levels of air quality, may highlight the role of the environment in optimizing states of well-being; further, policies may emphasize the connection between well-being and one's social and physical milieu (Stokols, 1992).

In the environmental approaches, healthfulness is seen as a multifaceted phenomenon incorporating physical health, emotional well-being, and social cohesion. Health may result from concurrent interventions in transactions between persons and environments over time (Stokols, 1992) and reflects the outcomes of joint approaches at multiple levels. Health care systems may also differ by their degrees of certainty and agreement among participants, necessitating both varied and variable approaches to achieving positive health outcomes over time (Plsek, 2001).

Social Ecology Model

Ecology pertains to the interrelationships between organisms and their environments (Hawley, 1950). The social ecology approach is grounded in a contextual view of human health and well-being (Moos, 1979). It attends to the social, institutional, and cultural contexts of person-environment relations. The model assumes that the healthfulness of a situation and the well-being of situation participants are influenced by multiple aspects of the environment—both physical (geography, architecture, and technology) and social (culture, economics, and politics). Characteristics of the environment interact with characteristics of the individual, such as genetic heritage, psychological predispositions, and behavioral patterns; health is a result of that interplay. Environments may vary, for example, in their lighting, temperature, noise levels, and land use or space arrangements; these are seen both as objective characteristics and as factors that can be perceived differently by each person (or subjective characteristics). The meshing of an environment and a particular person is unique.

The social ecology model incorporates components of systems theory, such as the dynamic states of interdependence, homeostasis, negative feedback, and a purposeful integration of separate parts (Cannon, 1932; Emery & Trist, 1972; Katz & Kahn, 1966; Maruyama, 1963). Person-environment interactions move through cycles of mutual influence, where each affects the other. The varied levels of human environments, such as worksites, are seen as complex systems in which each level is nested in more complex and distant levels. For example, the occupational health and safety of community work settings is directly influenced by state and local ordinances aimed at protecting public health and environmental quality (Stokols, 1992).

Environments differ in their relative scale and complexity, and the participants in these contexts may be studied as individuals, small groups, organizations, and populations. Interventions may be strengthened by the coordination of individuals and groups acting in different environments, such as corporate managers who shape organizational health policies alongside diverse teams of workers or health insurance (Green & Kreuter, 1990; Pelletier, 1984; Winett, King, & Altman, 1989). Further, individuals' physical and emotional well-being is enhanced when environments are personally controllable and predictable (Karasek & Theorell, 1990). Environments that are too predictable and controllable, however, can become so boring that they constrain opportunities for coping effectively with novel situations, thus impeding growth (Aldwin & Stokols, 1988; Schaefer & Moos, 1992).

The social ecology model recognizes the often contradictory influences of environments and persons. For example, a socially supportive family or organization may enable individuals to cope more effectively with physical constraints (e.g., overcrowding, drab surroundings). A well-designed physical environment may not, however, spur much health promotion if interpersonal or intergroup relations result in conflict and stress.

A focus on the impact of the physical, or "built environment," on health has received renewed attention by both health and design professionals (Jackson, Dannenberg, & Frumkin, 2013). A "sense of place" is a widely discussed concept in fields as diverse as geography, environmental psychology, and art (Frumkin, 2003); of late, it has become more influential in the health field, as empirical studies defining "good places" and research linking the space in which one lives to health outcomes across various diseases has emerged. Place includes geography (e.g., sprawl), aggregated group properties (such as census-tract level income), as well as broader political, cultural, or institutional effects (such as county-level physician supply; Krieger, 2001; Blalock, 1994; Diez-Roux, 1998; Berkman, Kawachi, Macintyre, & Ellaway, 2000; Kawachi, Subramanian, & Almeida-Filho, 2002).

Some places encourage walking, biking, and social interaction more than others do (Putnam, 2000; Saelens, Sallis, & Frank, 2003). Research on place has found that many traffic injuries can be prevented (Elvik, 2001); that increasing motor vehicle exhaust exacerbates pulmonary disease (Friedman, Powell, Hutwagner, Graham, & Teague, 2001); and that the presence of neighborhood liquor stores increases alcohol consumption and associated adverse health consequences (Rabow & Watts,

1983; Jackson, 2003). Adverse places increase the risk of various diseases and conditions (Pickett, Pearl, 2001; Kawachi & Berkman, 2003; Schootman, Andresen, Wolinsky, Malmstrom, Miller, & Miller, 2006; Stjarne, Fritzell, De Leon, & Hallqvist, 2006; Eschbach, Mahnken, & Goodwin, 2005; Schootman, Andresen, & Wolinsky, 2007), and worsen colorectal cancer prognosis (Gomez, O'Malley, Stroup, Shema, & Satariano, 2007; Du, Fang, Vernon, et al., 2007; Wrigley, Roderick, Smith, Mullee, & Goddard, 2003). The health impact of place (also including nature contact, buildings, public spaces, and urban form) may include physical, psychological, social, spiritual, and aesthetic outcomes (Frumkin, 2003), many of which have not yet been systematically examined.

Multilevel Approach

The multilevel approach, embedded in the ecological perspective, acknowledges that many levels of context directly and indirectly affect patients' health behaviors (Taplin et al., 2012, 2010; see Figure 3-1). Existing models consider three levels (the medical care system, the medical care organization, and the individual patient) or four levels (the system or environment in which medical care organizations are situated; the medical care organization; the provider group/team; and the individual clinician). Thus far, the multilevel perspective has been applied to the cancer continuum (Sheinfeld Gorin, Badr, Krebs, Prabhu Das, 2012; see Figure 3-2).

The continuum of cancer care (Figure 3-2) includes risk assessment, primary prevention, screening, detection, diagnosis, treatment, survivorship, and end-of-life care. Movement across the span of the cancer care continuum involves several *types* of needed care, as well as *transitions* between the types of care. *Type* refers to the care delivered to accomplish a specific goal, such as detection, diagnosis, or treatment. *Transition* refers to the set of interactions necessary to go from one type of care to another, such as from detection to diagnosis. Each type and each transition in care is subject to influences at multiple levels that can facilitate or impede successful achievement.

The multilevel approach expands upon the ecologic models to encompass additional relevant levels to the cancer care continuum: the *national health policy environment*, including such factors as national health reform, reimbursement policies or cancer programs; the *state health policy environment*, including

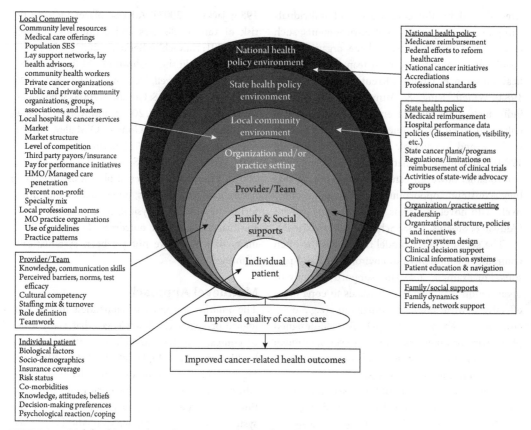

FIGURE 3-1: Multilevel Approaches to Prevention, with Special Emphasis on Cancer.

Source: Sheinfeld Gorin S, Badr H, Krebs P, Prabhu Das I. Multilevel Interventions and Racial/Ethnic Health Disparities. *J Natl Cancer Inst Monogr.* 2012;44:100–111. Reproduced with permission

state reimbursement policies or cancer programs; the *local community environment,* including local health care markets and professional norms; the *organization or practice setting,* including human and capital resources and processes designed to improve care; the *provider and provider team,* including skills and attitudes; *family and social supports,* including social networks; and the *individual patient,* including sociodemographic characteristics, risk factors, and beliefs and attitudes (Figure 3-1). The bottom panel of Figure 3-1 summarizes the ultimate effects of system/policy-level interventions: proactive provider teams, productive encounters, and activated patients.

Most simply, each successive level in Figure 3-1 may influence the adjacent or non-adjacent levels within it. For example, institutional theory describes how organizations are constrained by the technical (market, resource, technological) and institutional (social, political, legal) features of the community, state, and national contexts in which they operate. The relationships between levels may be more

complex, however. Actors may interact with one another *within* and *between* each contextual level. Network theory describes webs of linkages between organizations, with linkages across organizations of similar forms (such as hospitals linked to other hospitals), or linkages between organizations at different levels of the environment. In the context of cancer care, for example, we can envision an oncology practice embedded within a hospital, and linked to community-based or state-level cancer programs. Similarly, physicians who operate both within cancer programs and community hospitals, spanning the boundaries of multiple provider organizations, connect directly to patients as well as to multiple layers of the health care organization's environment.

The influences also may act in multiple directions. For example, while provider teams must live within the policies and regulations of their organizations on a daily basis, over time, providers and provider teams may interact with their organizations to influence policy changes. Furthermore,

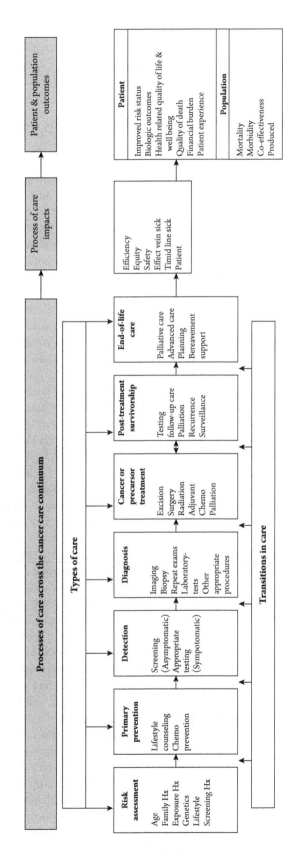

FIGURE 3-2: The Cancer Care Continuum.

Source: Taplin et al, 2012. Reproduced with permission

the influences of one contextual level may not be completely sequential (i.e., a change in one level having an impact on the adjacent level below it). Intervening levels may be skipped. For example, a change in national policy may directly influence the structures/process of health care organizations, without being "filtered" by intermediate levels of state health policies, or local community environments. Similarly, a change in health care organizational structure may directly influence patient-level outcomes, without intermediate effects on family or other social support systems. Because of the complexity of these interactions, perhaps it is important to ask whether addressing several levels simultaneously is necessary to achieve significant improvements to types and transitions of care, and thus individual progression across the cancer continuum to optimal care outcomes.

The multilevel model defines *level* to mean a conceptual construct that organizes and distinguishes different orders of hierarchically linked factors that influence the outcome of interest. In the current multilevel model, *levels* are the various contextual layers, such as the environment, organization, health care provider, family, and individual patient characteristics, which directly or indirectly influence a range of patient care outcomes.

Interventions are a set of specified strategies designed to change the knowledge, perceptions, skills, and/or behavior of individuals or organizations with the goal of improving patients' outcomes. A *multilevel* intervention addresses at least two levels of contextual influence, thereby targeting the individual patients whose behavior is intended to be changed and also some of the national, state, community, organizational, provider, and social/familial contexts in which those individuals exist and participate in health care.

To examine the impact of multilevel interventions (with three or more levels of influence) designed to reduce health disparities, the author conducted a systematic review and meta-analysis of interventions for ethnic/racial minorities (all except non-Hispanic whites) that were published between January 2000 and July 2011. The findings from this descriptive review suggest that multilevel interventions have positive effects on several health behavior outcomes, including cancer prevention and screening, as well improving the quality of health-care system processes. Enhanced application of theories to multiple levels of change, as suggested throughout

this Chapter, novel design approaches, and the use of cultural leveraging in intervention design and implementation are proposed for this nascent field (Sheinfeld Gorin, Badr, Krebs, & Prabhu Das, 2012).

COMPLEX ADAPTIVE SYSTEMS

Complex adaptive systems (CAS) are collections of individual agents that have the freedom to act in ways that are not always predictable and whose actions are interconnected such that one agent's actions changes the context for other agents (Plsek, 2001). Complexity is the pattern of behavior that emerges from the interaction of elements that respond to the limited information with which they are presented (Cilliers, 1998, Kernick, 2006; Waldrop, 1992; Lewin, 1993).

CAS have been the focus of intense study across a variety of scientific fields over the past 40 years (Plsek, 2001; see Waldrop, 1992; Lewin, 1992; Wheatley, 1992; Kelly, 1994; Gell-Mann, 1995; Zimmerman et al., 1998; Brown & Eisenhardt, 1998). Examples of systems that have been studied as a CAS include the human body's immune system (Varela and Coutinho, 1991); the mind (Morowitz and Singer, 1995); a colony of social insects such as termites or ants (Wilson, 1971); the stock market (Mandelbrot, 1999); and almost any collection of human beings (Brown & Eisenhardt, 1998; Stacey, 1996a,b; Zimmerman et al., 1998).

Viewing health care as complex adaptive systems, using complexity theory (Kernick, 2006), many issues rest in a "zone of complexity, where there are only modest levels of certainty and agreement "(p. 35. Kernick, 2004; Langton, 1989; Zimmerman et al., 1998; Varela, 1991; Zimmerman, 1993; 1999). Examples of such issues at the policy level might include: How should health care be financed? What is the best way to deliver primary care? For such issues only a modest level of "certainty" exists regarding what actions lead to what outcomes. Further, well-meaning, rational, intelligent people might not always agree as to the approach or outcome, meaning that there are only modest levels of agreement (Plsek, 2001).

Given both uncertainty and limited agreement among participants in the health care system, key elements in an approach to CAS design include: using biological metaphors to guide thinking (e.g., imagining a colony of social insects such as termites or ants; Wilson, 1971), rather than thinking of machines for control; and creating conditions in which the system can evolve naturally over time. Viewing the practice environment as a complex adaptive system, Miller et al. (1998, 2001) recommend tailoring interventions to account for differences in medical office culture, philosophy, and structure, as well as patient sociodemographic characteristics and medical acuity, to improve the provision of preventive services.

Complexity theory posits that relationships between individuals may be more important than individual attributes (Plsek & Wilson, 2001; Kernick, 2006). Thus, complex system design would rely on simple rules and minimum specifications, with a good enough vision that creates a wide space for natural creativity to emerge from local actions within the system (Plsek, 2001). The CAS approach to designing health care has undergirded many of the recommendations of the Institute of Medicine's influential *Crossing the Quality Chasm*.

THE CHRONIC CARE MODEL (CCM)

The CCM is among the most widely used health services intervention models in the field, having directed innovation throughout major integrated health care systems (e.g., Group Health Cooperative and the Veterans Health Administration) as well as federal agencies (e.g., Centers for Medicare and Medicaid Services Innovation Center). The CCM is based on the premise that improved chronic disease outcomes result from productive interactions among informed activated patients and a prepared proactive practice team.

Six components facilitate productive interchanges between physicians, the practice team, and patients in primary care: self-management support, delivery system design, decision support and clinical information systems, organized health care system, and community resources and policies (Rothman & Wagner, 2003).

The six components and their subcategories (Pearson et al., 2005; Grossman et al., 2008) include: (1) Self-management support, which is effected through the provider and patient working together to enhance patient self-management via patient education and activation (see Chapters 11 and 12); self-management support, tools, and resources; collaborative decision-making with patients; and making guidelines available to patients. (2) Delivery system design involves change in the organization of human resources through care management roles,

practice team, care delivery, proactive follow-up and a planned visit, and visit system changes. (3) Decision support includes guidance for provider behavior or decision-making, with the institutionalization of guidelines, protocols, or prompts; provider education; and expert consultation support. (4) Clinical information systems involve the gathering of information or improved use of information systems via a patient registry; the use of information for care management; and the provision of performance data. (5) Organized health system involves creating an organizational culture focused on quality through leadership support, provider participation, and coherent system improvement. (6) Community resources and policies are defined as accessing resources outside the center to facilitate linkages among patients and the community.

All six components of the CCM are considered necessary for improving health care in general (see Figure 3-3). The CCM was originally developed to apply widely across chronic illnesses, health care settings, and patient populations; interventions based on the CCM have been shown to improve myriad and varied chronic disease outcomes (Tsai, Morton, Mangione, Keeler, 2005; Glasgow, Orleans, Wagner, 2001).

SOCIAL NETWORK APPROACH

The social network approach is consonant with the core concepts of the social ecology model (Eng, 1993; Sheinfeld Gorin, 1997; Gotay & Wilson, 1998). The influence of social networks on health is well established. Within the context of nested systems—families, peer groups, organizations, and larger communities—the individual creates a network of unique relationships within which he or she exchanges emotional qualities (e.g., esteem, trust), appraisal (e.g., affirmation, social comparison), informational (e.g., advice, directives) and instrumental support (e.g., money, time; House, Landis, & Umberson, 1988; House & Kahn, 1985). These networks—including among health care providers—form the most salient norms and values to which the individual responds and also develop critical information convoys, subsequently influencing an individual's healthy behaviors (Fox, Murata, & Stein, 1991; Lane & Brug, 1990; Ashford et al., 2000; Mandelblatt & Yabroff, 1999).

Social networks affect health through a variety of mechanisms, including (a) the provision of social support (both perceived and actual), (b) social influence

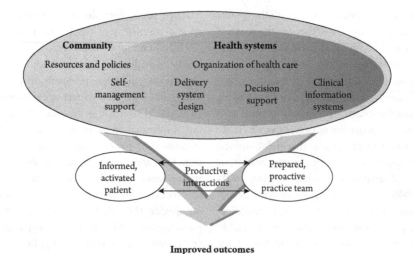

FIGURE 3-3: The Chronic Care Model.

Source: Rothman AA, Wagner EH. Chronic illness management: what is the role of primary care? *Ann Intern Med.* 2003;138:256–261.

(e.g., norms, social control), (c) social engagement, (d) person-to- person contacts (e.g., pathogen exposure, secondhand cigarette smoke), and (e) access to resources (e.g., money, jobs, information; Berkman & Glass, 2000). Some initial work has even begun to specify biological mechanisms by which social support flowing through a social network tie might affect morbidity and mortality (via cytokine functioning, Lutgendorf et al., 2002; Esterling et al., 1996; chronic stress and chronic inflammation, Miller et al., 2002; Pradhan et al., 2002; Ridker et al., 2000; Lindmark et al., 2001; global immune functioning, including a reduction in susceptibility to experimental rhinovirus inoculation, Cohen et al., 1997; and increased social complexity potentially associated with reduced risk for dementia, Cacioppo et al., 2000).

The early studies in this field focused primarily on social support, reporting on the existence of ties, their type, or number among individuals (Cohen & Syme, 1985; Stroebe & Stroebe, 1996). In these studies, social support was consistently linked to lower mortality (Berkman, 1985), lower prevalence and incidence of coronary heart disease (Seeman & Syme, 1987; Seeman, 2000), and faster recovery from heart disease and heart surgery (Ruberman, Weinblatt, Goldberg, & Chaudhary, 1984). Early studies found that those who have minimal psychosocial resources appear to be more prone to illness and mood disturbances when faced with increased stress levels than do individuals with considerable social support (DeLongis, Folkman, & Lazarus, 1988).

More recent research examines social networks, rather than social support individual by individual, by mapping individuals' networks and the impact of particular network components and kinds of ties on health outcomes (Kirsten, Smith, Christakis, 2008). Much of this research has used data from the Framingham Heart Study, and has linked social networks to obesity (Christakis & Fowler, 2007), smoking (Christakis & Fowler, 2008), diet (Pachucki et al., 2011); alcohol consumption (Rosenquist et al., 2010); spousal mortality after the hospitalization of a spouse (Christakis & Allison, 2006), loneliness (Cacioppo, Fowler & Christakis, 2009), and happiness (Fowler & Christakis, 2008). Social networks have been found to influence health screenings (Keating et al., 2011; Centola, 2010), and the use of complementary and alternative medicines, through lay referrals and word-of-mouth (Brown & Reingen, 1987).

A recent influential paper on obesity (Christakis & Fowler, 2007), using longitudinal data from the Framingham Heart Study, found that weight gain was similar between friends, and their influence was stronger than that of siblings or spouses. If this association reflects an underlying relationship, it implies that social norms, shared experiences, and similar environments may be as important in weight gain as genetic susceptibility, molecular pathways, and physiologic systems underlying the regulation of energy balance (e.g., leptin, insulin; Flier, 2004). The findings may also imply that new intervention strategies that use social marketing or peer-group efforts to reduce obesity might lead to successful weight control (Cohen-Cole & Fletcher, 2008).

While people are interconnected, and so their health is interconnected (Christakis & Fowler, 2007), other factors, including the social environment, as discussed previously in this Chapter (Coen-Fowler & Fletcher, 2008) and homophily, which is the tendency of people with similar attributes to form ties (McPherson, Smith-Lovin, and Cook, 2001), may be stronger influences on some health outcomes. These effects depend on the measures and analyses used, as well as the sample, and the specific health outcomes studied. Further, although the preponderance of the early evidence suggests that social support positively influences health-promoting behaviors, among some population subgroups social norms may discourage these behaviors (Sheinfeld Gorin, 1997). For example, African American women may have social networks that are fearful of orthodox medical care and thus are not able to encourage them to engage in health protective activities such as breast cancer screening (Burg & Seeman, 1994).

Social networks have been linked to happiness, as cited previously. A longitudinal analysis of 4,739 individuals followed from 1983 to 2003 in the Framingham Heart Study social network revealed clusters of happy and unhappy people, with the relationship between people's happiness extending up to three degrees of separation (e.g., to the friends of one's friends' friends; Fowler & Christakis, 2008). People who are surrounded by many happy people and those who are central in the network are more likely to become happy in the future than others. Longitudinal statistical models suggest that clusters of happiness result from the spread of happiness and not just a tendency for people to associate with similar individuals.

Applying these findings to the group level, people's happiness depends on the happiness of others with whom they are connected, suggesting a collective phenomenon (Fowler & Christakis, 2008), On an individual level, through the stability, predictability, and control that it provides, social support leads people to feel positively about themselves and their environment. These feelings, in turn, motivate people to want to take care of themselves, interact more positively with others, and demonstrate resilience in times of stress. Further, compared with those who are dour, individuals who are happy find it easier to develop a rich network of social support.

POSITIVE PSYCHOLOGY PERSPECTIVE

The primary building block of positive psychology is the hedonic quality of current experience (Kahnemann, 1999, p. 6), that which makes one moment "better" than another. Positive psychology is concerned with the study of the relationship between valued subjective experiences such as contentment and satisfaction (in the past), hope and optimism (for the future), and flow and happiness (in the present), as well as civic virtues at the group level: the elements of a meaningful life (Seligman & Csikszentmihalyi, 2000, p. 6).

Positive emotion has been most fully studied in relation to physical health (Salovey, Rothman, Detweiler, & Steward, 2000; Taylor, Kemeny, Reed, Bower, & Gruenewald, 2000), although the buffering function of resilience has been the focus of mental health prevention research (Masten, 2001). Taylor et al.'s work (2000) suggests that, although it is generally assumed that it is healthy to be rigorously objective about one's situation (Peterson, 2000; Schwartz, 2000; Vaillant, 2000), unrealistically optimistic beliefs about the future can protect people from illness, such as AIDS (acquired immune deficiency syndrome). The positive effects of optimism are mediated at the cognitive level, with optimistic individuals more likely than others to practice habits that enhance health and to enlist social support. Positive illusions may be adaptive in the face of life-threatening illnesses, in part because they help people to find meaning in the experience (Taylor, 1983). Further, people who are optimistic and hopeful are actually more likely than others to provide themselves with unfavorable information about their disease, thereby preparing themselves to face up to diagnostic, treatment, and curative realities (even though their positive outcome estimates may be inflated). It is also possible that positive affective states, like happiness, may have a direct physiological effect that retards the course of illness (Seligman & Csikszentmihalyi, 2000; Salovey et al., 2000).

There are initial indications in the work of Antoni and his colleagues (Antoni et al., 2009) that effective interventions might be designed to improve health and quality of life in seriously ill patients, based on several core constructs in positive psychology (e.g., benefit-finding, anxiety reduction and social support). Immune system functioning, cardiac reactivity, and other aspects of stress physiology are potential pathways through which positive phenomena may influence health. Mechanisms through which positive psychology may affect prevention include; social behavior, health-promoting and health-risk behavior, coping with adversity, and health-related decision-making (Aspinwall & Tedeschi, 2010).

Yet, a number of conceptual and methodological challenges to the development of knowledge in this field remain. Additional theory development, more applications of large prospective studies and use of registries, applying a wider range of outcome measures (e.g., survival), and refining instruments are warranted to understand the effects of positive constructs on health outcomes. While healthy communities were an early focus of the field of positive psychology, individuals have received the most attention thus far; ultimately, positive psychology interventions will need to address multilevel approaches, from policy to biology. These interventions could be more specific, as well, using Gordon Paul's (1967) (paraphrased) challenge to the early field of psychotherapy outcome measurement: What interventions, delivered by whom, are most effective for these individuals with those specific problems, under what set of conditions, and why?

Concerns remain about the "tyranny of positive thinking," (Holland & Lewis, 2000) that is, mandating positive thinking and the suppression of negative thoughts and feelings as the best way to manage serious illness. Attention to social justice questions is suggested in future studies as well, to assess the equity of the distribution of a higher quality of life across all socioeconomic groups (Sheinfeld Gorin, 2010, p. 45).

An important near-term contribution of this approach is the recognition that the health care professional can inspire hope in others. The health care professional's positive expectations (even when administering a placebo, a pharmacologically inert substance that yields symptom relief in about 35% of all patients; Hafen, Karren, Frandsen, & Smith, 1996) can have a concrete impact on the health of the patient (Salovey et al., 2000; Sheinfeld Gorin, 2010).

SOCIAL MARKETING MODEL

Social marketing is a framework frequently used in designing, targeting, refining, and implementing prevention and other public health programs (Lee & Kotler, 2012; Manoff, 1985). It adapts the approach used in commercial marketing to the arena of health behavior. The marketing framework revolves around four Ps: product, price, place, and promotion. The *product* is generally the program (e.g., weight reduction), as well as any attitudes, beliefs, ideas, additional behaviors, and practices connected with the program or the behavior (e.g., health as a value). *Price* refers to any psychological or social effort, opportunity, or monetary cost associated with the adoption and use of the product. *Place* is the distribution point for the product (e.g., an HMO). *Promotion* refers to the means of informing a target audience about the product and persuading them to use it (e.g., videos, brochures, and television spots). A fifth variable is *positioning*, which refers to the unique niche occupied by the product (e.g., a weight reduction program for seniors). Finally, a sixth variable, *politics*, describes the social and economic context (e.g., the reimbursement policies for weight control counseling) that can facilitate or hinder the marketing process.

POLITICAL ECONOMY APPROACH

As discussed in Chapter 2, fundamental to the relationships between organizations and their contexts is an exchange of resources, such as money, persons, information, space, and social legitimacy (or reputation). These exchanges create a set of political and economic interdependencies both within the organization (among staff and workgroups) and within its context (its funders, regulators, accreditors, and clients). An organization tends to be influenced by those who hold the political and economic resources that the organization needs. Thus the organization attempts to satisfy the demands of a given outside (or inside) group when that group holds a resource critical to organizational survival or has discretion over organizational use of the resource and when few alternative sources of that resource exist. For example, accreditors and the stamp of approval (or social legitimation) they give to a health care facility are increasingly important in competition for insured patients. As a result, major accrediting organizations, such as the Joint Commission on Accreditation of Healthcare Organizations (JCAHO), can demand significant changes in an organization by withholding a desired recognition (see Chapter 2).

BEHAVIORAL MODEL OF HEALTH CARE UTILIZATION

The behavioral model of utilization, developed by Andersen and Aday (1978; see Figure 3-4), is

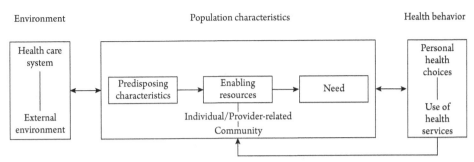

FIGURE 3-4: Behavioral Model of Health Care. Andersen RM. Revisiting the behavioral model and access to Medical Care: Does it Matter? *J Health Soc Behavior* 1995:36: 1–10.

frequently used to analyze the factors associated with patient use of health care services, to develop policies and programs to encourage appropriate use of services, and to promote cost-effective care (Aday, 1993). The model suggests that health care use patterns at the individual level are influenced by predisposing, enabling, and need-related factors as well as environmental conditions.

Individuals are predisposed to use health care services by their genes, sociodemographic factors such as age, social structure elements such as race or ethnicity, educational attainment, and knowledge of, beliefs about, or attitudes toward the use of health care. Factors that may enable or impede the use of health care services include family income, health insurance coverage, a regular source of care, and travel and waiting times; at the community level they include the location, size, and number of providers, as well as provider characteristics such as gender and age (Phillips, Morrison, Andersen, & Aday, 1998). The individual's need for care may be influenced by both perceived and evaluated illness (e.g., both self-rated health status and diagnosis).

Environmental variables such as health care delivery system characteristics, factors external to that system, and community-level enabling factors influence the individual's predisposing, enabling, and need factors (Andersen & Newman, 1973). Health care delivery system characteristics include policies, resources, organization, and financial arrangements influencing the accessibility, availability, and acceptability of medical care services (such as physician supply); these characteristics also reflect the economic climate, relative wealth, politics, level of stress and violence, and prevailing norms of the community.

PRECEDE-PROCEED FRAMEWORK

The PRECEDE-PROCEED framework, developed by Lawrence Green (1979), has been particularly influential in the planning of health education programs, a critical component of the health care professional's work. Health education planning generally proceeds in phases (Green & Kreuter, 1990). In phases 1 and 2, Social and Epidemiological Assessment, the health care professional begins by assessing the quality of life experienced by those whom the program might affect. For example, a program might focus on general social problems of concern to individuals or communities, such as diabetes among African Americans in East Baltimore (Gielen, McDonald, Gary, & Bone, 2008). The excess risk of diabetic nephropathy, including end stage renal disease (ESRD), is 2–5 times greater in African Americans than in whites, and the amputation rate is 1.2 times higher (Tull & Roseman, 1995). Interventions to promote foot care, blood glucose self-monitoring, medication adherence, and physical activity while reducing smoking and alcohol consumption may substantially reduce the excess burden of medical complications of diabetes in African Americans (Gielen, McDonald, Gary, & Bone, 2008).

In phases 3-4, Behavioral, Environmental, Educational, and Ecological Assessment, multilevel influences are identified. With diabetes, at the individual level, important enabling factors included patients' lack of skills to conduct glucose monitoring and foot care, and problems with access to necessary supplies. Factors at multiple levels are identified that contribute to poor metabolic control (HbA1c, as well as blood pressure and lipid control), which in turn, lead to diabetes complications.

As in the behavioral model of health care utilization, the health care professional then identifies predisposing, enabling, and reinforcing factors that have the potential for influencing a behavior (in this example, diabetes). Predisposing factors that affect an individual's willingness to change include knowledge, attitudes, values, and perceptions, such as those identified previously and those discussed in relation to the health belief model later in this Chapter. Enabling factors that may facilitate or present obstacles to change include the availability and accessibility of skills, resources, and barriers that help or hinder the desired behavior; the PRECEDE framework puts particular emphasis on barriers created by social forces or systems, such as insurance coverage, health care professional practices, and the location of or access to treatment resources. Reinforcing factors refer to rewards and feedback that are given to persons adopting a certain behavior and that influence the continuation of the behavior.

In the Administrative and Policy Assessment and Implementation phases 5-6, a program designed to combat the problem is developed and implemented. In this example, four intervention components were developed to address the multiple determinants that could affect individual and environmental factors to prevent medical complications of type 2 diabetes. These include (1) nurse case manager (NCM) clinical visits; (2) community health worker (CHW) home visits; (3) telephone follow-up; and (4) primary care physician feedback. All initial intervention visits focused on multiple domains: diet, physical activity, foot care, vision care, glucose self-monitoring, blood pressure control, medication and appointment adherence, referrals, and smoking cessation (Batts et al., 2001). In accord with the PRECEDE-PROCEED framework, the investigators considered the impact of new analyses on previous decisions (Gary, Bone, Hill, et al., 2003; Hill-Briggs, Gary, Baptiste-Roberts, & Brancati, 2005; Hill-Briggs et al., 2007; Batts et al., 2001; Gielen, McDonald, Gary, & Bone, 2008).

In phases 7-9, the program is evaluated, using process and outcome measures. In this project, they found that the nurse case manager/community health worker team intervention produced a 0.8% (P=NS) decline in HbA1c and moderate improvements in lipids and blood pressure, compared to usual care (control). Because this combined clinic and community-oriented approach seemed promising, but small numbers limited their statistical

power, they used the evaluation data to devise a larger and more focused study (Gary, Batts-Turner, Bone, Yeh, Wang, et al., 2004).

SOCIAL RESPONSIBILITY MODEL

The social responsibility model, so named because of the primacy attached to the value of government intervention on behalf of health and the model's focus on health as an end rather than as a means, is best expressed in the work of several British commissions (e.g., the Black Report and the Acheson Report) and in the writings of Downie, Fyfe, and Tannahill (1990). The definition of health promotion in this model is expansive and assumes that health is a value to be pursued in its own right.

At the microlevel, these reports and writings argue, individuals have a moral duty to do what they can to improve their own health. Well-being is a value of its own; positive pleasures accrue to the healthy. At the macrolevel, they contend that health is a value that governments should promote and that access to health is a fundamental right that government must implement. Their approach has influenced recent WHO initiatives that view health as a multisectoral responsibility.

LIFE CYCLE MODELS

Two general models are based on the concept of change over time: innovation diffusion and the stages of change. Life cycle is an appropriate metaphor for the patterns of change experienced by an individual, family, group, community, or larger social group over time. Transitions are met by social and cultural constructions around the meaning of health that change from one stage of life to another. For example, parenthood may be seen as a time when individuals reflect on "having no time" to keep healthy or physically fit (Backett & Davison, 1995, p. 635).

Demographics are also key to life cycle models. The relative proportions of the various groups in society can have enormous effects on societal definitions of health promotion and the value placed on them. This is evident in the demographic transitions that developed nations are experiencing as the result of increases in the numbers of elderly individuals and in their proportion relative to other parts of the population.

These transitions may also be characterized as sensitive or critical periods. In neurobiology, for example, considerable attention has been devoted to the impact of the environment (and experience) on behavior, by further understanding the mechanisms of plasticity in neural circuits. When the effect of experience on the brain is particularly strong during a limited period in development, this period is referred to as a sensitive period. Such periods allow experience to instruct neural circuits to process or represent information in a way that is adaptive for the individual. When experience provides information that is essential for normal development and alters performance permanently, such sensitive periods are referred to as critical periods.

There are strong biological reasons for believing that humans at specific periods in their early development may be especially sensitive to exposures to environmental agents. Fragility, speed, and the complexity of early development provide many targets for specific interactions with environmental agents that are not present at later life stages. For example, maternal smoking increases the risk for placenta previa (attachment of the placenta in an abnormal position in the uterus), placental abruption (premature separation of the placenta from the uterus), and stillbirth (Chelmow, 1996; DiFranza, 1995; Shiverick, 1999; Sibai, 1995).

As another example, epidemiologic research on the genesis of breast cancer suggests the importance of cumulative exposures to carcinogens, as well as early diet, infections in childhood, growth hormone levels, and genetic factors (as discussed more fully in Chapters 4 and 8) as influences on cancer risk later in life (Forman et al., 2005; e.g., relationship of adult height and breast cancer; Green et al., 2011). The Netherlands Cohort Study on Diet and Cancer, involving 62,573 women and 58,279 men who experienced puberty during the economic depression, the Second World War, and the hunger winter of 1944–1945, showed a weak inverse relation between energy restriction early in life and subsequent development of colon carcinoma (Pallavi et al., 2012; Dirx et al., 2003). With more understanding of the impact of these early influences on health, including the sensitive and critical periods for intervention, prevention could be timed for maximal impact on outcomes (Bornstein, 1989; Cacioppo et al., 2000; Knudsen, 2004).

INNOVATION DIFFUSION THEORY

The innovation diffusion theory addresses the contexts within which innovations are adopted and used. *Innovations* are defined as new and qualitatively different ideas over time. According to the late E.M. Rogers, diffusion of innovations is "the process by which an innovation is communicated through certain channels over time among the members of a social system" (Rogers, 1995). "Communication is a process in which participants create and share information with one another to reach a mutual understanding" (Rogers, 1995).

Innovation diffusion is influenced by four main elements: (1) the characteristics of the innovation itself, (2) communication channels (e.g., mass media, interpersonal; type and approach to decision-making), (3) time, and (4) the social system (e.g., type of decision, nature of the social system, and extent of the change agents' promotion efforts; see Figure 3-5). The characteristics of the innovation itself—its trialability, relative advantage, observability, compatibility, and complexity—influence the innovation's rate of adoption. Trialabiilty refers to whether the innovation can be tried on an experimental basis. The relative advantage of an innovation demonstrates its superiority over its replacement. Observability refers to whether the innovation will produce tangible results. Compatibility is an appropriate fit with the intended client. Complexity describes how simple the innovation is to implement (Rogers, 1995; 2003).

The second main element in the diffusion of new ideas is the communication channel. Communication is the process by which participants create and share information with one another in order to reach a mutual understanding. A communication channel is the means by which messages get from one individual to another (Rogers & Scott, 1997). Innovation-decisions differ by type (whether individual adoption or organizational decisions), and whether they are made by an authority or by consensus.

In a two-step process, new ideas, which are often first reported by the mass media, are mediated and modified through opinion leaders, who are often early adopters. The majority of persons are then influenced through interpersonal contact with opinion leaders who are seen as credible sources of information, as in academic detailing interventions (Sheinfeld Gorin et al., 2007; Soumerai, 1998). Collaboration among these leaders assists in both interpreting the needs of communities exposed to health promotion programs and encouraging the adoption of new ideas (Rogers, 1983; see

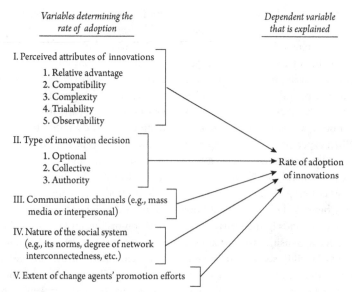

FIGURE 3-5: Influences on the Rate of Adoption of Innovations.
Source: Rogers, E. *Diffusion of Innovation.* New York: Free Press; 1983.

Figure 3-5). These leaders encourage adoption by eventually persuading the majority of persons, which may occur earlier or later in the process.

The diffusion of innovations requires some conceptual reorientation among participants over time (Delbecq, 1978; Sheinfeld Gorin & Weirich, 1995). An individual (or other decision-making unit) moves from initial knowledge of an innovation to forming an attitude toward the innovation, to a decision to adopt or reject, to implementation of the new idea, and to confirmation of this decision. An individual seeks information at various stages in the innovation-decision process in order to decrease uncertainty about an innovation's expected consequences (Rogers & Scott, 1997). Over time, an innovation may move through the stages of *program* adoption (from evaluation of the idea to initiation of the program to implementation and finally to routine use). Similarly, the use of a program may increase as the program continues (or decrease as it fails) to influence understanding among clients.

Time is involved in the degree to which an individual or other unit of adoption is relatively earlier in adopting new ideas than other members of a social system. There are five adopter categories, or classifications of the members of a social system on the basis on their innovativeness: (1) innovators, (2) early adopters, (3) early majority, (4) late majority, and (5) laggards. When an innovation is introduced, the majority of people will either be early majority adopters or late majority adopters; fewer will be early adopters or laggards; and very few will be innovators (the first people to use the innovation; Rogers, 2003).

The social system, a group of individuals who together adopt the innovation, is often influenced by a change agent (e.g., the academic detailer or practice facilitator, see Chapter 10). In addition, one health care system may differ from another in its norms, degree of interconnectedness, affluence, complexity, rate of change, extent of conflict, and degree of cooperation—all of which influence the adoption and use of new ideas and programs. For example, Carpenter and colleagues studied the impact of affiliations among organizations affiliated with the American College of Surgeons Oncology Group (ACOSOG) or other National Cancer Institute (NCI) cooperative groups and networks on the receipt of the then-innovative sentinel lymph node biopsy (SLNB) for the treatment of early-stage breast cancer. The study was conducted among patients, aged 65 and older, who were eligible for the SLNB, using linked claims data (from SEER-Medicare; http://healthservices.cancer.gov/seermedicare/), shortly after Medicare approved and began reimbursing for the procedure. The findings revealed that patients who received cancer treatment at an organization affiliated with cancer networks were more likely to receive SLNB, with improved patient outcomes, than those in unaffiliated centers. By identifying the characteristics of social systems, communication channels, and those of innovations themselves over time, providers can more effectively plan and implement strategies that are customized to their needs.

COMMUNICATION MODELS

Communication models explore "who says what, in which channels, to whom, and with what effects." Communication models explore how messages are created, transmitted, received, and assimilated; their concepts are embedded within a number of other theories and models, including innovation diffusion. *Persuasion* refers to any type of social influence, and is central to communication by the mass media. For persuasion to take place, a message must be conveyed, the person(s) must receive and comprehend the message and be convinced by it, the message must be retained, and there must be behavioral manifestations that change has taken place. The aim of persuasion is to introduce inconsistency in two related beliefs; that, according to social adaptation theory, will lead to a reinterpretation of social reality, and change (Fincham, 1992).

Every act of communication, whether intentional or not, involves some type of framing. "Framing" issues involves emphasizing one dimension of a complex issue over another, calling attention to certain considerations and certain arguments more so than other arguments. (Framing for individual decision-making is also discussed later in this Chapter.) Since most decisions in prevention are complex with uncertain causes and intervention outcomes, data can help to structure communication, and to clarify the frames of reference that are going to enable different publics to make effective judgments and decisions. In the process, evidence is used to help communicate why an issue may or may not be a problem, who or what is responsible for that problem, and then what should be done. Climate change, for example, has been reframed to emphasize its connections with fatalities and injuries from extreme weather events, to the increased incidence and severity of allergies and respiratory problems, and to an increased incidence of infectious disease and vulnerability to extreme heat. This reframing of the issue of climate change increases its applicability to older adults and children, increasing its short-term public relevance and importance.

RE-AIM

The *r*each, *e*ffectiveness, *a*doption, *i*mplementation, and *m*aintenance (RE-AIM) framework offers a comprehensive approach to considering five dimensions important for evaluating the potential public health impact of an intervention (Glasgow, Vogt, Boles, 1999; Glasgow, Lichtenstein, Marcus, 2003). The model includes (1) reach, the percent and representativeness of individuals willing to participate; (2) effectiveness, the impact of the intervention on targeted outcomes and quality of life; (3) adoption, the percent and representativeness of settings and intervention staff that agree to deliver a program; (4) implementation, the consistency and skill with which various program elements are delivered by various staff; and (5) maintenance, the extent to which individual participants maintain behavior change long term and, at the setting level, the degree to which the program is sustained over time within the organizations delivering it (www.re-aim.org). RE-AIM builds upon conceptual work by Rogers (2003) and Green and Kreuter (2005) and focuses attention on these five specific factors (Glasgow, Klesges, Dzewaltowski, Estabrooks & Vogt, 2006; see Figure 3-6). A recent synthesis of the use of the RE-AIM framework to review the published

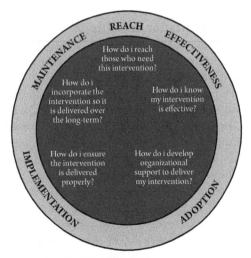

FIGURE 3-6: The RE-AIM Model.

Source: Glasgow RE, Vogt TM, Boles SM. Evaluating the public health impact of health promotion interventions: the REAIM framework. *Am J Public Health.* 1999;89:1322–1327. Reproduced with permission

literature from 1999 to 2010 in several databases revealed that the most frequent publications were on physical activity, obesity, and disease management. RE-AIM was broadly applied, but several criteria were not reported consistently (Gaglio, Shoup & Glasgow, 2013).

Implementation Science

Implementation science undergirds RE-AIM; implementation science is the scientific study of methods to promote the uptake of research findings, and hence to reduce inappropriate care. Implementation research is the last point along the diffusion to implementation continuum, in that it is research that supports the movement of evidence-based interventions and approaches from the experimental, controlled environment into the actual delivery contexts where the programs, tools, and guidelines will be used, promoted, and integrated into the existing operational culture (Rubenstein & Pugh, 2006). It includes the study of influences on clinicians' behavior, and interventions to enable them to use research findings more effectively (Bero, Grilli, Grimshaw, Harvey, Oxman, & Thomson, 1998; Effective Healthcare, 1999; Walker, Grimshaw, Johnston, Pitts, Steen, & Eccles, 2003). Two additional behavioral science constructs to the RE-AIM framework are central to implementation science: implementation intentions and self-regulation (Walker et al., 2003).

Implementation Intention

A goal intention is an intention to perform a behavior or achieve a goal (e.g., I intend to reduce the number of referrals i make for lumbar spine x-rays; Walker et al., 2003). This is conceptually close to the behavioral intention construct in the theory of planned behavior. By contrast, "implementation intentions" are explicit plans about when and where a goal intention will be achieved. Gollwitzer (1993) argues that by creating an implementation intention, people effectively transfer control of the behavior to the environment—establishing cues to action (as in the Health Belief Model, described previously in this Chapter)—for example, by saying that "When patients tell me about their low back pain, I will explain the pros and cons of an x-ray to them." Experimental studies suggest that people who

have formulated plans in advance of their actions are more likely to translate their intentions into action than those who have not (Orbell, Hodgkins, & Sheeran, 1997; Gollwitzer, 1996; Walker et al., 2003). This goal-setting approach is discussed further in Chapter 10.

Self-Regulation

In addition to plans and behavioral consequences, the actions that clinicians take may be influenced by their feelings about the patient's particular condition. Implementation-focused self-regulation proposes a unique application of a well-established psychologic model, self-regulation, found in both C-SHIP and protection motivation theory that are described in this Chapter.

Leventhal's self-regulatory model (1997) proposes that individuals attempt to make sense of illness by making use of preexisting knowledge or schemas (cognitive representations), and that these give rise to behavioral responses, in a dynamic process. For patients, behavioral responses may include going to see a doctor, stopping smoking, taking prescribed or non-prescribed medicines, for example. For clinicians, responses may include referring a patient for diagnostic tests, or prescribing a drug (Walker et al., 2003). Through self-regulation, people seek to restore their own (or their patient's) physical or emotional equilibrium; they monitor the success of the strategies they have adopted, and persist with those that enable them to reduce (or remove) the threat to their health (Leventhal, Benyamini, Brownlee, Diefenbach, Leventhal, Patrick-Miller, & Robitaille, 1997). Individuals' understandings (cognitive representation) of their situations are central to the self-regulatory approach, and influence how the individual responds to the problem (Leventhal, Benyamini, Brownlee, Diefenbach, Leventhal, Patrick-Miller, & Robitaille, 1997). Importantly, the self-regulatory theory proposes that people actively try to cope with the emotions that are associated with the illness (e.g., fear or distress), through approaches from information seeking to smoking. It is possible that health care professionals also experience emotional reactions to some conditions or patient groups, for example the emotional reaction embodied in the term, "heartsink" (challenging) patients (O'Dowd, 1988; Moscrop, 2011; Walker et al., 2003). Representations have been shown to influence the behavior of patients in coping with everyday living (Earll, Johnston, & Mitchell, 1993), taking prescribed medication (Myers, Midence, et al., 1998), and attending cardiac rehabilitation programs (Petrie et al., 1996).

STAGES OF CHANGE

The stages of change, or trans-theoretical, model is based on the assumption that individuals move through a series of predictable stages when changing a behavior, such as stopping smoking or beginning an exercise program. These changes include the following stages (DiClemente, 1991; Prochaska & DiClemente, 1983; Prochaska, Velicer, Guadagnoli, Rossi, & DiClemente, 1991; Prochaska & Velicer, 1997):

1. *Precontemplation* (considering the change);
2. *Contemplation* (starting to think about initiating change);
3. *Preparation* (seriously thinking about the change within a given time period [for example, the next 6 months] or taking early steps to change.) The individual has been unsuccessful in changing this behavior over the past year.
4. *Action* (making a change in or stopping the target behavior within a 6-month period): Individuals modify their behavior, experiences, or environment in order to overcome their problems. This requires a considerable commitment of time and energy.
5. *Maintenance of change* (maintaining the target behavior change for more than 6 months; preventing relapse);
6. *Relapse* (return of the behavior) or *Termination*: Overt behavior does not return, and the individual can cope without fear of relapse.

These stages are not necessarily linear. For example, the average smoker who quits reports at least several and often many relapses before achieving maintained abstinence (Fisher, Bishop, Goldmuntz, & Jacobs, 1988). The stages of change model may, however, suggest intervention points for different individuals at varied stages (Prochaska et al., 1991). In particular, it has been used to explain smoking cessation and physical activity changes in individuals.

The mechanisms that drive movement through the stages are called the *processes of change* (Prochaska & DiClemente, 1983). These processes draw heavily on components of other models, such as the health belief model.

The transtheoretical model also addresses the general element of decision making regarding adoption of a behavior, using a decisional balance approach. Decisional balance compares the strength of the target behavior's perceived pros with that of the perceived cons. The relative weights that people assign to a behavior's pros and cons influence their decisions about behavioral change (Janis & Mann, 1977), such as continuing or ceasing to smoke.

HEALTH ATTITUDE, BELIEF, AND BEHAVIORAL CHANGE APPROACHES

The following four major theories—the health belief model, the theory of planned behavior, prospect theory, and social learning theory—along with their corollaries and derivative models, identify different health-promotive paths for individuals or groups. Each model posits a trajectory for change in attitudes, beliefs, or behaviors.

Health Belief Model

The intention of one of the most prominent of these theories, the health belief model (modified by Becker, 1986), was to determine why some persons who are illness-free take actions to avoid illness, whereas others fail to take protective actions. Another aim of the health belief model was to predict the conditions under which people would engage in simple preventive behaviors, such as immunizations. The model was founded on the work of Kurt Lewin, who understood that the life space in which individuals live is composed of regions, some having a negative valence (one would seek to avoid), some a positive valence (one would seek to approach), and some a neutral valence (one would neither seek to approach nor avoid; Lewin, Dembo, & Festinger, 1944).

The health belief model suggests that before an individual takes action, he or she must decide that the behavior, whether it be smoking, eating fatty foods, or engaging in unprotected sexual activity, creates a serious health problem; that he or she is personally susceptible to this health harm; and that moderating or stopping the behavior will be beneficial. The perceived barriers to undertaking a behavior are considered most salient to health-promotive efforts (Janz & Becker, 1984). A person's perceived susceptibility to a disease and perceived severity of harm are based to a great extent on that person's knowledge of the disease and its potential outcome. Although the combination of perceived susceptibility to harm and severity of harm provides the force for action, and the perception of high benefits and low barriers provides a course of action, it is the *cues to action* that start the process of change (Rosenstock, 1974).

In an expansion of the health belief model, a separate construct of general health motivation (protection motivation theory) was added. Motives are viewed as dispositions within which individuals approach certain categories of positive incentives. For example, the desire to maintain a state of good health is a component of health motivation (Becker, Drachman, & Kirscht, 1974; Maiman & Becker, 1984; Curry & Emmons, 1994). In the last 10 years, the health belief model has subsumed the self-efficacy construct from social cognitive theory to better explain health behaviors (Rosenstock, Strecher, & Becker, 1988).

Protection Motivation Theory

Protection motivation theory uses health threats, or fear appeals, to change behavior by highlighting the harmful personal consequences of health-damaging behaviors. For example, a program to encourage substance safety among teens might use pictures of dead addicts under white sheets in the morgue and explicit warnings against drug use. The model identifies two parallel processes in health behavior change: (1) cognitive processes involving representation of the health threat and the efficacy of available coping responses (e.g., the perceived risks of lung cancer and the health benefits of quitting smoking); and (2) emotional or affective processes involving fear arousal (Orleans, Rotberg, Quade, & Lees, 1990; Velicer, DiClemente, Prochaska, & Brandenburg, 1985). The more personally salient the health risks are, the greater the motivational impact of the information. Empirical tests of the protection motivation theory further suggest that threat appeals, rather than the emotional state of fear itself, strengthen long-sustained cognitive structures (i.e., beliefs in the severity of the danger), as fear declines rapidly (Rogers, Deckner, & Mewborn, 1978). Generally, however, because of the difficulty of determining the appropriate timing and dose of fear, the promotion of healthy alternative behaviors is more effective (Job, 1988).

Cognitive-Social Health Information–Processing Model

The cognitive-social health information–processing model (C-SHIP) (Miller, Shoda, & Hurley, 1996) is a broad theoretical framework that incorporates both cognitive and affective responses to threats to health, primarily those responses related to cancer prevention and control (Leventhal, Safer, & Panagis, 1983; Miller, 1995; Shoda et al., 1998). According to the C-SHIP model, there are four distinctive cognitive-emotional processes that underlie the information processing of cancer risk information: (1) individuals' self-construals of their risk, including their knowledge levels and perceived risk; (2) their expectations about the benefits and limitations of specific cancer-related actions; (3) their health values (e.g., fatalistic attitudes about cancer); and (4) their cancer-specific emotional distress. A unique contribution of the model for health promotion is its description of *high monitors* (who scan for, and magnify, threatening cues) and *low monitors* (who distract from, and downgrade, threatening information) (Miller, 1995). Counseling strategies may be more effective when they are systematically tailored to the specific cognitive and affective profiles of individuals as they engage in health-promoting behaviors such as cancer screening (Miller, Shoda, & Hurley, 1996).

THEORY OF PLANNED BEHAVIOR

Ajzen and Fishbein (1980) developed the theory of reasoned action, later modified as the theory of planned behavior (TPB), which is a mathematical description of the relationship among beliefs (verbalized opinions), attitudes (judgments that a behavior is good or bad and that a person favors or is against performing the behavior), and intentions in determining action. The theory postulates that most volitional behavior can be predicted by beliefs, attitudes, and intentions; therefore efforts to change behavior should be directed at an individual's belief system. By altering the beliefs underlying attitudes or norms, changes in behavioral intentions, and subsequently in behavior, can also be induced (Ajzen & Fishbein, 1980). According to the TPB (Ajzen, 2002), perceived behavioral control, even when not particularly realistic, can affect behavior indirectly by its impact on intention.

According to the theory, first, the health care provider identifies and measures the behavior to be changed. Once the behavior is defined, he or she may specify the determinants. A person's intention to perform (or not perform) a behavior is the immediate determinant of the action. Second, the person's intention is a function of two other determinants: (a) the person's attitude toward the behavior; and (b) the person's subjective norm, or perception of the social pressures to perform or not perform the behavior in question (Ajzen & Fishbein, 1980). Individuals will intend to perform a behavior, such as brushing their teeth, when they evaluate it positively and when they believe that important others, such as parents, think they should perform it. The relative weights of the attitudinal and normative factors may vary from one person to another; thus one person may attach more weight to attitude, another to normative influences.

Further, attitudes are a function of behavioral and normative beliefs, perceived consequences of behavior, and the person's evaluation of these. The social or normative factor consists of the opinions of important referent individuals or groups (such as parents or peers). The person's motivation to comply with those opinions reflects a sense of the consequences of conforming (or not).

Specificity of intentions is highlighted in this theory. An action, such as exercising, is always performed with respect to a given target (e.g., walking rather than running), in a particular context (e.g., at work), and at a given time (e.g., during lunch) (Ajzen & Fishbein, 1980). The theory also considers external variables (e.g., access to family planning services for women using birth control) as influencing a person's beliefs or the relative importance that a person attaches to attitudinal and normative considerations. Finally, the individual controls the relationship between the intention to act and the behavior. If a female maintains a positive attitude toward using birth control pills, is supported by a set of family and community norms supporting the use of contraception, and intends to use birth control pills, ultimately she will use them (Fishbein, Jaccard, Davidson, Ajzen, & Loken, 1980).

PROSPECT THEORY

Prospect theory is a descriptive model that accounts for choice and decision-making strategies under conditions of risk (Kahneman & Tversky, 1984; Kahneman & Tversky, 1979). The assumptions of the theory are threefold. First, risk decisions are influenced by subjective evaluations of relative gains and losses, as opposed to objective evaluations of absolute outcomes. Second, persons tend to make risk-averse choices for sure *gain* and to make risk-seeking choices for a gamble over a sure *loss*. Third, the theory states that the degree to which a choice (or behavior) is seen as a gain or a loss can vary depending on how the consequences of the behavior are presented, or *framed* (Curry & Emmons, 1994, p. 309, as discussed previously in this Chapter).

When behavioral choices involve some risk or uncertainty, individuals will be more likely to take these risks when information is framed in terms of relative disadvantages (i.e., losses or costs) of the outcomes. When behavioral choices involve little risk or uncertainty, individuals prefer options for which information is framed by relative advantages (i.e., gains or benefits). Choosing to perform prevention behaviors (e.g., wearing a condom) is a risk-averse option for maintaining sexual health; these behaviors should be promoted with gain-framed messages (e.g., "using a condom during sexual intercourse can help to keep you healthy") (Salovey & Williams-Piehota, 2004). Behaviors involving an uncertain, potentially negative outcome (i.e., risk), including detection behavior for HIV (Human Immunodeficiency Virus) or breast self-examination among asymptomatic or low-risk individuals, should be promoted with loss-framed messages (e.g., "failing to use a condom during sexual intercourse exposes you to various sexually transmitted diseases such as AIDS") (Salovey & Williams-Piehota, 2004). Message framing approaches, derived from prospect theory, have been applied to breast cancer screening, sunscreen use, HIV testing, condom use, human papillomavirus vaccination, and dental mouthwashes, as well as to defining quality of life outcomes. These approaches are distinguished from the fear appeals of protection motivation theory that do not frame messages by the salience of the risk.

SOCIAL LEARNING THEORY

Social learning theory holds that behavior is determined by expectancies and incentives. Two approaches reflect this general theory: stimulus response theory and social cognitive theory. The role of cognition separates these two models. In social cognitive theory, expectancies are cognitive, or developed in the mind of the individual.

Cognitive expectations (e.g., feeling capable of stopping) influence the conduct of a behavior (e.g., stopping smoking). In stimulus response theory, cognitive mediators are not present.

Stimulus Response Theory

Stimulus response theory rests on the belief that learning results from events (called reinforcements or consequences of behavior) that reduce physiological drives (e.g., tension or anxiety) that activate behavior. Behavioral analysis underlies the application of the theory to behavior change. It involves objective definitions of the actions to be changed, measurable procedures for change, and an emphasis on antecedent and consequent events to change behavior. Over time, individuals may be conditioned to respond to cues in their environment by associating behaviors with them (e.g., associating smoking with a stimulus such as a cup of coffee in the morning). To extinguish such conditioned responses, the individual must be exposed to the conditioned stimulus (e.g., the coffee) without presentation of the unconditioned stimulus (e.g., a cigarette) (Rachlin, 1991). As rewarded behaviors are repeated, and may become "habitual," the frequency of past behavior can be a powerful predictor of future behavior (Oullette & Wood, 1998).

Similarly, several other principles of behavioral analysis (e.g., the use of contingency management, feedback and goal setting, sharing and successive approximation, modeling, and prompting) may be applied successfully to encourage healthy behaviors. Contingency management involves a system of attaching rewards (e.g., praise) to goal attainment (e.g., losing weight). The initiation and maintenance of behavioral change may be accomplished by providing feedback and rewards so that the positive behavior itself becomes reinforcing. For example, healthy eating practices may be reinforced by teaching individuals to prepare appealing, simple, and quick meals (Kelly et al., 1992). The likelihood of the behavior itself becoming reinforcing is increased when successive approximations (intermediate goals) are used with shaping tactics (Kazdin, 1994). In these procedures, individuals performing behaviors that are within their repertoires take the next step on a goal attainment gradient, with each (subgoal) behavior having a high likelihood of being reinforced. Programs teaching dieters how to lose weight begin with a low-fat variation of a meal dieters usually enjoy (such as vegetarian, rather than cheese,

pizza). Further, such programs make strategic use of models, such as successful program graduates.

Social Cognitive Theory

Social cognitive theory developed from the stimulus response and earlier classical conditioning theories. The cornerstone of the model is the *reciprocal determinism,* or a dynamic interaction among the person, behavior, and the environment in which behavior is performed (Bandura, 1986, p. 22). Social cognitive theory posits that the social environment, through the mechanism of social norms, affects a person's cognition and behavior. Rather than focusing on the automatic shaping of behavior by environmental forces, however, social cognitive theory emphasizes the importance of intervening thought processes (e.g., information acquisition, storage, and retrieval) and the importance of self-control for the performance of behavior. Most learning occurs through modeling, such as watching others prepare and eat meals, rather than trial and error. These vicarious and symbolic learning processes are affected by social influences, including reinforcements (responses to one's behavior that increase or decrease the likelihood of reoccurrence). Self-regulatory processes, including self-generated inducements and anticipated outcomes (expectations; for example, telling oneself to exercise daily so that one can climb a flight of stairs more easily) are also highlighted in the theory. Individual behavior change is similarly influenced by one's capacity (knowledge and skill to perform a given behavior).

Self-efficacy is a central concept in the application of social cognitive theory to health promotion. According to social cognitive theory (Bandura, 1986), self-efficacy is the conviction that one can execute a behavior successfully. Individuals high in self-efficacy, or more confident of their ability to maintain behavioral changes (e.g., smoking cessation or ideal weight), will attempt to execute it more readily, with greater intensity, and with greater perseverance in response to initial failure than will individuals with comparatively lower self-efficacy (Baer & Lichtenstein, 1988; Devins, 1992).

Social cognitive theory posits that change occurs in phases: (1) promotion and motivation of persons toward changing a target behavior; (2) skills training so that individuals can acquire specific behavioral change skills; (3) development of support networks so that a new behavior can be maintained;

(4) maintenance of the behavior through reinforcement; and (5) generalization to all levels of interaction, from the family to the community (Lefebvre, Lasater, Carleton, & Peterson, 1987).

Self-efficacy has been distinguished from locus of control, a similar concept. Locus of control is a generalized concept about the self, whereas self-efficacy is situation-specific or focused on one's beliefs about one's personal abilities in specific settings.

Overlapping Constructs in the Theory of Planned Behavior, Social Cognition Theory, and the Stages of Change Model

Several theories and models discussed so far have some overlapping constructs, suggesting the need for a more parsimonious understanding of the social psychological *pathways* by which beliefs, attitudes, values, and cognitions affect behavioral change. Perceived behavioral control, a feature of the theory of planned behavior, is considered conceptually similar to self-efficacy (Ajzen, 1991, 2002), which is also a concept in the stages of change (or trans-theoretical) model and social cognitive theory. It may be that the nature of the influence of intention and the nature of the influence of stage of change on behavior are similar. Given that *self-efficacy* refers to "beliefs in one's capabilities to organize and execute the course of action required to produce given levels of attainment" (Bandura, 1998, p. 624), both perceived behavioral control and self-efficacy are similarly concerned with one's perceived ability to perform a sequence of behaviors (Ajzen, 2002). Further, pros and cons in the stages of change model are considered conceptually similar to the behavioral beliefs that shape attitude toward a behavior in the theory of planned behavior (Ajzen, 1991).

HEALTH PROMOTION MATRIX

A novel, as yet untested practice-focused model for health promotion, the health promotion matrix (HPM; see Figure 3-7) (Sheinfeld Gorin & Arnold, 1998; Sheinfeld Gorin S, 2006), provides an organizing framework for assessing client systems and guiding them toward health. The matrix equips the health care professional with an understanding of the client's images of health, a means for working with those images, and specific behaviors with which the professional and client may work. It gives the clinician a means for understanding the client's view of health and a blueprint for maximizing health-promotive behaviors within varied contexts. Through the use of the matrix, the health care professional can assist the individual to modify his or her behavior, engage a group or family in altering a pattern of actions, or enlist the support of a community in changing health care policies.

At the core of the matrix is the notion of a health image. A *health image* is a picture, or concept, of health in the client's mind. The image is the client's representation of health; as such, it can serve as a motivating force for change. Health care professionals may examine the client's image of health from two perspectives: first, from the client's idealized picture of personal health and, second, relative to the client's current health. These two perspectives can then be juxtaposed in a dynamic comparison to reveal the discrepancies, or gaps, between them. Ultimately, the client's current health status will be altered through the adoption of health-promotive activities necessary to better realize the idealized picture.

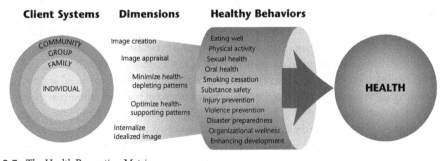

FIGURE 3-7: The Health Promotion Matrix.

Source: Sheinfeld Gorin S. Models of health promotion. In: Sheinfeld Gorin S, Arnold J. *The Health Promotion Handbook*, pp. 21–66. San Francisco, CA: Jossey-Bass, 2006. Reproduced with permission.

The HPM is a multicomponent model, along whose dimensions, client systems, and positive, or healthy, behaviors (discussed in Chapters 4 through 7) each client may be located. To some extent, all the models of change described earlier in this Chapter form the basis for the HPM. Applied as part of the clinical process, the matrix assists health care professionals to individualize client care by identifying clients' unique health images, strengths, and capabilities and to focus on specific behaviors appropriate to each client's need. Further, the matrix assumes a reorientation of the health care professional's thinking toward the multiplicity of forces—biological, psychological, social, political, economic, cultural, and spiritual—impinging on clients as they begin the change process (Butterfield, 1990).

An intervention using the health promotion matrix involves the following five processes.

Image Creation

The concept of the health image is unique to this model. Entry into the HPM begins with the client picturing, or creating, an idealized image of health; it is the client's snapshot of his or her desired self. These images are often rich and varied and may emphasize the totality of being (Woods et al., 1988). The health care professional assists the client in clarifying or detailing his or her definition of health and the relative value that health holds for him or her. In conjunction with the health care professional, the client crystallizes a positive and holistic image of health, one that is less encumbered by barriers and obstacles that he or she may have encountered in the past. This image becomes the aim of all subsequent intervention efforts.

For example, to assist the client in trying to create an image of himself or herself as a healthy person, the health care professional may ask the following: What do you see if you try to picture yourself as healthy? What would you like to be? or, How would you like to see yourself in relation to health? Questions such as these assist the client in visualizing an image of himself or herself as healthy. The sketch of one's healthy self may be made on paper or described verbally and may require more than one session to complete. The more specific and detailed the image, the more the health care professional can assist the client during image appraisal in recognizing what steps may be taken to achieve change.

Image Appraisal

During image appraisal, the health care professional and the client define the client's current health status. As the health care professional and the client begin to examine the client's idealized view of health relative to the client's present state, a gap often emerges.

Beginning with an attempt to determine the client's motivation for change, the health care professional may ask about any change attempts, with questions such as these: Have you ever made any changes in yourself or your behavior? When did you make those changes? and, Were you able to sustain those changes? To assist the client in identifying the gap between the image and present health practices (in relation to the health behaviors described in Chapters 4 through 7), the health care professional may direct a series of queries to the client, starting with, for example: How do you feel about being a cigarette smoker? or, more specifically, Do you have a car seat for your baby? The image appraisal step often ends with the health care professional asking the client about changing present health practices to match those of the idealized image, with a question such as, Are you interested in an educational program about taking care of your teeth during pregnancy? Once the gap has been identified and, often, a commitment to change made, both client and professional begin the next steps in the process of change.

Minimize Health-Depleting Patterns

The health care professional may now assist the client in identifying depleting and supporting behaviors for one or more of the healthy behaviors. The Matrix enables the client, in conjunction with the health care professional, to analyze patterns that are either health depleting or health promotive and to begin to change them. Often this proceeds in a problem-solving manner, moving from assessing the issues to developing choices, outlining alternatives, and evaluating each one, and then deciding on the optimal course of action.

Because the client may need assistance in altering a number of behaviors to narrow the gap between the ideal and the actual state, this process may take place over an extended time period. Together, the health care professional and the client prioritize the intervention areas.

To understand the depleting behaviors, the health care professional may ask the client to list behaviors that are damaging, such as eating a high-fat, high-sugar diet, or failing to engage in behaviors known to protect health, such as wearing a seat belt while driving. Barriers to behavioral change may rest in physiological forces, such as a craving; psychological attitudes, beliefs, or intentions toward change; social and cultural norms or patterns supporting certain behaviors; or economic, political, or spiritual factors. Lack of accessibility, few community resources, limited motivation to change, family members who support less healthy eating patterns, and a stressful job are examples of barriers that may prevent the client from taking the first step toward change. The health care professional seeks to specify the techniques or tools that may assist the client to change.

Optimize Health-Supportive Patterns

Optimizing supportive behaviors involves recognizing efforts toward undertaking healthy practices or those behaviors themselves. Often clients are given recognition only when a health goal is reached, as though health itself were a static and absolute state of being. A client who envisions a healthy ideal of weighing 50 pounds less than his or her present weight could, however, receive praise and encouragement for every effort made toward altering eating patterns, regularly monitoring his or her weight, or altering the meaning and purpose that food holds in his or her life. Every instance of success is then recognized as a gain, and the client is rewarded with support and encouragement by the health care professional. Similarly, the health care professional and the client may identify other health-promotive beliefs, attitudes, and behaviors in which the client already engages. For example, a client may wear a seat belt on a regular basis, a family may join together for a balanced meal at least once a day, or a community may lobby for additional bike paths—all of which are health promotive and have the potential to optimize health. These positive health actions provide the energy necessary to contend with depleting behaviors (i.e., to continue the process of change).

Internalize the Idealized Image

At this point in the change process, the client has begun to close the gap between the idealized image and his or her real health status. The health care professional now assists the client to strive for greater consistency in daily actions relative to the pictured image of health. These new patterns no longer require constant surveillance. The no-longer-idealized-but-realized behaviors become part of the client's health status.

The health care professional continues to praise the client for the changed behaviors but also reviews the plan for further modifications so that the behaviors might be maintained indefinitely. Any problems with the intervention are noted, and supports are bolstered. The health care professional asks the client how the professional may be of further help and reaffirms the client's plan (e.g., to remain at a healthy weight) for a specific length of time (e.g., 6 months). The health care professional's intent is to stabilize the altered health behaviors. As one set of behaviors is changed, the health care professional and the client may review the idealized image of health and the new present state, using the HPM, to determine the next starting point for change.

The process of moving from image creation and image appraisal, through minimizing depleting patterns and optimizing supportive patterns, toward internalizing an idealized image of health is repetitive, involving reevaluations and reformulations of intervention foci. With the continued support of the health care professional, the client needs to periodically formulate alternative strategies to move again toward an idealized image of health. In addition, as a client grows and develops, his or her ideals could change. It is also possible that a client might never reach the idealized state; nonetheless, the client may find success in the adoption of some health-sustaining patterns. The health care professional encounters clients in a multitude of states and contexts; the potential for supporting, protecting, and enhancing health is always a challenge.

SPIRITUALITY AS A HEALTH PROMOTION CONSTRUCT

Spirituality may be included as a construct in health promotion models; of late, it has been distinguished from religion (Larson et al., 1998). Until the 1960s and 1970s, religion was seen as a broad construct, encompassing individual and institutional elements as well as spirituality. Since that time, religion has become more narrowly defined, and spirituality has been distinguished from religiousness, or the practice of religious behavior (Peterman et al., 2002).

Recent definitions of spirituality include dimensions such as a person's search for meaning and purpose in life, connection with a transcendent dimension of existence, reliance on inner resources, a sense of within-person integration or connectedness, often to a higher power, a sense of life purpose and life satisfaction and the experience and feelings associated with that search and that connection (Ellison, 1983; Moberg, 1984; Peterman et al., 2002; Koenig et al., 2001; Zinnbauer et al., 1999; Chandler et al., 1992; Moberg, 2002; Miller et al., 2003).

Religion is seen, in contrast, as participation in the institutionally sanctioned beliefs and activities of a particular faith group and symbols designed to facilitate closeness to a higher power (Zinnbauer et al., 1997). Religiousness includes engaging in religious activities (e.g., religious service attendance), private and personal religious behaviors, and the extent to which religion is the primary motivating factor in people's lives, drives behavior, and decision-making (Monod et al., 2011; Allport & Ross, 1967; Koenig et al., 1997).

There is a growing body of research examining the relation between religion and health (Peterman et al., 2002). Studies have examined this relationship in community samples (Hummer et al., 1999; Musick et al., 1999; Strawbridge et al., 1997), among medical and surgical patients (Koenig et al., 1998; Oxman et al., 1995), and among cancer patients (Brady et al., 1999; Fehring et al., 1997; Holland et al., 1999; Mickley et al., 1992). Religious beliefs and practices have positive effects on illness prevention, recovery from surgery, mental illiness, and coping with physical illness (Matthews et al., 1998). As philosophies, most religions include preventive behaviors such as valuing ones body, not smoking, and not drinking in their theologies.[2]

Several interventions that explicitly use spirituality to promote health are found in the health promotion field; they include therapeutic touch (*laying-on of hands*), directed healing (by healers), distant healing (intercessory prayer), and spiritism (*espiritismo*, a healing system used with the aid of a spiritist). To bring the body, mind, and spirit together, meditation or mindfulness meditation (the attempt to achieve awareness without thought) is often practiced.

Clinical interest and research in the concept is rapidly growing, particularly as many as baby boomers seem to approach religion differently, defecting from organized religion to a more personal search for fulfillment (Roof, 1993; Wuthnow, 1998; Zinnbauer et al., 1997). At present, spirituality is considered a construct, or a mental image, however, rather than a fully developed model. To form a model of spirituality in prevention, more operational measures of spirituality are necessary (Monod et al., 2011), even though the widely cited functional assessment of chronic illness therapy–spiritual well-being scale (FACIT-Sp) has demonstrated good psychometric properties (Peterman et al., 2002). Interventions designed to assess the construct must be rigorously evaluated. The use of prayer in the practice of health care has been criticized as trivializing religion, however (Sloan et al., 2000). Yet clinical practice often moves ahead of the evidence. For example, the American College of Physicians suggested four simple questions designed to elicit a *spiritual history*, with which clinicians might ask seriously ill patients about their faith (Koening, 2000).

EMPOWERMENT AND COMMUNITY CAPACITY-BUILDING: CROSS-CUTTING CONSTRUCTS

The concepts of empowerment and community capacity-building, as central foundations of the field of health promotion, traverse all of the models. Both implement the principle of equity advanced in the World Health Organization agenda. Values, such as equity, are fundamental to these two constructs; to value something is to choose it for its own sake in preference to other alternatives.

Empowerment

Empowerment is a term with considerable weight and contested meanings. One's health is significantly affected by the extent to which one feels control or mastery over one's life or by the amount of power or powerlessness one feels (Wallerstein, 1992). From a political perspective, if health is seen as a

---

2 For example, in Judaism, the importance of good health is mentioned explicitly throughout numerous religious texts. The Torah (The Five Books of Moses or Jewish written law) says, "Guard yourself and guard your soul very carefully" (Deuteronomy 4:9–10). Jewish sages teach that when a doctor heals the sick, the doctor is performing the mitzva (good dead) of returning lost property: "And you shall return it to him" (Deuteronomy 22:2). Rambam [Moses Maimonides, a twelfth-century physician, philosopher, jurist, and major early Jewish intellectual figure] said that: "...if he [sic] is ill—therefore, he must avoid that which harms the body and accustom himself to that which is healthful and helps the body become stronger" (Rambam 4:1).

resource, health promotion implies advocacy for its equitable distribution. At the core of empowerment is power, which is found in the process of increasing personal, interpersonal, or political exchanges (Gutiérrez, 1990).

A set of moral values underpins the empowerment construct in health promotion. Moral values may be defined as the "humanly caused benefits that human beings provide to others.... By way of illustration, we may say that love and justice are moral goods" (Kekes, 1993, p. 44). Moral values at the base of the empowerment construct include promoting human diversity (promoting respect and appreciation for diverse social entities) and self-determination (promoting the ability of clients to pursue their chosen goals without excessive frustration and in consideration of other persons' needs) for individuals and marginalized groups, especially communities.

The concept embodies the larger political aspects of power. "Empowerment theory is based on a conflict model that assumes that a society consists of separate groups possessing different levels of power and control over resources" (Gutiérrez, 1990, p. 150). Questions of power are key to empowerment (e.g., Who has more power in a relationship? Are there attempts to share power?). Empowerment is thus attentive to rights and entitlements in relationships and to personal control over exchanges. Further, empowerment exists along a continuum— from personal power through community organization to political action (Labonte, 1986)—and implies potential conflict among differing views and interests.

Within the empowerment model of health promotion, however, Becker (1986) cautions that health may become a moral imperative. The pursuit of health may become more important than the pursuit of any other values, including distributive justice. Health could become more important as a value than seeking opportunities for the more vulnerable members of society to attain it.

Community Capacity-Building

Community, although an evolving concept subject to numerous interpretations, may be defined concretely as "a group of people living in the same defined area sharing the same basic values and organization," or abstractly as "a group of people sharing the same basic interests" (Rifkin, Muller, & Bichman, 1988, p. 933).

McKnight (1986) highlights the sense of connectedness among members of a community in describing its characteristics: (1) capacity- rather than deficiency-oriented; (2) informal; (3) rich in stories that "allow people to reach back into their common history and their individual experience for knowledge about truth and direction for the future;" and (4) incorporating celebration, tragedy, and fallibility "into the life of the community" (p. 58).

The emphasis that health promotion puts on the community is explicitly political, in that the community becomes a mediating structure between the domain of individuals' everyday life (microlevel) and the larger social, political, and economic context within which individuals live (macrolevel). Capacity is built as communities increase their abilities to participate in economic and political decisions, thereby enhancing health at the macrolevel (McKnight, 1990). Therefore, community health promotion often stresses the importance of structures and effective governance, service integration, efficiency and accountability, and information and management systems (Best et al., 2003).

Health care professionals must consider under what conditions individuals should sacrifice their personal uniqueness for the good of the community, as well as how many resources the community should provide to promote the health of a few. Further, it is important that as communities become more responsible for health promotion and confront complex, often multisectoral problems, such as mental illness, the broader health services continue to support them both politically and economically.

Encouaged by the Affordable Care Act of 2010, and modeled on the Patient Centered Medical Home, community-based health homes have been proposed to advocate for and coordinate indigenous resources—such as neighborhood walking trails or gardens—to improve health outcomes for diabetes, hypertension, and heart disease across both individuals and populations (Cantor et al., 2011). This approach has not yet been systematically implemented and evaluated, however.

EVIDENCE FOR THE EFFECTIVENESS OF HEALTH PROMOTION

The development of evidence for the effectiveness of health promotion has become more important as the push for evidence-based practice in medicine, nursing, and other health professions has grown (see Chapters 1 and 12 for more discussion of this topic). Evidence can be considered a fact or datum that is used, or could be used, in making a decision or judgement or in solving a problem. Such evidence, when used alongside good reasoning and principles of valuation, answers the question *why* (Butcher, 1998). Some consider evidence a culturally or geographically biased notion, borne of logical positivism, as delineated by such philosophers as Russell and Wittgenstein. In the philosophical tradition of logical positivism, meaning is verifiable only through rigorous observation and experiment. The randomized clinical trial and the quasi-experiment rest within this tradition. Anthropology and some branches of sociology have alternative approaches to assessing evidence and the effectiveness of interventions (see later in this Chapter and Chapter 12) that some feel are more relevant to health promotion in non-Western countries.

Health promotion is eclectic, multidisciplinary, and practice oriented. Many of its principal activities relate to advocacy, partnerships, and coalition building, functions that require more art than science; effectiveness studies may fail to capture the holistic focus of many health promotion activities (McQueen, 2001). Yet many practitioners and advocates of health promotion need to demonstrate that health promotion is a field with tangible benefits to offer the public.

A key challenge in health promotion is to foster and develop high-quality, widely recognized, and acceptable standards for evidence-based evaluation. Several approaches to developing evidence for the effectiveness of health promotion are described in detail in Chapter 2, including the work of the US Preventive Services Task Force and the Task Force on Community Preventive Services. Evidence of economic benefits from health promotion are important to many of these advisory groups; cost-effectiveness evaluation is described further in Chapters 1 and 12. In this Chapter, the program evaluation approach is applied to the development of evidence for the effectiveness of health promotion.

APPROACHES TO BUILDING EVIDENCE FOR HEALTH PROMOTION: PROGRAM EVALUATION

Program evaluation, or evaluation research, is the systematic application of social research procedures for assessing the conceptualization, design, implementation, and utility of social intervention and human service programs (Rossi & Freeman, 1993). Program evaluation generally is used for assessing program effectiveness and efficiency, for improving program and service delivery, and for guiding resource allocation and policy development.

The program evaluation process is shaped in part by a program's goals and is embedded in a definition of health promotion and a unique concept of health. To move from a concept of health to a theory of health promotion and finally to a test of one or more aspects of that model in an operating program, one must be able to measure key constructs.

Health may be measured subjectively (from the person's or community's own experience or sense of feeling *well, in touch,* or *empowered*). Yet health may also be measured objectively (e.g., by measuring resting heart rate or muscular strength). The data derived from interviews with clients or listening to their stories may be combined with data obtained from physical measures of client physiological functioning, observations of client behavior, or psychometrically sound assessments of clients' attitudes, beliefs, and behaviors. Qualitative and quantitative measures may together refine a more perfect picture of health.

The experience of health may vary both within and among clients. Yet consensus has developed around the use of several general instruments to measure health-related quality of life. One of the more widely used and translated instruments, the Short Form Health Survey (SF-36, reduced further to the SF-12), addresses six factors: physical, social, and role abilities; general mental health; general health perceptions; and symptoms (Fylkesnes & Forde, 1992; McHorney, Ware, & Raczek, 1993; Ware & Sherbourne, 1992). The instrument is composed of a series of questions, is easy to administer, and is comprehensible. Its psychometric, or measurement, properties are known and highly regarded.

Program evaluation, as an assessment of the processes and effects of a health promotion program or its components, begins with setting an evaluation agenda, including examining health promotion models and the program focus and design. The agenda generally is set in consideration of or in conjunction with those who will use the research and those who will be affected by it. Next, the research is formulated, planned, and implemented. As with other forms of social research, this process is systematic to ensure maximal construct validity (a strong relationship between the constructs and their measures) and reliability (constancy or consistency of measures over time, place, and person). Finally, the results are disseminated so that they may be used for program change. Generally, the findings are shared with key decision makers or client groups, or both.

Within this general framework, the health care professional may adopt one of the following four main models of evaluation, each of which implies a different understanding of the relationship between the program and its stakeholders (those with an interest in the program's processes and effects): evaluation as synonymous with applied research; evaluation as part of systems management, as an aid to program administration; evaluation as professional judgment; and evaluation as politics (Smith & Glass, 1987). Each is discussed in turn.

Evaluation as Social Research

The first model considers evaluation a form of social research, with the concomitant use of the scientific method, either in the positivist or constructivist tradition. The positivist scientific tradition assumes relationships within causal models. For example, the impacts of an intervention to reduce smoking among adolescents (the *cause*) are assessed relative to the effects on quit rates. Program goals are well specified and measurable. Rigorously designed comparative studies, true field experiments, randomized clinical trials, and quasi-experiments are implemented. Methodological rigor, including both internal validity (in testing for causality) and external validity (the generalizability of the evaluation), is critical. The evaluation is primarily summative (conducted at the outcome of the effort), comparative, and quantitative. Program success is judged relative to a comparison group in an experimentally controlled setting.

The constructivist tradition, as part of ethnomethodology, focuses on persons' lived experiences, with those experiences understood as being located in a particular sociohistorical context. In this methodology, the evaluator is a research instrument himself or herself and produces a type of narrative, text, or case report for the evaluation (Schwandt, 1990). For example, in a study of programs to increase community empowerment, the evaluator might use focus groups, intensive interviewing, and case studies. The evaluator is seeking to understand multiple discourses on how people experience becoming healthy (Labonte & Robertson, 1996;

Marlett, 1994). The evaluation may be either formative (providing information before the program is complete) or summative and qualitative. Program success is judged by criteria developed by the stakeholders or relative to other similar programs.

Evaluation as a Contributor to Systems Management

The second model incorporates evaluation into systems management, with the organization being viewed as an interrelated set of inputs, processes, and outputs. The evaluator describes these system parts and relates them to each other, relative to the stated goals. The program manager can then make decisions to regulate and improve the functions of the system. Research methods include program audits, performance appraisals, cost analyses, client satisfaction surveys, and continuous quality improvement programs. The evaluator is interested in the level of attainment on performance indicators of the given goals and in discrepancies between the stated objectives and performance (Thompson, 1992). The evaluation tends to be formative, in that information is conveyed to program administrators during the assessment process and is produced in a technically proficient manner.

Evaluation as Professional Judgment

A third model, evaluation as professional judgment, considers experts to be the appropriate persons to make judgments about the quality of a program. This model is found in accreditation approaches and assumes that peer review is objective, reliable, and valid. The experts' methods include direct observation, often using checklists and interviews with clients. Of late, these approaches have been integrated with evidence-based (using social research methods) standards of practice. The experts judge the program data against established standards, and program administrators and others in the profession generally are the audience for the evaluation. Other groups with an interest in the evaluation generally are not considered.

Evaluation as Politics

Evaluation as politics, the fourth general model, highlights the proposition that evaluation and politics are inextricably intertwined. Evaluation studies are not directed simply toward one decision maker but toward all major stakeholders who play a role in maintaining, modifying, or eliminating the program. In the evaluation-as-politics approach, each program has stakeholders and active partisans competing with each other for a greater share of authority over resources and social affairs. "At every stage, evaluation is only one ingredient in an inherently political process" (Rossi & Freeman, 1993, p. 417). The model uses a variety of methodological approaches, from controlled experiments to naturalistic case studies. Different reports or presentations are prepared for different audiences. The credible evaluation report is comprehensible, correct, complete, and reasonable to partisans on all sides (Cronbach, 1982).

CONCLUSIONS

The numerous health promotion models explored in this Chapter differ in their view of health, the outcome they wish to describe or explain. Each varies in its intended target, whether micro (individuals, groups, families) or macro (communities or populations). Further, the moral values implied by the cross-cutting constructs of empowerment and community capacity-building suggest different uses of these theoretical approaches. Each question that is asked about the process and outcome of health promotion calls for evidence, born of varied evaluation models and measurement approaches.

REFERENCES

Aday LA. Indicators and predictors of health services utilization. In: Williams S, Torrens P, eds. *Introduction to Health Services* (chap. 3). Albany, NY: Delmar; 1993.

Ajzen I. The theory of planned behavior. *Organ Behav Hum Dec.* 1991;50:179–211.

Ajzen I. Perceived behavioral control, self-efficacy, locus of control, and the theory of planned behavior. *Journal of Applied Social Psychology*, 2002;32:665–683.

Ajzen I, Fishbein M., eds. *Understanding Attitudes and Predicting Social Behavior.* Upper Saddle River, NJ: Prentice Hall; 1980.

Aldwin C, Stokols D. The effects of environmental change on individuals and groups: some neglected issues in stress research. *J Environ Psychol.* 1988;8:57–75.

Andersen RM, Aday LA. Access to medical care in the U.S.: realized and potential. *Medical Care.* 1978;16:533–546.

Andersen RM, Newman JF. Societal and individual determinants of medical care utilization in the United States. *Milbank Q.* 1973;51:95–124.

Antoni MH, Carver CS, Lechner SC. Enhancing positive adaptation: Example intervention during treatment for breast cancer. In: Park CL, Lechner SC, Antoni MH, Stanton AL, eds. *Medical Illness and Positive Life Change*, 197–214. Washington, DC: American Psychological Association; 2009.

Ashford A, Gemson D, Sheinfeld Gorin S, Bloch S, Lantigua R, Ahsan H, et al. Cancer screening and prevention practices of inner city physicians. *Am J Prev Med.* 2000;19:59–62.

Aspinwall LG, Tedeschi RG. The value of positive psychology for health psychology: progress and pitfalls in examining the relation of positive phenomena to health. *Ann Behav Med.* 2010;39(1):4–15.

Backett KC, Davison C. Lifecourse and lifestyle: the social and cultural location of health behaviors. *Soc Sci Med.* 1995;40(5):629–638.

Baer JS, Lichtenstein E. Cognitive assessment. In Donovan DM, Marlatt GA, eds. *Assessment of Addictive Behaviors*, 189–213. New York: Guilford Press; 1988.

Bandura A. *Social Foundations of Thought and Action.* Upper Saddle River, NJ: Prentice Hall; 1986.

Bandura A. Health promotion from the perspective of social cognitive theory. *Psychol Health.* 1988;13:623–649.

Batts ML, et al. Patient priorities and needs for diabetes care among urban African American Adults. *The Diabetes Educator.* 2001;27:405–412.

Bayes/Mendel Lab, Sidney Kimmel Comprehensive Cancer Center at Johns Hopkins University. 2004. BRCAPRO. Retrieved September 12, 2012, from http:/astor.som.jhmi.edu/BayesMendel/brcapro.html.

Becker M. The tyranny of health promotion. *Public Health Rev.* 1986;14:15–23.

Becker MH, Drachman RH, Kirscht JP. A new approach to explaining sick-role behavior in low-income populations. *Am J Public Health.* 1974;64:205–216.

Berkman LF. The relationship of social networks and social support to morbidity and mortality. In: Cohen S, Syme, SL, eds. *Social Support and Health*, 243–262. Orlando, FL: Academic Press; 1985.

Berkman LF, Glass T. Social integration, social networks, social support, and health. *See Berkman & Kawachi* 2000;137–173.

Bornstein MH. Sensitive periods in development: Structural characteristics and causal interpretations. *Psychological Bulletin.* 1989;105(2):179–197.

Brown SL, Eisenhardt KM. *Competing on the Edge: Strategy as Structured Chaos.* Cambridge, MA: Harvard Business School Press; 1998.

Brown JJ, Reingen P. Social ties and word-of-mouth referral behavior. *J Consumer Research.* 1987;14:350–362.

Burg MM, Seeman TE. Families and health: The negative side of social ties. *Ann Behav Med.* 1994;16(2):109–115.

Butcher RB. Foundations for evidence-based decision making. In: National Forum on Health, *Canada Health Action: Building on the Legacy*, Vol. 5, pp. 259–290. Quebec: Éditions MultiMondes; 1998.

Butterfield PG. Thinking upstream: Nurturing a conceptual understanding of the societal context of health behavior. *Adv Nurs Sci.* 1990;12(2):1–8.

Cacioppo JT, Berntson GG, Sheridan JF, McClintock MK. Multilevel integrative analyses of human behavior: Social neuroscience and the complementing nature of social and biological approaches. *Psychol. Bull.* 2000;126:829–843.

Cacioppo JT, Fowler JH, Christakis NA. Alone in the crowd: The structure and spread of loneliness in a large social network. *J Pers Soc Psychol.* 2009;97(6):977–991.

Calfas KJ, Hagler AS. Physical activity. In: Sheinfeld Gorin S, Arnold J. *Health Promotion in Practice*, 192–221. San Francisco, CA: Jossey-Bass; 2006.

Cannon WB. *The Wisdom of the Body.* New York: Norton; 1932.

Centola D. The spread of behavior in an online social network experiment. *Science.* 2010;329(5996): 1194–1197.

Christakis NA, Allison PD. Mortality after the Hospitalization of a Spouse. *N Engl J Med.* 2006;354:719–730.

Christakis NA, Fowler JH. The spread of obesity in a large social network over 32 years. *N Engl J Med.* 2007;357:370–379.

Christakis NA, Fowler JH. The collective dynamics of smoking in a large social network. *N Engl J Med.* 2008;358:2249–2258.

Cohen S. Psychosocial models of the role of social support in the etiology of physical disease. *Health Psychol.* 1988;7:269–297.

Cohen S, Doyle WJ, Skoner DP, Rabin BS, Gwaltney JM Jr. Social ties and susceptibility to the common cold. *JAMA.* 1997;277(24):1940–1944.

Cohen S, Syme SL. Issues in the study and application of social support. In: Cohen S, Syme SL, eds. *Social Support and Health*, 3–22. Orlando, FL: Academic Press; 1985.

Cohen S, Wills TA. Stress, social support, and the buffering hypothesis. *Psychol Bull.* 1985;98:310–357.

Cohen-Cole E, Fletcher JM. Is obesity contagious? Social networks vs. environmental factors in the obesity epidemic. *J Health Econ.* 2008;27(5):1382–1387.

Cousins E. Jewish spirituality: From the sixteenth-century revival to the present. In: Green A, ed. *World Spirituality: An Encyclopedic History of the Religious Quest*, Vol. 14, pp. ix–x. New York: Crossroad; 1987.

Crabtree BF, Miller WL, Aita VA, Flocke SA, Stange KC. Primary care practice organization and preventive services delivery: a qualitative analysis. *J Fam Pract.* 1998;46:403–409.

Cronbach LJ. *Designing Evaluations of Educational and Social Programs.* San Francisco, CA: Jossey-Bass; 1982.

Curry SJ, Emmons KM. Theoretical models for predicting and improving compliance with breast cancer screening. *Ann Behav Med.* 1994;16(4):302–316.

Delbecq AL. The social political process of introducing innovation in human services. In Sarri R,

DeLongis A, Folkman S, Lazarus RS. The impact of daily stress on health and mood: Psychological and social resources as mediators. *J Pers Soc Psychol.* 1988;54(3):486–495. doi: 10.1037/0022-3514.54.3 .486.

Devins GM. Social cognitive analysis of recovery from a lapse after smoking cessation: Comment on Haaga and Stewart. *J Consult Clin Psychol.* 1992;60(1):29–31.

DiClemente CC. Motivational interviewing and the stages of change. In Miller W, Rollnick R, eds. *Motivational Interviewing*, 191–203. New York: Guilford Press; 1991.

Downie RS, Fyfe C, Tannahill A. *Health Promotion: Models and Values.* New York: Oxford University Press; 1990.

Elvik R. Area-wide urban traffic calming schemes: A meta-analysis of safety effects. *Accid Anal Prev.* 2001;33:327–336.

Emery FE, Trist EL. *Towards a Social Ecology: Contextual Appreciations of the Future in the Present.* New York: Plenum; 1972.

Eng E. Save Our Sisters Project. *Cancer.* 1993;72:1071–1077.

Esterling BA, Kiecolt-Glaser JK, Glaser R. Psychosocial modulation of cytokine-induced natural killer cell activity in older adults. *Psychosom. Med.* 1996;58(3): 264–272.

Fawcet SB, Paine-Andrews A, Francisco VT, Schultz JA, Richter KB, Lewis RK, et al. Using empowerment theory in collaborative partnerships for community health and development. *Am J Commun Psychol.* 1995;23(5):677–697.

Fincham S. Community health promotion programs. *Soc Sci Med.* 1992;35(3):239–249.

Fishbein M, Jaccard JJ, Davidson AR, Ajzen I, Loken B. Predicting and understanding family planning behaviors: Beliefs, attitudes, and intentions. In Ajzen I, Fishbein M, eds. *Understanding Attitudes and Predicting Social Behavior*, 131–147. Upper Saddle River, NJ: Prentice Hall; 1980.

Fisher EB, Bishop DB, Goldmuntz J, Jacobs A. Implications for the practicing physician of the psychosocial dimensions of smoking. *Chest.* 1988;38:194–212.

Flier JS. Obesity Wars. *Cell.* 2004;116(2):337–350.

Fong GT, Rempel LA, Hall PA. Challenges to improving health risk communication in the 21st century: A discussion. *J Natl Cancer I.* 1999;25:173–176.

Fowler JH, Christakis NA. The dynamic spread of happiness in a large social network: Longitudinal analysis over 20 years in the Framingham Heart Study. *British Med J.* 2008;337:a2338.

Fox SA, Murata PJ, Stein JA. The impact of physician compliance on screening mammography by women. *Ann Behav Med.* 1991;151:50–56.

Friedman MS, Powell KE, Hutwagner L, Graham LM, Teague WG. Impact of changes in transportation and commuting behaviors during the 1996 Summer Olympic Games in Atlanta on air quality and childhood asthma. *JAMA.* 2001;285:897–905.

Frumkin H. Healthy places: Exploring the evidence. *Am J Public Health.* 2003;93(9):1451–1456.

Fylkesnes K, Forde H. Determinants and dimensions involved in self-evaluation of health. *Soc Sci Med.* 1992;35(3):271–279.

Gary TL, Batts-Turner M, Bone LR, et al. A randomized controlled trial of the effects of nurse case manager and community health worker team interventions in urban African-Americans with type 2 diabetes. *Controlled Clinical Trials.* 2004;25:53–66.

Gary TL, Bone LR, Hill MN, et al. Randomized controlled trial of the effects of nurse case manager and community health worker interventions on risk factors for diabetes-related complications in urban African Americans. *Prev Med.* 2003;37:23–32.

Gell-Mann M. *The Quark and the Jaguar: Adventures in the Simple and Complex.* New York: W. H. Freeman; 1995.

Gielen AC, McDonald EM, Gary TL, Bone LR. Using the precede-proceed model to apply health behavior theories, 407–434. In: Glanz K, Barbara K, Rimer BK, Viswanath K. *Health Behavior and Health Education Theory, Research, and Practice,* 4th ed. CA: Jossey-Bass; 2008.

Glasgow RE, Vogt TM, Boles SM. Evaluating the public health impact of health promotion interventions: the REAIM framework. *Am J Public Health.* 1999;89:1322–1327.

Glasgow RE, Lichtenstein E, Marcus AC. Why don't we see more translation of health promotion research to practice? Rethinking the efficacy to effectiveness transition. *Am J Public Health.* 2003;93:1261–1267.

Glasgow RE, Orleans CT, Wagner EH. Does the chronic care model serve also as a template for improving prevention? *Milbank Q.* 2001;79:579–612, iv–v.

Glasgow RE, Klesges LM, Dzewaltowski DA, Estabrooks PA, Vogt TM. Evaluating the impact of health promotion programs: using the RE-AIM framework to form summary measures for decision making involving complex issues. *Health Educ Res.* 2006;21(5):688–694.

Goodman S. Attributable risk in epidemiology: Interpreting and calculating population attributable fractions. In IOM Board on Population Health and Public Health Practice, *Estimating the contributions of lifestyle-related factors to preventable death: A workshop summary.* Washington, DC: National Academies Press; 2005.

Gordis L. *Epidemiology.* Philadelphia: Saunders; 2000.

Gotay CC, Wilson ME. Social support and cancer screening in African American, Hispanic, and Native American women. *Cancer Pract.* 1998;6:31–37.

Green L. *Health Education Today and the PRECEDE Framework.* Palo Alto, CA: Mayfield; 1979.

Green J, Cairns BJ, Casabonne D, Wright FL, Reeves, Beral V for the Million Women Study collaborators. Height and cancer incidence in the Million Women Study: Prospective cohort, and meta-analysis of prospective studies of height and total cancer risk. *The Lancet Oncology.* 2011;12(8):785–794.

Green LW, Kreuter MW. *Health Promotion Planning: An Educational and Environmental Approach,* 2nd ed. Palo Alto, CA: Mayfield; 1990.

Green LW, Kreuter MW. *Health Promotion Planning: An Educational and Ecological Approach.* New York: Mayfield Publishing, 2005.

Grossman E, Keegan T, Lessler AL, et al. Inside the health disparities collaboratives. A detailed exploration of quality improvement at community health centers. *Medical Care.* 2008;46:489–496.

Gutiérrez L. Working with women of color: An empowerment perspective. *Social Work.* 1990;35:149–154.

Hafen BQ, Karren KJ, Frandsen KJ, Smith NL. *Mind/Body Health: The Effects of Attitudes, Emotions, and Relationships.* Needham Heights, MA: Allyn & Bacon; 1996.

Harvard Center for Cancer Prevention. Harvard School of Public Health. *Your Disease Risk.* Retrieved September 2, 2012, from http://www.yourdiseaserisk.harvard.edu/index.htm.

Hawley AH. *Human Ecology: A Theory of Community Structure.* New York: Ronald Press; 1950.

Hill-Briggs F, et al. Training community health workers as diabetes educators for urban African Americans: Value added using participatory methods. *Progress in Community Health Partnerships: Research, Education, and Action.* 2007;1(2):185–193.

Hill-Briggs F, Gary TL, Baptiste-Roberts K, Brancati FL. Thirty-Six-Item short-form outcomes following a randomized controlled trial in Type 2 Diabetes. *Diabetes Care.* 2005;28:443–444.

Holland JC, Lewis S. eds. *The Human Side of Cancer: Living with Hope, Coping with Uncertainty.* New York: Harper Collins Publishers; 2000.

House JS, Kahn RI. Measures and concepts of social supports. In: Cohen S, Syme S, eds. *Social Support and Health,* 83–108. Orlando, FL: Academic Press; 1985.

House JS, Landis KR, Umberson D. Social relationships and health. *Science.* 1988;241:540–545.

Hummer RA, Rogers RG, Nam CB, Ellison CG. Religious involvement and U.S. adult mortality. *Demography.* 1999;36:273–285.

Hutchison GB. Evaluation of preventive services. In Schulberg HC, Sheldon A, Baker F, eds. *Program Evaluation in the Health Fields,* Vol. 1, pp. 59–72. New York: Human Sciences Press; 1969.

International Union for Health Promotion and Education. *The Evidence of Health Promotion Effectiveness: A Report for the European Commission by the International Union for Health Promotion and Education.* Brussels- Luxembourg: ES-EC-EAEC; 1999.

Jackson RJ. The impact of the built environment on health: An emerging field. *Am J Public Health.* 2003;93(9):1382–1384.

Jackson RJ, Dannenberg AL, Frumkin H. Health and the Built Environment: 10 Years After. *Am J Public Health.* 2013; e-View Ahead of Print.

Janis IL, Mann L. *Decision Making: A Psychological Analysis of Conflict, Choice and Commitment.* New York: Free Press; 1977.

Janz NK, Becker MH. The health belief model: A decade later. *Health Educ Q.* 1984;11:1–47.

Job RFS. Effective and ineffective use of fear in health promotion campaigns. *Am J Public Health.* 1988;78:163–167.

Judd CM, Smith EK, Kidder LH. *Research Methods in Social Relations,* 6th ed. Austin, TX: Holt, Rinehart & Winston; 1991.

Kahnemann D. Objective happiness. In: Kahnemann D, Diener E, Schwartz N, eds. *Well-being: The Foundations of Hedonic Psychology,* 3–25. New York: Russell Sage Foundation; 1999.

Kahneman D, Tversky A. Choices, values, and frames. *Am Psychol.* 1984;39:341–350.

Kahneman D, Tversky A. Prospect theory: An analysis of decision under risk. *Econometrica.* 1979;47(2):263–292.

Karasek R, Theorell T, eds. *Healthy Work: Stress, Productivity, and the Reconstruction of Working Life.* New York: Basic Books; 1990.

Katz D, Kahn RL. *The Social Psychology of Organizations.* New York: Wiley; 1966.

Kazdin AE. *Behavior Modification in Applied Settings,* 5th ed. Pacific Grove, CA: Brooks/Cole; 1994.

Keating NL, O'Malley AJ, Murabito JM, Smith KP, Christakis NA. Minimal social network effects evident in cancer screening behavior. *Cancer.* 2011;117(13):3045–3052.

Kekes J. *The Morality of Pluralism.* Princeton, NJ: Princeton University Press; 1993.

Kelly JA, St. Lawrence JS, Stevenson LY, Houth AC, Kuliehman AC, Diaz YE, et al. Community AIDS/ HIV risk reduction: The effects of endorsements by popular people in three cities. *Am J Public Health.* 1992;2:1483–1489.

Kernick D. Wanted—new methodologies for health service research. Is complexity theory the answer? *Family Practice* 2006;23:385–390.

Kernick D (Ed). Complexity and Healthcare Organization: A View from the Street. UK: Radcliffe Medical Press Ltd., 2004.

Knudsen EI. Sensitive periods in the development of the brain and behavior. *J Cognitive Neuroscience.* 2004;16(8):1412–1425.

Koening HG. Religion, spirituality, and medicine: Application to clinical practice. *JAMA.* 2000;284:1708.

Kotler P, Roberto E. *Social Marketing: Strategies for Changing Public Behavior.* New York: Free Press; 1989.

Labonte R. Social inequality and healthy public policy. *Health Promot.* 1986;1(3):341–351.

Labonte R, Robertson A. Delivering our goods, showing our stuff: The case for a constructivist paradigm for health promotion research and practice. *Health Educ Q.* 1996;23(4):431–447.

Lane DS, Brug MA. Breast cancer screening: Changing physician practices and specialty variation. *New York State J Med.* 1990;90:288–292.

Langton CG. Artificial Life. *Santa Fe Institute Studies in the Sciences of Complexity, Proceedings,* Vol. 6. Redwood City, CA: Addison-Wesley; 1989.

Leavell HR, Clark EG. *Textbook of Preventive Medicine.* New York: McGraw-Hill; 1953.

Lee NR, Kotler P. *Social Marketing Influencing Behaviors for Good,* 4th ed., 520. Thousand Oaks, CA: SAGE Publications; 2012.

Lefebvre RC, Lasater TM, Carleton RA, Peterson G. Theory and delivery of health programming in the community: The Pawtucket Heart Health Program. *Prev Med.* 1987;16:80–95.

Leventhal H, Safer MA, Panagis DM. The impact of communications on the self regulation of health beliefs, decisions, and behavior. *Health Educ Q.* 1983;10:3–29.

Lewin R. *Complexity: Life on the Edge of Chaos.* London: Phoenix; 1993.

Lewin K, Dembo T, Festinger L, Sears PS. Level of aspiration. In: Hunt J, ed. *Personality and the Behavioral Disorders: A Handbook Based on Experimental and Clinical Research,* 333–378. New York: Ronald Press; 1944.

Lilienfeld AM. *Foundations of Epidemiology.* New York: Oxford University Press; 1976.

Lindmark E, Diderholm E, Wallentin L, Siegbahn A. Relationship between interleukin 6 and mortality in patients with unstable coronary artery disease: effects of an early invasive or noninvasive strategy. *JAMA.* 2001;286(17):2107–2113.

Lipkus IM, Hollands JG. The visual communication of risk. *J Natl Cancer I.* 1999;25:149–163.

Llewellyn-Thomas H. Patients' health-care decision making: A framework for descriptive and experimental investigations. *Med Decis Making.* 1995;15:101–106.

Lutgendorf SK, Johnsen EL, Cooper B, Anderson B, Sorosky JI, et al. Vascular endothelial growth factor and social support in patients with ovarian carcinoma. *Cancer.* 2002;95(4):808–815.

Maiman LA, Becker MH. The health belief model: Origins and correlates in psychological theory. In: Becker MH, ed. *The Health Belief Model and Personal Health Behavior,* 9–26. Thorofare, NJ: Slack; 1984.

Mandelblatt JS, Yabroff KR. Effectiveness of interventions designed to increase mammography use: A meta-analysis of provider-targeted strategies. *Cancer Epidemiol Biomarkers Prev.* 1999;8:759–767.

Mandelbrot B. A fractal walk on Wall Street. *Scientific American*. 1999;*280*(2):70–73.

Manoff RK. *Social Marketing: Imperative for Public Health*. New York: Praeger; 1985.

Marlett N. *Partnerships and Communication in Health Promotion Research*. Paper presented at the Third Annual Health Promotion Research Conference, Calgary, Alberta, Canada; 1994.

Maruyama M. The second cybernetics: Decision-amplifying mutual causal processes. *Am Sci*. 1963;51: 164–179.

Masten AS. Ordinary magic: Resilience processes in development. *Am Psychol*. 2001;56:227–238.

McGinnis JM, Foege WH. Actual causes of death in the United States. *JAMA*. 1994;270:2207.

McGuire W. Theoretical foundations of campaigns. In Rice RE, Paisley WJ, eds. *Public Communication Campaigns*, 41–70. Thousand Oaks, CA: Sage; 1981.

McHorney CA, Ware JE, Raczek AE. The MOS 36-Item Short-Form Health Survey (SF-36): Psychometric and clinical tests of validity in measuring physical and mental constructs. *Medical Care*. 1993;31:247–263.

McKnight JL. Well-being: The new threshold of the old medicine. *Health Promot*. 1986;1:77–80.

McKnight J. Politicizing health care. In Conrad P, Kern R, eds. *The Sociology of Health and Illness: Critical Perspectives*, 432–436. New York: St. Martins Press; 1990.

McPherson M, Smith-Lovin L, Cook JM. Birds of a feather: homophily in social networks. *Ann Review of Sociology*. 2001;27:415–444.

McQueen DV. Strengthening the evidence base for health promotion. *Health Promot Int*. 2001;16:261–268.

Mensah GA. Attributing risks in preventable death: What metrics best inform health policy? In: Institute of Medicine, *Estimating the Contributions of Lifestyle-Related Factors to Preventable Death: A Workshop Summary*. Washington, DC: National Academies Press; 2005.

Miller SM. Monitoring versus blunting styles of coping with cancer influence the information patients want and need about their disease (implications for cancer screening and management). *Cancer*. 1995;76:167–177.

Miller GE, Cohen S, Ritchey AK. Chronic psychological stress and the regulation of proinflammatory cytokines: a glucocorticoid-resistance model. *Health Psychol*. 2002;21(6):531–541.

Miller WL, Crabtree BF, McDaniel R, Stange KC. Understanding change in primary care practice using complexity theory. *J Fam Pract*. 1998;46:369–376.

Miller WL, McDaniel RR Jr, Crabtree BF, Stange KC. Practice jazz: understanding variation in family practices using complexity science. *J Fam Pract*. 2001;50(10):872–878.

Miller SM, Shoda Y, Hurley K. Applying cognitive-social theory to health-protective behavior: Breast self-examination in cancer screening. *Psychol Bull*. 1996;119:70–94.

Moos RH. Social ecological perspectives on health. In Stone GC, Cohen F, Adler NE, eds. *Health Psychology: A Handbook*, 523–547. San Francisco: Jossey-Bass; 1979.

Morowitz HJ. Metaphysics, meta-metaphor, and magic. *Complexity*. 1998;3(4):19–20.

Morowitz HJ, Singer JL. *The Mind, the Brain, and Complex Adaptive Systems*. Reading, MA: Addison-Wesley Publishing; 1995.

Multilevel Interventions across the Cancer Care Continuum: Background Perspectives & Description of 2011 Conference and Journal Supplement, May 2010.

National Heart, Lung, and Blood Institute. *Framingham Heart Study: 50 Years of Research Success*. Retrieved September 2, 2012, from http://www.nhlbi.nih.gov/about/framingham/index.html.

O'Connor AM, Stacey D, Entwistle V, Llewellyn-Thomas H, Rovner D, Holmes-Rovner M, et al. Decision aids for people facing health treatment or screening decisions (Cochrane Review). *Cochrane Library*, 2004;2.

Oman D, Reed D. Religion and mortality among the community-dwelling elderly. *Am J Public Health*. 1988;88:1469–1475.

Orleans CT, Rotberg HL, Quade D, Lees P. A hospital quit-smoking consult service: clinical report and intervention guidelines. *Prev Med*. 1990;19(2):198–212.

Pachucki M, Jacques PF, Christakis NA. Social network concordance in food choice among spouses, friends, and siblings. *Am J Public Health*. 2011;101(11):2170–2177.

Parse R. *Nursing Science: Major Paradigms, Theories and Critiques*. Philadelphia: Saunders; 1987.

Paul GL. Strategy of outcome research in psychotherapy. *J Consult Psychol*. 1967;31:109–118.

Pearson ML, Wu S, Schaefer J, et al. Assessing the implementation of the Chronic Care Model in quality improvement collaboratives. *Health Serv Res*. 2005;40:978–996.

Pelletier KR. *Healthy People in Unhealthy Places: Stress and Fitness at Work*. New York: Dell; 1984.

Pender N. *Health Promotion in Nursing Practice*. Stamford, CT: Appleton & Lange; 1996.

Peterson C. The future of optimism. *Am Psychol*. 2000;55:68–78.

Phillips KA, Morrison KR, Andersen R, Aday LA. Understanding the context of healthcare utilization: Assessing environmental and provider-related variables in the behavioral model of utilization. *Health Serv Res*. 1998;33:571–596.

Plsek P. Appendix B: Redesigning health care with insights from the science of complex adaptive systems. In: Institute of Medicine. *Crossing the Quality Chasm: A New Health System for the 21st Century*

Committee on Quality of Health Care in America. Washington, DC: National Academy Press; 2001.

Plsek PE, Wilson T. Complexity, leadership, and management in healthcare organisations. *BMJ.* 2001;323:746–749.

Pradhan AD, Manson JE, Rossouw JE, Siscovick DS, Mouton CP, et al. Inflammatory biomarkers, hormone replacement therapy, and incident coronary heart disease: prospective analysis from the Women's Health Initiative observational study. *JAMA.* 2002;288(8):980–987.

Prochaska JO, DiClemente CC. Stages and processes of self-change of smoking: Toward an integrative model. *J Consult Clin Psychol.* 1983;51:390–395.

Prochaska JO, Velicer WF, Gaudagnoli E, Rossi JS, DiClemente CC. Patterns of change: Dynamic typology applied to smoking cessation. *Multivar Behav Res.* 1991;26:83–107.

Putnam R. *Bowling Alone: The Collapse and Revival of American Community.* New York: Simon and Schuster; 2000.

Rabow J, Watts RK. The role of alcohol availability in alcohol consumption and alcohol problems. *Recent Dev Alcohol.* 1983;1:285–302.

Rachlin H. *Introduction to Modern Behaviorism.* 3rd ed. San Francisco: Freeman; 1991.

Ridker PM, Rifai N, Stampfer MJ, Hennekens CH. Plasma concentration of interleukin-6 and the risk of future myocardial infarction among apparently healthy men. *Circulation.* 2000;101:1767–1772.

Rifkin SB, Muller F, Bichman W. Primary health care: On measuring participation. *Soc Sci Med.* 1988;29:931–940.

Rogers E. *Diffusion of Innovation.* New York: Free Press; 1983, 2003.

Rogers RW, Deckner CW, Mewborn CR. An expectancy-value theory approach to the long-term modification of smoking behavior. *J Clin Psychol.* 1978;34:562–566.

Rosenquist JN, Murabito J, Fowler JH, Christakis NA. The spread of alcohol consumption behavior in a large social network. *Ann Intern Med.* 2010;152(7):426–433.

Rosenstock IM. The health belief model and preventive health behavior. In Becker MH, ed. *The Health Belief Model and Personal Health Behavior,* 27–59. Thorofare, NJ: Slack; 1974.

Rosenstock IM, Strecher VJ, Becker MH. Social learning theory and the health belief model. *Health Educ Q.* 1988;15(2):175–183.

Rossi PH, Freeman IE. *Evaluation: A Systematic Approach,* 5th ed. Thousand Oaks, CA: Sage; 1993.

Rothman AA, Wagner EH. Chronic illness management: what is the role of primary care? *Ann Intern Med.* 2003;138:256–261

The Royal Society. *Risk Assessment: Report of a Royal Society Study Group.* London: The Royal Society; 1983.

Ruberman W, Weinblatt E, Goldberg JD, Chaudhary B. Psychosocial influences on mortality after myocardial infarction. *New Eng J Med.* 1984;311:552–559.

Saelens BE, Sallis JF, Frank LD. Environmental correlates of walking and cycling: findings from the transportation, urban design, and planning literatures. *Ann Behav Med.* 2003;25:80–91.

Sales A, Smith J, Curran G, Kochevar L. Models, strategies, and tools: theory in implementing evidence-based findings into health care practice. *J Gen Intern Med.* 2006;21(Suppl 2):S43–S49.

Salovey P, Rothman AJ, Detweiler JB, Steward WT. Emotional sates and physical health. *Am Psychol.* 2000;55:68–78.

Salovey P, Williams-Piehota P. Field experiments in social psychology: Message framing and the promotion of health protective behaviors. *Am Behav Sci.* 2004;47:488–505.

Schaefer JA, Moos RH. Life crises and personal growth. In: Carpenter BN, ed. *Personal Coping: Theory, Research, and Application,* 149–170. Westport, CT: Praeger Publishers/Greenwood Publishing Group; 1992; viii, 268 pp.

Schwandt T. Paths to inquiry in the social disciplines. In: Guba E, ed. *The Paradigm Dialog,* 258–276. Thousand Oaks, CA: Sage; 1990.

Schwartz B. Self determination: The tyranny of freedom. *Am Psychol.* 2000;55:79–88.

Schwartz LM, Woloshin S, Welch HG. Risk communication in clinical practice: Putting cancer in context. *J Natl Cancer I.* 1999;25:124–133.

Seeman TE. Health promoting effects of friends and family on health outcomes in older adults. *Am J Health Promot.* 2000;14(6):362–370.

Seeman TE, Syme SL. Social networks and coronary artery disease: A comparison of the structure and function of social relations as predictors of disease. *Psychosom Med.* 1987;49(4):341–354.

Seligman MEP, Csikszentmihalyi M. Positive psychology: An introduction. *Am Psychol.* 2000;55:5–14.

Sheinfeld Gorin S. The adoption and use of performance assessment systems. *Soc Work Res Abs.* 1982;18(3):74–75.

Sheinfeld Gorin S. Outcomes of social support for women survivors of breast cancer. In: Mullen E, Magnabosco, JL, eds. *Outcomes Measurement in the Human Services: Cross-Cutting Issues and Methods,* 276–289. Washington, DC: NASW Press; 1997.

Sheinfeld Gorin S, Arnold J. *The Health Promotion Handbook.* St. Louis, MO: Mosby; 1998.

Sheinfeld Gorin S, Weirich T. Innovation use: Performance assessment in a community mental health center. *Human Relat.* 1995;48(12):1427–1453.

Sheinfeld Gorin S. Models of health promotion. In: Sheinfeld Gorin S, Arnold J, eds. *The Health Promotion Handbook,* 21–66. San Francisco, CA: Jossey-Bass, 2006.

Sheinfeld Gorin S. Theory, measurement, and contro-versy in positive psychology, health psychology, and cancer: basics and next steps. *Ann Behav Med.* 2010;39(1):43–47.

Sheinfeld Gorin S, Badr H, Krebs P, Prabhu Das I. Multilevel interventions and racial/ethnic health disparities. *J Natl Cancer Inst Monogr.* 2012;44: 100–111.

Sheridan SL, Harris RP, Woolf SH. Shared decision mak-ing about screening and chemoprevention: A sug-gested approach from the US Preventive Services Task Force. *Am J Prev Med.* 2004;26:56–66.

Shoda Y, Mischel W, Miller SM, Diefenbach M, Daly MB, Engstrom PF. Psychological interventions and genetic testing: Facilitating informed decisions about BRCA1/2 cancer susceptibility. *J Clin Psychol Med S.* 1998;5:3–17.

Sloan RP, Bagiella E, VandeCreek L, Hover M, Casalone C, Hirsch TJ, et al. Should physicians prescribe religious activities? *New Engl J Med.* 2000;342:1913–1916.

Smith ML, Glass GV. *Research and Evaluation in Education and the Social Sciences.* Upper Saddle River, NJ: Prentice Hall; 1987.

Stacey RD. *Complexity and Creativity in Organizations.* San Francisco, CA: Berrett-Koehler; 1996a.

Stacey RD. *Strategic Management and Organizational Dynamics.* London: Pitmann Publishing; 1996b.

Stokols D. Establishing and maintaining healthy environ-ments: Toward a social ecology of health promotion. *Am Psychol.* 1992;47(1):6–22.

Stroebe M, Stroebe W. The role of lonliness and social support in adjustment to loss: A test of attach-ment versus stress theory. *J Pers Soc Psychol.* 1996;70(6):1241–1249.

Taplin SH, Clauser S, Rodgers AB, Breslau E, Rayson D. Interfaces across the cancer continuum offer oppor-tunities to improve the process of care. *J Natl Cancer I.* 2010;40:104–110.

Taplin SH, Price RA, Edwards H, Foster M, Breslau E, Chollette V, Prabhu-Das I, Clauser S, Fennell M, Zapka J. Understanding and influencing multilevel factors across the cancer care continuum. *J Natl Cancer I.* 2012;44:2–10.

Taylor SE. Adjustment to threatening events: A the-ory of cognitive adaptation. *Am Psychol.* 1983;38:1161–1173.

Taylor SE, Kemeny ME, Reed GM, Bower JE, Gruenewald TL. Psychological resources, positive illusions, and health. *Am Psychol.* 2000;55:99–109.

Thompson JC. Program evaluation within a health promotion framework. *Can J Public Health.* 1992;83(Suppl. 1):567–571.

Tsai AC, Morton SC, Mangione CM, Keeler EB. A meta-analysis of interventions to improve care for chronic illnesses. *Am J Manag Care.* 2005 Aug;11(8):478–488.

Tull ES, Roseman JM. Diabetes in African Americans. In: *National Institutes of Health, National Diabetes*

Data Group, National Institute of Diabetes and Digestive and Kidney Diseases, eds. Diabetes in America. (2nd ed.) NIH Publication No. 95–1468. Bethesda, Md.: National Institutes of Health, 1995.

Turner-McGrievy GM, Tate D Weight loss social support in 140 characters or less: use of an online social net-work in a remotely delivered weight loss intervention. *Translational Behavioral Medicine.* 2013 (published online).

US Preventive Services Task Force. *Guide to Clinical Preventive Services,* 3rd ed. 2004. Retrieved September 5, 2012, from http://www.ahrq.gov/clinic/uspstfix. htm

Vaillant GE. Adaptive mental mechanisms: Their role in a positive psychology. *Am Psychol.* 2000;55:89–98.

Varela F, Coutinho A. Second generation immune net-works. *Immunology Today.* 1991;12(5):159–166.

Varela F, Thompson E, Rosch E. *The Embodied Mind.* Cambridge, MA: MIT Press; 1991.

Velicer WF, DiClemente CC, Prochaska JO, Brandenburg N. Decisional balance measure for assessing and predicting smoking status. *J Pers Soc Psychol.* 1985;48(5):1279–1289.

Waldrop M. *Complexity: The Emerging Science at the Edge of Order and Chaos.* London: Penguin; 1992.

Wallerstein N. Powerlessness, empowerment, and health: Implications for health promotion programs. *Am J Health Promot.* 1992;6(30):197–205.

Ware JE, Sherbourne CD. The MOS 36-Item Short Form Health Survey (SF-36): Conceptual framework and item selection. *Medical Care.* 1992;30:473–483.

Wilson EO. *The Insect Societies.* Cambridge, MA: Harvard University Press; 1971.

Winett RA, King AC, Altman DG. *Health Psychology and Public Health: An Integrative Approach.* New York: Pergamon Press; 1989.

Woloshin S, Schwartz LM, Welch HG. Risk charts: Putting cancer in context. *J Natl Cancer I.* 2002;94:799–804.

Woods NE, Laffrey S, Duffy M, Lentz MJ, Mitchell ES, Taylor D, et al. Being healthy: Women's images. *Adv Nurs Sci.* 1988;11(1):36–46.

World Health Organization. *Health Promotion: A Discussion Document on the Concepts and Principles.* Copenhagen: WHO Regional Office for Europe; 1984.

World Health Organization. *From Alma-Ata to the Year 2000: Reflections at Midpoint.* Geneva: Author; 1988.

Zaltman G, Kotler P, Kaufman I. *Creating Social Change.* Austin, TX: Holt, Rinehart & Winston; 1972.

Zimmerman BJ. Chaos and nonequilibrium: the flip side of strategic processes. *Organizational Development Journal.* 1993;11(1):31–38.

Zimmerman BJ. Complexity science: a route through hard times and uncertainty. *The Health Forum Journal.* 1999;42(2):42–46, 96.

Zimmerman BJ, Lindberg C, Plsek PE. *Edgeware: Insights from Complexity Science for Health Care Leaders.* Dallas, TX: VHA Publishing; 1998.

4

Cancer Screening and Prevention

ZHIQIANG LU, ALANNA MURDAY,
AND CHARLES BENNETT

INTRODUCTION

Cancer has been and continues to be the second most common cause of death in the United States. In 2011, almost 1.6 million persons will be diagnosed with cancer (carcinoma *in situ* of any site, except urinary bladder; basal and squamous cell skin cancers) (ACS, 2011a). The most commonly occurring cancer in men is prostate cancer (about 25% of new cases), and in women, breast cancer (26%) and lung cancer.

All cancers involve the malfunction of genes that control cell growth or division. Epidemiologic studies have also identified environmental factors that contribute to the development of cancer, including environmental pollution, cigarette smoking, intensive alcohol consumption, physical inactivity, certain infectious diseases, obesity, and sun exposure. Further studies indicate that other risk factors, such as occupation and radiation exposure, contribute to the risk of some cancers. Many cancers can be prevented by the removal of such risk factors, or can be controlled if diagnosed at an early stage.

In public health, the best strategy is either to prevent the disease or detect it early by screening. Screening is the preliminary identification of unrecognized disease or defects through examinations, tests, or other procedures that can be applied rapidly and inexpensively. The first widely used screening test for cancer was the Pap test, developed in 1923 by George Papanicolaou as a research method in understanding the menstrual cycle and to identify cervical cancer in its early stages. Modern mammography methods were developed in the 1960s and then were officially recommended by the American Cancer Society (ACS) in 1976.

This chapter reviews the epidemiology of and the risk factors for cancer, in addition to evidence-based recommendations for screening for the most prevalent cancers in the United States.

EPIDEMIOLOGY

According to the American Cancer society, in 2011, one in four deaths in the United States was to cancer (ACS, 2011). In 2007, cancer was the second leading cause of death in the United States, accounting for 23% of all deaths annually, and it was the leading cause of death among women aged 35–74 and men aged 55–74 (Heron, 2011). About 1,660,290 new cancer cases are expected to be diagnosed in 2013; about 580,350 Americans are expected to die of cancer, almost 1,600 people per day (ACS, 2013; http://www.cancer.org). The most common cancer sites in men are prostate, lung and bronchus, and colon and rectum, accounting for approximately 50% of all newly diagnosed cancers. The most common cancer sites in women are breast, lung and bronchus, and colon and rectum, making up approximately 50% of all newly diagnosed cases. Prostate cancer accounts for 25% of newly diagnosed cancer cases in men, and breast cancer accounts for 26% of newly diagnosed cancer cases in women.

The Surveillance Epidemiology and End Results (SEER) program of the National Cancer Institute (NCI) reports that in 2001–2005, the median age of death for persons with cancer was 73 years old. Those within the age group of 75–84 years had the highest mortality rate, 29.9%. Morality rates due to cancer for other age groups were: for those under age 20 (0.4%), 20–34 (0.9%), 35–44 years (2.8%), 45–54 years (9%), 55–64 years (17.1%), 65–74 years (25.6%), and >85 years (14.4%) (SEER, 2011).

CANCER AND RISK FACTORS

Trends in cancer incidence and mortality have stabilized over the past 10 years and have decreased since 1990. The 5-year relative survival rate for all cancers diagnosed between 2002 and 2008 was 68%, up from 49% in 1975–1977 (ACS, 2013). Decreased rates of mortality from lung, prostate, and colorectal cancer accounted for the trend in men, and decreased rates of breast and colorectal cancer accounted for the decrease in women.

Estimated incidence rates of new cancer cases are highest in genital and digestive system cancers (both 19%), respiratory system cancers (16%), breast cancer (13%), and urinary system cancers (9%) in both sexes. Using 2013 estimates, more men will be diagnosed with new cases of cancer (excluding basal cell and squamous cell skin cancers and *in situ* carcinomas except urinary bladder) than women (ACS, 2013).

Cancer incidence and death rates vary among racial and ethnic subgroups. Factors associated with this racial disparity include genetics, culture, and access to health care and screening services (Kagawa-Singer et al., 2010). Across all cancers, African American men have a 14% higher rate of cancer incidence and 33% higher mortality rate compared to white men, while African American women have a 6% lower rate of cancer incidence but 17% higher mortality rate compared to white women. An exception is breast and lung cancer among women. White women have a higher incidence of both cancers and lower mortality in breast cancer but higher mortality in lung cancer (Siegel et al., 2011). Among men, cancer incidence is higher for all cancers among African American men; cancer mortality is higher in all types of cancer among African American men compared to whites except for kidney and renal pelvis cancers. Hispanic/Latino groups have the third highest rate of cancer incidence and the fourth highest rate of cancer mortality. Asian Americans and Pacific Islanders are the fourth highest group in cancer incidence rates and have the lowest rate of cancer mortality. Lastly, American Indians and Alaska Natives have the lowest rate of cancer incidence and the fourth highest rate of cancer mortality (Siegel et al., 2011).

There are variations by type of cancer within racial and ethnic groups. Uterine cervix cancer incidence is highest among Hispanic/Latino populations and mortality is highest among African American populations. Asian Americans and Pacific Islanders have the highest rate of liver and bile duct cancer, and the highest incidence of stomach cancer; they have the highest mortality rates due to liver and bile duct cancer in both males and females. For stomach cancer, Asian American and Pacific Islander females and African American males have the highest rate of mortality. Lastly, American Indians and Alaska Natives have the highest rates of mortality due to kidney and renal pelvis cancers (Jemal et al., 2008).

There is a close link between educational attainment and cancer mortality. For all cancer sites, men who report ≤12 years of education were twice as likely to die compared to those who had >12 years of education; similarly, women who reported having ≤12 years of education were approximately 1.5 times more likely to die compared to those with >12 years of education (ACS, 2008a). This stratification is seen within and between racial groups. For example, cancer mortality rates among both African American and non-Hispanic white men with 12 or fewer years of education are almost 3 times higher than those of college graduates for all cancers combined, and are 4–5 times higher for lung cancer. Furthermore, progress in reducing cancer death rates has been slower in persons with low SES (ACS, 2013). These results are also reflected in rates among Non-Hispanic white men and women. African American men and women have higher mortality than Non-Hispanic white men and women across all years of education, however. It is likely that there are multiple confounding factors that contribute to cancer mortality (Sorlie et al., 1992). Education is a reliable indicator of socioeconomic status for people aged 25 to 64 years; about 37% of the premature cancer deaths among people aged 25 to 64 years could have been avoided by elimination of educational and racial disparities in 2007 alone (Jemal et al., 2008).

SCREENING

Prevention, as defined by the National Cancer Institute, is a reduction in cancer mortality via a reduction in the incidence of cancer (NCI, 2011b). Cancer prevention in the primary care setting may include both *primary* prevention, consisting of health-promoting measures to reduce the development of disease, and *secondary* prevention, consisting of detection of disease when asymptomatic or mild, as discussed in Chapter 3. Prevention strategies, therefore, should include appropriate screening measures. Screening can reduce both the incidence and the mortality of cancer, by identifying and removing both pre-cancerous conditions and early-stage cancers (Atkin et al., 2010). Screening for colon cancer by endoscopy, for example, may result in detection and removal of pre-cancerous polyps. Likewise, screening for cervical cancer using Pap smears (Papanicolaou test; cytological screening) is a relatively inexpensive method and may result in identification and excision of pre-invasive lesions, although cervical cancer cells are difficult to detect or prevent (Ugboma and Aburoma, 2010).

As a general matter, in order for a screening test to be of value for routine use, several criteria should be met:

First, the disease or condition screened for must be common and must have sufficient impact on an individual's health to justify the risks and costs associated with the testing. Much of the interest and effort directed toward the development of cancer screening tests have been focused on the most common cancers, including breast, prostate, lung, colon, and cervical cancers. Estimates of the premature deaths that could have been avoided through cancer screening vary from 3% to 35%. Screening may reduce cancer morbidity since treatment for earlier-stage cancers is often less aggressive than that for more advanced-stage cancers (Soderstrom et al., 2005).

Second, effective prevention or treatment measures must be available for the condition, and earlier detection must improve clinical outcomes. As discussed below, although lung cancer is the most common cause of cancer death in the United States, until most recently, studies had not shown an improvement in clinical outcome from earlier detection through various imaging modalities. Most recently, the National Lung Screening Trial (NLST) reported a 20.0% decrease in mortality from lung cancer in the low-dose computed tomography (CT) group as compared with the radiography group (Aberle et al., 2011). However, the average risk of lung cancer among the participants of the NLST could be different from those that will be observed in the community due to the "healthy-volunteer" effect and thus bias the results.

Although prostate cancer screening with prostate-specific antigen (PSA, a serum biomarker) tests and/or digital rectal exam (DRE) have become commonplace, considerable controversy exists over whether they have improved clinical outcomes, and major cancer organizations report that there is insufficient evidence to recommend them in average-risk men. Results from the Prostate, Lung, Colorectal, and Ovarian (PLCO) Cancer Screening Trial revealed that annual screening for prostate cancer compared with community-based screening practices did not lead to fewer prostate cancer deaths up to 10 years after the start of screening (Barry, 2009).

Third, the screening and treatment benefits should outweigh any risks associated with testing and therapy. While most cancer screening tests are non-invasive or minimally invasive, some may involve risks of serious complications. Colonoscopies, for example, have a small but serious risk of bowel perforation. The odds ratios (ORs) for perforation from colonoscopy relative to perforation from sigmoidoscopy was 1.8 (95% CI = 1.2–2.8; Gatto et al., 2003). Moreover, the screening test must be accurate and readily available. False-positive tests results may lead to anxiety and unnecessary invasive diagnostic procedures, which may carry higher risks of serious complications than screening. More recently, concerns have been raised regarding the over-diagnosis of cancers (e.g., prostate, via PSA testing) that would not have become clinically significant in the absence of detection by screening. False-negative test results may falsely reassure individuals of the absence of cancer, thereby delaying diagnosis and treatment. The availability of screening tests may be limited in areas where patients have limited access to health care resources, however (Kramer, 2004).

Screening recommendations of several cancer organizations, including the US Preventive Services Task Force (USPSTF), the American Cancer Society (ACS), and the National Cancer Institute (NCI) are summarized in Table 4-4. The recommendations and underlying data for several of the more common cancers, including breast, cervical, colorectal, lung, and prostate cancers, are discussed more fully below.

BREAST CANCER

Breast cancer is the most common non-cutaneous cancer among women in the United States, and the

TABLE 4-1. PROBABILITY OF DEVELOPING BREAST CANCER BY FAMILY HISTORY (KERLIKOWSKE ET AL., 2000)

Ages	(+) Family History (# cases)	(-) Family History (# cases)
30–39	3.2 (per 1,000)	1.6 (per 1,000)
40–49	4.7	2.7
50–59	6.6	4.6
60–69	9.3	6.9

second leading cause of death from cancer. In 2011, 232,620 women in the United States were diagnosed with invasive breast cancer (and 53,360 with *in situ* disease), and 39,970 died of breast cancer (Siegel et al., 2011).

Breast cancer mortality increases with age. Women over 40 years have a very small (0.3%) chance of dying from breast cancer within the next ten years, while women over 65 years have a 1% chance. Women over 70 years have the highest risk of breast cancer mortality; however, they are most likely to die from other comorbidities instead (Kerlikowske et al., 1999).

Breast cancer risk factors include; prior history of invasive breast cancer, ductal carcinoma *in situ* (DCIS), or lobular carcinoma *in situ* (LCIS); a strong family history of breast or ovarian cancer, particularly among first-degree relatives (which may be associated with a genetic mutation in BRCA1 or BRCA2); early age at menarche and late age at first birth (reflecting estrogen exposure); and a history of breast biopsies, particularly those identifying proliferative benign breast disease (e.g., atypical ductal hyperplasia; London et al., 1992; McDivitt et al., 1992). The Gail Model approximates a person's individual risk over time based on each factor for women aged 40 or over who have received regular mammograms (Bondy et al., 1994; Gail et al., 1989; Spiegelman et al., 1994). This tool for estimating a woman's individual risk of developing breast cancer is available online (See: the National Cancer Institute's Breast Cancer Risk Assessment Tool [http://www.cancer.gov/bcrisktool]).

Radiological breast density, due to differences in tissue composition and differences in radiographic attenuation properties of fat, stromal, and epithelium, is a strong risk factor for breast cancer and also makes breast cancer more difficult to detect by mammography. Women who have extensive (≥75%) dense breast tissue on a mammography have a four- to sixfold increase in risk when compared to women with little or no dense breast tissue (Oza and Boyd, 1993). Women treated with radiation to the chest, particularly before age 30, have a 1% annual increased risk of breast cancer, starting 10 years after first exposure.

Behavioral and environmental factors such as hormone use, obesity, and alcohol consumption are associated with an increased risk of breast cancer. Risk for breast cancer incidence and mortality also vary with geographic region, culture, race, ethnicity, and socioeconomic status.

Screening Recommendations

All major North American expert groups recommend routine screening with mammography, with or without clinical breast examination (CBE), for women aged 50 and older. There is considerable controversy, however, about routine screening of women in their forties, based on analyses of the benefits versus the harms of screening in this age group. The literature documents great variation in benefits and harms associated with screening mammography among women between 40 and 49 years of age. The major benefit would be a potential decrease in breast cancer mortality. Potential harms could include, but are not limited to, increased anxiety due to false-positive results, diagnosis and treatment for cancer that would not be clinically evident, unnecessary radiation exposure, and procedure-associated pain. Therefore, individualized risk-benefit evaluation plays an important role when making decisions about screening mammography for this group of women (Qaseem et al., 2007).

The American Cancer Society, American College of Radiology, American Medical Association, and American College of Obstetrics and Gynecology all recommend starting routine screening at age 50. The US Preventive Services Task Force (USPSTF) recommends screening mammography every one to two years for women aged 50 and older (USPSTF, 2009). The American College of Physicians guidelines recommend individualized risk and benefit assessment, taking into account the woman's breast cancer risk profile and preferences, for women aged 40 to 49 (Qaseem et al., 2007). Most North American expert groups recommending breast cancer screening suggest a frequency of once a year for women over age 50 and once every one to two years for women aged 40 to 49.

There is less consensus among expert groups about teaching and promoting breast self-examination (BSE). The American College of Obstetricians and Gynecologists recommends routine teaching of BSE (ACOG, 2011). In 2003, the American Cancer Society changed its previous recommendation in favor of monthly BSE to a recommendation that women be educated about the benefits and limitations of BSE (Smith et al., 2003). The most current US Preventive Services Task Force found insufficient evidence to recommend for or against the procedure. The Advisory Committee on Cancer Prevention in the European Union states that there is "no convincing evidence for the effect of screening based on breast self-examination or clinical breast examination" (EC, 1999). The Canadian Task Force on Preventive Health Care concluded that "there is fair evidence to recommend that routine teaching of BSE be excluded from the periodic health examination of women aged 40–49 (grade D recommendation, "fair evidence against")," because of excessive work-ups for false-positive examinations and lack of firm evidence for decreasing breast cancer mortality (Baxter, 2001).

Much of the controversy surrounding breast cancer screening has focused on women aged 40 to 49. The benefits of screening mammography have been less clear and slower to appear for women in this age group. As noted above, results from RCTs (Randomized Clinical Trials) consistently showed no mortality benefit from screening for women aged 40 to 49 after 7 years of follow-up (Miller et al., 1992). As the period of follow-up has lengthened, however, meta-analyses have demonstrated a significant mortality benefit for women who began screening in their forties. A review by the USPSTF in 2002 found a 15% decrease in breast cancer mortality (RR 0.85, 95% CI 0.73–0.99) after 14 years of follow-up of women who started screening in their forties (Humphrey et al., 2002). Of note, the 95% confidence interval is wide and indicates that the mortality reduction could be as much as 27% or as little as 1% (Qaseem et al., 2007).

Special Populations
Women Ages 40 to 49

A review of the risks and benefits of mammographic screening in women ages 40 to 49 revealed that women between the ages of 40 and 49 who undergo routine mammograms will decrease their risk for breast cancer–related death (Armstrong et al., 2007). They will increase their risk for unnecessary procedures, anxiety, discomfort, and low-dose radiation, however. The review also noted that the incidence of breast cancer and the effectiveness of mammographic screening are lower in women in their forties than in women aged 50 or older. Thus, mammograms result in less benefit and greater risk for women aged 40 to 49 when compared to women aged 50 or older. Based on the above, the review concluded that women aged 40 to 49 with lower-than-average risks for breast cancer and higher-than-average concerns about false-positive results might reasonably delay screening.

In 2007, the American College of Physicians published clinical practice guidelines regarding mammographic screening for women aged 40 to 49 (Qaseem et al., 2007). The guidelines recommend that, for women in this age group, clinicians periodically perform an individualized assessment of a woman's risk for breast cancer to help guide decisions about screening, basing the decision on the benefits and harms of screening, as well as on a woman's breast cancer risk profile and her preferences. If a woman decides to forego mammography, the clinician should reassess this decision every one to two years.

Older Women

There are no clear data from RCTs for women older than 70; therefore, no conclusions can be made for this group of people (see Chapter 12).

Screening mammography in older women may result in a smaller tumor size and lower stage cancer at diagnosis, but the effect on mortality is unclear. While mammographic screening may yield a cancer diagnoses in 1% of older women, these cancers are usually low risk. A study of California Medicare beneficiaries aged 66 to 79 demonstrated this clearly (Smith-Bindman et al., 2000). The study found that *in situ*, local, and regional breast cancer were more likely to be detected among women who underwent screening mammography than comparable women who did not. For example, the relative risk of detecting local breast cancer in screened women was 3.3 (95% CI: 3.1–3.5). The risk of detecting metastatic breast cancer, on the other hand, was significantly reduced among women who underwent screening mammography (RR = 0.57, 95% CI: 0.45–0.72). These results suggest that there may be benefit of mammography screening in older women, although it comes with an increased risk of over-diagnosis (Smith-Bindman et al., 2000). Moreover, such screening is still accompanied by risks of unnecessary follow-up testing, diagnostic procedures, and attendant anxiety.

Looking at women older than age 65, a systematic review of cost-effectiveness analyses for the USPSTF concluded that extending biennial mammography screening to age 75 or 80 was estimated to cost between $34,000 and $88,000 (2002 U.S. dollars) per life-year gained, compared with stopping screening at age 65. The review concluded that biennial breast cancer screening after age 65 years reduces mortality at reasonable costs for women without clinically significant comorbid conditions (Mandelblatt et al., 2003).

According to the American College of Physicians, guiding screening among older women (above age 65) requires an evaluation of both quantitative factors relating to the benefits and harms of screening, such as life expectancy, risk of dying of cancer, the number needed to screen to prevent cancer death, and the likelihood of over-diagnosis; and qualitative factors, such as an individual patient's values and preferences (Walter & Covinsky, 2001). The authors noted that patients with life expectancies of less than five years are unlikely to derive any survival benefit from cancer screening.

Women with a Family History of Breast Cancer

Women with a known genetic predisposition to breast cancer (i.e., BRCA1 or BRCA2) should receive counseling for several options, including more intensive screening for breast cancer. As discussed above, the American Cancer Society recently released guidelines recommending annual breast cancer screening by MRI as an adjunct to mammography for women with approximately 20% or greater lifetime risk of breast cancer (Kerlikowske et al., 2000; see Table 4-1). It has been suggested that women without a known genetic syndrome who have a history of breast cancer in a first-degree relative should begin screening mammography at an earlier age, particularly if the family member had premenopausal breast cancer. One study compared the performance of mammography in almost 390,000 women aged 30 to 69 with and without a family history of breast cancer (Kerlikowske et al., 2000). The number of breast cancer cases increased with age and a positive family history of breast cancer. Detection rates in women with a positive family history of breast cancer were comparable to rates in women a decade older without a positive family history. However, the disparity of detection rates between positive and negative family history decreased with age.

Women with Thoracic Radiation

Breast cancer screening starting at an earlier age is recommended for women exposed to therapeutic radiation, particularly if exposed during youth. Mammographic screening and magnetic resonance imaging can identify early-stage cancers among these women as well, but the benefits and risks have not been clearly defined.

Males

It is estimated that 1% of all breast cancers occur in men. Most breast cancer cases are diagnosed during the evaluation of palpable lesions; treatment usually consists of surgery, radiation, and systemic adjuvant hormone therapy or chemotherapy. There is insufficient data on the benefits or risks of screening relative to survival.

CERVICAL CANCER

In 2008, 11,000 women in the United States were diagnosed with invasive cervical cancer and almost 4,000 died of this disease. The incidence of and mortality from cervical cancer have been decreasing steadily over time, from 70% between 1950 to 1970, to 40% between 1970 to 1999, largely due to screening with the Pap test.

Invasive squamous carcinoma of the cervix results from the progression of pre-invasive lesions called cervical intraepithelial neoplasia (CIN), or dysplasia. These dysplastic lesions are graded histologically as mild (CIN 1), moderate (CIN 2), or severe (CIN 3). A second classification system grades lesions based on cytologic findings as atypical squamous cells of undetermined significance (ASCUS), or cannot rule out low-grade squamous intraepithelial lesions (LSIL), LSIL (cytologic atypia and CIN 1), and high-grade squamous intraepithelial lesions (HSIL) (CIN 2, CIN 3, and carcinoma in situ). LSIL is used in reporting Pap smears; CIN 1 are used for defining changes in the tissue of the cervix; HSIL is the cytopatholgic designation, while CIN 2 and CIN 3 are the histopathologic diagnoses.

Many mildly and moderately dysplastic lesions regress rather than progress to invasive cancer. About 70% of ASCUS and CIN 1 lesions regress within 6 years; about 6% of CIN 1 lesions progress to CIN 3 or worse. About 10–20% of women with CIN 3 lesions progress to invasive cancer. Lesions that do progress to invasive cancer usually do so slowly, over years or decades, providing an opportunity for detection, treatment, and cure during the pre-invasive phase. At the same time, because many lesions would never have progressed to invasive cancer and were detected early due to routine screening, 33% of the women are treated unnecessarily due to over-diagnosis.

Virtually all cervical cancers are thought to result from human papillomavirus (HPV) infection, which is primarily transmitted by sexual contact. While approximately 95% of women with invasive cervical cancer have evidence of HPV infection, most HPV infections are transient, not leading to invasive cervical cancer. Sexual activity at an early age with multiple sexual partners is a strong risk factor (cervicalcancer.org, 2006).

Cervical cancer mortality increases with age (Howlader et al., 2011). Although the prevalence of CIN is highest among women in their twenties and thirties, mortality is rare among women younger than 30 years. The prevalence of HSIL is also low among women older than 65 years who have been previously screened, and mortality is rare among women of all ages who have had regular screening. The highest mortality for white women occurs from ages 45 to 70 years; for black women the highest mortality occurs in their seventies. Among women younger than 65 years, cervical cancer mortality is about 40% higher in black women that in white women; among women older than 65 years, this difference increases to more than 250% (Ries et al., 2003).

Screening Recommendations

All major North American expert groups recommend routine screening starting within 3 years after first vaginal intercourse, or no later than age 21 years. Recommendations differ regarding the method of screening and the appropriate screening interval, however (ACS, 2011b).

The American Cancer Society recommends screening initially be done annually with a conventional Pap test, or every 2 years with liquid-based cytology (e.g., *ThinPrep*); after age 30 years, women who have had three consecutive technically satisfactory screening tests with normal/negative results may be screened every 2 to 3 years with either technique, or every 3 years with a combination of HPV DNA testing plus either conventional Pap test or liquid-based cytology.

The USPSTF recommends screening with Pap smears at least every 3 years. In 2003, the organization found insufficient evidence to recommend for or against the routine use of liquid-based cytology or HPV testing to screen for cervical cancer.

Regarding the use of HPV DNA testing as a primary screening test, the NCI notes that the Hybrid Capture 2 (HC2), which detects the presence of 13 types of HPV that have been associated with cervical cancer, has been approved for use in conjunction with the Papanicolaou (Pap) test. In a randomized trial using both Pap and HPV testing in random order among women aged 30 to 69 years, sensitivity of HPV was higher than Pap testing, 95% and 55%, respectively. The combination of both HPV and Pap testing had a 100% sensitivity with a referral rate of 7.9% for further evaluation. However, the Pap test alone had a 97% specificity compared with 94% for HPV DNA testing only. Among women younger than 30 years, HPV DNA testing would be expected to have lower specificity because younger women may have asymptomatic, transient HPV infections that are of little clinical consequence. Thus, detecting HPV in these women could lead to unnecessary diagnostic workups (NCI, 2011a).

Special Populations: Older Women

As noted above, cervical cancer mortality increases with age, with the highest mortality for white women from ages 45 to 70 and for black women in their seventies. These are predominantly women who have not had recent screening, however. Mortality is rare at all ages among women who have recent negative screening. Accordingly, all of the major North American expert groups recommend discontinuing screening in older women who have had adequate recent negative screening. The NCI has concluded that women aged 60 years or older who have a negative test are very unlikely to have abnormal Pap tests on repeat screening, and therefore continued screening of these women is of minimal value. The USPSTF recommends against routinely screening women older than age 65 years, if they have had adequate recent screening (within 3 years) with normal Pap smears who are not otherwise at high risk for cervical cancer. The American Cancer Society has stated that women may safely discontinue screening after age 70 years, if they had no abnormal/positive cytology tests within the prior 10-year period, and if the three most recent Pap smears were technically adequate and normal.

Women with Total Hysterectomy for Benign Disease

Women who have undergone hysterectomy with removal of the cervix for benign disease rarely have important abnormalities found on Pap testing. According to the NCI, several studies have shown that the rate of high-grade vaginal lesions or vaginal cancer is less than 1 in 1,000 tests, and no study has shown that screening for vaginal cancer reduces mortality from this rare condition. Accordingly, all major North American groups recommend against routine screening in women who have had a total hysterectomy for benign disease. The American

Cancer Society does recommend continuing routine screening of women with a history of CIN 2/3, and women for whom it is not possible to document the absence of CIN 2/3 previously or as the indication for the hysterectomy, until they have a 10-year history of no abnormal/positive cytology tests. The American Cancer Society also recommends continuing routine screening of women with a history of in utero diethylstilbestrol (DES; a synthetic form of the hormone estrogen) exposure or a history of cervical carcinoma as long as they are in reasonably good health and would benefit from early detection and treatment. Women with a subtotal (supracervical) hysterectomy should continue to be screened following recommendations for average-risk women who have not undergone a hysterectomy.

COLORECTAL CANCER

Colorectal cancer is the third most common cancer type in the United States and is the second leading cause of death from cancer. Colorectal cancer makes up approximately 10% of all newly diagnosed cancer types. In 2008, over 148,000 people in the United States were diagnosed with colorectal cancer, and more than 24,000 men and 25,000 women died from it. The colorectal cancer death rate has been declining in both men and women over time with an average decline of 2% per year between 1978 and 2004.

The incidence of colorectal cancer increases linearly with age, with more than 80% of diagnosed cases occurring in patients older than 55 years. The estimated lifetime risk of developing colorectal cancer for men is 1 in 18 and for women is 1 in 19. In addition to disproportionately affecting males, colorectal cancer is more frequently diagnosed in African Americans, Native Alaskans, and those who have lower than 12 years of educational attainment than others. Although evidence shows that screening for colorectal cancer is effective in detecting early stage cancers and adenomatous polyps, colorectal cancer screening rates remain lower than screening rates reported for prostate, cervical, and breast cancer. Nationwide, colorectal cancer screening rates in the United States have been reported as less than 45%.

Screening Recommendations

The USPSTF recommends screening for colorectal cancer using fecal occult blood testing (FOBT), sigmoidoscopy, or colonoscopy in adults from ages 50 to 75 years. Current screening guidelines recommend (1) annual FOBT, (2) sigmoidoscopy every 5 years, combined with FOBT every 3 years, and (3) screening colonoscopy every 10 years. All these screening approaches have shown effectiveness in detecting early stage cancers and adenomatous polyps. Evidence shows that 100% adherence to any of the three guidelines will be equally effective in life-years gained. However, the USPSTF concluded that the net benefit gained from colorectal cancer screening for those aged 75 to 85 are small, and the risks of some screening procedures do not outweigh the benefits for those who are older than 85 years. The USPSTF recommends against routine screening for those aged 75 to 85 and against screening for those over 85 years. Lastly, the USPSTF has not made any screening recommendations concerning fecal DNA testing and computer tomographic (CT) colonography due to insufficient evidence regarding the risk-benefit ratio of these two novel test procedures.

Sensitivity and Harms

Currently, evidence shows that colonoscopy has the highest sensitivity and specificity of other colorectal cancer screening tests, although the risks associated with colonoscopy are higher than those for FOBT and sigmoidoscopy. The sensitivity and specificity of available colorectal cancer screening tests, according to the USPSTF, are detailed in Figure 4-1.

Although additional study is ongoing, the risk associated with fecal occult blood testing (FOBT) is small. Evidence shows that the risk of developing serious complications during flexible sigmoidoscopy testing is 3.4 in 10,000 procedures (USPSTF, 2008).

The risk of perforations of the colon in colonoscopy procedures is estimated at 3.8 cases per 10,000 procedures. Furthermore, the risk of developing serious complications with colonoscopy, including death or adverse events requiring hospital admission for perforation, major bleeding, diverticulitis, severe abdominal pain, and cardiovascular events, are estimated at 25 cases per 10,000 procedures (USPSTF, 2008).

CT colongraphy (a non-invasive imaging method that uses computed tomographic data combined with specialized imaging software to examine the colon) can image beyond the colon and therefore may be able to pick up extracolonic abnormalities. The clinical significance of these abnormalities

> Sensitivity: Hemoccult II < fecal immunochemical tests ≤ Hemoccult SENSA ≈ flexible sigmoidoscopy < colonoscopy
>
> Specificity: Hemoccult SENSA < fecal immunochemical tests ≈ Hemoccult II < flexible sigmoidoscopy < colonoscopy

FIGURE 4-1: USPSTF Sensitivity and Specificity of Available Colorectal Cancer Screening Tests (USPSTF 2008).

is unclear, so further evidence is needed to assess the benefits of this screening procedure. If such abnormalities turn out to have no clinical significance, wide use of extra procedures to probe the abnormalities will burden the patient and the health care system.

LUNG CANCER

Lung cancer is the second most common non-cutaneous cancer in the United States and the leading cause of death from cancer. About 222,520 new cases (15% of cancer diagnoses) of lung cancer were diagnosed in 2010, and more than 70,000 women and 90,000 men died of lung cancer. The lung cancer death rate increased rapidly for both sexes over several decades, but has been declining in men, from a high of 102.1 cases per 100,000 in 1984 to 71.3 cases in 2006. In women, lung cancer surpassed breast cancer as the leading cause of cancer in 1987 and will account for 26% of all female cancer deaths in 2011 (Siegel et al., 2011).

The incidence of lung cancer increases with age. The single most important risk factor for lung cancer is tobacco use. An unequivocal link between tobacco smoke and lung carcinogenesis has been established by molecular data. Tobacco smoking is estimated to cause 90% of lung cancers in men and 78% of lung cancers in women. Secondhand exposure to tobacco smoke also has been implicated as a cause of lung cancer. Unfortunately, although the overall prevalence rate of smoking in the United States has decreased over the past two decades, the prevalence of current adult smokers remains high at about 24%. Moreover, a high percentage of lung cancer cases occur in former smokers, because the risk of lung cancer does not decrease for many years following smoking cessation.

Occupational exposures to agents such as asbestos, arsenic, chromium, nickel, and radon also have been shown to be causally associated with lung cancer. Radon is relevant to the general public because of potential exposure in homes. However, even when combined together, the effect of these additional exposures is very small compared with cigarette smoking. Other risk factors include family history, chronic obstructive pulmonary disease, and idiopathic pulmonary fibrosis.

Lung cancer has a poor prognosis; it is the cause of death in over 90% of affected persons. Survival is directly related to the stage of lung cancer at the time of diagnosis; 5-year survival ranges from 70% for stage I disease to less than 5% for stage IV disease. Seventy-five percent of patients with lung cancer present with symptoms due to advanced or metastatic disease that is incurable. For this reason, screening for and treating early lung cancer is intuitively appealing.

Screening Recommendations

The US Preventive Services Task Force (USPSTF) has recently recommended annual screening for lung cancer with low-dose computed tomography (LDCT) in persons at high risk for lung cancer based on age and smoking history, as a Grade B recommendation, with moderate certainty that the net benefit is moderate for asymptomatic persons at high risk for lung cancer based on age, total cumulative exposure to tobacco smoke, and years since quitting. To form their recommendations, the USPSTF relied on the findings from the National Lung Screening Trial (NLST) that reported a 20.0% decrease in mortality from lung cancer, and 6.7% reduction in all-cause mortality in the low-dose CT group as compared with the radiography group (Aberle et al., 2011; Humphrey et al., 2013). The USPSTF found adequate evidence that annual screening for lung cancer with LDCT in current and former smokers ages 55 to 79 years who have significant cumulative tobacco smoke exposure can prevent a substantial number of lung cancer deaths. The absolute magnitude of benefit depends on the population screened and the screening program used. The USPSTF found insufficient evidence on the harms associated with incidental findings, and overdiagnosis. Radiation harms, including radiation-induced cancer resulting from cumulative scans over time, vary depending on the age at the start of screening and the number of scans received. The USPSTF concluded that, on balance, the benefits of screening for lung cancer were greater than the harms.

Data from the PLCO (Prostate, Lung, Colorectal, and Ovarian) Cancer Screening Trial reported a benefit of chest radiography among high-risk persons and possibly high-and average-risk women (Oken et al., 2011). This suggests that, if there is any benefit of chest radiography screening, the benefit of lung cancer screening with LDCT shown in the NLST may be even greater if applied to an unscreened population. New technologies are also being studied for potential use in lung cancer screening, including immunogenetic-based tests, molecular analysis of sputum, automated image sputum cytology, and fluorescence bronchoscopy.

PROSTATE CANCER

Prostate cancer is the most common malignancy in American men and the second leading cause of cancer-related death. The proportion of men diagnosed prior to age 70 increased from 38% in 1986 to 50% in 1993. In 2011, an estimated 240,890 men in the United States will be diagnosed with prostate cancer and 33,720 will die of prostate cancer. The median age of prostate cancer diagnosis is 67 years old.

Incidence and Mortality

The age-adjusted incidence of prostate cancer is lower in white males than in African American males, with African American males having an incidence of 258.3 per 100,000 and white males having an incidence of only 163.4 per 100,000 (Robbins et al., 1998). African American males have higher mortality rates from prostate cancer, even after adjusting for access-to-care factors (Steinberg et al., 1990). Cancer statistics from 2004 show that African American males go under-diagnosed compared to white males, with the percentage of disease diagnosed at a loco-regional stage and at a distant stage, 91% and 5% for whites, and 89% and 7% for African Americans, respectively (Ries et al., 2005). Stage distribution of prostate cancer is affected substantially by the intensity of early detection efforts.

The increase in incidence up to 1989 can be explained by an increase in tumor detection from the use of transurethral prostatectomy procedures (Bill-Axelson et al., 2005; Holmberg et al., 2002). Successive increases in incidence can be explained by the widespread use of PSA testing for screening (Gilbertsen, 1971; Stattin et al., 2010). Differences

in region-related, aggregate mortality have not been observed; however, a disparity in mortality rates exists across the United States between African American and white men (Chodak and Schoenberg, 1984; Jenson et al., 1960).

It is estimated that the lifetime risk of diagnosis of prostate cancer is about 17%, and the lifetime risk of mortality from prostate cancer is 2.9% (Siegel et al., 2011). The risk for developing invasive prostate cancer increases with age; the highest risk is in men over the age of 70 years (see Table 4-2).

Prostate cancer mortality also increases with age. From 2006–2010, the median age at death for cancer of the prostate was 80 years of age (Howlader et al., 2013). The majority (93%) of prostate cancers are discovered in the local or regional stages, for which the 5-year relative survival rate approaches 100% (ACS, 2013; Howlader et al., 2013). The 5-year survival rate for men diagnosed with distant stage prostate cancer is 27.9% and for unknown or unstaged across all races and ethnicities, 72.9% (Howlader et al., 2013).

Risk Factors

The biology of prostate cancer is not yet fully elucidated. However, men with a positive family history of prostate cancer have an increased risk compared to men without a family history (Matikainen et al., 1999; Steinberg et al., 1990). Other risk factors for prostate cancer include age, race, smoking, consumption of alcohol, interactions with minerals, obesity, and dietary habits (Eichholzer et al., 1996; Gann et al., 1994; Hayes et al., 1996; Morton et al., 1996; Platz et al., 2004; ACS, 2013). Studies indicate that a diet high in saturated and animal fat is related to a higher risk of prostate cancer (Clinton & Giovannucci, 1998; Fleshner & Klotz, 1998). Results from a nested case-control study, a case-control

TABLE 4-2. PROBABILITY OF DEVELOPING PROSTATE CANCER (SIEGEL ET AL., 2011)

Current Age (in Years)	Risk of Developing Invasive Prostate Cancer
0–39	0.01% (1 in 8,517)
40–59	2.52% (1 in 40)
60–69	6.62% (1 in 15)
70 and older	12.60% (1 in 8)
Lifetime risk	16.22% (1 in 6)

study, and a retrospective review of screened patients link higher plasma insulin-like growth factor-I levels with a higher risk of prostate cancer (J. M. Chan et al., 1998; Oliver et al., 2004; Turkes et al., 2000; Stattin et al., 2004). Unfortunately, other studies have not confirmed this link (Chen et al., 2005). Rigorous assessment of any prostate cancer procedure is needed due to the ambiguous etiology of the disease and current, unclear treatment.

Screening Recommendations Digital Rectal Examination and Prostate-Specific Antigen

Despite the identification of prostate cancer and pre-neoplastic lesions at autopsy, most lesions go clinically undetected (Sakr et al., 1993). Although the incidence of these lesions increases with age, routine administration of the prostate-specific antigen and the digital rectal exam to every age-eligible man has been met with controversy. Both the sensitivity and specificity of the test have been challenged. Most important, there is insufficient data to determine whether screening with prostate-specific antigen (PSA) or digital rectal exam reduces mortality from prostate cancer.

Since 1974, survival rates have increased for prostate cancer. Absolute disease-specific survival indicates crude disease-specific rates, while relative disease-specific survival reflects competing comorbidities for the given age group. Before interpretation, reported survival rates vary, depending on the

analytic methods. Interpreted survival data must account for both lead-time and length-bias effects , however (Pfister et al., 1990). However, interpreted survival data must account for both lead-time and length-bias effects (Pfister et al., 1990). Before interpretation, reported survival rates also vary, depending on analysis methods. Absolute disease-specific survival indicates crude disease-specific rates, while relative disease-specific survival reflects competing comorbidities for the given age group.

Benefits versus Risk

Evidence in some countries suggests a trend toward lower overall mortality for prostate cancer; however, the association between these trends and the intensity of screening is inconsistent. It is unclear whether these trends are the result of improved screening or improved treatment (Harris & Lohr, 2002).

In the midst of current studies, physicians and men are faced with uncertainty about whether to recommend or request a screening test. A qualitative study, based on small focus groups, was done to explore helpful information for men still uncertain about PSA screening (Chan & Sulmasy, 1998). Generally, men should be informed that screening has the possibility to yield false-positive and false-negative test results, that it has not been proven to reduce the number of deaths from prostate cancer, and that the recommendation for screening is still controversial (see Table 4-3). Results from the Prostate, Lung, Colorectal, and Ovarian

---

TABLE 4-3.[*]   PROSTATE CANCER SCREENING: PROS AND CONS

Pros of PSA Screening	Cons of PSA Screening
PSA screening may contribute to early detection of prostate cancer.	Some prostate cancers do not spread beyond the prostate gland, and therefore, early detection from PSC screening does not lead to clinical significance.
Cancer is easier to treat and is more likely to be controlled if diagnosed early.	Some prostate cancers do not need treatment. Urinary incontinence, erectile dysfunction, and bowel dysfunction are commonly seen risks and/or side effects due to treatment for prostate cancer.
PSA testing is inexpensive and easy to conduct.	Elevated PSA levels can be found in patients both with and without cancer.
Having the test may provide patients with some reassurance in terms of the presence of prostate cancer.	Concern that the cancer may not be life-threatening can make decision making complicated.
The number of deaths from prostate cancer has gone down since PSA testing became available.	Whether the decrease in deaths from prostate cancer is due to early detection and treatment based on PSA testing is unknown.

[*] Adapted from (Mayo Clinic, 2010)

(PLCO) Cancer Screening Trial revealed that annual screening for prostate cancer compared with community-based screening practices did not lead to fewer prostate cancer deaths up to 10 years after the start of screening.

Accuracy of Screening Tests

A 2002 review detailed the problems of using needle biopsy results as a standard reference to evaluate the accuracy of screening tests for prostate cancer. Biopsy detection rates increase with the number of biopsies performed during a single procedure. A saturation biopsy procedure ($\geq$20) tends to increase the validity of an elevated PSA level; however, this method can detect additional cancers that are clinically insignificant. The accuracy of the PSA test to detect clinically important prostate cancer cannot be consistently determined.

Active surveillance of PSA level has also been used as a standard reference. A retrospective study found the sensitivity of 4.0 μg/L or greater to be 91% for the detection of aggressive cases within 2 years of screening; the sensitivity was 56% for the detection of non-aggressive cases within the same 2 years. Conversely, 9% of men had an initial PSA level of 4.0 μg/L or higher and were not diagnosed with prostate cancer within the next 10 years (Gann et al., 1995).

How Does Evidence Fit with Biological Understanding?

PSA-level screening assumes that most asymptomatic prostate cancer cases will eventually become symptomatic cases. However, we have established that the etiology of prostate cancer is still poorly determined and that no prospective studies have been done to follow a cohort of patients with cancer detected from screening. Despite a lack of prospective studies, evidence from small, selected cohorts of men suggests a good prognosis for some men with cancer detected from screening; however, the longest of these studies only follows and reports cases 2 to 10 years after diagnoses (Lin et al., 2008).

THEORETICAL FOUNDATION(S) FOR CHANGING BEHAVIOR FOR CANCER PREVENTION

Ueland et al. conducted a quasi-experimental study and assessed the effects of colorectal cancer (CRC) education session on adult participants using a Health Belief Model (Ueland et al., 2006). The findings reported positive and significant improvement in the areas of diet (adding more fruits and vegetables to participants' diet and limiting the intake of red meat) and exercise (30 minutes of exercise at least three times per week). Maintenance of a healthy weight was also included in the study but did not change significantly over time. The study reported that participants found cancer to be either highly unlikely or impossible to prevent—thus reducing perceived susceptibility. When information about colorectal cancer and its risk factors was provided, along with information about what can be done to reduce these risk factors, the perceived severity and perceived benefits were positively improved. When this information was presented along with a screening method that provided a way in which the perceived susceptibility could be actively reduced, most people showed an increase in self-efficacy, that is, their desire to follow through with screening. Perceived barriers to screening were decreased when participants were educated about varied screening approaches, including the cheapest of the options at $4.50 for annual fecal occult blood test cards.

The theory of reasoned action and planned behavior was used in a study designed to identify motivating factors to using tanning salons (Joel Hillhouse et al., 2009). The objective of the study was to predict the use of tanning salons in young people who were motivated to improve their appearance and self-monitoring, based on the theory of planned behavior. Unlike many risk behaviors, in tanning, knowledge about the health risks associated with UV exposure has led to only minor changes in behavior. The perceived immediate benefits to UV exposure (i.e., looking tan for an improved appearance) outweigh the long-term risks associated with this behavior for most (generally the young) who participate in tanning.

When presented with the data that long-term effects would result in negative appearance near-term (rather than a cancer-related outcome), the use of tanning decreased. The best predictor of tanning was the intention to go to the salon and this in turn was influenced by the attitude toward tanning, subjective norms, and perceived behavioral control. Thus the study found the most effective approach to behavior change was to emphasize tanning attitudes and beliefs (i.e., appearance-related concerns), rather than health-related risks.

TABLE 4-4. ACS GENERAL CANCER SCREENING GUIDELINES

USPSTF		NCI
SCREENING		
Bladder Recommend against screening		Inadequate evidence of screening impact on mortality.
Breast The USPSTF recommends biennial screening mammography for women aged 50 to 74 years. Insufficient evidence for/against screening w/CBE alone, or for/against teaching or performing BSE. The USPSTF recommends that women whose family history is associated with an increased risk for deleterious mutations in BRCA1 or BRCA2 genes be referred for genetic counseling and evaluation for BRCA testing.	Average risk: CBE at least every 3 years, ages 20–39; CBE, then mammo, every year, starting age 40, no specific upper age. High risk (known BRCA, 1st-degree relative w/BRCA, 20–25% or greater lifetime risk (based on, e.g., Gail model), mantle chest XRT (radiotherapy) between ages 10 and 30, mutation carriers or 1st-degree relatives of other high-risk genetic syndromes:	NCI recommends that women age 40 or older have screening mammograms every 1 to 2 years. Mammography in women ages 40 to 70 years decreases breast cancer mortality. The benefit is higher for older women, in part because their breast cancer risk is higher.
Cervical Pap with history of sexual activity, start with 3 years of onset of sexual activity or by age 21, at least every 3 years. Insufficient evidence for/against HPV screening Recommend against screening >age 65, if adequate recent screening w/normal Pap, not otherwise at high risk. Recommend against screening after total hysterectomy for benign disease.	Starting 3 years after first vaginal intercourse, or no later than age 21, conventional Pap every year, or liquid-based Pap every 2 years. At age ≥30, if 3 consecutive normal Paps, may screen every 2–3 years w/Pap alone, or every 3 years w/HPV DNA test + Pap. At age ≥70, if 3 most recent Paps were normal, and no abnormal Pap in prior 10 years, may stop screening. If total hysterectomy or removal of cervix for benign disease, may stop screening.	Screening is effective when started within 3 years after first vaginal intercourse.Based on solid evidence, continued screening in older women (≥60 years) who have had negative Pap tests is of minimal value. Based on solid evidence, screening is not helpful in women who do not have a cervix as a result of a hysterectomy for a benign condition.
Colorectal FOBT, sigmoidoscopy, or colonoscopy, ages 50–75 (see clinical considerations sections for comparisons of different screening regimens, as well as specific intervals). Recommend against routine screening ages 76–85; considerations may support screening in an individual patient. Recommend against routine screening age 85. Insufficient evidence for/against CT colonography or fecal DNA testing as screening modalities.	Beginning at age 50: FOBT or FIT (fecal immunochemical test) w/high sensitivity, every year, OR Stool DNA test, interval uncertain, OR Flexible Sigmoidoscopy, DCBE (double-contrast barium enema), or CT colonography every 5 years, OR Colonoscopy every 10 years.	Based on solid evidence, screening for colorectal cancer (CRC) reduces CRC mortality, but there is little evidence that it reduces all-cause mortality, possibly because of an observed increase in other causes of death.

(continued)

TABLE 4-4. (CONTINUED)

	USPSTF		NCI
Endometrial		Insufficient evidence to recommend screening women at average risk, or at somewhat increased risk due to history of unopposed estrogen, tamoxifen, late menopause, nulliparity, infertility or failure to ovulate, obesity, diabetes, or HTN (hypertension).	There is inadequate evidence that screening by ultrasonography or endometrial sampling would reduce mortality from endometrial cancer. Most cases are diagnosed because of symptoms, are nonetheless "early" stage, and have high survival rates.
Esophageal			Based on fair evidence, screening would result in no (or minimal) decreased mortality from esophageal cancer in the U.S.
Gastric			Based on fair evidence, screening would not result in decreased mortality from gastric cancer in the U.S.
Hepatocellular			Based on fair evidence, screening would not result in decreased mortality from hepatocellular cancer.
Lung	The USPSTF found adequate evidence that annual screening for lung cancer with LDCT (low-dose computed tomography) in current and former smokers ages 55 to 79 years who have significant cumulative tobacco smoke exposure can prevent a substantial number of lung cancer deaths. Direct evidence from a large, well-conducted randomized, controlled trial provides moderate certainty of the benefit of lung cancer screening with LDCT in this population (Abele et al., 2011). The absolute magnitude of benefit depends on the population screened and the screening program used.	The American Cancer Society does not recommend tests to screen for lung cancer in people who are at average risk of this disease. However, the ACS does have screening guidelines for individuals who are at high risk of lung cancer due to cigarette smoking, meeting all of the following criteria: • 55 to 74 years of age • In fairly good health • Have at least a 30 pack-year smoking history AND are eithers till smoking or have quit smoking within the last 15 years	CXR (chest x-ray) and/or sputum cytology: Based on solid evidence, screening with chest x-ray and/or sputum cytology does not reduce mortality from lung cancer in the general population or in ever-smokers. LDCT: There is evidence that screening persons aged 55 to 74 years who have cigarette smoking histories of 30 or more pack-years and who, if they are former smokers, have quit within the last 15 years reduces lung cancer mortality by 20% and all-cause mortality by 6.7%.
Oral	Insufficient evidence for/ against screening.		There is inadequate evidence to establish that screening would result in a decrease in mortality from oral cancer.

(continued)

TABLE 4-4. (CONTINUED)

	USPSTF		NCI
Ovarian	Recommend against screening.		There is inadequate evidence to determine whether routine screening for ovarian cancer with serum markers such as CA-125 (Cancer Antigen 125) transvaginal ultrasound, or pelvic exams would result in decreased mortality from ovarian cancer.
Pancreatic	Recommend against screening.		
Prostate	The USPSTF recommends against PSA-based screening for prostate cancer.	Insufficient evidence to recommend screening average risk men. Recommend shared decision making (with discussion of potential benefits, limitations, and harms); PSA and DRE. should be offered every year, starting at age 50, for men w/life expectancy of at least 10 years. In high-risk men (sub-Saharan African descent, 1st-degree relative diagnosed <65 years), start testing age 45; in higher risk men (more than one 1st degree relative diagnosed <65 years), start testing age 40. If PSA >1.0 ng per milliliter but <2.5 ng per milliliter, test annually; if PSA ≥2.5 ng per milliliter, consider biopsy.	There is insufficient data to determine whether screening with prostate-specific antigen (PSA) or digital rectal exam (DRE) reduces mortality from prostate cancer. Screening tests are able to detect prostate cancer at an early stage; however, it is not clear whether earlier detection and treatment lead to any change in the disease's etiology and eventual patient outcome. Recent evidence suggests a trend toward lower mortality for prostate cancer in some countries; however, the relationship between these trends and the intensity of screening is still unclear. Screening patterns remain inconsistent. These trends may be due to screening, or to other medical or environmental factors such as new treatments or improved diets.
Skin (cutaneous melanoma, basal cell, squamous cell)	Insufficient evidence for/against counseling Insufficient evidence for/against screening w/total body skin exam.		In asymptomatic populations, the effect of visual skin exam on mortality from nonmelanomatous skin cancers is unknown. Further, in asymptomatic individuals, evidence is inadequate to determine whether visual skin exam would lead to a reduction in mortality from melanomatous skin cancer.

(continued)

TABLE 4-4. (CONTINUED)

	USPSTF	NCI
Testicular	Recommend against screening.	Based on fair evidence, screening for testicular cancer would not result in an appreciable decrease in mortality, in part because therapy at each stage is so effective.
Thyroid	[Currently being updated]	

CHEMOPREVENTION AND VACCINES

	USPSTF	NCI
Breast	SERM (tamoxifen/raloxifene) — recommend discussing with women with high risk family histories (FH; based on, e.g., Gail model) with low risk adverse effects; — recommended against in women with low/average risk FH.	Based on solid evidence for tamoxifen and fair evidence for raloxifene, treatment reduces the incidence of breast cancer in postmenopausal women. Tamoxifen also reduces the risk of breast cancer in high-risk premenopausal women. Effects were observed for tamoxifen and persistence several years after discontinuing active treatment.
Cervical	Routine HPV vaccination for females ages 11–12; as young as age 9; recommended for females age 13–18; insufficient evidence to recommend for or against universal vaccination of females ages 19–26, or for males of any age.	Based on fair evidence, vaccination against HPV-16/HPV-18 is effective to avoid HPV infection, and thus cervical cancer.
Colorectal	Recommend against ASA (acetylsalicylic acid or aspirin)/NSAID for prevention in average risk.	
Gastric		Based on solid evidence, *Helicobacter pylori* infection is associated with increased risk of gastric cancer; however, evidence is inadequate to determine if treatment with antibiotics reduces risk of gastric cancer. Evidence is inadequate to determine if dietary or antibiotic interventions will reduce the risk of gastric cancer. A chemoprevention trial in China reported statistically significant reduction of gastric cancer mortality after supplementation with beta carotene, vitamin E, and selenium (Blot et al., 1993).

(continued)

TABLE 4-4. (CONTINUED)

USPSTF	NCI
Hepatocellular	Based on solid evidence, immunization against hepatitis B would decrease the incidence of hepatocellular cancer (HCC).
Prostate	Based on solid evidence, chemoprevention with finasteride reduces the incidence of prostate cancer, but the evidence is inadequate to determine whether chemoprevention with finasteride reduces mortality from prostate cancer. Men in finasteride group had statistically significantly more erectile dysfunction, loss of libido, and gynecomastia than men in placebo group. Men in finasteride group had a statistically significant incidence of high-grade (Gleason 8–10) cancers. Whether this was histological artifact or not is uncertain.

Sources: Recommendations. US Preventive Services Task Force.
http://www.uspreventiveservicestaskforce.org/recommendations.htm;
http://www.uspreventiveservicestaskforce.org/prostatecancerscreening.
http://www.uspreventiveservicestaskforce.org/adultrec.htm;
http://www.cancer.org/healthy/findcancerearly/cancerscreeningguidelines/american-cancer-society-guidelines-for-the-early-detection-of-cancer.
http://www.cancer.gov/cancertopics/screening.

CANCER PREVENTION ACCORDING TO SUBSTANCE EXPOSURE

Tobacco

About one-third of all cancer deaths in developed countries are attributed to tobacco exposure (Peto & Lopez, 2001). Half of all those who continue to smoke will die from smoking-related diseases (Peto et al., 2004). Tobacco use represents the single largest preventable cause of cancer deaths in the United States (ACS, 2013), and is responsible for nearly 1 in 5 deaths (Mokdad et al., 2004; CDC, 2008; CDC, 2003; ACS, 2013). In addition, an estimated 8.6 million people suffer from chronic conditions related to smoking, such as chronic bronchitis, emphysema, and cardiovascular disease (CDC, 2003).

Secondhand smoke exposure has been classified as a known carcinogen by the US Environmental Protection Agency (EPA), the US National Toxicology Program (NPT), the US Surgeon General, and the International Agency for Research on Cancer (IARC). There is no safe level of secondhand smoke exposure. It is estimated that a non-smoker's risk of lung cancer is increased 20–30% by living with a smoker. Many state and local governments have banned smoking from public places such as hospitals, airports, and schools, as well has private workplaces such as restaurants and bars (NCI, 2000).

Alcohol

Drinking two or more drinks a day is associated with an increased risk of cancers of the mouth, throat, larynx, liver, and esophagus. Alcohol-associated risks are more pronounced among smokers than non-smokers. Some studies have demonstrated that heavy drinking is associated with increased risks of developing breast and colon cancers (IARC, 2010, 2012; Nelson et al., 2013; Baan et al., 2007; Hashibe et al., 2009; Grewal & Viswanathen, 2012; Hamajima et al., 2002; Allen et al., 2009; Fedirko et al., 2011; Bellocco et al., 2012; Tramacere et al., 2012; Turati et al., 2013; Druesne-Pecollo et al., 2009; Kanda et al., 2009; Yokoyama & Omori, 2005; Athaar et al., 2007; Patel et al., 2011; Rehm et al., 2007).

Ultraviolet (UV) Radiation Exposure

Skin cancer represents the most common type of cancer in the United States (NCI, http://www.cancer.gov/cancertopics/wyntk/skin). Sun exposure (ultraviolet [UV] radiation) leads to DNA damage that leads to melanoma and other forms of skin cancer (NCI, http://www.cancer.gov/cancertopics/wyntk/skin/page5). Findings from the National Information National Trends Survey (HINTS, 2005) indicate that sun safety behavior increases with age, and more women than men reported using sunscreen regularly. To avoid skin cancer, the CDC recommends that people seek shade, cover up, wear a hat, use at least SPF 15 sunscreen, and wear sunglasses with UV-B and UV-A protection (HINTS, 2005). The American Academy of Dermatology recommends the use of sunless tanning products as a substitute for tans induced by harmful UV rays (hints.cancer.gov).

Viruses, Medical Drugs, and Solvents

Hepatitis B (HBV) and hepatitis C (HCV) viral infections are a major cause of liver cancer; long-term infection with HCV increases the risk for certain types of non-Hodgkin lymphoma (http://www.cancer.gov/dictionary). Almost all cervical cancers are caused by persistent infections with oncogenic, or high-risk, types of human papillomavirus (HPV; Munoz et al.,2003); HPV is a major risk factor for anal cancers (http://www.cancer.gov/cancertopics/pdq/treatment/anal/Patient). HBV and HCV are spread by sharing needles with an infected person and being stuck accidentally by a needle contaminated with the virus. Infants born to infected mothers may also become infected with these viruses (http://www.cancer.gov/dictionary). HPV is transmitted most frequently via penetrative vaginal or anal intercourse, and is classified as a sexually transmitted infection (STI). In fact, HPV is one of the most common STIs in the US (review in: Sheinfeld Gorin, Glenn, & Perkins, 2011).

Some medical drugs are associated with increased risks of cancer. Estrogens, a hormonal replacement therapy following menopause, have been shown to increase the risk of endometrial cancer; the combination of estrogen/progesterone use is reported to be associated with increased risks of breast cancer; long-term use of combination oral contraceptives can increase the risk of early onset of breast and liver cancers. (Lemons & Goss, 2001; Henderson, Ross, & Bernstein, 1988).

Benzene, a solvent used in gasoline and cigarette smoke and used commonly by pharmaceutical, rubber, and leather industries, is known to cause leukemia in humans (Lan et al., 2004; http://dceg.cancer.gov/research/what-we-study/environment). Other solvents used as paint thinners, paint and grease removers and by the dry cleaning industry have shown to promote cancer in animal studies (Brown et al., 2002; Blair et al., 2003; Vaughan et al., 1997).

Fibers, Fine Particles, Dust, and Metals

Asbestos fiber exposure is known to cause mesothelioma and lung cancer and accounts for the largest percentage of occupational-related cancer (Rice & Heinemann, 2003; Agency for Toxic Substances and Disease Registry, 2009; National Toxicology Program, 2005; USEPA, 1984; IARC, 2013). Construction workers, electricians, and carpenters may experience high levels of asbestos exposure during renovations, repairs, and building demolitions (Rice & Heinemann, 2003; Agency for Toxic Substances and Disease Registry, 2009; National Toxicology Program, 2005; USEPA, 1984; IARC, 2013). Individuals involved in the rescue, recovery, and cleanup at the site of the September 11, 2001, attacks on the World Trade Center (WTC) in New York City are another group at risk of developing an asbestos-related disease. Because asbestos was used in the construction of the North Tower of the WTC, when the building was attacked, hundreds of tons of asbestos were released into the atmosphere (Landrigan et al., 2004; Herbert et al., 2006). In addition, occupational exposures such as arsenic, nickel, and chromium are causally associated with lung cancer (Agency for Toxic Substances and Disease Registry, 2013).

Ceramic fibers, used to line furnaces and kilns, and silica dusts, found in industrial settings such as coal mines and granite quarrying industries, are associated with increased risk of lung cancer (Baccarelli et al., 2006; Agency for Toxic Substances and Disease Registry, 2013). Moreover, wood dust exposure, common among sanding operations and furniture industries, is related to increased nasal cavity and sinus cancers (Agency for Toxic Substances and Disease Registry, 2013). See Table 4-5 for a description of metals as risk factors for cancer.

PREVENTIVE THERAPIES FOR HIGH-RISK PATIENTS
Chemoprevention

A number of trials have shown that 5 years of adjuvant tamoxifen, an estrogen receptor modulator, safely reduces 15-year risks of breast cancer recurrence and death. A recent meta-analysis strengthened the evidence that substantially reduced mortality rates for breast cancer continue well beyond year 10, as a delayed effect of the greatly reduced recurrence rates during years 0–9. The effect is substantial even in disease that was only weakly ER positive, although not in disease that was wholly ER negative. The meta-analysis also confirmed that tamoxifen increases the risks of uterine cancer and of blood clots in the lungs (Early Breast Cancer Trialists' Collaborative Group [EBCTCG], 2011). The results of the Study of Tamoxifen and Raloxifene (STAR) program revealed that, for postmenopausal women at increased risk of breast cancer, raloxifene (another type of selective estrogen receptor modulator [SERM]). is just as effective as tamoxifen, without some of the serious side effects (Vogel et al., 2006; Land et al., 2006).

Chemoprevention among prostate cancer patients with finasteride and dutasteride reduces the incidence of prostate cancer, but the evidence is inadequate to determine whether chemoprevention with finasteride or dutasteride reduces mortality (Andriole et al., 2010) Further, finasteride appears to be associated with a statistically significant increase of high-grade (Gleason sum 8–10) prostate cancers (Thompson et al., 2003).

Gene Therapy

Gene therapy encompasses a wide range of treatment types in which genetic materials are used to modify cells (either in vitro or in vivo) for cancer treatment (Mulligan, 1993). Mutated genes that cause disease are replaced with a healthy copy of the gene; a mutated gene is "knocked out" or inactivated if it is functioning improperly; or a new gene is introduced into the body to help fight disease (http://ghr.nlm.nih.gov/handbook/therapy/genetherapy).

Recent advances in the molecular and cellular biology of gene transfer have led gene therapy to

TABLE 4.5. METALS AS A RISK FACTOR FOR CANCER

Metal	Related Cancers	Present In	Workers Exposed
Arsenic	Skin, lung, bladder, kidney, liver	Wood preservatives, glass, pesticides	Ore smelting, pesticide application, wood preservation
Beryllium	Lung	Nuclear weapons, rocket fuel, ceramics, glass, plastic, fiber optic products	Ore miners, alloy makers, phosphor manufacturers, ceramic workers, missile technicians, nuclear reactor workers, electric and electric equipment workers, and jewelers
Cadmium	Lung	Metal coatings used to prevent erosion, plastics, batteries and fungicides	Smelting zinc and lead ores, and producing, processing and handling cadmium powders
Chromium	Lung	Anti-corrosive metal plating for automotive parts, pigments for floor covering and glass, paper, cement, and asphalt roofing	Stainless steel production, welding, chrome plating, and leather tanning
Lead	Kidney, brain	Cotton dyes, metal coatings, paint varnish and pigment drying agents, certain hair dyes, explosives, poison ivy washes	Construction and smelter workers
Nickel	Nasal cavity, lung, possibly larynx	Steel, dental fillings, copper and brass, storage batteries, permanent magnets	Battery makers, ceramic makers, jewelers, nickel mine workers, smelters, paint-related workers, electroplaters, enamelers

TABLE 4.6.[*] AMERICAN CANCER SOCIETY (ACS) GENERAL NUTRITION AND PHYSICAL ACTIVITY RECOMMENDATIONS FOR CANCER PREVENTION

Nutrition:	- Maintain a healthy weight - Balance caloric intake with physical activity - Avoid excessive weight gain throughout life - Achieve and maintain a healthy weight if currently overweight/obese - Eat 5 or more servings of a variety of fruits and vegetables each day - Choose whole grains over processed grains - Limit intake of processed and red meats Being overweight or obese is clearly linked with the following cancer types: - breast (post-menopausal women) - colon - endrometrium (uterus) - esophagus - kidney
Physical Activity:	- Adults: Engage in at least 30 minutes (45–60 minutes is preferable) of moderate to vigorous activity, 5 or more days of the week. - Children and adolescents: Engage in at least 60 minutes/day of moderate to vigorous physical activity, at least 5 days/week. Physical activity may reduce the following cancer types: - breast - colon - endrometrium - prostate
Alcohol:	- Women: Limit intake to no more than 1 drink/day - Men: Limit intake to no more than 2 drinks/day Alcohol is known to cause the following cancer types: - mouth - pharynx (throat) - larynx - esophagus - liver - breast

[*] Adapted from (ACS, 2011c)

play an increasing role in the treatment of cancer. For example, recently, scientists identified 10 mutations in the genome of a woman that led to her development of leukemia (Grady, 2008); some of these could begin to inform her treatment.

To increase information about the myriad of disease-specific tests that are now available, in 2012, the NIH created a Genetic Testing Registry, a database of genetic tests that are voluntarily submitted by test producers (http://www.ncbi.nlm.nih.gov/gtr/). Genetic testing for individuals with high risk of breast cancer or colon cancer may be the most widely used in oncology (Keogh et al., in press; Sherman et al., in press; Gerber & Offit, 2005; Lindor et al., 2008; Riley et al., 2012; Robson et al., 2010). Over the next decade, findings from genetic (as well as genomic and proteomic) testing and additional technological developments may lead to new gene therapies based on a detailed, individualized genetic picture of each cancer patient in clinical practice (see chapters 8 and 12 on "personalized medicine").

Nutrition Therapy

Over 50% of the patients with cancer will eventually need surgery, which in turn would impact patients' digestive functions. Nutrition also contributes to patients' recovery from surgery, and is critical for those malnourished patients with cancer. See Tables 4-6 and 4-7 for recommendations regarding nutrition and physical activity.

Diet
Breast Cancer

Diet has been linked with risk reduction among women with breast cancer, although the data are inconsistent. Women who had completed their initial therapy <70 years of age, who ate a low-fat diet rich in fruits, vegetables, and fiber, did not reduce their risk of recurrence, compared with women who ate 5 or more fruits and vegetable servings a day (Pierce et al., 2007). The Women's Intervention Nutrition Study (WINS) suggests that a low-fat diet may help prevent breast cancer recurrence in some women (Hoy et al., 2009). The interim data from 2,437 women ages 48 to 79 report breast cancer recurrences in 9.8% of the women eating low-fat diets, and 12.4% of women eating a standard diet. (This is a 24% decreased relative risk reduction for women on the low-fat diet.) The largest risk reduction, 42%, was among women on the low-fat diet with ER- tumors (with only a 15% reduction among women with ER+ tumors). Other studies have suggested that

TABLE 4-7.* AMERICAN CANCER SOCIETY (ACS) NUTRITION AND PHYSICAL ACTIVITY RECOMMENDATIONS FOR CANCER PREVENTION: REDUCING RISK ACCORDING TO CANCER TYPE

Breast Cancer	- Engage in moderate to vigorous physical activity 45–60 minutes, 5 or more days/week - Reduce lifetime weight gain by limiting calories and maintaining regular physical exercise. - Avoid or limit intake of alcoholic beverages
Colorectal Cancer	- Regular physical activity - Limit intake of processed and red meats - Maintain recommended calcium intake - Eat at least 5 servings of fruits and vegetables per day - Avoid obesity - Avoid excess alcohol
Kidney Cancer	- Maintain a healthy weight and avoid alcohol
Lung Cancer	- Avoid tobacco use and secondhand smoke - Avoid radon exposure - Eat at least 5 servings of fruits and vegetables per day
Mouth, throat, and esophagus cancers	- Avoid all forms of tobacco - Restrict alcohol intake - Avoid obesity - Eat at least 5 servings of fruits and vegetables per day
Prostate Cancer	- Eat at least 5 servings of fruits and vegetables per day - Limit intake of red meats and dairy products - Maintain an active lifestyle and healthy weight
Stomach Cancer	- Eat at least 5 servings of fruits and vegetables per day - Reduce intake of foods preserved with salt - Maintain a healthy weight

* Adapted from (ACS, 2011c)

lower levels of fat intake are associated with lower breast cancer recurrence and better survival.

Colon Cancer

The findings for dietary influences on colorectal cancer prevention are similarly inconsistent. The Polyp Prevention Trial examined the effect of diet on the growth of new colorectal polyps of men or women (n = 2,079) who had one or more polyps removed within the prior 6 months. Participants were randomized to counseling for low-fat, high fiber, fruit- and vegetable-enriched eating versus a standard brochure on healthy eating. Dietary changes did not reduce the number of new polyps the participants developed (Schatzkin et al., 2000). In the Wheat Brain Fiber Study (n = 1,429 men and women), those who had one or more polyps removed within the prior 3 months were randomized to a high wheat bran fiber cereal supplement or low wheat bran fiber cereal supplement. Subjects were given supplements for at least 3 years. The results found that a low-fat, high-fiber, fruit- and vegetable-enriched eating plan did not reduce the recurrence of colorectal polyps.

According to the American Cancer Society, a high-fat diet, heavy with red meat, fatty foods, and desserts, can raise a person's risk of developing colon cancer. For example, individuals diagnosed with Stage III colon cancer on a "prudent" diet of fish, poultry, fruits and vegetables were compared with those eating a "Western" diet that was high in meat, fat, processed grains, French fries, and desserts (Meyerhardt et al., 2007). Participants were asked about their eating habits 6 months after chemotherapy; participants were followed for an average of 5 years post-chemotherapy. People who ate the most Western diets had almost 3 times the risk of their colon cancer returning compared to those whose diets were least Western (Meyerhardt et al., 2007).

People with a family history of colon cancer may reduce their chances of developing the disease by taking folate (Fuchs et al., 2002). Of 88,758 women in the Nurses Health Study, people with familial history were twice as likely to develop the disease as those without. However, among those with a family history of colon cancer, those who consumed 400 mcg of folate daily were half as likely to get colon cancer as those who took 200 mcg or less. Folate decreases methylation (that is key to the production of working normal genes).

Prostate Cancer

Older men with early-stage prostate cancer are actually at higher risk of death from heart disease than from prostate cancer. The Selenium and Vitamin E Cancer Prevention Trial (SELECT) found that taking selenium and vitamin E supplements daily did not prevent prostate cancer (Dunn et al., 2010). The trial was halted due to concerns from preliminary results that suggested a higher incidence of diabetes mellitus in men who took selenium.

Pancreatic Cancer

In addition to smoking (Iodice et al., 2008; Anderson et al., 2006; Lynch et al., 2009; Bosetti et al., 2012), being overweight, especially in the mid-section, increases the risk of pancreatic cancer (Patel et al., 2005). Researchers suspect that this distribution of body weight is a factor because weight influences insulin production and the chance of developing diabetes, which is also a risk factor for pancreatic cancer (Pannala et al., 2008; Chari et al., 2008; Huxley et al., 2005). Obese individuals have a 20% higher risk of developing pancreatic cancer than those who are normal weight (Berrington et al., 2003; Michaud et al., 2001; Arslan et al., 2010). Obesity during adolescence may confer increased risk for pancreatic cancer (Li et al., 2009).

CONCLUSIONS

Cigarette smoking causes an estimated 443,000 deaths each year, including approximately 49,000 deaths due to exposure to secondhand smoke (CDC, 2012; NCI, 2013). It has been estimated by the World Cancer Research Fund that one-quarter to one-third of the cancers that occur in high-income countries like the US are due to poor nutrition, physical inactivity, and excess weight, and thus could be prevented (ACS, 2013). Cancer screening is one of the most important preventive health services. The US National Cancer Institute reports that about 35% of premature cancer deaths could have been prevented through screening tests. Being adherent to screening recommendations can prevent the development of cancer through the identification and removal or treatment of pre-malignant abnormalities in early stages and therefore can improve survival and decrease mortality. Systematic efforts such as decreasing cigarette smoking, reducing obesity, improving diet, increasing physical activity, and adhering to screening test recommendations can both prevent cancer and reduce deaths from cancer.

REFERENCES

Aberle DR, et al. Reduced lung-cancer mortality with low-dose computed tomographic screening. *N Engl J Med.* 2011;*365*(5):395–409.

Aberle DR, Adams AM, Berg CD, Black WC, Clapp JD, Fagerstrom RM, et al. National Lung Screening Trial Research Team. Reduced lung-cancer mortality with low-dose computed tomographic screening. *N Engl J Med.* 2011; *365*:395–409.

ACOG, American College of Obstetricians-Gynecologists. Practice bulletin no. 122. Breast cancer screening. *Obstet Gynecol.* 2011;*118*(2 Pt 1):372–382.

ACS, American Cancer Society. *Cancer Prevention & Early Detection Facts & Figures 2011.* 2011a. Retrieved October 1, 2011, from http://www.cancer.org/acs/groups/content/@epidemiologysurveilance/documents/document/acspc-029459.pdf.

ACS, American Cancer Society. *Cervical Cancer: Prevention and Early Detection.* 2011b. Retrieved October 1, 2011, from http://www.cancer.org/acs/groups/cid/documents/webcontent/003167-pdf.pdf.

ACS, American Cancer Society. *American Cancer Society Guidelines on Nutrition and Physical Activity for Cancer Prevention.* 2011c. Retrieved October 1, 2011, from http://www.cancer.org/acs/groups/cid/documents/webcontent/002577-pdf.

Agency for Toxic Substances and Disease Registry. Cancer and the Environment. Accessed April 13, 2013 from: http://www.atsdr.cdc.gov/risk/cancer/cancer-substances2.html

Agency for Toxic Substances and Disease Registry. Toxicological Profile for Asbestos. September 2001. Retrieved April 10, 2013, from: http://www.atsdr.cdc.gov/toxprofiles/tp61.pdf

Allen NE, Beral V, Casabonne D, et al. Moderate alcohol intake and cancer incidence in women. *J National Cancer Institute.* 2009;*101*(5):296–305.

American Cancer Society. Cancer Facts & Figures 2013. Atlanta: American Cancer Society; 2013. http://www.cancer.org/acs/groups/content/@epidemiologysurveilance/documents/document/acspc-036845.pdf

Anderson K, Potter JD, Mack TM. Pancreatic cancer. In: Schottenfeld D, Fraumeni JF, eds. *Cancer Epidemiology and Prevention,* pp. 721–762. New York: Oxford University Press; 2006.

Andriole GL, Bostwick DG, Brawley OW, et al. Effect of dutasteride on the risk of prostate cancer. *N Engl J Med.* 2010;*362*(13):1192–1202.

Armstrong K, et al. Screening mammography in women 40 to 49 years of age: a systematic review for the American College of Physicians. *Ann Intern Med.* 2007;*146*(7):516–526.

Arslan AA, Helzlsouer KJ, Kooperberg C, et al. Anthropometric measures, body mass index, and pancreatic cancer: a pooled analysis from the Pancreatic Cancer Cohort Consortium (PanScan). *Arch Intern Med.* 2010;*170*(9): 791–802.

Athar M, Back JH, Tang X, et al. Resveratrol: a review of preclinical studies for human cancer prevention. *Toxicology and Applied Pharmacology.* 2007; *224*(3):274–283.

Atkin WS, et al. Once-only flexible sigmoidoscopy screening in prevention of colorectal cancer: a multicentre randomised controlled trial. *Lancet.* 2010;*375*(9726):1624–1633.

Baan R, Straif K, Grosse Y, et al. Carcinogenicity of alcoholic beverages Exit Disclaimer. *Lancet Oncology.* 2007;*8*(4):292–293.

Baccarelli A, Khmelnitskii O, Tretiakova M, Gorbanev S, Lomtev A, Klimkina I, Tchibissov V, Averkina O, Rice C, Dosemeci M. Risk of lung cancer from exposure to dusts and fibers in Leningrad Province, Russia. *Am J Ind Med.* 2006;*49*(6):460–467.

Barry MJ. Screening for Prostate Cancer—The Controversy That Refuses to Die. *N Engl J Med* 2009;*360*:1351–1354.

Baxter N. Preventive health care, 2001 update: should women be routinely taught breast self-examination to screen for breast cancer? *CMAJ.* 2001;*164*(13): 1837–1846.

Bellocco R, Pasquali E, Rota M, et al. Alcohol drinking and risk of renal cell carcinoma: results of a meta-analysis. *Annals of Oncology.* 2012;*23*(9):2235–2244.

Berrington de Gonzalez A, Sweetland S, Spencer E. A meta-analysis of obesity and the risk of pancreatic cancer. *Br J Cancer* 2003;*89*(3):519–523.

Bill-Axelson A, et al. Radical prostatectomy versus watchful waiting in early prostate cancer. *N Engl J Med.* 2005;*352*(19):1977–1984.

Blair A, Petralia SA, Stewart PA. Extended mortality follow-up of a cohort of dry cleaners. *Ann Epidemiol.* 2003;*13*(1):50–56.

Blot WJ, Li J-Y, Taylor PR, et al. Nutrition Intervention Trials in Linxian, China: Supplementation with specific vitamin/mineral combinations, cancer incidence, and disease-specific mortality in the general population. *J Natl Cancer Inst.* 1993;*85*:1483–1492.

Bondy ML, et al. Validation of a breast cancer risk assessment model in women with a positive family history. *J Natl Cancer Inst.* 1994;*86*(8):620–625.

Bosetti C, Lucenteforte E, Silverman DT, et al. Cigarette smoking and pancreatic cancer: an analysis from the International Pancreatic Cancer Case-Control Consortium (Panc4). *Ann Oncol.* 2012;*23*(7):1880–1888.

Brown LM, Moradi T, Gridley G, Plato N, Dosemeci M, Fraumeni JF Jr. Exposures in the painting trades and paint manufacturing industry and risk of cancer among men and women in Sweden. *J Occup Environ Med.* 2002;*44*(3):258–264.

Centers for Disease Control and Prevention. Cigarette smoking: attributable morbidity—United States, 2000. *MMWR Morb Mortal Wkly Rep.* 2003;*52*(35):842–844.

Centers for Disease Control and Prevention. Smoking: attributable mortality, years of potential life lost, and productivity losses—United States, 2000–2004. *MMWR Morb Mortal Wkly Rep.* Nov 14 2008;*57*(45):1226–1228.

CervicalCancer.org. *Risk Factors for Cervical Cancer.* 2006. Retrieved October 1, 2011, from http://www.cervicalcancer.org/riskfactors.html.

Chan EC, Sulmasy DP. What should men know about prostate-specific antigen screening before giving informed consent? *Am J Med.* 1998;*105*(4): 266–274.

Chan JM, et al. Plasma insulin-like growth factor-I and prostate cancer risk: a prospective study. *Science.* 1998;*279*(5350):563–566.

Chari ST, Leibson CL, Rabe KG, et al. Pancreatic cancer-associated diabetes mellitus: prevalence and temporal association with diagnosis of cancer. *Gastroenterology.* 2008;*134*(1):95–101.

Chen C, et al. Prostate carcinoma incidence in relation to prediagnostic circulating levels of insulin-like growth factor I, insulin-like growth factor binding protein 3, and insulin. *Cancer.* 2005;*103*(1):76–84.

Chodak GW, Schoenberg HW. Early detection of prostate cancer by routine screening. *JAMA.* 1984;*252*(23):3261–3264.

Clinton SK, Giovannucci E. Diet, nutrition, and prostate cancer. *Annu Rev Nutr.* 1998;*18*:413–440.

Druesne-Pecollo N, Tehard B, Mallet Y, et al. Alcohol and genetic polymorphisms: effect on risk of alcohol-related cancer. *Lancet Oncology.* 2009;*10*(2):173–180.

Dunn BK, et al. A nutrient approach to prostate cancer prevention: The Selenium and Vitamin E Cancer Prevention Trial (SELECT). *Nutr Cancer.* 2010;*62*(7):896–918.

Early Breast Cancer Trialists' Collaborative Group (EBCTCG), Davies C, Godwin J, Gray R, Clarke M, Cutter D, Darby S, McGale P, Pan HC, Taylor C, Wang YC, Dowsett M, Ingle J, Peto R. et al. Collaborators (693). Relevance of breast cancer hormone receptors and other factors to the efficacy of adjuvant tamoxifen: patient-level meta-analysis of randomised trial. *Lancet.* 2011;*378*(9793):771–784.

EC, European Commission. *Recommendations on Cancer Screening in the European Union.* 1999. Retrieved October 1, 2011, from http://ec.europa.eu/health/ph_determinants/genetics/cancer_screening_en.pdf.

Eichholzer M, et al. Prediction of male cancer mortality by plasma levels of interacting vitamins: 17-year follow-up of the prospective Basel study. *Int J Cancer.* 1996;*66*(2):145–150.

Fedirko V, Tramacere I, Bagnardi V, et al. Alcohol drinking and colorectal cancer risk: an overall and dose-response meta-analysis of published studies. *Annals of Oncology.* 2011;*22*(9):1958–1972.

Fleshner NE, Klotz LH. Diet, androgens, oxidative stress and prostate cancer susceptibility. *Cancer Metastasis Rev.* 1998;*17*(4):325–330.

Fuchs CS, et al. The influence of folate and multivitamin use on the familial risk of colon cancer in women. *Cancer Epidemiol Biomarkers Prev.* 2002;*11*(3):227–234.

Gail MH, et al. Projecting individualized probabilities of developing breast cancer for white females who are being examined annually. *J Natl Cancer Inst.* 1989;81(24):1879–1886.

Gann PH, Hennekens CH, Stampfer MJ. A prospective evaluation of plasma prostate-specific antigen for detection of prostatic cancer. *JAMA.* 1995;273(4):289–294.

Gann PH, et al. Prospective study of plasma fatty acids and risk of prostate cancer. *J Natl Cancer Inst.* 1994;86(4):281–286.

Garber J, Offit K. Hereditary cancer predisposition syndromes. *J Clinical Oncology.* 2005;23(2):276–292.

Gatto NM, et al. Risk of perforation after colonoscopy and sigmoidoscopy: a population-based study. *J Natl Cancer Inst.* 2003;95(3):230–236.

Gilbertsen VA. Cancer of the prostate gland. Results of early diagnosis and therapy undertaken for cure of the disease. *JAMA.* 1971;215(1):81–84.

Grady D. Scientists decode set of cancer genes. 2008. Retrieved October 1, 2011, from http://www.nytimes.com/2008/11/06/health/research/06cancer.html?ref=health.

Grewal P, Viswanathen VA. Liver cancer and alcohol. *Clinics in Liver Disease* 2012;16(4):839–850.

Hamajima N, Hirose K, Tajima K, et al. Alcohol, tobacco and breast cancer: collaborative reanalysis of individual data from 53 epidemiological studies, including 58,515 women with breast cancer and 95,067 women without the disease. *British J Cancer* 2002;87(11):1234–1245.

Harris R, Lohr KN. Screening for prostate cancer: an update of the evidence for the U.S. Preventive Services Task Force. *Ann Intern Med.* 2002;137(11):917–929.

Hashibe M, Brennan P, Chuang SC, et al. Interaction between tobacco and alcohol use and the risk of head and neck cancer: pooled analysis in the International Head and Neck Cancer Epidemiology Consortium. *Cancer Epidemiology, Biomarkers & Prevention.* 2009;18(2):541–550.

Hayes RB, et al. Alcohol use and prostate cancer risk in US blacks and whites. *Am J Epidemiol.* 1996;143(7): 692–697.

Henderson BE, Ross R, Bernstein L. Special Lecture. Estrogens as a cause of human cancer: The Richard and Hinda Rosenthal Foundation Award Lecture. *Cancer Res.* 1988;48:246–253.

Herbert R, Moline J, Skloot G, et al. The World Trade Center disaster and the health of workers: five-year assessment of a unique medical screening program. *Environmental Health Perspectives.* 2006;114(12):1853–1858.

Heron M. Deaths: leading causes for 2007. *Natl Vital Stat Rep.* 2011;59(8):1–95.

Holmberg L, et al. A randomized trial comparing radical prostatectomy with watchful waiting in early prostate cancer. *N Engl J Med.* 2002;347(11):781–789.

Howlader N, et al. *SEER Cancer Statistics Review, 1975–2008.* 2011. Retrieved October 1, 2011, from http://seer.cancer.gov/csr/1975_2008/.

Howlader N, Noone AM, Krapcho M, Garshell J, Neyman N, Altekruse SF, Kosary CL, Yu M, Ruhl J, Tatalovich Z, Cho H, Mariotto A, Lewis DR, Chen HS, Feuer EJ, Cronin KA (eds). *SEER Cancer Statistics Review, 1975-2010, National Cancer Institute.* Bethesda, MD, http://seer.cancer.gov/csr/1975_2010/, based on November 2012 SEER data submission, posted to the SEER web site, 2013.

Hoy MK, et al. Implementing a low-fat eating plan in the Women's Intervention Nutrition Study. *J Am Diet Assoc.* 2009;109(4):688–696.

Humphrey LL, Johnson M, Teutsch S. *Lung Cancer Screening: An Update for the U.S. Preventive Services Task Force. Systematic Evidence Review No. 31* (2010/08/20 ed.). Rockville, MD: Agency for Healthcare Research and Quality; 2004.

Humphrey LL, et al. Breast cancer screening: a summary of the evidence for the U.S. Preventive Services Task Force. *Ann Intern Med.* 2002;137(5 Part 1):347–360.

Humphrey, LL, Deffebach, M, Pappas, M, Baumann, C, Artis, K, Mitchell, JP, Zakher, B, Fu, R, Slatore, CG. Screening for lung cancer with low-dose computed tomography: a systematic review to update the U.S. Preventive Services Task Force Recommendation. *Ann Intern Med.* 2013.

Huxley R, Ansary-Moghaddam A, Berrington de Gonzalez A, Barzi F, Woodward M. Type-II diabetes and pancreatic cancer: a meta-analysis of 36 studies. *British J Cancer.* 2005;92(11):2076–2083.

IARC Working Group on the Evaluation of Carcinogenic Risks to Humans. Alcohol consumption and ethyl carbamate Exit Disclaimer. *IARC Monographs on the Evaluation of Carcinogenic Risks in Humans.* 2010;96:3–1383.

IARC Working Group on the Evaluation of Carcinogenic Risks to Humans. Personal habits and indoor combustions. Volume 100 E. A review of human carcinogens. Exit Disclaimer. *IARC Monographs on the Evaluation of Carcinogenic Risks in Humans.* 2012;100(Pt E):373–472.

International Agency for Research on Cancer. Asbestos. IARC Monographs on the Evaluation of Carcinogenic Risks to Humans, vol. 14. Lyon, France. Retrieved April 10, 2013, from: http://monographs.iarc.fr/ENG/Monographs/vol14/volume14.pdf Exit Disclaimer.

Iodice S, Gandini S, Maisonneuve P, Lowenfels AB. Tobacco and the risk of pancreatic cancer: a review and meta-analysis. *Langenbecks Arch Surg.* 2008; 393(4):535–545.

Jemal A, et al. Cancer statistics, 2008. *CA Cancer J Clin.* 2008;58(2):71–96.

Jenson CB, Shahon DB, Wangensteen OH. Evaluation of annual examinations in the detection of cancer: special reference to cancer of the gastrointestinal tract, prostate, breast, and female generative tract. *JAMA.* 1960;174:1783–1788.

Joel Hillhouse GC, et al. Investigating the role of appearance-based factors in predicting sunbathing and tanning salon use. *J Behav Med.* 2009;32(6): 532–544.

Kagawa-Singer M, et al. Cancer, culture, and health disparities: time to chart a new course? *CA Cancer J Clin.* 2010;60(1):12–39.

Kanda J, Matsuo K, Suzuki T, et al. Impact of alcohol consumption with polymorphisms in alcohol-metabolizing enzymes on pancreatic cancer risk in Japanese. *Cancer Science.* 2009;100(2):296–302.

Keogh LA, Fisher D, Sheinfeld Gorin S, Schully SD, Lowery JT, Ahnen DJ, Maskiell JA, Lindor NM, Hopper JL, Burnett T, Holter S, Arnold JL, Gallinger S, Laurino M, Esplen MJ, Sinicrope PS, Colon Cancer Family Registry. How do researchers manage genetic results in practice? The experience of the multinational Colon Cancer Family Registry. *J Community Genetics* (in press).

Kerlikowske K, et al. Continuing screening mammography in women aged 70 to 79 years: impact on life expectancy and cost-effectiveness. *JAMA.* 1999;282(22):2156–2163.

Kerlikowske K, et al. Performance of screening mammography among women with and without a first-degree relative with breast cancer. *Ann Intern Med.* 2000;133(11):855–863.

Kramer BS. The science of early detection. *Urol Oncol.* 2004;22(4): 344–347.

Lan Q, Zhang L, Li G, et al. Hematotoxicity in workers exposed to low levels of benzene. *Science.* 2004;306(5702):1774–1776.

Land SR, Wickerham DL, et al. Patient-reported symptoms and quality of life during treatment with tamoxifen or raloxifene for breast cancer prevention: the NSABP Study of Tamoxifen and Raloxifene (STAR) P-2 Trial. *JAMA.* 2006;295:2742–2751.

Landrigan PJ, Lioy PJ, Thurston G, et al. Health and environmental consequences of the World Trade Center disaster. *Environmental Health Perspectives.* 2004; 112(6):731–739.

Lemons MC, Goss P. Estrogen and the risk of breast cancer. *New Engl J Med.* 2001;344:276–285.

Li D, Morris JS, Liu J, et al. Body mass index and risk, age of onset, and survival in patients with pancreatic cancer. *JAMA.* 2009;301(24):2553–2562.

Lin K, et al. Benefits and harms of prostate-specific antigen screening for prostate cancer: an evidence update for the U.S. Preventive Services Task Force. *Ann Intern Med.* 2008;149(3):192–199.

Lindor NM, McMaster ML, Lindor CJ, Greene MH. Concise handbook of familial cancer susceptibility syndromes. 2nd ed. *J National Cancer Institute Monographs.* 2008;38:1–93.

London SJ, et al. A prospective study of benign breast disease and the risk of breast cancer. *JAMA.* 1992;267(7):941–944.

Lynch SM, Vrieling A, Lubin JH, et al. Cigarette smoking and pancreatic cancer: a pooled analysis from the pancreatic cancer cohort consortium. *Am J Epidemiol.* 2009;170(4): 403–413.

Mandelblatt J, et al. The cost-effectiveness of screening mammography beyond age 65 years: a systematic review for the U.S. Preventive Services Task Force. *Ann Intern Med.* 2003;139(10):835–842.

Matikainen MP, et al. Detection of subclinical cancers by prostate-specific antigen screening in asymptomatic men from high-risk prostate cancer families. *Clin Cancer Res.* 1999;5(6):1275–1279.

Mayo Clinic. Prostate cancer screening: should you get a PSA test? 2010. Retrieved October 1, 2011, from http://www.mayoclinic.com/health/prostate-cancer/HQ01273.

McDivitt RW, et al. Histologic types of benign breast disease and the risk for breast cancer: The Cancer and Steroid Hormone Study Group. *Cancer.* 1992;69(6):1408–1414.

Meyerhardt JA, et al. Association of dietary patterns with cancer recurrence and survival in patients with stage III colon cancer. *JAMA.* 2007;298(7):754–764.

Michaud DS, Giovannucci E, Willett WC, Colditz GA, Stampfer MJ, Fuchs CS. Physical activity, obesity, height, and the risk of pancreatic cancer. *JAMA.* 2001;286(8):921–929.

Miller AB, et al. Canadian National Breast Screening Study: 1. Breast cancer detection and death rates among women aged 40 to 49 years. *CMAJ.* 1992;147(10):1459–1476.

Mokdad AH, Marks JS, Stroup DF, Gerberding JL. Actual causes of death in the United States, 2000. *JAMA.* 2004;291(10):1238–1245.

Morton MS, Griffiths K, Blacklock N. The preventive role of diet in prostatic disease. *Br J Urol.* 1996;77(4):481–493.

Mulligan RC. The basic science of gene therapy. *Science.* 1993;260(5110):926–932.

Muñoz N, Bosch FX, de Sanjosé S, et al. Epidemiologic classification of human papillomavirus types associated with cervical cancer. *N Engl J Med.* 2003;348:518–527.

National Cancer Institute. Surveillance, Epidemiology and End Results (SEER) Program. http://seer.cancer.gov/

National Cancer Institute. *State and Local Legislative Action to Reduce Tobacco Use. Smoking and Tobacco Control Monograph No. 11.* Bethesda, M: US Department of Health and Human Services, National Institutes of Health, National Cancer Institute NIH Pub. No. 00-4804; 2000.

National Cancer Institute. *Cervical Cancer Screening (PDQ®).* 2011a. Retrieved October 1, 2011, from http://www.cancer.gov/cancertopics/pdq/screening/cervical/HealthProfessional/page2.

National Cancer Institute. *Cancer Prevention Overview.* 2011b. Retrieved October 1, 2011, from http://

www.cancer.gov/cancertopics/pdq/prevention/ overview/HealthProfessional.

National Toxicology Program. Asbestos. In: Report on Carcinogens. Eleventh Edition. U.S. Department of Health and Human Services, Public Health Service, National Toxicology Program, 2005.

NCI Fact Sheet. *Secondhand Smoke and Cancer.* Accessed April 13, 2013, from http://www.cancer.gov/ cancertopics/tobacco/statisticssnapshot#2.

Nelson DE, Jarman DW, Rehm J, et al. Alcohol-attributable cancer deaths and years of potential life lost in the United States. *Am J Public Health.* 2013;*103*(4): 641–648.

Oken MM, Hocking WG, Kvale PA, et al; PLCO Project Team. Screening by chest radiograph and lung cancer mortality: the Prostate, lung, colorectal, and ovarian (PLCO) randomized trial. *JAMA.* 2011;*306*:1865–1873.

Oliver SE, et al. Serum insulin-like growth factor-I is positively associated with serum prostate-specific antigen in middle-aged men without evidence of prostate cancer. *Cancer Epidemiol Biomarkers Prev.* 2004;*13*(1):163–165.

Oza AM, Boyd NF. Mammographic parenchymal patterns: a marker of breast cancer risk. *Epidemiol Rev.* 1993;*15*(1):196–208.

Pannala R, Leirness JB, Bamlet WR, Basu A, Petersen GM, Chari ST. Prevalence and clinical profile of pancreatic cancer-associated diabetes mellitus. *Gastroenterology.* 2008;*134*(4): 981–987.

Patel AV, et al. Obesity, recreational physical activity, and risk of pancreatic cancer in a large U.S. Cohort. *Cancer Epidemiol Biomarkers Prev.* 2005;*14*(2):459–466.

Patel KR, Scott E, Brown VA, et al. Clinical trials of resveratrol. *Annals of the New York Academy of Sciences.* 2011;*1215*:161–169.

Peto R, Lopez AD. Future worldwide health effects of current smoking patterns. In Koop CE, Pearson CE, Schwarz MR, eds. *Critical issues in global health.* San Francisco, CA: Jossey-Bass, 2001.

Peto R, Lopez A, Boreham J, Thun M, Heath CJ. *Mortality from Smoking in Developed Countries, 1950–2000.* New York: Oxford University Press; 1994.

Pfister DG, et al. Classifying clinical severity to help solve problems of stage migration in nonconcurrent comparisons of lung cancer therapy. *Cancer Res.* 1990;*50*(15):4664–4669.

Pierce JP, et al. Influence of a diet very high in vegetables, fruit, and fiber and low in fat on prognosis following treatment for breast cancer: the Women's Healthy Eating and Living (WHEL) randomized trial. *JAMA.* 2007;*298*(3):289–298.

Platz EA, et al. Alcohol intake, drinking patterns, and risk of prostate cancer in a large prospective cohort study. *Am J Epidemiol.* 2004;*159*(5):444–453.

Qaseem A, et al. Screening mammography for women 40 to 49 years of age: a clinical practice guideline from the American College of Physicians. *Ann Intern Med.* 2007;*146*(7):511–515.

Rehm J, Patra J, Popova S. Alcohol drinking cessation and its effect on esophageal and head and neck cancers: a pooled analysis. *Int J Cancer* 2007;*121*(5):1132–1137.

Rice C, Heineman EF. An asbestos job exposure matrix to characterize fiber type, length, and relative exposure intensity. *Appl Occup Environ Hyg.* 2003;*18*(7):506–512.

Ries LAG, et al. *SEER Cancer Statistics Review, 1975–2002.* 2005. Retrieved October 1, 2011, from http:// seer.cancer.gov/csr/1975_2002/.

Ries LAG, et al. *SEER Cancer Statistics Review, 1975–2000.* 2003. Retrieved October 1, 2011, from http:// seer.cancer.gov/csr/1975_2000.

Riley BD, Culver JO, Skrzynia C, et al. Essential elements of genetic cancer risk assessment, counseling, and testing: updated recommendations of the National Society of Genetic Counselors. *J Genetic Counseling.* 2012;*21*(2):151–161.

Robbins AS, Whittemore AS, Van Den Eeden SK. Race, prostate cancer survival, and membership in a large health maintenance organization. *J Natl Cancer Inst.* 1998;*90*(13):986–990.

Robson M, Storm C, Weitzel J, et al. American Society of Clinical Oncology Policy Statement update: genetic and genomic testing for cancer susceptibility. *J Clinical Oncology* 2010;*28*(5):893–901.

Sakr WA, et al. The frequency of carcinoma and intraepithelial neoplasia of the prostate in young male patients. *J Urol.* 1993;*150*(2 Pt 1):379–385.

Schatzkin A, et al. Lack of effect of a low-fat, high-fiber diet on the recurrence of colorectal adenomas. Polyp Prevention Trial Study Group. *N Engl J Med.* 2000;*342*(16):1149–1155.

SEER, Surveillance Epidemiology and End Results. 2011. Retrieved October 1, 2011, from http://seer. cancer.gov/.

Sheinfeld Gorin S, Glenn B, Perkins RB. The human papillomavirus (HPV) vaccine and cervical cancer: uptake and next steps. *Advances in Therapy.* 2011;(28)8:615–639.

Sherman KA, Miller SM, Shaw L, Cavanagh K, Sheinfeld Gorin S. Psychosocial approaches to participation in BRCA1/2 genetic risk assessment among African American women: a systematic review. *J Community Genetics* (in press).

Siegel R, et al. Cancer statistics, 2011: the impact of eliminating socioeconomic and racial disparities on premature cancer deaths. *CA Cancer J Clin.* 2011;*61*(4):212–236.

Smith-Bindman R, et al. Is screening mammography effective in elderly women? *Am J Med.* 2000;*108*(2): 112–119.

Smith RA, et al. American Cancer Society guidelines for breast cancer screening: update 2003. *CA Cancer J Clin.* 2003;*53*(3):141–169.

Soderstrom L, et al. Health and economic benefits of well-designed evaluations: some lessons from evaluating neuroblastoma screening. *J Natl Cancer Inst.* 2005;97(15):1118–1124.

Sorlie PD, Rogot E, Johnson NJ. Validity of demographic characteristics on the death certificate. *Epidemiology.* 1992;3(2):181–184.

Spiegelman D, et al. Validation of the Gail et al. model for predicting individual breast cancer risk. *J Natl Cancer Inst.* 1994;86(8):600–607.

Stattin P, et al. High levels of circulating insulin-like growth factor-I increase prostate cancer risk: a prospective study in a population-based nonscreened cohort. *J Clin Oncol.* 2004;22(15):3104–3112.

Stattin P, et al. Outcomes in localized prostate cancer: National Prostate Cancer Register of Sweden follow-up study. *J Natl Cancer Inst.* 2010;102(13):950–958.

Steinberg GD, et al. Family history and the risk of prostate cancer. *Prostate.* 1990;17(4):337–347.

Thompson IM, Goodman PJ, Tangen CM, et al. The influence of finasteride on the development of prostate cancer. *N Engl J Med.* 2003; 349(3):215–224.

Tramacere I, Pelucchi C, Bonifazi M, et al. A meta-analysis on alcohol drinking and the risk of Hodgkin lymphoma. *European J Cancer Prevention.* 2012;21(3):268–273.

Turati F, Garavello W, Tramacere I, et al. A meta-analysis of alcohol drinking and oral and pharyngeal cancers: results from subgroup analyses. *Alcohol and Alcoholism.* 2013;48(1):107–118.

Turkes A, Peeling WB, Griffiths K. Serum IGF-1 determination in relation to prostate cancer screening: possible differential diagnosis in relation to PSA assays. *Prostate Cancer Prostatic Dis.* 2000; 3(3):173–175.

Ueland AS, Hornung PA, Greenwald B. Colorectal cancer prevention and screening: a Health Belief Model-based research study to increase disease awareness. *Gastroenterol Nurs.* 2006;29(5):357–363.

Ugboma HAA, Aburoma HLS. Pap smear: an important screening technique for preventing and detecting cervical cancer. *Continental J Medical Research.* 2010;4:13–17.

U.S. Environmental Protection Agency. Health Effects Assessment for Asbestos. September 1984. EPA/540/1-86/049 (NTIS PB86134608). Retrieved April 10, 2013, from: http://cfpub.epa.gov/ncea/cfm/recordisplay.cfm?deid=40602.

USPSTF. *Screening for Colorectal Cancer.* 2008. Retrieved October 1, 2011, from http://www.uspreventiveservicestaskforce.org/uspstf/uspscolo.htm.

USPSTF. *Screening for Breast Cancer.* 2009. http://www.uspreventiveservicestaskforce.org/uspstf/uspsbrca.htm.

Vaughan TL, Stewart PA, Davis S, Thomas DB. Work in dry cleaning and the incidence of cancer of the oral cavity, larynx, and oesophagus. *Occup Environ Med.* 1997; 54(9):692–695.

Vogel VG, Constantino JP, et. al., for the National Surgical Adjuvant Breast and Bowel Project (NSABP). Effects of tamoxifen vs raloxifene on the risk of developing invasive breast cancer and other disease outcomes: the NSABP Study of Tamoxifen and Raloxifene (STAR) P-2 Trial. *JAMA.* 2006;295:2727–2741.

Walter LC, Covinsky KE. Cancer screening in elderly patients: a framework for individualized decision making. *JAMA.* 2001;285(21):2750–2756.

Yokoyama A, Omori T. Genetic polymorphisms of alcohol and aldehyde dehydrogenases and risk for esophageal and head and neck cancers Exit Disclaimer. *Alcohol.* 2005;35(3):175–185.

5

Cardiovascular Disease Prevention

SANDRA A TSAI, JOSEPH RAVENELL, SENAIDA FERNANDEZ, ANTOINETTE
SCHOENTHALER, KATHLEEN KENNY, AND GBENGA OGEDEGBE

INTRODUCTION

Affecting more than 80 million Americans at an estimated cost of $312.6 billion annually, cardiovascular
disease (CVD), which includes coronary heart disease
(CHD) and stroke, is easily one of the most important public health problems of our time (Go et al.,
2013). While significant therapeutic advances have
contributed to four decades of decline in death rates
from CVD, it remains the number one killer of men
and women, responsible for nearly 800,000 deaths
per year in 2009 (Go et al., 2013). Unfortunately,
increases in body mass index (BMI) and prevalence
of diabetes have partially offset reductions in CHD
mortality (Ford et al., 2007). Thus, CVD prevention is paramount to fulfilling the national health care
goals to reduce preventable deaths (US Department
of Health and Human Services, 2008).

Longitudinal studies (including the Framingham
Heart Study, the National Health and Nutrition
Examination Survey [NHANES], and the Nurses
Health Study) have established that CVD is not a
categorical disease, but rather a spectrum of risk
(Mosca et al., 2011). Risk factors can be classified as
modifiable and non-modifiable. Non-modifiable risk
factors include age, sex, and family history and are
beyond the scope of this Chapter. Traditional modifiable risk factors include smoking, elevated blood
pressure, diabetes, dyslipidemia, overweight and
obesity, physical inactivity, and diet and nutrition.
More recently, the metabolic syndrome has emerged
as a significant and modifiable contributor to cardiovascular risk (Grundy et al., 2005). Because these
risk factors are largely primary care-amenable conditions, the vital role of the primary care physician in
prevention of CVD cannot be overstated. Preventing
morbidity and mortality from CVD requires timely
risk factor assessment, accurate risk stratification,
and institution of appropriate therapies to prevent or

optimize risk factors. In this Chapter, we present an
overview of CVD primary prevention, with a focus
on the epidemiology, assessment, prevention, and
management of the major modifiable CVD risk factors in the primary care setting.

CVD RISK FACTORS: DEFINITIONS, EPIDEMIOLOGY, AND ASSESSMENT IN THE PRIMARY CARE SETTING

Cigarette Smoking

Epidemiology and Associated Risks

Over 91 million US adults (43%) have smoked
more than 100 cigarettes in their lifetime, and nearly
45 million (21%) are current smokers. Cigarette
smoking accounts for over 440,000 deaths per year
in the United States and accounts for approximately
20% of deaths from CVD (Cigarette smoking, 2005;
Go et al., 2013; Surgeon General, 2004). Those who
smoke at least a pack of cigarettes a day have more
than twice the risk of having a cardiovascular event
than non-smokers, and quitting smoking is associated with a 50% reduction in risk of CHD after just
1 year of abstinence (Surgeon General, 2004). Its
role as a risk factor for heart disease, stroke, and a
number of cancers makes it an especially salient public health issue and the leading preventable cause of
death in the United States (Surgeon General, 2004;
US Public Health Service, 2008).

The addictive nature of smoking is largely
due to the presence of nicotine in tobacco products, and evidence-based counseling and pharmacologic interventions for nicotine dependence
can increase abstinence and lead to increased life
expectancy and improved quality of life (American
Psychiatric Association Work Group on Substance
Use Disorders, 2006; Fiore et al., 2008; US Public

Health Service, 2008). Given the chronic and relapsing nature of nicotine dependence, patients may make five to seven quit attempts before they are successful (Centers for Disease Control and Prevention [CDC], 1990). Thus, a patient's motivation for re-initiating or continuing with interventions after relapse may be enhanced through a strong alliance between clinician and patient, as well as a supportive, empathic, and non-judgmental communication style (American Psychiatric Association Work Group on Substance Use Disorders, 2006).

Assessing Tobacco Use

Tobacco use is often a chronic and relapsing condition. Therefore, clinicians are advised to inquire about tobacco use at each encounter with patients. This recommendation is underscored by the fact that 70% of smokers will visit a physician within a given year, and 70% of this group state that they are interested in quitting. Smokers who have attempted to quit report clinician advice to quit as a primary motivator for making such an attempt (US Public Health Service, 2008).

One key strategy for implementing such an effort is to add tobacco use assessment to current vital signs. Assessing tobacco use is the initial step in a counseling framework known as known as "the 5As": ask, advise, assess, assist, and arrange (see Table 5-1) (Fiore et al., 2008). Clinicians who identify patients who use tobacco via the *ask* portion of the paradigm are encouraged to *advise* patients to quit in language that is clear, strong, and personalized. Following this step, clinicians then *assess* patients' current level of interest in quitting. An assessment of current level of nicotine addition can be quickly performed with a brief instrument such as the Fagerström Test for Nicotine Dependence to determine the appropriate intensity of intervention. A smoker's dependence on nicotine predicts the difficulty a smoker will have with quitting and the level of intensity required to help the smoker quit. Smoking duration, number of cigarettes smoked daily, and how soon after awakening the smoker smokes the first cigarette help to determine nicotine dependence. More dependent smokers smoke a greater number of years, smoke more cigarettes daily, and smoke within 30 minutes of awakening (Fagerstrom & Schneider, 1989; Heatherton et al., 1991). The first three As (ask, advise, assess) should be performed at every visit with current smokers.

TABLE 5-1. THE 5 AS MODEL FOR ASSESSMENT AND TREATMENT OF TOBACCO USE AND DEPENDENCE

Ask about tobacco use
- *Identify and document tobacco use status for every patient at every visit.*

Advise to quit
- *In a clear, strong, and personalized manner, urge every tobacco user to quit.*

Assess willingness to make a quit attempt
- *Is the tobacco user willing to make a quit attempt at this time?*

Assist in quit attempt
- *For the patient willing to make a quit attempt, offer medication and provide or refer for counseling or additional treatment to help the patient quit.*
- *For patients unwilling to quit at the time, provide interventions designed to increase future quit attempts.*

Arrange follow-up
- *For the patient willing to make a quit attempt, arrange for follow-up contacts, beginning within the first week after the quit date.*
- *For patients unwilling to make a quit attempt at the time, address tobacco dependence and willingness to quit at next clinic visit.*

Adapted from Fiore MC, Jaén CR, Baker TB, et al. *Treating Tobacco Use and Dependence: 2008 Update.* Clinical Practice Guideline. Rockville, MD: US Department of Health and Human Services. Public Health Service. May 2008.

Physical Activity
Epidemiology and Associated Risks

Physical activity is associated with a reduction in cardiovascular risk and CVD risk factors. For example, physical activity is linked to weight loss, lower blood pressure, improved glycemic control, improved insulin sensitivity, and improved lipid parameters (World Health Organization [WHO], 2007). Prospective investigations have consistently demonstrated an inverse relationship between physical activity and cardiovascular risk. This relationship appears to be independent of other factors that might mediate the relationship between physical activity and CVD, such as obesity or elevated blood pressure (Haskell et al., 2007). Additionally, the effect appears to be dose-dependent; the higher the level of exercise, the lower the cardiovascular risk. It is estimated that physical inactivity results in 250,000 deaths per year (Meriwether et al., 2008). As a result, physical inactivity and sedentary lifestyle are considered important risk factors for CVD.

Unfortunately, 51% of American adults do not meet recommended physical activity goals. According to the National Health Interview Survey (NHIS), in 2011 32% of US adults ≥18 years old reported no leisure-time physical activity (Go et al., 2013). Women are more likely to report no leisure-time activity than men, and younger adults are more likely than older adults to report meeting physical activity goals. Non-whites without a college degree are least likely to fulfill recommended physical activity levels (Haskell et al., 2007).

Assessing Physical Activity in the Primary Care Setting

Level of physical activity should be assessed and physical activity goals should be promoted for nearly all ambulatory patients. Physical activity recommendations from the US Department of Health and Human Services for healthy adults are 150 minutes per week of moderate-intensity physical activity or 75 minutes of vigorous physical activity per week plus 2 non-consecutive days per week of muscle strengthening activity (Haskell et al, 2007) (see Table 5.8).

Similar to the paradigm for smoking cessation, a 5As model has been proposed for physical activity counseling: (1) *assess* level of physical activity, including the frequency, intensity, duration, and types of physical activity; (2) *advise* patients on current recommendations and patient-oriented benefits; (3) *agree* on a plan of action based on the patient's readiness to increase physical activity; (4) *assist* the patient with resources to facilitate a change in physical activity (e.g., a written prescription, behavioral contract, pedometer, useful websites); and (5) *arrange* for frequent in-person or collateral follow-up. (Whitlock et al., 2002) Several tools to assess physical activity in the primary care setting have been developed, including the Patient-Centered Assessment and Counseling for Exercise and Nutrition (PACE) (Calfas & Hagler, 2006) and the Physical Activity Assessment Tool (PAAT). The PAAT was specifically designed to help physicians assess patients quickly to reserve time during the medical encounter for counseling (Meriwether et al., 2008).

Diet
Epidemiology and Associated Risks

Over the last half-century, several studies have documented the association between diet and CVD risk. Epidemiologic, experimental, and clinical trial data support an adverse relationship between sodium intake and blood pressure, saturated fatty acids and lipid levels, and trans-fatty acids and CHD (Van Horn et al., 2008). Many studies demonstrate that reducing sodium intake reduces blood pressure, and reducing total and saturated fat intake reduces cardiovascular events (Estruch et al., 2013; Sacks et al., 2001). Observational studies have shown that individuals consuming a diet high in fruits and vegetables, such as the Mediterranean diet, and adhering to a healthy lifestyle had reduced CVD mortality (Knoops et al., 2004; Sofi et al., 2008). Based on such evidence, the American Heart Association (AHA) recommends that healthy Americans consume no more than 7% of daily caloric intake from saturated fat and less than 2,300 mg of sodium in a day, with special populations (e.g., patients with hypertension, chronic kidney disease, or diabetes) having less than 1,500 mg of sodium in a day (see Table 5-2). Unfortunately, the 2005–2006 NHANES survey revealed that the average American derives more than 11% of daily calories from saturated fat, and consumes 278 mg of cholesterol and more than 3,400 mg of sodium (US Department of Agriculture [USDA], 2008).

Assessing Dietary Behaviors in the Primary Care Setting

Dietary patterns should be assessed periodically in primary care, though the optimal screening interval is not known. The US Preventive Services Task Force (USPSTF) specifically recommends intensive behavioral assessment and lifestyle counseling, which includes nutrition counseling for patients with dyslipidemia and other risk factors for CVD (USPSTF, 2003a, 2003b). Several brief, validated dietary assessment instruments have been developed and recently reviewed. While they are subject to bias (e.g., patients over-reporting healthy dietary behaviors), assessment tools can identify counseling needs and guide intervention. The Food Frequency Questionnaire used in the Nurses Health Study is a quick, comprehensive, and well-studied instrument that can be easily administered in the primary care setting. Other modalities to assess dietary behavior include dietary records (food diaries) and 24-hour dietary recall, though recent studies have found that they may not accurately reflect usual dietary behavior. Regardless of which modality the provider chooses, the aim is to assess targets for intervention, including total caloric intake and consumption of plant proteins (fruits and vegetables), omega-3 fatty acids, and dietary fiber and whole grains (Olendzki, Speed, & Domino, 2006).

TABLE 5-2. AMERICAN HEART ASSOCIATION DIETARY GUIDELINES AND FOOD SELECTION FOR HEALTHY AMERICAN ADULTS, BASED ON A 2,000 CALORIE DIET

Dietary Guidelines	Food Selection Recommendations
Total fat intake should range between 25–35% of energy; the majority of fats should be monounsaturated and polyunsaturated.	
Limit saturated fat to <7% of energy, trans fat to <1% of energy, and cholesterol to <300 mg per day.	Eat fish, especially oily fish like salmon, twice a week.
Choose whole grains (three 1-oz servings per day).	Choose lean meats and vegetable alternatives. Minimize intake of partially hydrogenated fats.
Limit the amount of added sugars (on average for women <100 calories/day, for men <150 calories/day).	Limit sugar-sweetened beverages, no more than 450 calories (36 ounces) a week.
Choose diet rich in fruits and vegetables.	9–10 servings (4.5 cups) of fruits and vegetables per day
Select fat-free (skim), 1%-fat, and low-fat dairy products.	2 to 4 servings of non-fat or low-fat milk and dairy products per day.
Cholesterol intake should be no more than 300 mg/d.	No more than 3–4 egg yolks per week.
Sodium intake should be no more than 2,300 (2.3 g) per day for most adults and no more than 1,500 mg (1.5 g) per day for adults with CVD risk factors.	Choose foods with little or no salt.

A behavioral assessment should also be part of the initial diet assessment. Inquiring about the patient's eating behavior will help tailor counseling and highlights the factors that influence a patient's food choice. Questions about time constraints, stress at home or work, regularity of eating out/getting take-out, age and number of children, who cooks, who purchases food, and timing of food intake should be part of this assessment. Like cigarette smoking and physical activity, assessment and counseling approaches to dietary change can be organized into the 5As framework: *assess* dietary practices; *advise* on dietary goals and needed changes; *agree* on a plan to change diet based on patient readiness; *assist* to change dietary behavior by addressing barriers; and *arrange* for regular follow-up or referral to a nutritionist.

Overweight and Obesity
Epidemiology and Associated Risks

The prevalence of overweight (BMI 25–29.9) and obesity (BMI >30) in the United States is escalating at a rapid rate. Data from the NHANES 2007–2010 show that over 154 million adults are considered overweight and obese; 73% of adult men and 64% of adult women are overweight and 34% of adult men and 36% of adult women are obese (Go et al., 2013). Overweight and obesity are major contributors to preventable deaths and substantially raise the risk of morbidity from hypertension, dyslipidemia, type 2 diabetes, CHD, stroke, gallbladder disease,

osteoarthritis, sleep apnea and respiratory problems, and certain cancers. Higher body weights are also associated with an increased risk in all-cause mortality (National Task Force, 2000).

Obese individuals may also suffer from a lower quality of life and social functioning due to social stigmatization and discrimination (Puhl & Brownell, 2001). Medical costs attributed to both overweight and obesity accounted for 9.1% of total US medical expenditures in 1998 and were estimated to be $147 billion in 2008 (in 2008 dollars) (Finkelstein, Fiebelkorn, & Wang, 2003; Go et al., 2013).

Obesity is a complex multifactorial chronic disease that develops from an interaction of genetics and the environment (National Heart, Lung and Blood Institute [NHLBI], 2002). However, the significant increase in obesity rates over the past 30 years cannot be explained by genetics alone. Rather, changes in lifestyle factors, such as decreased fruit and vegetable intake, higher fat intake, and decreased physical activity, account for a substantial portion of the rising rates. Environmental factors such as increased portion sizes and the number of individuals eating out of the home are also key contributors to the obesity epidemic (NHLBI, 2002).

Overweight and obesity are especially evident in some minority groups, as well as in those with lower incomes and less education. Approximately half of non-Hispanic black women and Mexican American women in the 2005–2006 survey were obese, compared to 39% of non-Hispanic white women of the same age (Ogden et al., 2007). This relationship between obesity and race was even more pronounced in non-Hispanic black women aged 60 years and older (61% obese vs. 32% of non-Hispanic white women and 37% of Mexican American women) (Ogden et al., 2007). Among men, the prevalence of obesity did not differ by racial/ethnic group or age. Despite these significant racial gaps in obesity, only 65% of obese adults are ever told by their primary care provider that they are overweight. Compared to other racial groups, non-Hispanic black men are least likely to be told they were overweight (Ogden et al., 2007). South Asians in the United States have the highest rates of overweight/obesity (25% of men and 37% of women) among all US Asians. South Asians also tend to develop insulin resistance and increased cardiovascular risk at a lower BMI (Ye et al., 2009). In response to the mounting evidence, the WHO in 2002 recommended lower BMI standards for Asians: normal (BMI 18.5 to <23 kg/m^2), moderate risk (BMI at or above 23 kg/m^2), and high risk (BMI at or above 27.5 kg/m^2) (Shiwaku et al., 2004).

Assessment of Overweight and Obesity and Associated Health Risks

According to the National Heart, Lung, and Blood Institute Guidelines on Overweight and Obesity, the first step in treating overweight and obese patients is assessment. Assessment includes determination of body mass index (BMI), waist circumference, and overall risk status. The BMI (calculated as weight in kilograms divided by height in meters squared) is the most commonly used test to screen for obesity and is the measure used to define obesity. The BMI is an easy-to-use and reliable measure that is highly correlated with percentage of body fat and body fat mass (USPSTF, 2012). Waist circumference should be measured because visceral and abdominal adiposity is an independent predictor of risk factors and morbidity (National Institutes of Health [NIH], 1998). A waist circumference greater than 102 cm (40 in.) for men and 88 cm (35 in.) for women magnifies the increased cardiovascular risk associated with elevated BMI. Assessment of overall health risk should include clinical evaluation for CHD and other atherosclerotic diseases, hypertension, other CVD risk factors, and sleep apnea. This comprehensive assessment is critical because if the patient desires a weight management program, this information will guide the provider's selection of

the safest and most appropriate management strategy (see Table 5-3). The USPSTF recommends that clinicians offer or refer patients with a BMI of 30 kg/m^2 or greater to an intensive, multicomponent behavioral intervention (USPSTF, 2012).

Since national weight loss guidelines are designed for healthy adults, providers should also screen for pregnancy, binge eating or other eating disorders, psychiatric disorders, and medical conditions such as diabetes that might be exacerbated by alterations in energy intake and shifts in nutrient distribution. Laboratory studies should generally include screening for diabetes, hypertension, renal disease, liver disease, and thyroid function and a complete lipid panel (Lyznicki et al., 2001).

Hypertension
Definition, Epidemiology, and Associated Risks

Currently defined as systolic blood pressure (BP) greater than or equal to 140 mm Hg or diastolic BP greater than or equal to 90 mm Hg, hypertension is

---

TABLE 5-3. AMERICAN HEART ASSOCIATION SUMMARY OF ESSENTIAL COMPONENTS OF AN EFFECTIVE WEIGHT MANAGEMENT PROGRAM FOR ADULTS 18 YEARS AND OLDER

1. Participant/patient information (informed consent)
2. Screening of all persons beginning a weight management program using an appropriate medical history form to identify people who require a physician's supervision
3. Guidelines for who needs to be evaluated by a physician before beginning a weight management program
4. Staffing by individuals qualified by education, training, and experience to provide these services
5. Identification of reasonable weight loss goals: Is weight loss needed to reduce risk for cardiovascular disease (e.g., improve blood pressure or diabetes) or to improve general health (e.g., improved fitness)?
6. Individualized nutritional, exercise, and behavioral components
7. A maintenance program for at least 2 years
8. Evaluation of the long-term effectiveness and safety of the program: Review weight loss and health status of all participants after completion of the program and at 1, 2, and 5 years after program completion.
9. Most weight loss programs initially meet weekly, which generally lasts from 12 to 24 weeks.

a global public health problem. It is a leading cause of preventable death in the world, affecting 1 billion people worldwide (Chobanian et al., 2003). In the United States, hypertension affects one in three US adults ≥20 years of age (an estimated 77.9 million people), is the leading outpatient diagnosis by physicians, and is arguably the most important treatable risk factor for stroke, myocardial infarction, heart failure, peripheral vascular disease, and end-stage renal disease (Go et al., 2013; Victor, 2004). In the overwhelming majority (90–95%) of hypertensive patients, a single reversible cause of the elevated BP cannot be identified; this is classified as *primary hypertension*.The remaining 5–10% of cases are classified as *secondary* or *identifiable hypertension*, where a more discrete mechanism can be identified (Victor & Kaplan, 2007).

In general, the prevalence of hypertension increases with age. The age-adjusted prevalence of hypertension (diagnosed and undiagnosed) was 75% for older (≥65 years of age) women and 65% for older men. The prevalence of hypertension is greater in men than women until 45 years of age, equal from 45 to 64 years of age, and then greater in women than men at and above 65 years of age. Hypertension is two to three times more common in women taking oral contraceptives, especially older obese women (Go et al., 2013).

The prevalence of hypertension among blacks in the United States is among the highest in the world. Among US adults, hypertension is present in over 40% of blacks compared with 25% of whites and Latinos (Hertz et al., 2005). Blacks who are middle-age or older, have less education, are overweight or obese, are physically inactive, and have diabetes tend to have higher rates of hypertension (Go et al., 2013).

Chen et al. found that coexisting hypertension with diabetes was the major contributor to cardiac morbidity and mortality. More than half of the Framingham cohort at the time of diabetes diagnosis had coexisting hypertension defined as ≥140/90. They found an estimated two-fold increased risk of CV events in diabetics with hypertension than diabetics without hypertension (Chen et al., 2011).

Hypertension is a consistent risk factor of cardiovascular disease independent of other risk factors. For those 40–89 years of age, every increment of 20 mm Hg systolic or 10 mm Hg diastolic over 115/75 doubles the risk of mortality from CHD and stroke (Chobanian et al., 2003). In addition, the estimated direct and indirect cost of hypertension for 2009 was $51.0 billion dollars. Unfortunately, projections show that by 2030 this cost may rise more than six-fold (Go et al., 2013).

Assessment of Hypertension in the Primary Care Setting

The goal of the initial evaluation for hypertension is three-fold: (1) to accurately stage the BP, (2) to assess global cardiovascular risk, and (3) to detect secondary (i.e., potentially reversible) forms of hypertension (Victor, 2004). Accurate BP assessment is one of the most important procedures performed by the primary care physician, yet it is done poorly in most primary care offices (Victor, 2004). The importance of proper BP measurement technique and properly calibrated and accurate equipment cannot be overstated. Flawed technique and/or equipment can result in BP measured on the same patient that varies by 40 mm Hg or more (Campbell, Culleton, & McKay, 2005). In general, BP should be measured in the office at least twice after 5 minutes of rest with the patient seated in a chair with legs uncrossed, both feet on the floor, the back supported, and the arm bare and at heart level. Most overweight adults will require a "large-adult" cuff, so using a standard-sized cuff that is too small for a large arm will almost always produce spuriously elevated readings. Tobacco and caffeine should be avoided for at least 30 minutes prior to the BP measurement (Victor & Kaplan, 2007).

Currently, BP is staged as normal, prehypertension, or stage 1 or stage 2 hypertension based on the average of two or more readings taken at two or more office visits (see Table 5-4) (Chobanian et al., 2003). Wherever possible, the use of oscillometric electronic monitors designed for clinic BP measurement and validated according to British Hypertension Society validation protocol (see www.dableducational.com) is recommended. Electronic monitors overcome many of the pitfalls of office measurement, including operator errors (faulty technique, digit preference) and alerting ("white coat") reactions. Twenty-four-hour ambulatory BP monitoring provides the most accurate assessment of a patient's usual BP and has been shown to be superior to standard office measurement in predicting cardiovascular death (Dolan et al., 2005).

All patients with hypertension should be assessed for additional cardiovascular risk factors and important comorbid diseases such as diabetes

TABLE 5-4. JNC-7 BLOOD PRESSURE CLASSIFICATION FOR THE DIAGNOSIS
OF HYPERTENSION

BP Classification	SBP mm Hg		DBP mmHg
Normal	<120	and	<80
Prehypertension	120–139	or	80–89
Stage 1 Hypertension	140–159	or	90–99
Stage 2 Hypertension	≥160	or	≥100

Adapted from *Seventh Report of the Joint National Committee on Prevention, Detection, Evaluation, and Treatment of High Blood Pressure (JNC 7 Express)*. http://www.nhlbi.nih.gov/guidelines/hypertension/jncintro.htm. Accessed June 24, 2013.

and chronic kidney disease (CKD). Evaluation for target organ damage, including hypertensive retinopathy, cerebrovascular disease, CHD, left ventricular hypertrophy, and congestive heart failure, is critical to selecting treatment targets and ancillary therapies. The initial laboratory evaluation should include blood electrolytes, fasting glucose, a fasting lipid panel, hematocrit, serum creatinine (with calculated glomerular filtration rate), urinalysis, urine microalbumin, and a resting 12-lead electrocardiogram (Victor, 2004). In addition, obtaining an echocardiogram to detect left ventricular hypertrophy (LVH) in asymptomatic patients with hypertension as evidence of target organ damage is reasonable (Greenland et al., 2010).

In patients with hypertension requiring hospitalization or hypertension that is refractory to intensive pharmacologic treatment, a prudent search for secondary causes, including renovascular disease, primary hyperaldosteronism, hypercortisolism, pheochromocytoma, or obstructive sleep apnea, may be indicated. The evaluation of resistant or suspected hypertension may require referral to a hypertension specialist and is beyond the scope of this Chapter but is reviewed excellently in an AHA consensus statement (Calhoun et al., 2008).

Diabetes Mellitus
Epidemiology and Associated Risks

Diabetes mellitus (DM) comprises a group of disorders characterized by abnormally high levels of serum glucose due to defects in insulin production, insulin action, or both (National Institute of Diabetes and Digestive and Kidney Diseases [NIDDK], 2007). DM affects 8% of the total US population. More than 26 million adults aged 20 years or older have diabetes; of these over 8 million people are unaware that they have the condition. Type 2 DM accounts

for 90–95% of all diagnosed DM cases. Prediabetes (impaired fasting glucose, impaired glucose tolerance, or both), the precursor to type 2 DM, affects another 38%, an estimated 87.3 million adults. DM rates vary by ethnicity/race. National survery data from 2007–2009 adjusted for population age differences found 7.1% of non-Hispanic whites, 8.4% of Asian Americans, 11.8% of Hispanics, and 12.6% of non-Hispanic blacks had diagnosed DM (Go et al., 2013). In 2004–2006, a two-fold increased prevalence was seen in Asian Indians (14%) compared with Chinese (6%) and Japanese (5%) adults (Go et al., 2013).

There were 1.9 million new adult cases of diabetes (type 1 or type 2) in 2010, and with the rising prevalence of overweight and obesity, a critical risk factor for type 2 DM, the incidence and prevalence will continue to increase. The total national cost of diabetes in the United States was estimated to be $174 billion in 2007 (Economic costs of diabetes, 2008). In addition to the economic burden, diabetes increases CVD risk and mortality. DM increases CVD risk 2.5-fold in women and 2.4-fold in men. Diabetics have two- to four-fold higher CHD death rates than non-diabetics and have a significantly higher prevalence of hypertension and dyslipidemia (Go et al., 2013).

Assessment of Diabetes in the Primary Care Setting: Screening, Diagnosis, and Classification

Patients at high risk, such as those with excess weight, family history of diabetes, personal history of gestational diabetes, dyslipidemia, impaired fasting glucose/impaired glucose tolerance, and certain ethnic groups (Asians, Hispanic, black), should be screened for DM. The fasting plasma glucose (FPG), 2-hour oral glucose tolerance (OGTT), and hemoglobin A1c

(A1c) are the most common screening tests. Diabetes is defined as FPG at or above 126 mg/dL, A1c at or above 6.5%, a 2-hour value in an OGTT at or above 200 mg/dL, or a random plasma glucose concentration at or above 200 mg/dL in the presence of symptoms (see Table 5-5). Confirmation is recommended on a separate day. Once patients are diagnosed, DM is classified into one of four groups, usually based on clinical presentation: (1) type 1 diabetes, due to pancreatic beta-cell destruction leading to insulin deficiency; (2) type 2 diabetes, resulting from insulin resistance; (3) gestational DM, which occurs in women who have diabetes only during pregnancy and normal blood glucose otherwise; and (4) other types of diabetes due to specific causes, such as cystic fibrosis or certain medications (i.e., prednisone).

Dyslipidemia
Epidemiology and Associated Risks

Dyslipidemia is a disorder of lipoprotein metabolism, including lipoprotein overproduction or defiency, that results in elevated total serum cholesterol, elevated low-density lipoprotein cholesterol (LDL-C) and triglycerides (TG), and reduced high-density lipoprotein cholesterol (HDL-C). Epidemiologic data has documented a continuous graded relationship between serum total cholesterol and coronary risk; thus high serum cholesterol is a major modifiable risk factor for CVD (Grundy et al., 2004). Approximately one-third of all Americans (>100 million people) have high total cholesterol levels (>200 mg/dL) and more than 31 million adults have levels in excess of 240 mg/dL with a prevalence of 13.8% (Go et al., 2013). Seventy-one million US adults (33.5%) have high LDL-C (>130 mg/dL). Some improvement was noted between the periods 1988–1994 to 1999–2002 (NHANES data) for adults aged 20 years or older; mean total cholesterol decreased from 206 to 203 mg/dL, mean HDL-C increased from 50.7 to 51.3 mg/dL, and mean LDL-C decreased from 129 to 123 mg/dL (Schober et al., 2007). Thirty-one percent of the US adult population have high triglycerides (≥150 mg/dL), with no appreciable change from NHANES 1988–1994 and 1999–2008. Elevated triglycerides are associated with low HDL-C as risk factors for metabolic syndrome, but the relationship of elevated triglycerides as an independent risk factor for CVD remains unclear (Miller et al., 2011).

Assessing Dyslipidemia in the Primary Care Setting

Recommendations include screening for dyslipidemia with a standard fasting lipoprotein profile (which generally includes direct measurement of serum total cholesterol, HDL-C, and TG and a calculated LDL-C) once every 5 years for adults, beginning at the age of 20 years (National Cholesterol Education Program [NCEP], 2002). Alternatively, the USPSTF recommends screening for dyslipidemia in all adults, starting at the age of 35 in men and 45 in women. Screening should begin earlier for patients at risk for CVD; screen men aged 20–35 and women aged 20–45 for dyslipidemia if they have increased CHD risk (USPSTF, 2008).

TABLE 5-5. CLASSIFICATION OF BLOOD GLUCOSE AND CRITERIA FOR DIAGNOSIS OF DIABETES MELLITUS

Blood Glucose Classification	Fasting Plasma Glucose	Hemoglobin A1c	2-hour OGTT	Random Plasma Glucose
Normal	<100 mg/dl	<5.7%	—	
Pre-diabetes		5.7–6.4%		
Impaired Fasting Glucose (IFG)	100–125 mg/dl		—	
Impaired Glucose Tolerance (IGT)	—		140–199 mg/dl	
Diabetes	≥126 mg/dl	≥6.5%	≥200 mg/dl	≥200 mg/dL with classic symptoms of hyperglycemia

OGTT = oral glucose tolerance test.

*Symptoms of hyperglycemia (polyuria, polydipsia, and unexplained weight loss) plus a casual glucose ≥200 mg/dl also meet criteria for diagnosis of diabetes.
Adapted from American Diabetes Association. Standards of medical care in diabetes, *2011. Diabetes Care.* 2011;34:S11.

Optimal lipid parameters are total cholesterol <200 mg/dL, LDL-C <100 mg/dL, HDL-C >40 mg/dL (men) and >50 mg/dL (women), and TG <150 mg/dL (see Table 5-6). Though an optimal screening interval has not yet been established, repeating a fasting lipoprotein profile every 1–2 years in adults with increased CVD risk and/or abnormal lipid parameters is reasonable.

In some cases, dyslipidemia is genetic, resulting from either an overproduction or defective clearance of TG and LDL-C, or an underproduction or excessive clearance of HDL-C. To identify patients with genetic predisposition, primary care providers should inquire about the following: (1) a family history of premature CHD (CHD in first-degree male relative <55 years old, first-degree female relative <65 years old); (2) a family history of very high LDL-C; and (3) a serum cholesterol level above 240 mg/dL (>6.2 mmol/L). More often, elevated LDL-C levels associated with dyslipidemia are a result of poor lifestyle behaviors, with up to 80% of cases due to excessive intake of dietary fats, smoking, and physical inactivity (Knoops et al., 2004; Stampfer et al., 2000). Elevated TG and low HDL-C levels associated with dyslipidemia can also be a result of comorbid conditions such as DM, alcoholism, obesity, and hypothyroidism (NCEP, 2002).

TABLE 5-6. NATIONAL CHOLESTEROL EDUCATION PROGRAM–ADULT TREATMENT PANEL III (ATP III) CLASSIFICATION OF LDL, TOTAL, AND HDL CHOLESTEROL (MG/DL)

LDL Cholesterol, mg/dL	
<100	Optimal
100–129	Near optimal/above optimal
130–159	Borderline high
160–189	High
≥190	Very high

Total Cholesterol, mg/dL	
<200	Desirable
200–239	Borderline high
≥240	High

HDL Cholesterol, mg/dL	
<40	Low
≥60	High

As such, it is important that primary care providers identify patients at increased risk for cardiovascular events and properly manage their serum cholesterol levels by recommending therapeutic lifestyle changes or prescribing lipid-lowering medications.

Metabolic Syndrome Pathogenesis, Epidemiology, and Associated Risks

The metabolic syndrome is a cluster of risk factors of metabolic origin that are associated with an increased risk for CVD and type 2 diabetes. Risk factors included in the metabolic syndrome are atherogenic dyslipidemia, elevated BP, elevated plasma glucose, a prothrombotic state, and a pro-inflammatory state. The pathogenesis of metabolic syndrome is thought to be related to abdominal obesity and insulin resistance (Grundy et al., 2005). According to NHANES 2003–2008 data, ~34% of adults aged ≥20 years in the United States met the criteria for metabolic syndrome (as defined by ATP III, discussed below). The prevalence increases with age and, according to 2003–2008 NHANES data, is greatest among non-Hispanic black (38.8%) and Mexican American (40.6%) women (Ford, Giles, & Dietz, 2002; Go et al., 2013). The prevalence of metabolic syndrome also increased among pregnant women to 26.5% during 1999–2004, from 17.8% during 1988–1994 (Go et al., 2013).

Clinical Diagnosis of the Metabolic Syndrome

In 2001, the ATP III introduced a set of diagnostic criteria for the metabolic syndrome to facilitate identification and intervention for patients at higher risk for CHD (NCEP, 2002). ATP III required the presence of any three of the five following risk factors for diagnosis: (1) abdominal obesity, defined as a waist circumference of 102 cm (40 in.) or more in men or 88 cm (35 in.) or more in women; (2) a high TG level (≥150 mg/dL); (3) a low HDL-C level (<40 mg/dL in men, <50 mg/dL in women); (4) elevated BP, defined as at least 135 mm Hg systolic or at least 85 mm Hg diastolic; and (5) fasting glucose of at least 110 mg/dL (or diabetes). The AHA and NHLBI endorsed the ATP III guidelines, with minor modifications (Grundy et al., 2005). The AHA/NHLBI diagnostic criteria are summarized in Table 5-7.

TABLE 5-7. DIAGNOSTIC CRITERIA
FOR METABOLIC SYNDROME

Any Three of the Five Criteria Below Constitute a
Diagnosis of Metabolic Syndrome

Measure	Categorical Cut Points
Elevated waist circumference	≥102 cm (≥40 inches) in men ≥88 cm (≥35 inches) in women
Elevated triglycerides	≥150 mg/dl or drug treatment for elevated triglycerides
Reduced HDL-C	<40 mg/dl in men <50 mg/dl in women or drug treatment for reduced HDL-C
Elevated blood pressure	≥130 mm Hg systolic blood pressure or ≥85 mm Hg diastolic blood pressure or drug treatment for hypertension
Elevated fasting glucose	≥100 mg/dl or drug treatment for elevated glucose

Adapted from Grundy S. Diagnosis and management of the metabolic syndrome. An American Heart Association/National Heart, Lung, and Blood Institute Scientific Statement. Executive summary. *Cardiol Rev.*2005;13 (6):322–327.

CVD RISK STRATIFICATION: APPROACH TO ASSESSING GLOBAL CVD RISK

As emphasized above, assessing individual risk factors is critically important to identifying targets for intervention, because any major risk factor, if left untreated, has the potential to lead to CVD. However, it is also important to assess total (global) risk based on the summation of risk factors to identify high-risk patients who deserve immediate attention and intervention, and to guide the intensity of risk-reduction efforts. In 2013, the American College of Cardiology (ACC) and the American Heart Association (AHA) released updated guidelines for the treatment of blood cholesterol which were designed to be easily used in the clinical setting and a significant change from the prior guidelines introduced by NCEP/ATPIII in 2002 (Stone et al., 2013). The new guidelines focused on estimating risk of atherosclerotic cardiovascular disease (ASCVD) rather than CHD alone, identifying and treating individuals most likely to benefit from statin treatment, and intensity of statin treatment rather than continued use of specific LDL-C and/or non-HDL-C treatment targets (Stone et al., 2013).

Several risk prediction models have been developed and are available for use in clinical practice in the form of "risk calculators." The best-known and most widely used tool is the Framingham Risk Score (FRS). The new guidelines introduced and recommended the Pooled Cohort Equation which estimates 10-year risk for first hard ASCVD event (defined as first occurrence of nonfatal myocardial infarction or CHD death, or fatal or nonfatal stroke); this is felt to be more relevant to patients and providers than estimating hard CHD outcome alone. A web-based calculator is available at: http://www.cardiosource.org/science-and-quality/practice-guidelines-and-quality-standards/2013-prevention-guideline-tools.aspx. This risk should be estimated for individuals without evidence of clinical ASCVD or diabetes with LDL-C between 70–190 mg/dL not already on statin therapy. The risk should guide the initiation of moderate to high intensity statin therapy. The new guidelines specified four statin benefit groups for which moderate to high intensity statin therapy should be initiated. See page 140 Table 5-12a for the other ASCVD Statin Benefit Groups and Table 5-12b for High-Moderate- Low-Intensity Statin Therapy (Stone et al., 2013)

Risk stratification algorithms based on traditional risk factors have well-known limitations for individual risk assessment. Global risk scores, such as FRS, classify more than 90% of women as low risk, with few women assigned as high risk before the age of 70 (Greenland et al., 2010). One study of 2,447 non-diabetic asymptomatic women found 84% of women with significant coronary artery calcium (≥75th percentile) were classified as low risk using the FRS (Michols et al., 2006). One potential way to enhance risk prediction in women and young low-risk patients is to estimate 30-year risk because some patients will have substantially higher 30-year risk compared to their 10-year risk. Pencina et al. developed a tool for estimating 30-year risk of "hard" CVD events, using data from the Framingham Offspring cohort and advanced statistical techniques that allowed them to utilize standard risk factors while adjusting for competing non-CVD death (Pencina et al., 2009). The calculator is available online (http://www.framingham-heartstudy.org/risk/cardiovascular30.html).

A number of studies have also investigated the use of additional risk factors, such as lipoprotein (a) [Lp(a)] and hsCRP, for improving risk prediction. However, recent recommendations by the ACC and the AHA do not recommend using lipid parameters, including lipoprotein, apolipoprotein, particle size, and density beyond a standard fasting lipid profile for cardiovascular risk assessment in asymptomatic adults because the data to support improved risk prediction above traditional risk factors are lacking. For certain populations, including men ≥50 years old and women ≥60 years old with LDL <130 mg/dL not on lipid-lowering therapy and without CHD, diabetes, CKD, or severe inflammatory conditions, hsCRP can help with the selection of patients for statin therapy. In asymptomatic intermediate-risk men ≤50 years old and women ≤60 years old, hsCRP measurement is reasonable for cardiovascular risk assessment (Greenland et al., 2010). Risk scores such as the Reynold's risk score improved risk classification in low-risk non-diabetic women and men by incorportating high sensitivity C-reactive protein (hsCRP) and family history of premature CHD (Ridker et al., 2007; Ridker et al., 2008). This calculator is available online (http://www.reynoldsriskscore.org/home.aspx).

The coronary artery calcium (CAC) score as a measure of coronary artery plaque burden has also been shown to improve individual cardiovascular risk assessment. The majority of published data reveal that the total amount of coronary artery calcium (expressed as an Agatston score) predicts future CAD events beyond what is predicted through traditional risk factors alone. Thus, recommendations from the ACC and AHA state measurement of CAC are reasonable in asymptomatic intermediate risk (10–20% 10-year risk) adults and may be reasonable in low to intermediate risk (6–10%) adults for cardiovascular risk assessment. It is important to remember that the utility of CAC testing as a risk assessment tool is in guiding clinical management of patients, such as in the use of preventive measures (Greenland et al., 2010).

It is crucial to remember that global risk scores, such as the FRS and the Pooled Cohort Equations, only apply to patients without a history of CVD or diabetes, and are therefore only useful for guiding primary prevention in non-diabetics. Patients with a known history of CVD, diabetes, or CKD constitute a special group who on average are at much higher risk of future CVD events and therefore almost always warrant the most aggressive management of individual risk factors.

IMPACT OF RISK FACTOR MODIFICATION INTERVENTIONS

Risk factor modification is rarely an easy undertaking for patients or primary care physicians. Successful implementation of interventions to improve individual risk factors requires dedication and motivation by both parties. Having a concrete sense of the cardiovascular benefits of modifying each risk factor may aid in increasing motivation.

Impact of Smoking Cessation

Several prospective cohort studies demonstrate a significant effect of smoking cessation on CVD risk (WHO, 2007). In the first 1–2 years after cessation, smokers who quit reduce their excess risk of a coronary event by 50%. Studies suggest that 3 to 10 years after cessation, ex-smokers reduce their CHD risk to that of never-smokers (Gaziano et al., 2007; WHO, 2007). Although there are cardiovascular benefits from cessation for smokers of all age, some studies suggest that there is a significant benefit to smoking cessation at a younger age. A 50-year follow-up of a physician cohort demonstrated those who quit before age 45 had identical survival to never-smokers (Doll et al., 2004). Patients who quit smoking before age 50 compared to persistent smokers have one-half the risk of dying in the next 15 years (Surgeon General, 2004).

Impact of Physical Activity and Healthy Diet

Abundant epidemiologic evidence suggests that a higher level of leisure-time physical activity is associated with reduced CVD risk, lower cardiovascular mortality, and lower all-cause mortality. In the MRFIT trial, a prospective study of 12,138 middle-aged men with CVD risk factors, men who averaged 5 minutes a day of leisure-time physical activity had 29% higher CHD mortality rates compared to those who averaged 23 minutes a day of predominantly light and moderate activity (Leon, Myers, & Connett, 1997). A recent meta-analysis demonstrates a similar dose-response relationship between physical activity and CVD for women as well (Oguma & Shinoda-Tagawa, 2004). The Nurses Health Study involving over 72,000 women showed a dose-associated reduction in coronary events, with the highest quintile achieving an age-adjusted relative risk of 0.66 compared to the lowest quintile (Manson et al., 1999). The Women's Health Study also showed a dose relationship; among 40,000 healthy women, the time spent walking correlated with reduced CV risk, with a relative risk of 0.48 in those walking 2 or more hours per week (Lee et al., 2001). In another study of male runners, each 10-mile increase in distance run per week up to 40–50 miles per week was associated with further gains in HDL and improvements in weight and triglycerides (Williams, 1997).

Much of the data showing the benefit of exercise are from observational studies. In general, the most active individuals have about 30–40% lower risk of developing CHD compared to the least active. This relationship is consistent across different age ranges, gender, and ethnicities. Such observational data are subject to confounders, but randomized trials of exercise are difficult due to high dropout rates. Most randomized controlled studies are small and of limited duration. Exercise can dramatically impact the most important cardiovascular risk factors by improving lipid parameters, blood pressure, type 2 diabetes, and inflammatory markers that correlate with CVD (Hamer et al, 2012; Swardfager et al., 2012).

Accumulating evidence supports the beneficial impact of dietary modification on cardiovascular health. In clinical trials, healthy dietary changes including increased fresh fruits and vegetables, reduced dietary saturated fat, reduced sodium intake, and increased potassium intake were associated with lowering blood pressure (WHO, 2007). Randomized trials that focused on weight reduction, dietary modification, and physical activity reduced the incidence of type 2 diabetes in those at risk for developing diabetes (Knowler et al., 2002; Norris et al., 2005). Randomized trials that focused on reduction of saturated fat with partial replacement with unsaturated fats improved dyslipidemia (Hu et al., 2001). A systematic review of 27 interventions to reduce or modify dietary fat intake, comprising 30,902 person-years of observation, found a 16% reduction in combined cardiovascular events and a 9% reduction in cardiovascular mortality (Hooper et al., 2000). Dietary interventions such as reducing salt and saturated fat intake and increasing consumption of fruits and vegetables can potentially reduce the risk of coronary heart disease by 12% and stroke by 11% (WHO, 2007). An overall healthy diet should help a patient achieve a healthy body weight, desirable lipid profile, and desirable blood pressure.

Impact of Weight Loss

While there are several trials linking overweight and obesity to cardiovascular morbidity and mortality, there are few data linking weight loss directly to improved cardiovascular risk. There is, however, myriad evidence that weight loss directly affects major CVD risk factors and therefore indirectly lowers CVD risk (WHO, 2007). Weight-loss interventions that combine dietary change with exercise are associated with improvements in systolic BP of at least 4 mmHg as well as significant reductions in LDL-C and triglycerides (Gaziano et al., 2007; WHO, 2007).

Weight loss has a significant impact on a person's risk for developing diabetes. One study found that for each kilogram of weight lost annually over 10 years, there was a 33% lower risk of diabetes in the subsequent 10 years (Resnick et al., 2000).

Impact of Treating Hypertension

The potential impact of treating hypertension is large, due to its high prevalence and its association with cardiovascular events; hypertension accounts for an estimated 54% of all strokes and 27% of all ischemic heart events globally. Treating raised blood pressure has been associated with a 35–40% reduction in stroke risk and a 16% reduction in risk of myocardial infarction. Observational and clinical trial data confirm the reduction in cardiovascular events with lowering BP for patients with BP above140/90 mm Hg (WHO, 2007). In diabetics without known CHD or cerebrovascular disease, reaching a goal BP <140/90 within the first year of hypertension diagnosis reduced major CVD events within 3 years compared with not reaching this goal within the first year of hypertension diagnosis (O'Connor et al., 2013). The incidence of hypertension is incredibly high among diabetics, so timely hypertension treatment is important.

A lower BP goal (<130/80) was recommended for diabetics until recently, when the ADA revised their guidelines to recommend a less restrictive BP goal of <140/80 based on recent evidence that cast doubt on the evidence supporting more intensive BP control (ADA, 2013). The Action to Control Cardiovascular Risk in Diabetes (ACCORD) trial investigated the effects on CVD events of treating to a normal systolic BP (<120 mmHg) in type 2 diabetes (Cushman et al., 2010). The investigators found that targeting a systolic BP <120 mm Hg compared with targeting a systolic BP <140 did not reduce major cardiovascular events.

Impact of Treating Diabetes

Large studies of type 1 diabetics and type 2 diabetics demonstrate a direct relationship between hyperglycemia and cardiovascular events and risk reduction with more aggressive glucose control. Among 1,441 young adults with type 1 diabetes in the Diabetes Control and Complications Trial, those who had their glucose more aggressively controlled had a 57% reduction in serious cardiovascular events (Diabetes Control and Complications Trial Research Group, 1993). In the United Kingdom Prospective Diabetes Study (UKPDS), intensive glucose control in type 2 diabetics resulted in a 16% decrease in myocardial infarction that was of borderline significance (p=0.052) (WHO, 2007; UKPDS Group, 1998). However, results of the 10-year follow-up of the UKPDS survivor cohort revealed risk reductions for myocardial infarction (15%, p=0.01) and death from any cause (13%, p=0.007) (Holman et al., 2008).

Impact of Treating Dyslipidemia

The enormous impact of LDL-C lowering for both primary and secondary prevention is well established. A meta-analysis of over 200 randomized trials evaluating LDL-C lowering with statins (regardless of which statin or dose was used) demonstrated a 37% reduction of LDL-C, associated with a 61% reduction in CHD events and a 17% reduction in stroke (Law, Wald, & Rudnicka 2003; WHO, 2007). The benefit of statin use in primary prevention, which initially seemed less clear, has gained increasing support. A recent Cochrane Collaboration review, which included 18 randomized control trials with 59,934 participants found reductions in all-cause mortality (OR 0.86, 95% CI 0.79–0.94), major vascular events (CHD OR 0.73, 95% CI 0.67–0.80; stroke OR 0.78, 95% CI 0.68–0.89) and revascularizations (RR 0.62, 95% CI 0.54–0.72) with no excess adverse events among people without evidence of CVD treated with statins (Taylor et al., 2013). Thus, men and women of all ages, with or without CVD, appear to benefit from statin therapy for dyslipidemia.

STRATEGIES FOR PREVENTING CVD
Non-pharmacologic Approaches to Managing Risk Factors
Counseling for Smoking Cessation

Physician counseling, including brief clinical interventions, is a critical part of getting smokers to quit. Brief clinical interventions are especially well suited to practices in which clinicians see a variety of patients and have a limited amount of time to intervene. Interventions as brief as 3 minutes have been shown to be effective in increasing cessation rates (West et al., 2000). Brief interventions like the 5As are effective with three types of patients: those who are current users and willing to quit; those who are former users and have quit recently; and those who are current users and unwilling to quit.

Counseling for tobacco cessation includes elements such as problem solving, skills training to promote cessation and avoid relapse, and social support. Problem solving and skills training should provide education about tobacco use and components of the quitting process, help patients recognize smoking triggers, and develop coping skills for trigger situations. Quit lines (1-800-QUIT-NOW or 1-800-784-8669) that provide supportive counseling by phone have been instituted in all 50 states and were included in the *Treatment of Tobacco Use and Dependence 2008 Update* as an additional effective intervention for tobacco use and dependence (Fiore et al., 2008).

For those who are not interested in quitting, clinicians can employ motivational enhancement strategies, or motivational interviewing, which include expressing empathy; developing the discrepancy between patients' current behavior and their goals; "rolling with resistance"; and supporting patients' self-efficacy, or belief that they can be successful in a quit attempt. The content of motivational interviewing intervention includes a discussion of "the 5Rs": relevance, risks, rewards, roadblocks, and repetition around quitting. (For a more in-depth discussion of these techniques and content areas, see Rollnick, Mason, & Butler, 1999, and Rollnick, Miller, & Butler, 2008.)

Physical Activity

In light of the increasingly sedentary lifestyle of American adults, the CDC and the American College of Sports Medicine (ACSM) in 1995 issued a "public health recommendation" to increase participation in regular physical activity (Haskell et al., 2007). Current preventive recommendations issued by the US Department of Health and Human Services for healthy adults aged 18–65 include a minimum of 150 minutes per week of moderate-intensity aerobic exercise (e.g., walking at a brisk pace, water aerobics, riding a bike on level ground, playing doubles tennis, or ballroom dancing) or a minimum of 75 minutes per week of vigorous aerobic exercise (e.g., jogging, riding a bike fast or on hills, swimming laps, playing singles tennis, or hiking at moderate grade). An important update to this recommendation is that the exercise does not have to be continuous but can be achieved in 10-minute bouts. Muscle-strengthening activities such as progressive weight training, weight-bearing calisthenics, or other resistance exercises that work all major muscle groups (legs, hips, back, abdomen, chest, shoulders, and arms) should be performed at least 2 days per week on non-consecutive days. Only moderate intensity exercise is necessary to attain the cardiovascular benefits, whereas higher intensities may be needed for significant gains in aerobic fitness. Physical activity beyond the minimum recommendations has additional health benefits of further lowering the risks of unhealthy weight gain and chronic health conditions such as diabetes and

promoting and maintaining skeletal health (Haskell et al., 2007). Physical activity recommendations from the US Department of Health and Human Services for healthy adults are summarized in Table 5-8.

Diet and Nutrition

The importance of diet in the prevention and management of CVD risk factors and other chronic diseases cannot be overstated. Lifestyle modification begins with diet and nutrition modification. The AHA considers diet a critical component of cardiovascular risk reduction for the general population. The AHA and the US Department of Health and Human Services (DHHS) have published dietary guidelines with similar themes (Table 5.2). The recommendations include the following: (1) achieve or maintain a healthy body weight through caloric balance (ensuring intake of calories does not exceed expenditure through exercise); (2) modify diet so

---

TABLE 5-8. PHYSICAL ACTIVITY RECOMMENDATIONS FOR HEALTHY ADULTS

How Much Physical Activity Do Adults Need?

Physical activity is anything that gets your body moving. According to the *2008 Physical Activity Guidelines for Americans*, you need to do two types of physical activity each week to improve your health–aerobic and muscle-strengthening.

For Important Health Benefits

Adults need at least:

2 hours and 30 minutes (150 minutes) of *moderate-intensity aerobic activity* (i.e., brisk walking) every week **and**

muscle-strengthening activities on 2 or more days a week that work all major muscle groups (legs, hips, back, abdomen, chest, shoulders, and arms).

1 hour and 15 minutes (75 minutes) of *vigorous-intensity aerobic activity* (i.e., jogging or running) every week **and**

muscle-strengthening activities on 2 or more days a week that work all major muscle groups (legs, hips, back, abdomen, chest, shoulders, and arms).

An equivalent mix of moderate- and vigorous-intensity *aerobic activity* **and**

muscle-strengthening activities on 2 or more days a week that work all major muscle groups (legs, hips, back, abdomen, chest, shoulders, and arms).

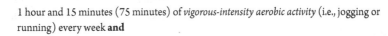

Source: Centers for Disease Control and Prevention. http://www.cdc.gov/physicalactivity/everyone/guidelines/adults.html

that a core component is the intake of a variety of fruits and vegetables; (3) when consuming grains, choose whole grains and include many high-fiber foods in the diet; (4) consume fish, especially oily fish, at least twice weekly; (5) limit intake of fat and cholesterol so that each day less than 7% of energy comes from saturated fat, less than 1% of energy comes from trans fats, and less than 300 mg of cholesterol is consumed (this can be accomplished by choosing lean meats, consuming vegetables as a substitute for meats, choosing fat-free or low-fat dairy products, and limiting intake of partially hydrogenated fats); (6) limit consumption of sugary beverages and foods; (7) use salt sparingly or not at all when preparing foods, and choose foods with little or no salt, with the goal of limiting sodium consumption to less than 2.3 g/day; (8) moderate intake of alcohol, if one chooses to drink (no more than 2 glasses wine-equivalent/day for men, no more than 1 glass wine-equivalent/day for women); and (9) follow all of these lifestyle and dietary guidelines both at home and when eating outside the home (Lichtenstein et al., 2006).

The USDA issued a "food pyramid" in 2005, which was replaced in 2010 by a simpler construct termed a "food plate." The plate is divided into four sections, with approximately one-quarter each for fruits, vegetables, grains, and protein, and a small side of dairy. The new food plate image reflects the 2010 Dietary Guidelines for Americans, which promote measures like switching to fat-free or low-fat milk and opting for water over sugary drinks. The guidelines also recommend ensuring that half your plate is filled with fruits and vegetables (USDA, 2011).

Primary and Secondary CVD Prevention

A recent randomized trial from Spain sought to investigate whether a Mediterranean diet would prove to reduce cardiovascular events in those with high cardiovascular risks. The study enrolled almost 7,500 participants. Those randomized to the Mediterranean diet were instructed to eat five or more fruits and vegetables daily, fish three times per week, high legume intake; one subgroup also supplemented with 50 g of olive oil daily and another 50 g of nuts daily. This was compared to the third group, who were advised to eat a low-fat diet. The trial was stopped early, at almost 5 years, due to finding an approximately 30% reduction in CV events in both of the Mediterranean diet subgroups

compared to the low-fat diet group (Estruch et al., 2013). An earlier study by Dean Ornish, MD, in patients with preexisting CHD showed that progression of coronary disease could be prevented, and that existing atherosclerosis might be reversed with an anti-inflammatory, vegetarian diet. The intervention consisted of intensive dietary and lifestyle changes: a low-fat, whole-food vegetarian diet with 10% of energy from fat; aerobic exercise; stress management training; smoking cessation; and social support. At 5-year follow-up, a relative improvement in diameter stenosis of 7.9% was observed compared with a 27.7% worsening in the control group (p=0.001). The risk ratio for a cardiac event in the control group compared with the experimental group was 2.47 (95% CI 1.48–4.20). (Ornish et al., 1998). Dietary guidelines for the prevention and management of hypertension, diabetes, dyslipidemia, and overweight and obesity all strongly overlap with the above recommendations. Risk factor–specific diet recommendations are discussed briefly below.

Hypertension

The Dietary Approaches to Stop Hypertension (DASH) diet (e.g., decreased sodium consumption, increased potassium consumption, increased intake of fruits and vegetables, consumption of fat-free or low-fat dairy products and lean meats) is a rigorously studied eating plan that was shown to lower blood pressure by 5/3 mm Hg in as little as 2 weeks. In one randomized control trial evaluating the effects of different levels of sodium intake on participants consuming a typical American diet and the DASH diet, blacks and females, compared with other ethnic/racial groups and males, respectively, had significantly greater blood pressure–lowering effects with reduced salt intake (Sacks et al., 2001). The DASH diet is recommended by the JNC-7 report and the DHHS as an important part of initial therapy for adults with hypertension, and by AHA/ NHLBI for treating the elevated BP component of the metabolic syndrome (Chobanian et al., 2003; Grundy et al., 1999).

Diabetes

The ADA recommends dietary modification, known as medical nutrition therapy (MNT), as first-line treatment in the management of type 2 diabetes. General diet principles of MNT are similar to the TLC diet described below, but the ADA recommends that (1) MNT be individualized for adults with prediabetes and diabetes, and (2) such therapy is best provided by a registered dietitian familiar with the components of diabetes MNT (ADA, 2008). MNT focuses on caloric intake, weight loss, increased physical activity, carbohydrate consistency, nutritional content, and timing of meals/snacks (ADA, 2013). The nutrition prescription for patients with type 2 DM should optimize the "ABCs" of diabetes: A1c, blood pressure, and LDL-C. Referring your patient to a diabetic educator to begin this process is important.

Dyslipidemia, Overweight and Obesity, and Metabolic Syndrome

To enhance LDL lowering and reduce the risk for CHD, NCEP/ATP III recommends that patients adopt the following TLC plan: reduced intake of saturated fats (<7% of total calories) and cholesterol (<200 mg/day), increased intake of plant stanols/sterols (2 g/day) and viscous (soluble) fiber (10–25 g/day), weight loss, and increased physical activity (NCEP, 2002). In addition, the guidelines recommend that total fat represent 25–35% of an individual's total daily caloric intake, with the lowest intake coming from saturated fats and *trans* fatty acids (NCEP, 2002). While the US Department of Agriculture guidelines recommend a lower intake of total fat, a higher intake of unsaturated fat can help reduce triglycerides and raise HDL-C in individuals with evidence of insulin resistance and metabolic syndrome. An additional emphasis on avoiding very high carbohydrate foods, replacing refined grains with whole grains, fruits, and vegetables, and eliminating high-glycemic beverages may improve their lipid derangements (NCEP, 2002).

Several trials have attempted to determine whether one diet type might be superior to another in achieving weight loss goals. One recent study investigated four different diet types with varying combinations of high and low carbohydrate, fat, and protein and found that at 24 months there were no differences in the amount of weight loss between groups. The average weight loss achieved in all the diet groups was about 4 kg at the end of the trial (Sacks et al., 2009). The A to Z study compared four different diet plans (Ornish, Atkins, Zone, and LEARN diets) and in this study it was noted that at 1 year the Atkins diet had slightly more weight loss (~6% vs. ~4%), but there was no statistically different weight loss among the Zone, Ornish, and LEARN groups (Gardener et al.,

2007). Another study suggested that insulin-resistant patients, as defined by their measured fasting insulin, may have particularly poor dietary response to low fat/high carb diets. Thus, adherence to this type of diet, as compared to their insulin-sensitive counterparts, may be more difficult (McClain et al., Diab Obes Metab, 2013).

It is likely that diets need to be individualized in order to be most effective. With this in mind, we need to be flexible in our recommendations, but also mindful that the *types* of proteins and carbohydrates must be chosen wisely, with healthy selections to optimize not just weight but overall cardiovascular health. Dietary adherence is one of the most important predictors of weight loss, irrespective of the type of diet. Thus it is probably best to tailor a diet to the individual's preference in terms of macronutrient predominance, so as to improve long-term adherence.

Behavioral Change Strategies for Primary Care Providers

For individuals to achieve their weight loss goals, the AHA recommends several behavioral change strategies that can be used when counseling primary care patients about dietary intake and physical activity. Effective principles of behavioral management strategies include self-monitoring, stimulus control, stress management, cognitive-behavioral strategies, problem solving, use of rewards, and relapse prevention approaches.When counseling patients about weight loss and physical activity, it is important to build their self-efficacy so that patients feel confident that they have the behavioral skills to overcome weight loss barriers and to successfully manage high-risk situations. To build self-efficacy, primary care providers can encourage patients to self-monitor by keeping diaries of their dietary intake and physical activity. To help with patient tracking, tools are available online and using smart phone applications (e.g. www.myfitnesspal.com/iphone, www.loseit.com/, www.sparkpeople.com/). Stimulus control involves helping patients identify and modify environmental cues associated with poor eating or physical inactivity. Similarly, stress management techniques can be used to help people cope with negative emotions or events that interfere with healthy eating. (For patients who enjoy mobile applications, one is available at www.t2health.org/apps/breathe2relax.) By discussing attitudes, beliefs, and perceptions about healthy eating and physical activity, primary care providers can assist patients in adopting and maintaining a healthy lifestyle. When patients confront barriers or experience setbacks, providers can use problem-solving and relapse-prevention approaches to help them get back on track. Finally, rewards can be used when habits are changed (e.g., increasing the number of minutes exercised).

The AHA has identified specific goals to improve health and decrease CVD risk, providing a set of evidence-based diet and lifestyle recommendations to achieve these goals (Lichtenstein et al., 2006). These Seven Cardiovascular Health Metrics, which incorporate the non-pharmacologic strategies for CVD prevention discussed to this point, include the following:

1. *Consume an overall healthy diet.* As maintaining a healthy diet is significantly related to a decreased risk of CVD and improvement in individual CVD risk factors, the AHA recommends consuming a diet rich in variety of fruits, vegetables, and grains (especially whole grains). In addition, the patient should choose fat-free or low-fat dairy products, lean meats, legumes, and poultry and should eat fish, especially oily fish, twice per week.

2. *Aim for a healthy body weight.* A BMI of 18.5–24.9 is recommended, given that obesity serves as an independent risk factor for CVD. Greater emphasis should be placed on preventing weight gain, given that this is a less difficult task than losing weight once it has been gained.

3. *Aim for a desirable lipid profile.* This goal includes maintaining recommended levels of LDL-C (optimal <100 mg/dL; near or above optimal 100–129 mg/dL), total cholesterol (optimal <200 mg/dL), and achieving appropriate levels of HDL-C (HDL-C<50 mg/dL in women and <40 mg/dL in men), and TG (<150 mg/dL).

4. *Aim for a normal blood pressure (BP).* Normal BP is defined as systolic BP less than 120 mm Hg and diastolic BP less than 80 mm Hg. BP above these normal levels is significantly associated with an increased risk of CVD.

5. *Aim for a normal blood glucose level.* A fasting blood glucose level of 100 mg/dL

or less is considered normal. Achieving and maintaining such a level reduces the risk of multiple negative health outcomes such as stroke and heart failure.

6. *Be physically active.* Regular physical activity reduces the risk of developing diseases such as diabetes, depression, and cancer, improves fitness, and is a central component in maintaining a healthy weight.

7. *Avoid use of and exposure to tobacco products.* Adults should quit use of tobacco products, given their links to multiple diseases, including cancer and CVD.

Pharmacologic Strategies to CVD Prevention

When managing individual risk factors for the prevention of CVD, pharmacotherapy should be added to lifestyle modification if optimization is not possible with non-pharmacologic therapies alone.

Pharmacologic Approaches to Smoking Cessation

Pharmacotherapy for nicotine dependence currently includes both nicotine replacement therapy (NRT) and non-NRT approaches (i.e., bupropion SR, varenicline), and both can be safely used in patients with a history of CVD (Fiore et al., 2008; US Public Health Service, 2008). NRTs can be delivered as a patch (i.e., nicotine patch), in which nicotine is delivered transdermally; as a vapor inhaler, in which nicotine is delivered through the lining of the mouth; orally (i.e., nicotine lozenge, nicotine gum), in which nicotine is absorbed through the buccal mucosa; or as a nasal spray, in which nicotine is absorbed through the nasal membranes. In individuals with a high degree of nicotine dependence, nicotine patches can be combined safely with the other four NRTs to provide a higher intensity of treatment. While nicotine patches, lozenges, and gum are available over the counter, nicotine inhalers and nasal sprays are available by prescription only.

Bupropion SR, a non-NRT medication, was originally introduced as an antidepressant and may be an effective choice for patients who wish to quit smoking and have a history of depression. Originally marketed as Wellbutrin SR, it has recently been introduced as Zyban for the treatment of nicotine dependence. Varenicline (Chantix) was formulated specifically for treatment of nicotine dependence and acts as a nicotine receptor partial agonist, mimicking the effects of nicotine to reduce cravings while reducing the pleasurable effects of smoking (Fiore et al., 2008; US Public Health Service, 2008). The addition of varenicline as a first-line treatment is based on evidence reviewed in the recent US Public Health Service Clinical Practice Guideline (Fiore et al., 2008; US Public Health Service, 2008). Both of these medications are available by prescription only. Bupropion SR is contraindicated for patients with a history of seizures or eating disorders. For varenicline, contraindications include current dialysis or a significant history of kidney disease.

Table 5-9 summarizes the dosage, treatment schedule, and side effects for each of these first-line treatments. Of note, though information on dosage and duration of treatment is presented for monotherapy inpatients with a moderate level of addiction, patients with a high level of nicotine addiction may need prolonged treatment or combinations of pharmacologic approaches to achieve and sustain abstinence (Fiore et al., 2008; US Public Health Service, 2008).

Pharmacologic Approaches to Weight Loss

Drug therapy is used as an adjunct to the behavioral change strategies for patients who, after 6 months of lifestyle changes, remain at increased medical risk and have not met reasonable weight loss goals. The decision to start drug therapy should be made after careful discussion of risks and benefits with patients. The

TABLE 5-9. SUMMARY OF PHARMACOTHERAPY FOR NICOTINE DEPENDENCE

Pharmacotherapy	Possible Side Effects	Dosage	Treatment Duration
Nicotine Replacement Therapy (NRT)			
Patch	Skin irritation, Insomnia	Example: Patient who smokes 1 pack (20 cigarettes) per day 21 mg/24 hrs patch every day for first 4 weeks 14 mg/24 hrs patch every day for next 2 weeks 7 mg/24 hrs patch every day for next 2 weeks	8 weeks
Gum	Sore mouth, Indigestion	Up to 24 pieces/day 2 mg piece for those who smoke 1–24 cigarettes/day 4 mg piece for those who smoke ≥ 25 cigarettes/day	Up to 12 weeks
Lozenge	Nausea, Heartburn	Between 4–20 lozenges/day 2 mg lozenge for those who smoke 1st cigarette within >30 minutes of waking 4 mg lozenge for those who smoke 1st cigarette within ≤30 minutes of waking	Up to 12 weeks
Inhaler	Irritation of mouth, throat	6–16 inhaler cartridges/day	Up to 6 months
Nasal Spray	Nasal Irritation	8–40 doses/day (suggested limit of 5 doses per hour)	3–6 months
Non-NRT			
Bupropion SR	Dry mouth, Insomnia, Seizures	Every morning, first three days = 150 mg/day Then 150 mg 2x/day Begin treatment 1-2 weeks prior to quit date	7–12 weeks initial; Up to 6 months maintenance
Varenicline	Nausea, Insomnia, Unusually vivid dreams, Depressed mood	First three days = 0.5 mg/day Next four days = 0.5 mg 2x/day Then 1mg 2x/day Begin treatment 1 week prior to quit date	3–6 months

Adapted from Fiore MC, Jaen CR, Baker TB, et al. Treating tobacco use and dependence: 2008. Update.Rockville, MD: USDHHS, US Public Health Service, 2008.

decision should be made after calculating a patient's BMI and assessing for comorbid illness such as diabetes, heart disease, hypertension, hyperlipidemia, sleep apnea, and others. Medical therapy should be considered in addition to lifestyle change in patients with a BMI over 30 alone, or in patients with a BMI of 27–29.9 with comorbid illness or in whom surgery is being considered (Bray & Ryan, 2012).

It is important to set realistic outcome goals with patients, recognizing that most patients will not achieve optimal body weight, even with drug therapy. Success has been defined as 2 kg or more of weight loss in the first month, and greater than 5% of baseline weight reduction at 6 months with *maintenance* of the weight loss (Bray & Ryan, 2012). Assessment of improvement in cardiovascular risks, diabetes outcomes, and so on, should also be performed in making a decision to continue medical therapy. Achieving more than 15% weight loss is considered an excellent response and is associated with lower blood pressure, decreased insulin resistance, and improved serum lipids. In terms of maintaining weight loss, it is important to recognize that the weight will tend to return to baseline when medication is discontinued, and patients need proper education that these medications do not *cure* obesity.

The following drugs are available for use in the treatment of obesity (see Table 5-10):

(1) Orlistat, which decreases fat absorption by inhibition of pancreatic lipases;

approximately 30% of fat in diet will not be digested, and physician must watch for depletion of fat-soluble vitamins and supplement accordingly;

(2) Lorcaserin, a newly approved serotonin 2C receptor agonist that suppresses appetite; the drug's affinity for 2C receptors is 100 times greater than for 2B receptors. The latter is associated with the prior "fen-phen" (fenfluramine, a non-selective serotonin agonist) epidemic with cardiac valvular toxicity and pulmonary hypertension; no such toxicities have been reported with this newer serotonergic drug;

(3) Phentermine alone, which stimulates norepinephrine release and increases satiety; only approved for short-term use or as a newly approved drug combination phentermine-topiramate (the latter used as an anti-epileptic and migraine drug, and also found to produce weight loss). These drugs should not be used in pregnancy and should not be used in patients with cardiovascular disease or hypertension;

(4) Other sympathomimetics (diethylproprion, benzphetamine, phendimetrazine) are rarely used, are subject to abuse, and are approved only for short-term use up to 12 weeks, like phentermine. It should also be noted

TABLE 5-10. PHARMACOLOGIC OPTIONS IN THE TREATMENT OF OBESITY

Generic Name	FDA Approval for Weight Loss	Drug Type	Common Side Effects
Phentermine	Yes; short term (up to 12 weeks) for adults	Appetite Suppressant	Increased blood pressure and heart rate, sleeplessness, nervousness
Diethylpropion	Yes; short term (up to 12 weeks) for adults	Appetite Suppressant	Dizziness, headache, sleeplessness, nervousness
Phendimetrazine	Yes; short term (up to 12 weeks) for adults	Appetite Suppressant	Sleeplessness, nervousness
Lorcaserin	Yes; long term (up to 1 year) for adults	Appetite Suppressant	Serotonin syndrome, headaches, dizziness, fatigue, constipation
Orlistat	Yes; long term (up to 1 year) for adults and children age 12 +	Lipase Inhibitor	Gastrointestinal issues (cramping, diarrhea, oily spotting)
Phentermine/ topiramate	Yes; long term (up to 1 year) for adults	Appetite Suppressant/ anti-epileptic	Tingling hands and feet, dizziness, altered taste sensation, insomnia

Adapted from National Institute of Diabetes and Digestive and Kidney Diseases. Weight-control Information Network: Prescription Medications for the Treatment of Obesity. Updated from Bray et al., 2012.

that certain diabetes medications may be useful for weight loss and should be considered for treatment of obese diabetics, including metformin, pramlintide, exanatide, and liraglutide.

In terms of efficacy, lorcaserin and orlistat have similar weight loss effects. Weight loss over placebo with orlistat was noted to be 3 kg at 1 year based on meta-analysis of 12 trials; trials with lorsaserin showed 3–4 kg excess weight lost over placebo. The phentermine-topiramate studies showed about 4–9 kg excess weight loss over placebo at 1–2 years (Bray & Ryan, 2012). Weight-loss drugs should be stopped if patients have not achieved a 5% weight loss at 12 weeks.

Weight-loss drugs must be prescribed with discretion as they may have serious adverse effects. A careful discussion must include review of risks, lack of long-term safety and efficacy data, temporary nature of the weight loss from such drugs, and the importance of maintaining a healthy lifestyle and changing unhealthy eating habits.

Pharmacologic Approaches to Treating Hypertension

All patients with hypertension who do not reach recommended BP targets (<140/90 mm Hg for non-diabetics and <140/80 mm Hg for diabetics) with lifestyle modification alone should be treated with antihypertensive medications. The pathogenesis of hypertension is multifactorial, and the available medications target one or more pathologic mechanisms (for a comprehensive review, see Victor, 2004). Commonly used classes of medications include diuretics, calcium channel blockers (CCBs), angiotensin-converting enzyme (ACE) inhibitors, angiotensin receptor blockers (ARBs), beta-adrenergic antagonists, and aldosterone antagonists. According to the JNC-7 guidelines published in 2003, diuretics should be the cornerstone of antihypertensive management for most adults without compelling indications for other therapies (see Figure 5-1) (Chobanian et al., 2003). This recommendation was based on the ALLHAT trial, in which diuretics were comparable to or better than other antihypertensive drugs at preventing cardiovascular

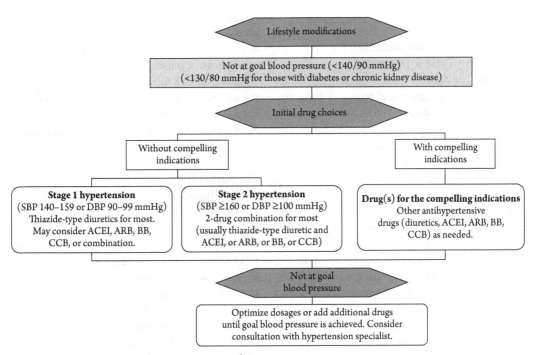

FIGURE 5-1: JNC-7 Algorithm for the Management of Hypertension.

Source: Adapted from *Seventh Report of the Joint National Committee on Prevention, Detection, Evaluation, and Treatment of High Blood Pressure (JNC 7 Express).* http://www.nhlbi.nih.gov/guidelines/hypertension/jncintro.htm. Accessed June 24, 2013. *New recommendations from the ADA include a less restrictive BP target of <140/80 for diabetes, and <130/80 for certain diabetics who can achieve this goal without undue treatment burden.

events, particularly among African American participants (ALLHAT, 2002). Since publication of JNC-7, it has become more apparent that the major determinant of cardiovascular risk reduction is the degree of BP lowering rather than the choice of antihypertensive drug (Rosendorff et al., 2007). In addition, the ADA recently recommended a less restrictive BP goal of <140/80 for diabetics and a BP goal <130/80 for certain diabetics such as younger patients who can achieve this goal without undue treatment burden (ADA, 2013). The AHA practice guidelines for the treatment of hypertension in the prevention of ischemic heart disease concluded that there is sufficient evidence to support use of a diuretic, calcium channel blocker, ACE inhibitor, or ARB as first-line therapy, supplemented by a second drug if BP goals are not achieved with one drug. Most patients with BP >20/10 mm Hg above goal will require two or more medications, and in most patients without CHD, any combination of diuretic, CCB, ACE inhibitor, or ARB should be explored before considering other antihypertensive classes (Rosendorff et al., 2007). Patients requiring more than three antihypertensive classes should be considered for referral to a hypertension specialist, as they may have refractory or secondary hypertension.

Pharmacologic Approaches to Managing Type 2 Diabetes

The ADA has developed a consensus algorithm for the metabolic management of type 2 diabetes (see Table 5-11) (Nathan et al., 2009). There are several pharmacologic options for lowering glucose, including but not limited to (1) insulin therapy (analogues of endogenous insulin that come in many forms; for full review see Hirsch et al., 2003); (2) metformin (a medication that lowers hepatic glucose output and improves insulin resistance); (3) sulfonylureas (a class of medications that increase pancreatic insulin secretion); and (4) glitazones (a class of medications that increase insulin sensitivity of muscle, fat, and liver). Step 1 in the algorithm is to initiate lifestyle modification plus metformin to achieve a goal HbA1C below 7%. Achieving the HbA1C goal usually requires a patient's fasting plasma glucose between 70–130 mg/dL and postprandial glucose (90–120 minutes after eating) to be <180 mg/dL. If the goal HbA1C <7% is not achieved after 3 months on step 1 therapy, step 2 includes the addition of basal insulin (intermediate-acting insulin at bedtime or long-acting insulin at bedtime or in morning; start with 10 units

TABLE 5-11. SIMPLIFIED ALGORITHM FOR MEDICAL MANAGEMENT OF HYPERGLYCEMIA IN TYPE 2 DIABETES

Step 1: After accurate diagnosis of type 2 diabetes and assessment of other CVD risk factors:
- Lifestyle modification plus metformin
- Assess HbA1C in 3 months

Step 2: If HbA1C <7% not achieved:
- Add sulfonylurea or glitazone if HbA1C is less than 8.5%
- Add basal insulin if HbA1C ≥8.5% or if symptoms of hyperglycemia present
- Assess HbA1C in 3 months

Step 3: If HbA1C <7% still not achieved with Step 2 interventions:
- Start or intensify insulin therapy
- A third oral agent can be added to Step 2 if HbA1C < 8%

Adapted from Nathan DM, Buse JB, Davidson MB, Heine RJ, et al. Management of hyperglycemia in type 2 diabetes: A consensus algorithm for the initiation and adjustment of therapy: a consensus statement from the American Diabetes Association and the European Association for the Study of Diabetes. *Diabetes Care.* 2009 Jan;32(1):193–203.

or 0.2 units/kg daily; increase by 2 every 3 days until fasting glucose in target range), a sulfonylurea, or a glitazone. If HbA1C is still 7% or more on step 2 therapy, basal insulin should be intensified or added to the sulfonylurea or glitazone. Each of these therapies has advantages and disadvantages and important potential adverse effects. For an excellent review of these considerations, see the consensus statement from the ADA and the European Association for the Study of Diabetes (Nathan et al., 2009).

Pharmacologic Management of Dyslipidemia

Despite the many benefits of TLC, statin benefit groups at high risk for short-term or long-term CVD will benefit from moderate to high intensity statin therapy (see Table 5-12 A and B). The LDL-C goal is determined after risk assessment and stratification. When medication is needed, it is typically prescribed after two visits (3–6 months) have targeted TLC. However, even when lipid-lowering agents are prescribed, providers should reinforce the need for patients to maintain their TLC behaviors to maximize the benefits of lipid-lowering therapies and to avoid repeated escalations in medication dosage.

Drugs that affect lipoprotein metabolism work by improving and preventing, slowing, or

TABLE 5-12. LDL CHOLESTEROL GOALS AND CUTPOINTS FOR THERAPEUTIC LIFESTYLE CHANGES (TLC) AND DRUG THERAPY IN DIFFERENT RISK CATEGORIES

A: ASCVD Statin Benefit Groups

Individuals with clinical ASCVD

Individuals with primary elevations of LDL-C ≥190 mg/dL

Individuals with diabetes aged 40–75 years with LDL-C 70–189 mg/dL and without clinical ASCVD

Individuals without clinical ASCVD or diabetes with LDL-C 70–189 mg/dL and estimated 10-year ASCVD risk ≥7.5%

B: High- Moderate- and Low-Intensity Statin Therapy

High-Intensity Statin Therapy	Moderate-Intensity Therapy	Low-Intensity Therapy
Daily dose lowers LDL-C on average, by approximately ≥50%	Daily dose lowers LDL-C on average, by approximately 30%–50%	Daily dose lowers LDL-C on average by <30%
Atorvastatin 40–80 mg	Atorvastatin 10–20 mg	Simvastatin 10 mg
Rosuvastatin 20–40 mg	Rosuvastatin 5–10 mg	Pravastatin 10–20 mg
	Simvastatin 20–40 mg	Pravastatin 10–20 mg
	Pravastatin 40–80 mg	Fluvastatin 20–40 mg
	Lovastatin 40 mg	Pitavastatin 1 mg
	Fluvastatin XL 80 mg	
	Fluvastatin 40 mg bid	
	Pitavastatin 2–4 mg	

Adapted from 2013 *ACC/AHA Guidelines on the Treatment of Blood Cholesterol to Reduce Atherosclerotic Cardiovascular Risk in Adults: A Report of the American College of Cardiology/American Heart Association Task Force on Practice Guidelines.* J Am Coll Cardiol. 2013.

reversing atherosclerotic lesions (Nissen et al., 2004). Currently, statins (HMG CoA reductase inhibitors) are the most widely prescribed cholesterol-lowering medications and have been shown to reduce LDL by 60% in high-risk patients. Reductions by 30–40% in CHD mortality and major cardiovascular events have also been achieved through statin use (Cannon et al., 2004; Colhoun et al., 2004; LIPID Study Group, 1998; MRC/BHF, 2002; Pedersen et al., 2004; Sacks et al., 1996; Shepherd et al., 2002).

Statins are generally safe; rare adverse side effects include rhabdomyolysis and renal failure. The most common side effects reported by patients are muscle-related problems such as cramps and myalgias (1–7%) and less frequently gastrointestinal symptoms. The lipophilic statins (simvastatin, lovastatin, atorvastatin, and fluvastatin) seem to have a greater association with muscle-related problems than the hydrophilic statins (pravastatin and rosuvastatin). Choosing a hydrophilic statin in a patient with a known history of myalgias should be considered (Rosenson, 2004). Increased age, being female, certain concomitant medications, and hepatic dysfunction may also increase the risk for muscle-related problems. Elevated liver enzymes as a result of statin

therapy are often a concern of patients, but the incidence is low and dose-dependent. An increased risk for type 2 diabetes has also been reported (RR 1.18, 95% CI 1.01–1.39), so this may be a consideration in primary prevention of CVD (Taylor et al., 2013).

Recently, several cholesterol-lowering drugs have become available over the counter (e.g., nicotinic acid) in immediate and sustained release; however, patients who wish to take these medications should continue to consult with their primary physicians about the need for the medication, potential side effects, details of the dosing regimen, and goals of therapy. The extended release requires a prescription and is reported to reduce the side effect of flushing. Table 5.13 gives more information on commonly prescribed lipid-lowering medications and their effects on cholesterol.

After a minimum of 6 weeks of drug therapy, the individual's response to the medication should be assessed to determine if cholesterol goals have been met; if so, the current dosage can be maintained. If the treatment goal has not been met, LDL-lowering therapy should be intensified, usually by increasing the dose of statin. If this is not tolerated, the statin can be combined with a bile acid sequestrant or nicotinic acid. Ezetimibe, a

TABLE 5-13. SUMMARY OF LIPID-LOWERING MEDICATIONS

Drug Class, Agents and Daily Doses	Lipid/ Lipoprotein Effects	Side Effects	Contraindications	Clinical Trial Results
HMG CoA reductase inhibitors (statins)*	LDL 18–55% HDL 5–15% TG 7–30%	Myopathy Increased liver enzymes	Absolute: • Active or chronic liver disease Relative: • Concomitant use of certain drugs†	Reduced major coronary events, CHD deaths, need for coronary procedures, stroke, and total mortality
Bile acid Sequestrants‡	LDL 15–30% HDL 3–5% TG No change or increase	Gastrointestinal distress Constipation Decreased absorption of other drugs	Absolute: • dysbetalipoproteinemia • TG >400 mg/dL Relative: • TG >200 mg/dL	Reduced major coronary events and CHD deaths
Nicotinic acid¥	LDL 5–25% HDL 15–35% TG 20–50%	Flushing Hyperglycemia Hyperuricemia (or gout) Upper GI distress Hepatotoxicity	Absolute: • Chronic liver disease • Severe gout Relative: • iabetes • yperuricemia • Peptic ulcer disease	Reduced major coronary events, and possibly total mortality
Fibric acids§	LDL 5–20% (may be increased in patients with high TG) HDL 10–20% TG 20–50%	Dyspepsia Gallstones Myopathy Unexplained non-CHD deaths in WHO study	Absolute: • Severe renal disease • Severe hepatic disease	Reduced major coronary events
Cholesterol absorption inhibitors◊	LDL 18%	Increased transaminases in combination with statins	Relative: Hepatic impairment	

* Lovastatin (20–80 mg), pravastatin (20–40 mg), simvastatin (20–40 mg), fluvastatin (20–80 mg), atorvastatin (10–80 mg), rosuvastatin (5–40 mg), pitavastatin (1–4 mg).
† Cyclosporine, macrolide antibiotics, various antifungal agents and cytochrome P-450 inhibitors (fibrates and niacin should be used with appropriate caution).
‡ Cholestyramine (4–24 g), colestipol (5–30 g), colesevelam (2.6–3.8 g).
¥ Immediate release (crystalline) nicotinic acid (1.5–3 g starting with 250 mg qhs), extended release nicotinic acid (Niaspan ®) (1–2 g), sustained release nicotinic acid (1–2 g).
§ Gemfibrozil (600 mg BID), fenofibrate (40–200 mg).
◊ Ezetimibe (10 mg).

new class of cholesterol absorption inhibitors, may be used as monotherapy or in combination with statins. Ezetimibe 10 mg daily reduced LDL-C by an estimated 17% (Knopp et al., 2003). When ezetimibe was co-administered with simvastatin, a 13.8% incremental reduction in LDL-C was found (Davidson et al., 2002).

Response to therapy should be assessed at regular intervals until the treatment goal has been met. Note that periodic liver function testing is no longer recommended for patients taking statins if the liver function tests were normal prior to starting therapy. Liver function tests should be repeated as clinically indicated. If the LDL goal cannot be attained by standard lipid-lowering therapy, the patient should be referred to a lipid specialist. Once the goal for LDL-C has been reached, other important components of the lipid panel should be optimized (i.e., lowering TG or increasing HDL) with continued TLC. Cholesterol levels can be monitored every 4–6 months, as indicated, to ensure that treatment goals are maintained.

Aspirin Use

Although the benefits of aspirin use in reducing CVD risk in men and women with known CVD are well-established, its use in primary prevention is less clear. In 2002, the USPSTF strongly recommended that clinicians discuss aspirin chemoprevention with adults who are at increased risk of CHD. This recommendation was based on a meta-analysis of five studies (which included mostly middle-aged men) that demonstrated a significant reduction in cardiovascular events, but no mortality benefit (Wolff et al., 2009). Subsequent studies, including the Women's Health Study, a randomized control trial that prospectively examined aspirin for primary prevention in women, found a benefit from aspirin use for the reduction of strokes (RR 0.83, 95% CI 0.69–0.99) but no statistically significant benefit in reduction of combined cardiovascular events or all-cause mortality (Ridker et al., 2005). Also, a good quality sex-specific meta-analysis suggested sex-specific differences in aspirin use; men benefit from myocardial infarction reduction and women benefit from ischemic stroke reduction (Berger et al., 2006). Because the CVD risk reduction appears to differ by sex, the AHA developed aspirin guidelines specifically for women, recommending that women with a 10-year CVD risk (not just CHD risk) of 10% or more be considered for aspirin 75–325 mg per day in the absence of contraindications (Mosca et al., 2011). In 2009, the USPSTF reissued recommendations that focused on a balanced benefit-risk profile. Aspirin is recommended for women aged 55–79 years when the potential benefit in ischemic stroke reduction outweighs the potential harm of an increase in GI hemorrhage. Aspirin is recommended for men aged 45–79 years when the potential benefit of myocardial infarction reduction outweighs the potential harm of an increase in GI hemorrhage (USPSTF, 2009). Increased risk of bleeding with aspirin must be taken seriously, so we advocate ensuring that patients have BP controlled below 180/110 mm Hg before initiating aspirin to avoid hemorrhagic stroke.

SURGICAL APPROACHES TO CVD PREVENTION
Bariatric Surgery for the Treatment of Obesity

Bariatric surgery should be considered only for patients who are at a high risk for future cardiovascular events due to extreme obesity and who have been unsuccessful with behavioral modifications and drug

therapies (NHLBI, 2002). Bariatric surgeries, including vertical-banded gastroplasty and Roux-en-Y gastric bypass, have been shown to improve or eradicate obesity-related conditions such as type 2 diabetes, dyslipidemia, hypertension, and obstructive sleep apnea, as well as reducing mortality in the majority of patients (Buchwald et al., 2004; Kushner & Noble, 2006). Patients who follow the recommended lifestyle changes following surgery can expect to lose 50–60% of excess body weight (Mayo Clinic, 2008). The NHLBI recommends that surgery be considered for those with clinically severe obesity (BMI ≥ 40) or a BMI of at least 35 with serious medical comorbidities (see Table 5-14) (NHLBI, 2002). The American College of Physicians recommends that surgery be considered for those with a BMI of at least 40 with comorbidities (Snow et al., 2005).

Bariatric surgery poses major risks, and patients should be closely monitored for complications and lifestyle modifications throughout their lives (NHLBI, 2002). In addition to surgical complications of infection, bleeding, adverse reaction to the anesthesia, anastomotic leak, subphrenic abscess, splenic injury, pulmonary embolism, blood clots, and stoma stenosis, later complications can include incisional hernias, gallstones, and dumping syndrome (NHLBI, 2002; Snow et al., 2005). One study reported a significant increase in the hospitalization rate following the first year of gastric bypass surgery compared to the prior year (19.3% vs. 7.9%, respectively). These rates were not significantly reduced in the second year or third year after gastric bypass (18.4% and 14.9%, respectively) and most likely represented late complications of the procedure (Zingmond, McGory, & Ko, 2005). The total 30-day mortality rate has been reported to be 0.33–1.9%, with higher risks among Medicare recipients due to a greater burden of comorbid disease (Flum et al., 2005; MayoClinic, 2008). As with drug therapy, primary care providers should discuss with patients the potential short- and long-term adverse effects associated with bariatric surgery and the importance of maintaining a healthy lifestyle.

CONCLUSIONS

From 1980 to 2000, nearly half of the reduction in cardiac mortality may be explained by improvements in cardiovascular risk factors, such as systolic blood pressure control and cholesterol lowering (Ford et al., 2007). Primary care physicians play a key role in these cardiovascular risk factor

TABLE 5-14. NHLBI GUIDE TO SELECTING TREATMENT FOR OVERWEIGHT AND OBESITY

Treatment	BMI Category				
	25–26.9	27–29.9	30-34.9	35–39.9	≥40
Diet, physical activity, and behavior therapy	With comorbidities	With comorbidities	*	*	*
Pharmacotherapy		With comorbidities	*	*	*
Surgery				With comorbidities	

The * represents the use of indicated treatment regardless of comorbidities.

modifications. By being familiar with cardiovascular risk factors and their epidemiology, method of assessment, and treatment strategies, primary care physicians can deliver early intervention and education on cardiovascular disease prevention at timely and regular intervals. Behavior change is difficult, so utilizing behavior change techniques such as motivational interviewing, goal setting, problem solving, and promoting patient self-efficacy is important in helping patients to succeed. If primary care physicians successfully engage their patients to improve their cardiovascular risk factors, improved cardiovascular health is possible.

REFERENCES

ACCORD Study Group, Cushman WC, Evans GW, Byington RP, Goff DC Jr, Grimm RH Jr, Cutler JA, Simons-Morton DG, Basile JN, Corson MA, Probstfield JL, Katz L, Peterson KA, Friedewald WT, Buse JB, Bigger JT, Gerstein HC, Ismail-Beigi F. Effects of intensive blood-pressure control in type 2 diabetes mellitus. N Engl J Med. 2010;362(17):1575–1585.

ALLHAT. Major outcomes in high-risk hypertensive patients randomized to angiotensin-converting enzyme inhibitor or calcium channel blocker vs diuretic: The Antihypertensive and Lipid-Lowering Treatment to Prevent Heart Attack Trial (ALLHAT). JAMA. 2002;288(23):2981–2997.

American Diabetes Association. Standards of medical care in diabetes—2013. Diabetes Care. 2013;Suppl 1:S11–66.

American Psychiatric Association Work Group on Substance Use Disorders. Practice Guideline for the Treatment of Patients with Substance Use Disorders. Arlington, VA: American Psychiatric Publishing; 2006.

Berger JS, Roncaglioni MC, Avanzini F, Pangrazzi I, Tognoni G, Brown, DL. Aspirin for the primary prevention of cardiovascular events in women and men: a sex-specific meta-analysis of randomized controlled trials. JAMA. 2006;295(3):306–313.

Bray GA, Ryan DH. Medical Therapy for the Patient with Obesity. Circulation. 2012;125(13):1695–1703.

Buchwald H, Avidor Y, Braunwald E, Jensen MD, Pories W, Fahrbach K, Schoelles K. Bariatric surgery: a systematic review and meta-analysis. JAMA. 224;292(14):1724–1737.

Calfas KJ, & Hagler AS. Physical Aactivity. (pp. 192–221). In: Sheinfeld Gorin S & Arnold J. Health Promotion in Practice,. pp. 192–221. San Francisco, CA: Jossey-Bass;, 2006

Calhoun DA, Jones D, Textor S, Goff DC, Murphy TP, Toto RD, White A, Cushman WC, White W, Sica D, Ferdinand K, Giles TD, Falkner B, Carey RM. Resistant hypertension: diagnosis, evaluation, and treatment: a scientific statement from the American Heart Association Professional Education Committee of the Council for High Blood Pressure Research. Circulation. 2008;117(25):e510–e526.

Campbell NR, Culleton BW, McKay DW. Misclassification of blood pressure by usual measurement in ambulatory physician practices. Am J Hypertens. 225;18(12 Pt 1):1522–1527.

Cannon CP, Braunwald E, McCabe CH, Rader DJ, Rouleau JL, Belder R, Joyal SV, Hill KA, Pfeffer MA, Skene AM. Intensive versus moderate lipid lowering with statins after acute coronary syndromes. N Engl J Med. 2004;350(15):1495–1504.

CDC. National trends in smoking cessation. In The Health Benefits of Smoking Cessation: A Report of the Surgeon General. Washington, DC: US Government Printing Office; 1990.

Chen G, McAlister FA, Walker RL, Hemmelgarn BR, Campbell N. 2011. Cardiovascular outcomes in Framingham participants with diabetes: the importance of blood pressure. Hypertension 57: 891–897.

Chobanian AV, Bakris GL, Black HR, Cushman WC, Green LA, Izzo JL Jr, Jones DW, Materson BJ, Oparil S, Wright JT Jr, Roccella EJ. Seventh report of the Joint National Committee on Prevention, Detection, Evaluation, and Treatment of High Blood Pressure. Hypertension. 2003;42(6):1206–1252.

Colhoun HM, Betteridge DJ, Durrington PN, Hitman GA, Neil HA, Livingstone SJ, Thomason MJ, Mackness MI, Charlton-Menys V, Fuller JH. Primary prevention of cardiovascular disease with atorvastatin in type 2 diabetes in the Collaborative Atorvastatin Diabetes Study (CARDS): multicentre randomised placebo-controlled trial. *Lancet.* 2004;364(9435):685–696.

Davidson MH, McGarry T, Bettis R, Melani L, Lipka LJ, LeBeaut AP, Suresh R, Sun S, Veltri EP. Ezetimibe coadministered with simvastatin in patients with primary hypercholesterolemia. *J Am Coll Cardiol.* 2002;40(12):2125–2134.

Diabetes Control and Complications Trial Research Group. The effect of intensive treatment of diabetes on the development and progression of long-term complications in insulin-dependent diabetes mellitus. *N Engl J Med.* 1993;329(14):977–986.

Dolan E, Stanton A, Thijs L, Hinedi K, Atkins N, McClory S, Den Hond E, McCormack P, Staessen JA, O'Brien E. Superiority of ambulatory over clinic blood pressure measurement in predicting mortality: the Dublin outcome study. *Hypertension.* 2005;46(1):156–161.

Doll R, Peto R, Boreham J, Sutherland I. Mortality in relation to smoking: 50 years' observations on male British doctors. *BMJ.* 2004;328(7455):1519.

Economic costs of diabetes in the U.S. in 2007. *Diabetes Care.* 2008;31(3):596–615.

Estruch R, Ros E, Salas-Salvadó J, Covas MI, Corella D, Arós F, Gómez-Gracia E, Ruiz-Gutiérrez V, Fiol M, Lapetra J, Lamuela-Raventos RM, Serra-Majem L, Pintó X, Basora J, Muñoz MA, Sorlí JV, Martínez JA, Martínez-González MA; PREDIMED Study Investigators. Primary prevention of cardiovascular disease with a Mediterranean diet. *N Engl J Med.* 2013;368(14):1279–1290.

Fagerstrom KO, Schneider NG. Measuring nicotine dependence: a review of the Fagerstrom Tolerance Questionnaire. *J Behav Med.* 1989;12(2):159–182.

Finkelstein EA, Fiebelkorn IC, Wang G. National medical spending attributable to overweight and obesity: how much, and who's paying? *Health Aff (Millwood).* 2003;Suppl Web Exclusives:W3-219–226.

Fiore MC, Jaen CR, Baker TB, et al. *Treating Tobacco Use and Dependence: 2008 Update.* Rockville, MD: US Department of Health and Human Services, US Public Health Service; 2008.

Flum DR, Salem L, Elrod JA, Dellinger EP, Cheadle A, Chan L. Early mortality among Medicare beneficiaries undergoing bariatric surgical procedures. *JAMA.* 2005;294(15):1903–1908.

Ford ES, Giles WH, Dietz WH. Prevalence of the metabolic syndrome among US adults: findings from the third National Health and Nutrition Examination Survey. *JAMA.* 2002;287(3):356–359.

Ford ES, Ajani UA, Croft JB, Critchley JA, Labarthe DR, Kottke TE, Giles WH, Capewell S. Explaining the decrease in U.S. deaths from coronary disease, 1980–2000. *N Engl J Med.* 2007;56(23):2388–2398.

Gaede P, Vedel P, Larsen N, Jensen GV, Parving HH, Pedersen O. Multifactorial intervention and cardiovascular disease in patients with type 2 diabetes. *N Engl J Med.* 2003;348(5):383–393.

Gaziano JM, Manson JE, Ridker PM. Primary and Secondary Prevention of Coronary Heart Disease. In: Libby PB, Bonow R, Mann D, Zipes D, eds. *Braunwald's Heart Disease: A Textbook of Cardiovascular Medicine.* Philadelphia: Saunders Elsevier; 2007.

Gardner CD, Kiazand A, Alhassan S, Kim S, Stafford RS, Balise RR, Kraemer HC, King AC. Comparison of the Atkins, Zone, Ornish, and LEARN diets for change in weight and related risk factors among overweight premenopausal women: the A TO Z Weight Loss Study: a randomized trial. *JAMA.* 2007;297(9):969–977.

Go AS, Mozaffarian D, Roger VL, Benjamin EJ, Berry JD, Borden WB, Bravata DM, Dai S, Ford ES, Fox CS, Franco S, Fullerton HJ, Gillespie C, Hailpern SM, Heit JA, Howard VJ, Huffman MD, Kissela BM, Kittner SJ, Lackland DT, Lichtman JH, Lisabeth LD, Magid D, Marcus GM, Marelli A, Matchar DB, McGuire DK, Mohler ER, Moy CS, Mussolino ME, Nichol G, Paynter NP, Schreiner PJ, Sorlie PD, Stein J, Turan TN, Virani SS, Wong ND, Woo D, Turner MB; American Heart Association Statistics Committee and Stroke Statistics Subcommittee. Executive summary: heart disease and stroke statistics--2013 update: a report from the American Heart Association. *Circulation.* 2013;127(1):143–152.

Greenland P, Alpert JS, Beller GA, Benjamin EJ, Budoff MJ, Fayad ZA, Foster E, Hlatky MA, Hodgson JM, Kushner FG, Lauer MS, Shaw LJ, Smith SC Jr, Taylor AJ, Weintraub WS, Wenger NK, Jacobs AK; American College of Cardiology Foundation/American Heart Association Task Force on Practice Guidelines. 2010 ACCF/AHA guideline for assessment of cardiovascular risk in asymptomatic adults: executive summary: a report of the American College of Cardiology Foundation/American Heart Association Task Force on Practice Guidelines. *Circulation.* 2010;122(25):2748–2764.

Grundy SM, Cleeman JI, Daniels SR, Donato KA, Eckel RH, Franklin BA, Gordon DJ, Krauss RM, Savage PJ, Smith SC Jr, Spertus JA, Costa F. Diagnosis and management of the metabolic syndrome. An American Heart Association/National Heart, Lung, and Blood Institute Scientific Statement. Executive summary. *Cardiol Rev.* 2005;13(6):322–327.

Grundy SM, Cleeman JI, Merz CN, Brewer HB Jr, Clark LT, Hunninghake DB, Pasternak RC, Smith SC Jr, Stone NJ; National Heart, Lung, and Blood Institute; American College of Cardiology Foundation; American Heart Association. Implications of recent clinical trials for the National Cholesterol Education Program Adult Treatment Panel III guidelines. *Circulation*. 2004;*110*(2):227–239.

Grundy SM, Pasternak R, Greenland P, Smith S Jr, Fuster V. AHA/ACC scientific statement: assessment of cardiovascular risk by use of multiple-risk-factor assessment equations: a statement for healthcare professionals from the American Heart Association and the American College of Cardiology. *J Am Coll Cardiol*. 1999a;*34*(4):1348–1359.

Grundy SM, Pasternak R, Greenland P, Smith S Jr, Fuster V. Assessment of cardiovascular risk by use of multiple-risk-factor assessment equations: a statement for healthcare professionals from the American Heart Association and the American College of Cardiology. *Circulation*. 1999b;*100*(13):1481–1492.

Hamer M, Sabia S, Batty GD, Shipley MJ, Tabák AG, Singh-Manoux A, Kivimaki M. Physical activity and inflammatory markers over 10 years: follow-up in men and women from the Whitehall II cohort study. *Circulation*. 2012;*126*(8):928–933.

Haskell WL, Lee IM, Pate RR, Powell KE, Blair SN, Franklin BA, Macera CA, Heath GW, Thompson PD, Bauman A. Physical activity and public health: updated recommendation for adults from the American College of Sports Medicine and the American Heart Association. *Circulation*. 2007;*116*(9):1081–1093.

Heatherton TF, Kozlowski LT, Frecker RC, Fagerstrom KO. The Fagerstrom Test for Nicotine Dependence: a revision of the Fagerstrom Tolerance Questionnaire. *Br J Addict*. 1991;*86*(9):1119–1127.

Hertz RP, Unger AN, Cornell JA, Saunders E. Racial disparities in hypertension prevalence, awareness, and management. *Arch Intern Med*. 2005;*165*(18):2098–2104.

Holman RR, Paul SK, Bethel MA, Matthews DR, Neil HA. 10-year follow-up of intensive glucose control in type 2 diabetes. *N Engl J Med*. 2008;*359*(15):1577–1589.

Hu FB, Manson JE, Willett WC. Types of dietary fat and risk of coronary heart disease: a critical review. *J Am Coll Nutr*. 2001;*20*(1):5–19.

Knoops KT, de Groot LC, Kromhout D, Perrin AE, Moreiras-Varela O, Menotti A, van Staveren WA. Mediterranean diet, lifestyle factors, and 10-year mortality in elderly European men and women: the HALE project. *JAMA*. 2004;*292*(12):1433–1439.

Knopp RH, Gitter H, Truitt T, Bays H, Manion CV, Lipka LJ, LeBeaut AP, Suresh R, Yang B, Veltri EP, Ezetimibe Study Group. Effects of ezetimibe, a new cholesterol absorption inhibitor, on plasma lipids in patients with primary hypercholesterolemia. *Eur Heart J*. 2003;*24*(8):729.

Knowler WC, Barrett-Connor E, Fowler SE, Hamman RF, Lachin JM, Walker EA, Nathan DM; Diabetes Prevention Program Research Group. Reduction in the incidence of type 2 diabetes with lifestyle intervention or metformin. *N Engl J Med*. 2002;*346*(6):393–403.

Kushner RF, Noble CA. Long-term outcome of bariatric surgery: an interim analysis.*Mayo Clin Proc*. 2006;*81*(10 Suppl):S46–S51.

Law MR, Wald NJ, Rudnicka AR. Quantifying effect of statins on low density lipoprotein cholesterol, ischaemic heart disease, and stroke: systematic review and meta-analysis. *BMJ*. 2003;*326*(7404):1423.

Lee IM, Rexrode KM, Cook NR, Manson JE, Buring JE. Physical activity and coronary heart disease in women: is "no pain, no gain" passé? *JAMA*. 2001;*285*(11):1447–1454.

Leon AS, Myers MJ, Connett J. Leisure time physical activity and the 16-year risks of mortality from coronary heart disease and all-causes in the Multiple Risk Factor Intervention Trial (MRFIT). *Int J Sports Med*. 1997;*18*(Suppl 3):S208–S215.

Lichtenstein AH, Appel LJ, Brands M, Carnethon M, Daniels S, Franch HA, Franklin B, Kris-Etherton P, Harris WS, Howard B, Karanja N, Lefevre M, Rudel L, Sacks F, Van Horn L, Winston M, Wylie-Rosett J. Diet and lifestyle recommendations revision 2006: a scientific statement from the American Heart Association Nutrition Committee. *Circulation*. 2006;*114*(1):82–96.

Long-Term Intervention with Pravastatin in Ischaemic Disease (LIPID) Study Group. Prevention of cardiovascular events and death with pravastatin in patients with coronary heart disease and a broad range of initial cholesterol levels. *N Engl J Med*. 1998;*339*(19):1349–1357.

Lyznicki JM, Young DC, Riggs JA, Davis RM. Obesity: assessment and management in primary care. *Am Fam Physician*. 2001;*63*(11):2185–2196.

Manson JE, Hu FB, Rich-Edwards JW, Colditz GA, Stampfer MJ, Willett WC, Speizer FE, Hennekens CH. A prospective study of walking as compared with vigorous exercise in the prevention of coronary heart disease in women. *N Engl J Med*. 1999;*341*(9):650–658.

Mayo Clinic. *Gastric bypass surgery: What can you expect?* [cited October 25, 2008]. Available from http://www.mayoclinic.com/health/gastric-bypass/HQ01465.

Meriwether RA, Lee JA, Lafleur AS, Wiseman P. Physical activity counseling. *Am Fam Physician*. 2008;*77*(8):1129–1136.

McClain AD, Otten JJ, Hekler EB, Gardner CD. Adherence to a low-fat vs. low-carbohydrate diet differs by insulin resistance status. *Diabetes Obes Metab*. 2013;*15*(1):87–90.

Michos ED, Nasir K, Braunstein JB, Rumberger JA, Budoff MJ, Post WS, Blumenthal RS. Framingham risk equation underestimates subclinical atherosclerosis risk in asymptomatic women. *Atherosclerosis*. 2006;*184*(1):201–206.

Miller M, Stone NJ, Ballantyne C, Bittner V, Criqui MH, Ginsberg HN, Goldberg AC, Howard WJ,

Jacobson MS, Kris-Etherton PM, Lennie TA, Levi M, Mazzone T, Pennathur S; American Heart Association Clinical Lipidology, Thrombosis, and Prevention Committee of the Council on Nutrition, Physical Activity, and Metabolism; Council on Arteriosclerosis, Thrombosis and Vascular Biology; Council on Cardiovascular Nursing; Council on the Kidney in Cardiovascular Disease. Triglycerides and cardiovascular disease: a scientific statement from the American Heart Association. *Circulation.* 2011;*123*(20):2292–2333.

Mosca L, Benjamin EJ, Berra K, Bezanson JL, Dolor RJ, Lloyd-Jones DM, Newby LK, Piña IL, Roger VL, Shaw LJ, Zhao D, Beckie TM, Bushnell C, D'Armiento J, Kris-Etherton PM, Fang J, Ganiats TG, Gomes AS, Gracia CR, Haan CK, Jackson EA, Judelson DR, Kelepouris E, Lavie CJ, Moore A, Nussmeier NA, Ofili E, Oparil S, Ouyang P, Pinn VW, Sherif K, Smith SC Jr, Sopko G, Chandra-Strobos N, Urbina EM, Vaccarino V, Wenger NK; American Heart Association. Effectiveness-based guidelines for the prevention of cardiovascular disease in women—2011 update: a guideline from the American Heart Association. *J Am Coll Cardiol.* 2011;*57*(12):1404–1423.

MRC/BHF Heart Protection Study of cholesterol lowering with simvastatin in 20,536 high-risk individuals: a randomised placebo-controlled trial. *Lancet.* 2002;*360*(9326):7–22.

Nathan DM, Buse JB, Davidson MB, Ferrannini E, Holman RR, Sherwin R, Zinman B. 2009. Medical management of hyperglycemia in type 2 diabetes: a consensus algorithm for the initiation and adjustment of therapy: a consensus statement of the American Diabetes Association and the European Association for the Study of Diabetes. *Diabetes Care.* 2009;*32*(1):193–203.

National Cholesterol Education Program Expert Panel. Third Report of the National Cholesterol Education Program (NCEP) Expert Panel on Detection, Evaluation, and Treatment of High Blood Cholesterol in Adults (Adult Treatment Panel III) final report. *Circulation.* 2002;*106*(25):3143–3421.

National Institutes of Health. *Clinical Guidelines on the Identification, Evaluation, and Treatment of Overweight and Obesity in Adults: The Evidence Report.* Bethesda (MD). National Heart Lung and Blood Institute; 1998.

National Task Force on the Prevention and Treatment of Obesity. Overweight, obesity, and health risk. *Arch Intern Med.* 2000;*160*(7):898–904.

NHLBI. *The Practical Guide: Identification, Evaluation, and Treatment of Overweight and Obesity.* Bethesda, MD; 2002. NIH Publication No. 02-4084.

NIDDK. *National Diabetes Statistics, 2007.* NIH; 2002.

Nissen SE, Tuzcu EM, Schoenhagen P, Brown BG, Ganz P, Vogel RA, Crowe T, Howard G, Cooper CJ, Brodie B, Grines CL, DeMaria AN. Effect of intensive compared with moderate lipid-lowering therapy on progression of coronary atherosclerosis: a randomized controlled trial. *JAMA.* 2004;*291*(9):1071–1080.

Norris SL, Zhang X, Avenell A, Gregg E, Schmid CH, Lau J. Long-term non-pharmacological weight loss interventions for adults with prediabetes. *Cochrane Database Syst Rev.* 2005; *18*;(2):CD005270.

O'Connor PJ, Vazquez-Benitez G, Schmittdiel JA, Parker ED, Trower NK, Desai JR, Margolis KL, Magid DJ. Benefits of early hypertension control on cardiovascular outcomes in patients with diabetes. *Diabetes Care.* 2013;*36*(2):322–327.

Ogden CL, Carroll MD, McDowell MA, Flegal KM. *Obesity among Adults in the United States—No Statistically Significant Changes since 2003–2004.* US Department of Health and Human Services: National Center for Health Statistics Data Brief; 2007.

Oguma Y, Shinoda-Tagawa T. Physical activity decreases cardiovascular disease risk in women: review and meta-analysis. *Am J Prev Med.* 2004;*26*(5):407–418.

Olendzki B, Speed C, Domino FJ. Nutritional assessment and counseling for prevention and treatment of cardiovascular disease. *Am Fam Physician.* 2006;*73*(2):257–264.

Ornish D, Scherwitz LW, Billings JH, Brown SE, Gould KL, Merritt TA, Sparler S, Armstrong WT, Ports TA, Kirkeeide RL, Hogeboom C, Brand RJ. Intensive lifestyle changes for reversal of coronary heart disease. *JAMA.* 1998;*280*(23):2001–2007.

Pedersen TR, Kjekshus J, Berg K, Haghfelt T, Faergeman O, Faergeman G, Pyorala K, Miettinen T, Wilhelmsen L, Olsson AG, Wedel H. Randomised trial of cholesterol lowering in 4444 patients with coronary heart disease: the Scandinavian Simvastatin Survival Study (4S). 1994. *Atheroscler.* 2004; Suppl 5(3):81–87.

Pencina MJ, D'Agostino RB Sr, Larson MG, Massaro JM, Vasan RS. Predicting the 30-year risk of cardiovascular disease: The Framingham Heart Study. *Circulation.* 2009;*119*(24):3078–3084.

Pescatello LS, Franklin BA, Fagard R, Farquhar WB, Kelley GA, Ray CA. American College of Sports Medicine position stand: exercise and hypertension. *Med Sci Sports Exerc.* 2004;*36*(3):533–553.

Puhl R, Brownell KD. Bias, discrimination, and obesity. *Obes Res.* 2001;*9*(12):788–805.

Resnick HE, Valsania P, Halter JB, Lin X. Relation of weight gain and weight loss on subsequent diabetes risk in overweight adults. *J Epidemiol Community Health.* 2000;*54*(8):596–602.

Ridker PM, Buring JE, Rifai N, Cook NR. Development and validation of improved algorithms for the assessment of global cardiovascular risk in women: the Reynolds Risk Score. *JAMA.* 2007;*297*(6):611–619.

Ridker PM, Cook NR, Lee IM, Gordon D, Gaziano JM, Manson JE, Hennekens CH, Buring JE. A randomized trial of low-dose aspirin in the primary prevention of cardiovascular disease in women. *N Engl J Med.* 2005;*352*(13):1293–1304.

Ridker PM, Paynter NP, Rifai N, Gaziano JM, Cook NR. C-reactive protein and parental history improve global cardiovascular risk prediction: the Reynolds Risk Score for men. *Circulation.* 2008;*118*(22):2243–2251.

Rollnick S, Mason P, Butler C. *Health Behavior Change: A Guide for Practitioners.* Edinburgh; New York: Churchill Livingstone; 1999.

Rollnick S, Miller WR, Butler C. *Motivational Interviewing In Health Care: Helping Patients Change Behavior, Applications of Motivational Interviewing.* New York: Guilford Press; 2008.

Rosendorff C, Black HR, Cannon CP, Gersh BJ, Gore J, Izzo JL, Jr, Kaplan NM, O'Connor CM, O'Gara PT, Oparil S. Treatment of hypertension in the prevention and management of ischemic heart disease: a scientific statement from the American Heart Association Council for High Blood Pressure Research and the Councils on Clinical Cardiology and Epidemiology and Prevention. *Circulation.* 2007;*115*(21):2761–2788.

Sacks FM, Pfeffer MA, Moye LA, Rouleau JL, Rutherford JD, Cole TG, Brown L, Warnica JW, Arnold JM, Wun CC, Davis BR, Braunwald E. 1996. The effect of pravastatin on coronary events after myocardial infarction in patients with average cholesterol levels. Cholesterol and Recurrent Events Trial investigators. *N Engl J Med.* 1996;*335*(14):1001–1009.

Sacks FM, Svetkey LP, Vollmer WM, Appel LJ, Bray GA, Harsha D, Obarzanek E, Conlin PR, Miller ER, 3rd, Simons-Morton DG, Karanja N, Lin PH. Effects on blood pressure of reduced dietary sodium and the Dietary Approaches to Stop Hypertension (DASH) diet. DASH-Sodium Collaborative Research Group. *N Engl J Med.* 2001;*344*(1):3–10.

Sacks FM, Bray GA, Carey VJ, Smith SR, Ryan DH, Anton SD, McManus K, Champagne CM, Bishop LM, Laranjo N, Leboff MS, Rood JC, de Jonge L, Greenway FL, Loria CM, Obarzanek E, Williamson DA. Comparison of weight-loss diets with different compositions of fat, protein, and carbohydrates. *N Engl J Med.* 2009;*360*(9):859–873.

Schober SE, Carroll MD, Lacher DA, Hirsch R. *High Serum Total Cholesterol—An Indicator for Monitoring Cholesterol Lowering Efforts: U.S. Adults, 2005–2006.* US Department of Health and Human Services: National Center for Health Statistics; 2007.

Shepherd J, Blauw GJ, Murphy MB, Bollen EL, Buckley BM, Cobbe SM, Ford I, Gaw A, Hyland M, Jukema JW, Kamper AM, Macfarlane PW, Meinders AE, Norrie J, Packard CJ, Perry IJ, Stott DJ, Sweeney BJ, Twomey C, Westendorp RG. Pravastatin in elderly individuals at risk of vascular disease (PROSPER): a randomised controlled trial. *Lancet.* 2002;*360*(9346):1623–1630.

Shiwaku K, Anuurad E, Enkhmaa B, Kitajima K, Yamane Y. Appropriate BMI for Asian populations. *Lancet.* 2004;*363*(9414):1077.

Snow V, Barry P, Fitterman N, Qaseem A, Weiss K. Pharmacologic and surgical management of obesity in primary care: a clinical practice guideline from the American College of Physicians. *Ann Intern Med.* 2005;*142*(7):525–531.

Sofi F, Cesari F, Abbate R, Gensini GF, Casini A. Adherence to Mediterranean diet and health status: meta-analysis. *BMJ.* 2008;*337*:a1344.

Stampfer MJ, Hu FB, Manson JE, Rimm EB, Willett WC. Primary prevention of coronary heart disease in women through diet and lifestyle. *N Engl J Med.* 2000;*343*(1):16–22.

Stone NJ, Robinson J, Lichtenstein AH, Bairey Merz CN, Lloyd-Jones DM, Blum CB, McBride P, Eckel RH, Schwartz JS, Goldberg AC, Shero ST, Gordon D, Smith SC Jr, Levy D, Watson K, Wilson PW. 2013 ACC/AHA Guideline on the Treatment of Blood Cholesterol to Reduce Atherosclerotic Cardiovascular Risk in Adults: A Report of the American College of Cardiology/American Heart Association Task Force on Practice Guidelines. *J Am Coll Cardiol.* 2013. S0735–1097(13)06028–2.

Surgeon General. *The Health Consequences of Smoking: A Report of the Surgeon General.* Atlanta, GA: DHHS, Center for Disease Control and Prevention, National Center for Chronic Disease Prevention and Promotion; 2004.

Swardfager W, Herrmann N, Cornish S, Mazereeuw G, Marzolini S, Sham L, Lanctôt KL. Exercise intervention and inflammatory markers in coronary artery disease: a meta-analysis. *Am Heart J.* 2012;*163*(4):666–676.

Taylor F, Huffman MD, Macedo AF, Moore TH, Burke M, Davey Smith G, Ward K, Ebrahim S. Statins for the primary prevention of cardiovascular disease. *Cochrane Database Syst Rev.* 2013.

UK Prospective Diabetes Study (UKPDS) Group. Intensive blood-glucose control with sulphonylureas or insulin compared with conventional treatment and risk of complications in patients with type 2 diabetes (UKPDS 33). *Lancet.* 1998;*352*(9131):837–853.

USDA Research Service. *What We Eat In America,* NHANES. 2008. Available from http://www.ars.usda.gov/Services/docs.htm?docid=17041.

USDA. *Development of 2010 Dietary Guidelines for Americans: Consumer Messages and New Food Icon.* Retrieved June 14, 2013, from http://www.choosemyplate.gov/food-groups/downloads/MyPlate/ExecutiveSummaryOfFormativeResearch.pdf.

US Department of Health and Human Services. Healthy People 2010. 2008. Available from http://www.healthypeople.gov/.

US Public Health Service. A clinical practice guideline for treating tobacco use and dependence: 2008 update. *Am J Prev Med.* 2008;35(2):158–176.

USPSTF. *Counseling for a Healthy Diet, Topic Page.* Rockville, MD: US Preventive Services Task Force. Agency for Healthcare Research and Quality; 2003a.

USPSTF. *Screening and Interventions to Prevent Obesity in Adults, Topic Page.* Rockville, MD: US Preventive Services Task Force. Agency for Healthcare Research and Quality; 2003b.

USPSTF. *Screening for Lipid Disorders in Adults, Topic Page.* Rockville, MD: US Preventive Services Task Force. Agency for Healthcare Research and Quality; 2008.

USPSTF. Aspirin for the prevention of cardiovascular disease: US Preventive Services Task Force Recommendation Statement. *Ann Intern Med.* 2009;150:396–404.

USPSTF. Screening for and management of obesity in adults: US Preventive Services Task Force recommendation statement. *Ann Intern Med.* 2012;157(5):373–378.

VanHorn L, McCoin M, Kris-Etherton PM, Burke F, Carson JA, Champagne CM, Karmally W, Sikand G. The evidence for dietary prevention and treatment of cardiovascular disease. *J Am Diet Assoc.* 2008;108(2):287–331.

Vasan RS, Beiser A, Seshadri S, Larson MG, Kannel WB, D'Agostino RB, Levy D. Residual lifetime risk for developing hypertension in middle-aged women and men: The Framingham Heart Study. *JAMA.* 2002;287(8):1003–1010.

Victor RG. Arterial hypertension. In Goldman D., ed. *Cecil Textbook of Medicine.* Philadelphia: Saunders; 2004.

Victor RG, Kaplan NM. Systemic hypertension: mechanisms and diagnosis. In: Libby PM, Zipes D. eds. Braunwald's Heart Disease: A Textbook of Cardiovascular Medicine. Philadelphia: Saunders Elsevier; 2007.

West R, McNeill A, Raw M. Smoking cessation guidelines for health professionals: an update. *Thorax.* 2000;55(12):987–999.

WHO. *Prevention of Cardiovascular Disease: Guidelines for Assessment and Management of Cardiovascular Risk.* Geneva: World Health Organization; 2007.

Whitlock EP, Orleans CT, Pender N, Allan J. Evaluating primary care behavioral counseling interventions: an evidence-based approach. *Am J Prev Med.* 2002;22(4):267–284.

Williams PT. Relationship of distance run per week to coronary heart disease risk factors in 8283 male runners. The National Runners' Health Study. *Arch Intern Med.* 1997;157(2):191–198.

Wolff T, Miller T, Ko S. Aspirin for the primary prevention of cardiovascular events: an update of the evidence for the US Preventive Services Task Force. *Ann Intern Med.* 2009;150(6):405–410.

Ye J, Rust G, Baltrus P, Daniels E. Cardiovascular risk factors among Asian Americans: results from a National Health Survey. *Ann Epidemiol.* 2009;19(10):718–723.

Zingmond DS, McGory ML, Ko CY. Hospitalization before and after gastric bypass surgery. *JAMA.* 2005;294(15):1918–1924.

6

Stroke Prevention

FRED RINCON AND CLINTON WRIGHT

INTRODUCTION

Stroke is a leading cause of morbidity and mortality in the United States (Roger et al., 2011). In 2011 the American Heart Association (AHA) estimated that there were 610,000 new stroke cases in the United States, 185,000 recurrent strokes, and 7 million Americans who have suffered a stroke, many of whom required long-term health care with an estimated cost to the economy of $40.9 billion dollars annually (Roger et al., 2011). In the same year, at least 1 in 18 deaths in the United States were attributed to stroke (Roger et al., 2011). Based on these facts and the limited number of effective acute therapies to lower morbidity and mortality, clinicians and epidemiologists have focused on primary and secondary prevention strategies through risk factor assessment and treatment.

Non-modifiable risk factors include age, sex, race/ethnicity, and genetic predisposition. Although these risk factors are non-modifiable, they help to identify those patients at higher risk of stroke and those who may benefit from more aggressive interventions that modify the risk of stroke.

Modifiable risk factors of stroke include hypertension (high blood pressure), diabetes mellitus (diabetes), dyslipidemia, cigarette smoking, obesity, alcohol use, physical inactivity, and atrial fibrillation (AF), among others. Fortunately, the list of modifiable risk factors is larger than those that are non-modifiable, such as advanced age and male gender. Effective counseling approaches by primary care providers can modify these lifestyle factors including; cigarette smoking, obesity, alcohol use, and physical inactivity; these approaches are discussed throughout *Prevention Practice in Primary Care*.

In this Chapter, we will summarize the most current evidence for the prevention of stroke or transient ischemic attack (TIA) and we have categorized the recommendations based on the AHA grading of evidence (AHA, 2000) (see Table 6-1).

NON-MODIFIABLE RISK FACTORS
Age

Epidemiological studies have confirmed the effects of age on the risk of cardiac and cerebrovascular disease. The risk of stroke or TIA doubles for each decade after 55 years of age (Brown et al., 1996; Wolf et al., 1992). Older patients should be screened for treatable risk factors.

Gender

Men are at greater risk of stroke and TIA, with greater age-adjusted incidence rates than women, except for two age groups: those 35–44 years old and those >85 years (Brown et al., 1996; Sacco et al., 1998). The explanation for this phenomenon is that young women have a higher incidence of stroke, perhaps due to the use of oral contraceptives and pregnancy (Kittner et al., 1996). In addition, men die earlier, of cardiovascular disease, and these earlier deaths contribute to the apparently higher age-adjusted incidence rates for stroke in older women.

Race/Ethnicity

Certain groups such as blacks and Hispanics may be at greater risk of stroke and TIA (Sacco et al., 1998; Sacco et al., 2001). Possible reasons for the higher incidence of stroke and mortality rates in blacks include a higher prevalence of known risk factors such as hypertension and diabetes (Gillum, 1999). Additionally, epidemiological studies have identified certain Asian groups at higher risk of stroke (He et al., 1995). These higher risk groups should be evaluated for risk factors that can be treated.

Genetic Predisposition

Several studies have demonstrated the association of family history and the risk of stroke (Kiely et al., 1993; Liao et al., 1997). The higher risk of stroke in those with affected family members may be mediated

TABLE 6-1. DEFINITION OF CLASSES AND LEVELS OF EVIDENCE USED IN AHA
RECOMMENDATIONS

Class I	Conditions for which there is evidence for and/or general agreement that the procedure or treatment is useful and effective
Class II	Conditions for which there is conflicting evidence and/or a divergence of opinion about the usefulness/efficacy of a procedure or treatment
Class IIa	Weight of evidence or opinion is in favor of the procedure or treatment
Class IIb	Usefulness/efficacy is less well established by evidence or opinion
Class III	Conditions for which there is evidence and/or general agreement that the procedure or treatment is not useful/effective and in some cases may be harmful
Level of Evidence A	Data derived from multiple randomized trials
Level of Evidence B	Data derived from a single randomized trial or non-randomized trials
Level of Evidence C	Expert Opinion or case studies

by shared heritability of modifiable risk factors as well as susceptibility to the effects of those risk factors, familial or cultural lifestyles that increase stroke risk (i.e., poor diet), and the interaction between genetic predisposition and these environmental factors. In addition, a limited group of rare genetic diseases have been associated with stroke: cerebral autosomal dominant arteriopathy with sub-cortical infarcts and leukoaraiosis (CADASIL), Marfan syndrome, Fabry disease, neurofribromatosis I and II, hereditary cerebral hemorrhage with amyloidosis–Dutch type, and mithochondrial inherited diseases. Genetic counseling should be considered for patients with rare genetic causes of stroke. However, there is insufficient data to recommend genetic screening for the primary prevention of stroke (Goldstein et al., 2006).

MODIFIABLE RISK FACTORS
Hypertension

According to recent reports, about 43 million men and women in the United States are afflicted by hypertension (Wolz et al., 2000). Overwhelming evidence suggests that hypertension increases the risk of developing either a fatal or a non-fatal stroke (Mzimba, Beevers, & Lip, 1998). In the Framingham study, which defined hypertension as systolic blood pressure (SBP) >160 mmHg or diastolic blood pressure (DBP) >95 mmHg, or both, the age-adjusted relative risk (RR) of stroke among those with hypertension was 3.1 for men and 2.9 for women (Danneberg, Garrison, & Kannel, 1988). Similarly, several randomized trials looking at the treatment of patients with hypertension have consistently demonstrated the benefits of anti-hypertensive treatment by reduction of the risk of incident stroke and reduction of the overall mortality.

For example, the Swedish Trial on Old Patients with Hypertension (STOP), which randomized patients to receive either a beta-blocker, diuretic, or placebo, showed a 47% relative reduction in the risk of incident stroke in the treatment group (Dahlof et al, 1991). The European Systolic Hypertension (SYST-EUR) trial, which randomized patients to receive a calcium channel blocker (CCB), enalapril, or placebo showed a 42% relative reduction in stroke incidence in the treatment group (Staessen et al., 1997), and the British Medical Research Council Trial of Treatment of Hypertension in Older Adults (MRC) study showed similar results (MRC, 1992). Although the results of these studies support the treatment of hypertension for primary cardiovascular disease prevention, only limited studies have directly addressed the role of blood pressure reduction for the secondary prevention of stroke or TIA. Evidence from randomized controlled trials supports the use of anti-hypertensive agents for the prevention of vascular events in patients with previous stroke or TIA and is consistent with the hypothesis that the prevention of vascular events is associated with the magnitude of blood pressure reduction (Rashid, Leonardi-Bee, & Bath, 2003).

Treatment with anti-hypertensive medications has been associated with significant reductions in recurrent fatal and non-fatal strokes, myocardial infarction (MI), and combined vascular events (stroke, MI, and vascular death), even in patients without hypertension (Rashid, Leonardi-Bee, & Bath, 2003), but whether a particular class of anti-hypertensive drug or a particular drug within a given class offers a particular advantage for use in patients after ischemic stroke remains unknown. Several studies, however, have shown beneficial effects from angiotensin converting enzyme inhibitor (ACE-I) and angiotensin receptor blockers (ARBs) (Yusuf et al., 2000; Randomised trial, 2001), and these agents are recommended for blood pressure control.

In the Heart Outcomes Prevention Evaluation (HOPE) Study, the effects of the Angiotensin Converting Enzyme Inhibitor (ACEI) ramipril were compared against placebo in 1,013 high-risk patients with a history of stroke or TIA and a 24% relative risk reduction for stroke, MI, and vascular death was found (Yusuf et al., 2000). Similarly, in the Perindopril Protection Against Recurrent Stroke Study (PROGRESS) (PROGRESS Collaborative Group, 2001), 6,105 patients with stroke or TIA within 5 years were randomized to the ACE-I perindopril versus the combination of perindopril plus the diuretic indapamide. The combination resulted in a 43% relative reduction of risk of recurrent stroke and a 40% relative reduction in vascular events without significant difference in the ACE-I alone group. Based on this, the JNC-7 report concluded that stroke rates are lowered by the combination of ACE-I and thiazide-type diuretics (Chobanian et al., 2003).

In the Acute Candesartan Cilexetil therapy in stroke Survivors Study (ACCESS) (Schrader et al., 2003), patients were randomized to the use of candesartan versus placebo. Though no significant difference was found in blood pressure reduction or mortality between treatment groups at one year, the stroke recurrence was lower in the candesartan group (9.7% vs. 18.7%, p = 0.026).

The benefit of hypertension treatment for primary prevention of stroke is clear. Regular screening for hypertension every 2 years is an appropriate primary prevention strategy (Class I, Level of Evidence A; see Table 6-1), along with dietary changes, lifestyle modification, particularly smoking cessation,, and pharmacological interventions as summarized by the JNC-7 (Chobanian et al., 2003). Anti-hypertensive therapy is also recommended for both prevention of recurrent stroke and other vascular events beyond the hyperacute period (Class I, Level of Evidence A; see Table 6-1). As shown in the PROGRESS study, this benefit extends to patients with and without hypertension so this recommendation should be considered for all ischemic stroke and TIA patients (Class IIA, Level of Evidence B; see Table 6-1). The BP goal should be individualized, but a benefit has been associated with average reductions of 10/5 mmHg, and normal blood pressure levels have been identified as <120/80 mmHg by the JNC-7 (Chobanian et al., 2003) (Class IIA,

Level of Evidence B; see Table 6-1). Lifestyle modifications have been associated with blood pressure reductions and should be included as part of a comprehensive anti-hypertensive therapy (Class IIB, Level of Evidence C; see Table 6-1).

Diabetes Mellitus

Diabetes is an established risk factor for cardiovascular disease and stroke (Kannel & McGee, 1979). Similar to the interventions for hypertension, most of the evidence on stroke prevention in patients with diabetes is focused on primary rather than on secondary prevention. Nevertheless, multidisciplinary interventions of aggressive control of hyperglycemia, hypertension, dyslipidemia, and microalbuminuria, such as the use of ACEI, ARB, and/or anti-platelet medications as indicated, have demonstrated reductions in the risk of cardiovascular events (Gaede et al., 2003).

Primary stroke prevention guidelines have emphasized the more rigorous control of BP among type 1 and type 2 diabetics (Goldstein et al., 2006) and tight control of BP in these groups has been associated with significant reductions in the incidence of stroke (UKPDS, 1998a). In the United Kingdom Prospective Diabetes Study (UKPDS), diabetic patients with controlled hypertension (mean BP, 144/82mmHg) had a 44% RR of stroke compared with diabetic patients with uncontrolled hypertension (mean BP, 154/87mmHg, p = 0.013) (UKPDS, 1998a).

The current guidelines support a long-term BP goal target of less than 130/80 mmHg in diabetic patients (Chobanian et al., 2003), and the American Diabetes Association (ADA) recommends that all patients with diabetes and hypertension should be treated with a regimen that includes either an ACEI or ARB (ADA, 2004). Thiazide diuretics, beta-blockers (BB), ACEI, and ARBs are beneficial for reducing cardiovascular events and stroke incidence in patients with diabetes (UKPDS, 1998B; ALLHAT, 2002; Weber et al., 2004). Several studies have demonstrated the favorable effects of ACE-I and ARBs on stroke and other cardiovascular outcomes (PROGRESS Collaborative Group, 2001; Heart Outcomes, 2000; Shindler et al., 1996). In the Anti-hypertensive and Lipid-Lowering Treatment to Prevent Heart Attack Study (ALLHAT), which included more than 12,000 diabetic patients, no difference in the number of coronary events was found between ACEI and diuretics, regardless of diabetic status. However, for other vascular end points such as stroke, the diuretic chlorthalidone was found to be superior to the ACE-I lisinopril and CCB amlodipine (ALLHAT, 2002). The results of the Valsartan Antihypertensive Long-Term Use Evaluation (VALUE) study, which included diabetic and non-diabetic patients, found no differences in event rates in the groups treated with CCB or the ARB valsartan. However, the LIFE trial found beneficial effects of the ARB irbesartan in stroke reduction in black patients with left ventricular dysfunction, suggesting a race-specific benefit (Julius et al., 2004).

More rigorous control of hypertension and lipids should be considered in patients with diabetes (Class IIA, Level of Evidence B, see Table 6-1). Although all major classes of anti-hypertensives are suitable for BP control, most patients require more than one agent, but ACEI and ARBs are more effective in reducing the progression of renal disease and are recommended as the first choice for patients with diabetes (Heart Outcomes, 2000) (Class I, Level of Evidence A; see Table 6-1). Glucose control to near normoglycemic levels is recommended among diabetics with ischemic stroke and TIA to reduce microvascular complications (Class I, Level of Evidence A; see Table 6-1), and possibly to reduce macrovascular complications as well (Class IIB, Level of Evidence B; see Table 6-1). The goal of Hemoglobin A1c should be < 7% (Class IIA, Level of Evidence B; (see Table 6-1).

Dyslipidemia

The abnormalities of serum lipids (dyslipidemia) such as hypertryglyceridemia, high total cholesterol, high low-density lipoprotein (LDL-C), and low high-density lipoprotein (HDL-C) have been found to be risk factors more for coronary artery disease (CAD) than cerebrovascular disease. Cholesterol level and LDL-C have a direct relationship with the incidence of heart disease (CHD), whereas HDL-C has an inverse relationship.

Hypercholesterolemia and hyperlipidemia are not well-established risk factors for first or recurrent stroke in contrast to what is seen in cardiac disease. In general, observational epidemiological studies have shown a weak or no association between cholesterol level and the risk of ischemic stroke. Moreover, the reduction of stroke risk in the statin trials may be primarily for non-fatal stroke (MCR/BHF, 2002). The Medical Research Council/British Heart Foundation (HPS) addressed the effect of administration of simvastatin in those with or without prior cerebrovascular disease (Collins et al.,

2004). In this study, 20,536 patients with a history of CAD, peripheral vascular disease (PVD) or vascular disease in other beds, diabetes, or hypertension were enrolled to receive either 40 mg of simvastatin or placebo. Overall, there was a significant RR reduction of 25% in the end point of stroke (p <0.0001). The HPS showed that among those with prior history of stroke, the addition of statin therapy resulted in a significant reduction in coronary events and revascularization regardless of the baseline cholesterol level. Interestingly, among those with a prior history of stroke, the risk of recurrent stroke was not different among treatment groups. Based on the results of HPS, stroke patients with a history of CAD or diabetes had no benefit from statin therapy to reduce the risk of recurrent stroke. However, the more recent results of the Stroke Prevention by Aggressive Reduction in Cholesterol Levels Study (SPARCL) showed that in patients with recent stroke or TIA and without known coronary heart disease, 80 mg of atorvastatin per day reduced the overall incidence of strokes and of cardiovascular events for over 5 years, despite a small increase in the incidence of hemorrhagic stroke (Amarenco et al., 2006).

The National Cholesterol Education Program (NCEP) Expert Panel on Detection, Evaluation, and Treatment of High Cholesterol (Adult Treatment Panel ATP III) emphasizes LDL-C lowering with two major modalities: therapeutic lifestyle change and drug-specific therapy (Executive Summary, 2001). Lifestyle modification encompasses a reduction of saturated fat and cholesterol intake, weight reduction, and an increase in physical activity. LDL-C goals for patients with CHD, or the CHD equivalents (diabetes or symptomatic carotid disease) is <100 mg/dL. More rigorous control of lipids is now recommended for diabetic patients with target goals for LDL of <70 mg/dL. The HPS demonstrated a beneficial effect of cholesterol-lowering therapy among diabetic patients. Addition of simvastatin was associated with a 28% RR reduction in ischemic strokes (p = 0.01) and 22% RR reduction in first coronary events (MI), strokes, and revascularization procedures (MCR/BHF, 2002). Similarly, for very high-risk patients (established cardiovascular disease, diabetes, poorly controlled risk factors, ongoing cigarette smoking, metabolic syndrome, and patients with acute coronary syndromes) the LDL-C goal should be <70 mg/dL.

Patients with ischemic stroke or TIA with elevated cholesterol levels, comorbid CAD, or evidence of atherosclerotic disease should be managed according to the NCEP III guidelines, which include lifestyle modification, dietary guidelines, and medications (Class I, Level of Evidence A; see Table 6-1). Statin agents are recommended, and the target goal for cholesterol lowering in those with CHD or symptomatic atherosclerotic disease is an LDL-C level of <100 mg/dL and LDL-C level of <70 mg/dL for very high-risk patients (Class I, Level of Evidence A; see Table 6-1). Patients with ischemic stroke or TIA due to atherosclerosis origin but with no preexisting indications for statins (normal cholesterol levels, no CAD, no evidence of atherosclerosis) are reasonable candidates for treatment with a statin to reduce risk of vascular events (Class I, Level of Evidence B; see Table 6-1) (Adams et al., 2008). Patients with ischemic stroke or TIA with low HDL-C may be considered for treatment with niacin or gemfibrozil (Class IIB, Level of Evidence B;see Table 6-1).

Smoking

Cigarette smoking is the leading preventable cause of death in the United States. Smoking is an independent determinant of stroke based on epidemiological studies, even after controlling for known risk factors (Lightwood & Glantz, 1997). The risk is present in all ages, both sexes, and across different race-ethnic groups. From epidemiologic data the risk of stroke due to smoking is thought to disappear after about 5 years of abstinence (Wolf et al., 1988). Moreover, growing evidence supports the association of passive smoking with the risk of cardiovascular disease and ischemic stroke (You et al., 1999). For obvious ethical reasons, no randomized trial has been conducted.

Smoking cessation is strongly encouraged to reduce the risk of stroke. Every patient with stroke or TIA should be advised to stop smoking, using the 5 As: Ask, Advise, Assess, Assist, and Arrange (Fiore et al., 2000; see Chapters 5 and 11; Class I, Level of Evidence C; see Table 6-1). Avoidance of environmental tobacco smoke is recommended (Fiore et al., 2000; Class IIA, Level of Evidence C; see Table 6-1).

Alcohol Consumption

The association between alcohol and consumption and stroke or TIA is controversial. Recent large epidemiological studies have confirmed the association of chronic alcohol abuse and heavy drinking as risk factors for all stroke sub-types (Gorelick, 1987; Gill et al., 1991; Mazzaglia et al., 2001). For ischemic strokes, several studies have shown a J-shaped association, with a protective effect in light or moderate drinkers, and elevated stroke risk in heavy drinkers (Djousse et al., 2002; Elkind et al., 2006; Sacco et al., 1999). In the recent meta-analysis of 35 observational studies by Reynolds et al. (2003), alcohol consumption was categorized into 0, <1, 1, 1–2, 2–5 or >5 drinks/day; an average drink contained 12 g, 15 ml, 0.5 ounces of alcohol (found in 1 bottle of beer, one small glass of wine, or one alcoholic cocktail). Compared to non-drinkers, those who consumed more than five drinks per day had a 69% higher risk of stroke. Similarly, recurrent stroke was significantly increased among those with prior ischemic strokes and history of alcohol abuse in the Northern Manhattan Study (Sacco et al., 1994).

Current guidelines from the American Heart Association/American Stroke Association Council on Stroke (AHA/ASA; Jauch, Saver, Adams, Bruno, Conners, Demaerschalk et al., 2013) support the elimination or reduction of alcohol consumption in patients with ischemic stroke or TIA who are heavy drinkers (Class I, Level of Evidence A; see Table 6-1). Light to moderate levels of no more than two drinks per day for men and one drink per day for non-pregnant women may be considered beneficial, although the AHA does not recommend that alcohol abstainers begin drinking to lower their risks (Class IIB, Level of Evidence C; see Table 6-1).

Obesity

Obesity is an independent risk factor for CHD and premature mortality (Fontaine et al., 2003), and it has been strongly associated with several of the major risk factors for cardiovascular disease including hypertension, diabetes, and dyslipidemia (Turcato et al., 2000). The causal relationship of obesity with stroke, however, is complex. In men, findings from the Physician's Health Study have shown that an elevated body mass index (BMI) is associated with an steady increase in the risk of ischemic stroke, independent of the effects of other cardiovascular risk factors (Kurth et al., 2003). For women, however the data are inconsistent. Several studies have suggested that abdominal obesity (defined as waist circumference >102 cm [40 in.] in men and 88 cm [35 in.] in women), rather than general obesity, is associated with an increased risk of stroke (Suk et al., 2003). In the Northern Manhattan Stroke Study, investigators found an independent association between abdominal obesity and incident ischemic stroke in all racial/ethnic groups (Suk et al., 2003). No epidemiological study has demonstrated that weight reduction is associated with reduced risk of stroke. However, weight loss is significantly associated with improvement of BP, fasting glucose levels, serum lipids, and physical endurance (Anderson & Konz, 2001).

Weight reduction should be considered for all overweight patients, especially after ischemic stroke or TIA, to maintain the goal of a BMI 18.5–24.9 kg/m^2 and a waist circumference of <35 for women and <40 for men (Class IIB, Level of Evidence C; see Table 6-1). Some suggested counseling approaches are discussed in Chapters 5 and 11.

Physical Activity

Physical activity exerts a beneficial effect on multiple cardiovascular risk factors, including those for stroke (Lee, Folsom, & Blair, 2003). Physical activity may lower stroke risk by reducing BP and weight, enhancing vasodilatation, improving glucose tolerance, and promoting cardiovascular health (improving the fitness of the heart and lungs). In a recent meta-analysis, individuals who were moderately and highly active had a lower risk of stroke and death than those with low activity. Moderately active men and women had a 20% lower risk, and those who were highly active had a 27% lower risk than less active individuals (Lee, Folsom, & Blair, 2003).

Current guidelines from the American Heart Association/American Stroke Association Council on Stroke (Jauch, Saver, Adams, Bruno, Connors, Demaerschalk et al., 2013) support engaging in physical activity for patients with risk factors and ischemic stroke or TIA. At least 30 minutes of moderate intensity physical exercise most days may be considered to reduce the risk factors and comorbid conditions that increase the likelihood of recurrence of stroke (Class IIB, Level of Evidence C; see Table 6-1). Counseling approaches for physical activity are discussed briefly in Chapters 5 and 11. For stroke survivors with disability, a supervised therapeutic physical regimen is recommended.

LARGE VESSEL ASSOCIATED STROKE OR TIA
Extra-cranial Atherosclerotic Carotid Disease
Carotid Endarterectomy (CEA) in Asymptomatic Patients

Natural history studies reflect an annual stroke risk of 1–3% per year in patients with asymptomatic carotid artery stenosis (Chambers & Norris, 1986; Hennerici et al, 1987; Mackey et al., 1997). The Toronto Asymptomatic Cervical Bruit Study followed a group of 500 patients for a mean of 23 months. In this study, stroke or TIA was more frequent in patients with high-grade stenosis (>75%), progressing carotid stenosis, history of heart disease, and in men, but only 0.4% of the events corresponded to the high-grade side (2 of 8, or 25%, of incident strokes) suggesting that these patients would benefit from aggressive medical intervention targeted at other stroke risk factors (Mackey et al., 1997). In a sub-group analysis of the North American Symptomatic Carotid Endarterectomy Trial (NASCET), patients with 60–99% asymptomatic carotid stenosis contralateral to the symptomatic side (Inzitari et al., 2000) had a 3% annual risk of stroke over 5 years that increased to 3.7% per year in the 75–94% stenosis group. Overall, 45% of these events were attributed to lacunes or cardio-embolism suggesting the importance of screening these patients for other modifiable risk factors.

The Asymptomatic Carotid Atherosclerosis Study (ACAS) and the Asymptomatic Carotid Surgery Trial (ACST) addressed the use of CEA in asymptomatic patients. The degree of benefit seen from these studies is substantially less than in studies of symptomatic carotid disease. Both studies demonstrated a 5.4–5.9% absolute risk reduction over 5 years, but peri-procedural risks are relevant to the decision analysis for the treatment of this patient group, with a risk >3% minimizing any benefit. In ACAS, the benefit in women was less clear due to the small sample size of women recruited. However, in ACST an adequate number of women were enrolled, and a benefit was seen for both sexes.

For the above mentioned reasons, it is recommended that patients with asymptomatic carotid stenosis be screened for other treatable causes of stroke and TIA, and that aggressive therapy be initiated to reduce the burden of known risk factors (Class I, Level of Evidence C; see Table 6-1). Prophylactic CEA may be recommended in highly selected cases with high-grade asymptomatic carotid stenosis if performed by surgeons with <3% morbidity/mortality rates (Class I, Level of Evidence A; see Table 6-1). Carotid endarterectomy is not recommended for asymptomatic patients with stenosis <60%.

Carotid Endarterectomy (CEA) in Symptomatic Patients

For patients with stroke or TIA and carotid stenosis, several randomized controlled trials have demonstrated the benefits of endarterectomy over medical therapy alone. In the NASCET, patients with symptomatic carotid stenosis of >70% randomized to the surgical arm had impressive relative and absolute risk reductions (NASCETC, 1991). The European Carotid Surgery Trial (ECST) (Randomised trial, 1998; European Carotid Surgery, 1991) and the Veterans Affairs Cooperative Study (Mayberg et al., 1991) demonstrated similar results.

For patients with symptomatic carotid stenosis of 50–69%, there is still some uncertainty about the optimal treatment approach. From the NASCET, the 5-year risk of fatal or non-fatal stroke was 22% in the medical arm versus 15% in the surgical arm (p = 0.045) (NASCETC, 1991). The relative and absolute risk reductions were less impressive than in those patients with critical stenosis of more than 70%. However, several conditions can affect the benefit-to-risk ratio for CEA in the moderate carotid stenosis sub-group. Benefits were greatest in patients older than 75 years of age, in men, in those with recent stroke rather than TIA, and in patients with hemispheric symptoms rather than transient monocular blindness (Rothwell et al., 2004). Other factors, such as the presence of intracranial stenosis, the absence of leukoaraiosis, and the presence of good collateral blood supply, favored a better outcome in multiple NASCET post hoc analyses (Henderson et al., 2000; Kappelle et al., 1999). For patients with carotid stenosis of less than 50%, the trials showed no significant differences between surgery and medical treatment (NASCETC, 1991; Randomised trial, 1998).

For patients with recent TIA or stroke and ipsilateral severe (70–99%) carotid stenosis, CEA by a surgeon with a peri-operative risk less than 6% is recommended (Class I, Level of Evidence A; see Table 6-1). For patients with recent TIA/stroke and moderate (50–69%) stenosis, CEA is recommended depending on patient-specific factors such as age, gender, comorbidities, and the severity of the initial symptoms (Class I, level of Evidence A; see Table 6-1). Carotid endarterectomy is not recommended for patients with symptomatic stenosis of <50% (Class III, Level of Evidence A; see Table 6-1).

Carotid Artery Stenting (CAS)

For high-risk surgical patients with asymptomatic high-grade carotid stenosis, stenting is a reasonable alternative to CEA (Class IIB, Level of Evidence B; see Table 6-1; Goldstein et al., 2006). In the symptomatic carotid stenosis group, the data are derived from case series and a few randomized studies

comparing CEA to CAS. In the Wallstent Trial, which randomized 219 symptomatic patients with carotid stenosis of 60–90%, a higher risk of stroke and death at one year was observed in the CAS group. The trial was halted due to early adverse results in the CAS arm. This trial allowed inexperienced operators and used no distal protection device (e.g., small umbrellas that are distal to the site of angioplasty; http://www.ev3.net/peripheral/us/embolic-protection/spiderfxtrade-embolic-protection-device.htm), however.

In the Carotid and Vertebral Artery Transluminal Angioplasty Study (CAVATAS), 504 symptomatic patients with carotid stenosis were randomized to surgery or CAS. Major outcomes at 30 days did not differ between treatment arms (Endovascular versus surgical treatment, 2001).

In the Stenting and Angioplasty with Protection in Patients at High Risk for Endarterectomy (SAPPHIRE) Trial (68), 334 patients were randomized to CEA versus CAS with the use of an embolic-protection device. The trial attempted to test the hypothesis that CAS was not inferior to CEA. In this study, operators for CAS had a peri-procedural risk of stroke of 4% or less. The 30-day risk (composite end point of incident stroke, MI, or death) for CAS was 5.8% vs. 12.6% (p = <0.004 for non-inferiority). Most of this benefit was detected in the lower risk of MI for the stent group compared with the high-surgical risk endarterectomy cases.

Recent reports from randomized trials of CAS versus CEA in symptomatic patients have failed to demonstrate non-inferiority of the stenting procedure. In the Stent-Supported Percutaneous Angioplasty of the Carotid Artery versus Endarterectomy (SPACE) study (Ringleb et al., 2006), a slightly higher rate of ipsilateral ischemic stroke and death at 30 days was seen in the patients undergoing stenting. Similarly, the Endarterectomy versus Angioplasty in Patients with Symptomatic Severe Carotid Stenosis (EVA-3S) trial (Mas et al., 2006) failed to meet non-inferiority criteria in patients with symptomatic stenosis of 60% or more. At both 1 and 6 months after the procedure, death and stroke rates were lower with CEA. The results of these trials do not justify the widespread use of carotid-artery stenting for treatment of carotid-artery stenosis.

The National Institute of Neurological Diseases and Stroke (NINDS)–sponsored Carotid Revascularization with Endarterectomy or Stent

Trial (CREST) compared the efficacy of CEA versus CAS in patients with symptomatic severe stenosis (>70% by ultrasound or >50% by NASCET angiographic criteria) (Brott et al., 2010). The study showed that CEA or CAS performed by highly qualified surgeons and interventionists is effective and safe, as the study did not find any difference in the composite end point of stroke, myocardial infarction, or death. However, during the periprocedural period, there was a higher risk of stroke with stenting and a higher risk of myocardial infarction with endarterectomy (Brott et al., 2010). The decision to pursue CAS or CEA should depend on patient characteristics such as age, comorbidities, and the physician's experience.

In patients with extracranial vertebrobasilar disease and repeated TIA/strokes despite optimal medical therapy, endovascular revascularization with angioplasty and stenting to prevent recoil or re-stenosis can be performed. However, supportive data are derived from case series (Class IIB, Level of Evidence C; see Table 6-1).

Intra-cranial Atherosclerotic Artery Disease

Patients with symptomatic intracranial atherosclerosis have a high relative risk of recurrent stroke of about 20–25%. In the Extra-Cranial/Intra-Cranial (EC/IC) bypass study, patients with middle cerebral artery stenosis were randomized to surgical intervention and medical treatment with aspirin; no benefit was found for the surgical group (EC/IC, 1985). A newer clinical trial using more specific techniques to select patients with perfusion failure due to hemodynamic compromise was also negative (Powers et al., 2011).

In the recent Warfarin Aspirin Symptomatic Intracranial Disease (WASID) study, 569 patients with symptomatic intracranial stenosis were prospectively randomized to aspirin or warfarin, but the study was halted prematurely because of increased bleeding in the Warfarin arm and no difference between groups was detected for the end point of recurrent ischemic stroke. Importantly, this study demonstrated that patients with intracranial stenosis who fail anti-platelet therapy may be at higher risk of recurrent stroke (Chimowitz et al., 2005). However, it is unclear if warfarin and aspirin are equivalent in those who have "failed" anti-platelet therapy.

Endovascular management of intracranial stenosis by either angioplasty or stent, or both, provides an opportunity to rapidly improve cerebral blood flow in affected patients. Nevertheless, only a few large randomized prospective controlled trials have addressed this issue. Results from single-center studies suggest that these procedures can be achieved with a high level of technical success in those patients with recurrent symptoms despite optimal medical therapy. The Guidant-sponsored multicenter Stenting of Symptomatic Atherosclerotic lesions in the Vertebral or Intracranial Arteries (SSYLVIA) study was a prospective non-randomized feasibility study of stenting for the treatment of intracranial artery stenosis (SSYLVIA, 2004). In this study, 43 intracranial vessels and 18 extracranial vertebral arteries were treated. Successful stent deployment occurred in 95% of the cases. The 30-day stroke incidence was 6.6% with no deaths. Late (more than 30-day) stroke incidence was 7.3%. Recurrent stenosis occurred in 32% of intracranial vessels treated and 43% of those extracranial vessels treated.

In the recent Stenting versus Aggressive Medical Management for Preventing Recurrent Stroke in Intracranial Stenosis (SAMMPRIS) trial (Chimowitz et al., 2011), the investigators indicated that medical therapy was superior than stenting, which was associated with a higher risk of peri-procedural stroke or death. Moreover, the essential elements of the medical regimen used in this trial can readily be adopted in clinical practice.(Chimowitz et al., 2011).

Arterial Dissection

Spontaneous cervico-cerebral dissections account for approximately 2% of all ischemic strokes, especially among young adults and middle-aged patients. Population-based studies have determined that the incidence of dissections is about 2.6–2.9 cases per 100,000 persons per year. The annual incidence of extra-cranial internal carotid (ICA) dissection is 3.5 cases per 100,000 in a case series from Rochester, Minnesota (Schievink, Mokri, & O'Fallon, 1994). Extracranial vertebral artery (VA) dissection is more common, accounting for up to 15% of reported cases, whereas intracranial VA dissection accounts for 5% of cases (Zweifler & Silverboard, 2004).

The treatment of spontaneous extracranial cerebrovascular dissections is controversial, and there are no controlled clinical trials to guide us. In 2003 a Cochrane Review of the use of antithrombotic drugs for carotid artery dissection found no evidence to support routine use of anticoagulation or antiplatelet agents in this setting (Lyrer & Engelter,

2003). Therefore, treatment is based on clinical observations and expert opinions. We manage most acute symptomatic extracranial dissections with full dose heparin anticuoagulation (target aPTT 2.0–2.5 times normal) followed by warfarin (target INR 2.0–3.0) therapy for 3–6 months (Class IIB, Level of Evidence C; see Table 6-1). However, in those with extracranial carotid dissections with minimal flow limitation, we prefer anti-platelet therapy. Those treated with warfarin are monitored every 3 months with non-invasive tests such as vascular ultrasound or magnetic resonance angiography (MRA). If at 3 months non-invasive tests show resolution of dissection, then anti-platelet (usually acetylsalicylic acid or Aspirin®; ASA) therapy is substituted for warfarin. If non-invasive testing shows no reconstitution of the dissection, we often continue warfarin for an additional 3 months (Zweifler & Silverboard, 2004). At 6 months, a new assessment of the involved vessel is performed, and if there is a persistent filling defect, lifelong anti-platelet therapy is initiated. Clear contraindications to the initial approach are intracranial arterial dissections with aneurysmatic dilatations, especially VA dissections due to the risk of aSAH (aneurysmal subarachnoid hemorrhage) in up to 50% of cases (Connolly et al., 2013), and similarly, large embolic infarcts with mass effect and/or hemorrhagic transformation. In those patients, a single anti-platelet agent can be used as an alternative (Zweifler & Silverboard, 2004).

CARDIOEMBOLIC SOURCES
Atrial Fibrillation (AF)

Atrial fibrillation is present in approximately 1% of the US population and the incidence increases with age, with a prevalence of 6% in individuals older than 65 years, and of 10% in those older than 75 years (Feinberg et al, 1995). Both persistent and paroxysmal AF are potent predictors of first and recurrent stroke. The annual risk of stroke in untreated

individuals with non-valvular AF is about 5% per year (Risk factors, 1994). Atrial fibrillation related stroke is associated with higher severity, disability, and mortality than stroke due to other causes (Lin et al., 1996) and the risk of stroke is even higher in patients with concomitant hypertension, diabetes, prior stroke or TIA, CAD, or CHF (Risk factors, 1994).

Warfarin is more effective than aspirin for reducing the risk of first and recurrent stroke or TIA in patients with *either* paroxysmal or chronic AF, and in patients with valvular and non-valvular heart disease. For non-valvular heart disease, the absolute stroke risk varies among AF patients, according to age and associated vascular diseases. The 2001 American College of Cardiology (ACC)/AHA/European Society of Cardiology (ESC) guideline recommends anti-coagulation for patients with AF who are 60 years or older and have history of either hypertension, diabetes, CAD, impaired LV function, CHF, or prior thromboembolism, or for those with AF who are 75 years or older. Though the individuals factors have been validated as independent predictors of thromboemblic disease, the scheme has not. A recently validated stratification scheme CHADS$_2$ score (see Table 6-2) has been proposed as an alternative tool for the assessment of stroke risk in these patients (CHADS is an acronym for CHF, Hypertension, Age >75 years, Diabetes mellitus, and Stroke or TIA; Gage et al., 2001). The score gives 1 point for each independent predictor and 2 points for prior stroke or TIA and treatment recommendations are based on the score (see Table 6-2). The CHA2DS2VASC2 is a newer score with more vascular variables involved in the model calculation (Camm et al., 2010).

The efficacy of warfarin compared to placebo in the prevention of thromboembolic events among patients with non-valvular AF has been shown in multiple studies (Risk factors, 1994). The relative risk reduction of stroke with warfarin is 68% with

TABLE 6-2. CHADS$_2$ SCORE*

Score	Risk	Stroke Rate (%/year)	Treatment Recommendations
0	Low	1	ASA 75–325 mg/d
1	Low-Moderate	1.5	Warfarin INR 2-3 or ASA 75–325 mg/d
2	Moderate	2.5	Warfarin INR 2-3
3	High	5	Warfarin INR 2-3
>4	Very high	>7	Warfarin INR 2-3

* CHADS = C, CHF; H, Hypertension; A, Age; D, Diabetes mellitus; S, Stroke or TIA

an absolute RR of 1.4–4.5% per year. The optimal intensity of oral anti-coagulation for stroke prevention in these patients appears to be an INR of 2.0–3.0. Evidence supporting the efficacy of aspirin is substantially weaker than that of warfarin. In the Atrial Fibrillation Clopidogrel Trial with Ibesartan for Prevention of Vascular Events (ACTIVE), evidence of benefit in favor of warfarin over clopidogrel plus aspirin therapy was found, leading to the early termination of the study in September 2005 (Atrial Fibrillation, 2007).

Newer alternatives to warfarin for stroke prevention and with fewer side effects such as symptomatic hemorrhage include thrombin inhibitors and direct factor Xa inhibitors, based on the results of recent clinical trials (Connolly et al., 2009; Patel et al., 2011; Granger et al., 2011). However, lack of reversibility in patients with hemorrhagic complications is a concern with the use of the newer agents.

For patients with valvular and those with chronic AF, anti-coagulation with adjusted-dose warfarin (Target INR, 2.5, range 2.0–3.0) or direct factor Xa inhibitor or thrombin inhibitor is recommended (Class I, Level of Evidence A; see Table 6-1). For patients unable to tolerate oral anti-coagulants, aspirin 325mg/day is recommended (Class I, Level of Evidence A; see Table 6-1). The CHADS$_2$ score may be used to assess the risk of stroke or TIA in patients with non-valvular paroxysmal or chronic AF.

Cardiomyopathy

Dilated cardiomyopathy of ischemic or non-ischemic origin causing left ventricular (LV) systolic dysfunction may produce blood stasis within the LV, predisposing to thrombus formation and leading to thrombo-embolism. Two large studies found an increased incidence of stroke proportional to a decrease in systolic ejection fraction (EF) in those patients with ischemic cardiomyopathy (Granger et al., 2011; Pfeffer et al., 1992). In the Survival and Ventricular Enlargement (SAVE) study (Granger et al., 2011), patients with an EF of 29–35% (mean 32%) has a stroke incidence of 0.8%/year versus 1.7%/year in patients with EF of <28% (mean, 23%). There was an 18% increment in the risk of stroke for every 5% decline in EF in the male participants, and such an effect was not seen in the women. Conversely, in a retrospective analysis of the Studies of Left Ventricular Dysfunction (SOLVD) study (Shindler et al., 1996), there was a 50% increase in risk of thrombo-embolic events for every 10%

decrease of EF among women, but the difference was not seen in men (Shindler et al., 1996).

Sometimes anti-coagulation with warfarin is prescribed for patients with dilated cardiomyopathy to prevent the risk of cardioembolic phenomena including TIA or stroke. However, no randomized controlled trial has addressed this issue. The Warfarin versus Aspirin for Reduced Cardiac Ejection Fraction (WARCEF) study comparing these two agents with a primary end point of stroke and death in patients with reduced EF (<35%) and no AF found no overall difference between the therapies. However, the trial found a lower risk of ischemic stroke for those in the warfarin arm. This was offset by a higher risk of systemic bleeding (Homma et al., 2012).

Current recommendations support the use of aspirin or warfarin to achieve INR 2.0–3.0 for the secondary prevention of TIA/stroke in patients with dilated cardiomyopathy (Class IIB, level of Evidence C; see Table 6-1; Sacco et al., 2006).

Acute Myocardial Infarction (MI) and Left Ventricular (LV) Thrombus

Stroke or systemic cardioembolism may be a complication after MI, especially for those patients with anterior wall rather than inferior wall infarctions (Visser et al., 1984). For patients with TIA/stroke in the setting of acute MI in whom LV mural thrombus is identified by echocardiography, oral anti-coagulation with warfarin (INR 2.0–3.0) is recommended for 3 months to up to 1 year (Class IIA, Level of Evidence B; see Table 6-1).

Patent Foramen Ovale (PFO)

A persistent embryonic defect in the inter-atrial septum is present in up to 27% of the general population. Atrial septal aneurysms (ASA) are less common, affecting at least 2% of the population. The presence of a large right to left shunt and/or ASA appears to increase the risk of stroke (Mas & Zuber, 1995). There is a reported association between PFO and cryptogenic stroke (DiTullio et al., 1992; Homma et al., 2002), and estimates for the rate of annual stroke recurrence among PFO patients vary from 1.5% to 12% (DiTullio et al., 1992; Homma et al., 2002).

Preventive therapies for recurrent TIA/stroke in patients with PFO are controversial. Medical therapy with an anti-platelet agent is the first choice. The only randomized comparison of anti-platelet agent (ASA) versus warfarin in patients with PFO comes from the Patent Foramen Ovale in Cryptogenic

Stroke Study (PICSS) (Homma et al., 2002), which demonstrated that there was no difference in recurrent stroke for the 2-year period of follow-up between the two treatment arms. Although PICSS was a pre-planned analysis of the Warfarin versus Aspirin in Recurrent Stroke Study (WARSS) (Mohr et al., 2001), the sub-study was not powered to answer the question of which agent is superior.

The recent CLOSURE-II trial demonstrated that in patients with cryptogenic stroke or TIA who had a PFO, closure with a device did not offer a greater benefit than medical therapy alone for the prevention of recurrent stroke or TIA (Furlan et al., 2012). The interesting observation from CLOSURE-I was that a cause other than paradoxical embolism was usually apparent in patients with recurrent neurologic events. In these patients, look for additional causes of stroke, or TIA may be indicated.

For patients with TIA/stroke and PFO, anti-platelet therapy is a reasonable approach to prevent recurrences (Class IIA, Level of Evidence B; see Table 6-1). Oral anti-coagulation with warfarin is recommended for those patients who have failed anti-platelet therapy or with other indications for long-term anti-coagulation such as a history of hypercoagulable state or evidence of deep venous thrombosis (DVT) (Class IIA, Level of Evidence C; see Table 6-1; Sacco et al., 2006).

The closure of PFO via surgical or endovascular techniques for the prevention of recurrent TIA/stroke is a relatively safe approach. However, randomized trials demonstrated that this approach was not associated with lower stroke recurrence (Furlan et al., 2012). Current recommendations support PFO closure for patients with a recurrent event despite anti-coagulation with warfarin (Class IIB, Level of Evidence C; see Table 6-1; Sacco et al., 2006).

ANTI-THROMBOTIC THERAPY FOR NON-CARDIOEMBOLIC STROKE OR TIA

Four anti-platelet agents have been approved by the FDA for secondary prevention of stroke or TIA: aspirin (ASA), ticlopidine, clopidogrel, and the combination of extended-release dipyridamole and ASA. In the Antithrombotic Trialists' Collaborative meta-analysis of randomized trials of anti-platelet therapy for prevention of cardiovascular events, anti-platelet therapy was associated with 28% relative odds reduction of non-fatal strokes

and 16% reduction in fatal strokes (Antithrombotic Trialists' Collaboration, 2002).

Aspirin in doses ranging 50–1300 mg/day are efficacious in preventing recurring stroke or TIA. The Dutch TIA trial and the UK-TIA trial demonstrated that high and low dose ASA had similar efficacy in preventing recurrent vascular events, but higher doses were associated with greater risk of gastrointestinal hemorrhage (Dutch-TIA, 1988; Farrell et al., 1991).

Ticlopidine has been studied in three randomized trials: the Canadian American Ticlopidine Study (CATS), the Ticlopidine ASA Stroke Study (TASS), and the African American Stroke Prevention Study (AAASPS). The CATS and TASS trials found significant reductions in stroke recurrence, but AAASPS failed to find an association. Ticlopidine use has been associated with neutropenia in up to 2% of patients and with thrombotic thrombocytopenic purpura (TTP) in less than 1% of patients (Gent et al., 1989; Gorelick et al., 2003; Hass et al., 1989).

Clopidogrel was compared to ASA in the Clopidogrel versus ASA in Patients at Risk of Ischemic Events (CAPRIE, 1996) study. In this study more than 19,000 patients received either 325 mg of ASA or 75 mg of clopidogrel. A relative RR of 8.7% was seen in patients taking clopidrogel for the composite end point of stroke, MI, or vascular death, but in patients with prior stroke the benefit of clopidogrel was non-significant. However, a secondary analysis of CAPRIE demonstrated that in diabetics with prior strokes, clopidogrel was more beneficial than ASA alone (Bhatt et al., 2002; Ringleb et al., 2004). Another problem with generalizing the results of CAPRIE to stroke patients is that the benefit in this study was among those who were enrolled based on a history of peripheral arterial disease rather than stroke. Clopidogrel has a better safety profile than ticlopidine with less incidence of side effects and/or TTP.

The combination of ASA and extended-release dipyridamole has been evaluated in several trials (ESPS, 1987; Bousser et al., 1983; Diener et al., 2001; Guiraud-Chaumiel et al., 1982; Halkes et al., 2006; Sacco et al., 2008). The ESPS-2 trial randomized 6,602 patients with prior stroke or TIA to different dipyridamole and ASA combinations. The combination ASA/dipyridamole was associated with 37% RR in stroke versus 18% in the ASA alone group. Similarly, in the recent European/Australasian Stroke Prevention in Reversible Ischemia (ESPRIT)

Trial, 2,763 patients were randomized to ASA 30–325 mg/day with or without dipyridamole 200 mg twice daily. The risk for the primary outcome (death from vascular causes, non-fatal stroke, non-fatal MI, or major bleeding complication) was lower in the combination group (HR 0.80, 95% CI 0.66–0.98) and the combination conferred an ARR of 1% per year (Halkes et al., 2006).

The recent Prevention Regimen For Effectively avoiding Second Strokes (PROFESS) Trial included more than 20 thousand stroke patients and found that ASA/dipyridamole and clopidogrel were equivalent, however. There was no evidence that either of the two treatments was superior to the other in the prevention of recurrent stroke (Sacco et al., 2008), but combination therapy with ASA/dipyridamole was associated with a greater risk of bleeding than clopidogrel.

The combination of clopidogrel and ASA was recently analyzed in the Management of Atherothrobosis with Clopidogrel in High Risk Patients with TIA or Stroke (MATCH) trial (Diener et al., 2004) that randomized 7,599 patients to clopidogrel 75 mg/day or the combination clopidrogel 75 mg/day + ASA 75 mg/day. There was no significant benefit of the combination in reducing the primary outcome (stroke, MI or vascular death). However, the risk of symptomatic hemorrhage was significantly higher in the combination group. Similarly, in the recent Clopidogrel and ASA versus ASA Alone for the Prevention of Atherthrombotic Events (CHARISMA) Trial (Bhatt, 2006), 15,603 patients were randomized to either clopidogrel 75 mg/day + ASA 75–162 mg/day or placebo + ASA 75–162 mg/day, but no significant difference in the rates of non-fatal stroke was found between treatment arms. The combination therapy was not associated with symptomatic severe or fatal bleeding complications, and a non-significant trend toward benefit was seen in those patients with prior stroke in the combination therapy group.

For patients with non-cardoembolic ischemic stroke or TIA, anti-platelet agents rather than oral anti-coagulants are recommended to reduce the risk of recurrence (Class I, Level of Evidence A; see Table 6-1). Aspirin (50–325 mg/day) or combination ASA + extended release dipyridamole or clopidogrel monotherapy are acceptable options for initial therapy as well (Class I, Level of Evidence A; see Table 6-1). The combination of ASA + extended release dipyridamole is recommended over ASA

alone in the new update to the AHA/ASA guidelines (Class I, Level of Evidence B; see Table 6-1; Adams et al., 2008). However, based on the results of PROFESS, we feel that aspirin, ASA/dipyridamole, and clopidogrel are equivalent. Patients with ASA or dipyridamole intolerance may benefit of clopidogrel alone (Class IIB, Level of Evidence B; see Table 6-1). The addition of ASA to clopidogrel may increase the risk of symptomatic bleeding, so this combination is not recommended for secondary prevention of stroke/TIA (Class III, Level of Evidence B; see Table 6-1), unless there is a specific cardiac indication for its use (coronary stent, acute coronary syndrome) (see Table 6-1).

SUMMARY

Fortunately, most of the risk factors for stroke and TIA are modifiable through therapeutic and counseling interventions that are proven to reduce the risk of recurrence. Among these, blood pressure control, aggressive blood sugar management in diabetes, optimization of cholesterol levels, and lifestyle modification (particularly smoking cessation), as well as the appropriate use of anti-platelet therapy, are considered strategic targets for medical intervention after stroke or TIA.

For blood pressure control, a regimen of ACEI, ARB, and/or thiazide diuretic is recommended for both prevention of stroke or TIA and other vascular events. Goals for the management of diabetes in survivors of stroke and TIA include a regimen of anti-hypertensive agents such as ACEI, ARB, or thiazide diuretic to a target level of <130/80 mm Hg. Recently, the SPARCLE trial demonstrated that aggressive cholesterol lowering therapy with atorvastatin 80 mg was beneficial in the prevention of recurrent stroke among long-term survivors of stroke or TIA, making this particular intervention an important tool in the armamentarium (Amarenco et al., 2006). Long-term anti-coagulation with warfarin or newer agents, such as thrombin or factor Xa inhibitors, is the intervention of choice to reduce the risk of recurrent stroke or TIA in patients with *either* paroxysmal or chronic AF. If long-term anti-coagulation is contraindicated, an antiplatelet may be substituted, but with a more modest stroke risk reduction. Based on the results of recent trials, CEA for severe carotid stenosis is the treatment of choice for symptomatic patients.

Finally, over the next few years, several clinical trials may clarify the roles for interventional procedures that are alternatives to medical therapy for lowering stroke risk in specific conditions. The Watchman trial (WATCHMAN, 2007 will compare occlusion of the left atrial appendage with a device to anti-thrombotic therapy.)

CONCLUSIONS

Stroke is a common neurological disorder, more often disabling than lethal. Thus far, treatment of stroke has been limited to a few acute therapies that lower morbidity and mortality. Therefore, clinicians and researchers have focused on primary and secondary prevention strategies. The targets for prevention include; identification of people at higher risk and aggressive treatment of risk factors such as hypertension, diabetes mellitus, dyslipidemia, cigarette smoking, obesity, alcohol use, and physical inactivity, among others.

REFERENCES

Adams RJ, Albers G, Alberts MJ, Benavente O, Furie K, Goldstein LB, et al. Update to the AHA/ASA Recommendations for the Prevention of Stroke in Patients with Stroke and Transient Ischemic Attack. *Stroke.* 2008.

AHA. Measuring and improving quality of care: a report from the American Heart Association/American College of Cardiology First Scientific Forum on Assessment of Healthcare Quality in Cardiovascular Disease and Stroke. *Circulation.* 2000;101(12):1483–1493.

ALLHAT Officers and Coordinators for the ALLHAT Collaborative Research Group. The Antihypertensive and Lipid-Lowering Treatment to Prevent Heart Attack Trial. Major outcomes in high-risk hypertensive patients randomized to angiotensin-converting enzyme inhibitor or calcium channel blocker vs diuretic: The Antihypertensive and Lipid-Lowering Treatment to Prevent Heart Attack Trial (ALLHAT). *JAMA.* 2002;288(23):2981–2997.

Amarenco P, Bogousslavsky J, Callahan A, 3rd, Goldstein LB, Hennerici M, Rudolph AE, et al. High-dose atorvastatin after stroke or transient ischemic attack. *N Engl J Med.* 2006;355(6):549–559.

American Diabetes Association. ADA clinical practice recommendations. *Diabetes Care.* 2004;27:S1–S143.

Anderson JW, Konz EC. Obesity and disease management: effects of weight loss on comorbid conditions. *Obesity Res.* 2001;9 Suppl 4:326S–334S.

Antithrombotic Trialists' Collaboration. Collaborative meta-analysis of randomised trials of antiplatelet therapy for prevention of death, myocardial infarction, and stroke in high risk patients. *BMJ.* 2002;324(7329):71–86.

Atrial Fibrillation Clopidogrel Trial with Irbesartan for Prevention of Vascular Events (ACTIVE). [May 1st 2007]; Available from: http://www.strokecenter.org/trials/TrialDetail.aspx?tid=699.

Bhatt DL, Fox KA, Hacke W, Berger PB, Black HR, Boden WE, et al. Clopidogrel and aspirin versus aspirin alone for the prevention of atherothrombotic events. *N Engl J Med.* 2006;354(16):1706–1717.

Bhatt DL, Marso SP, Hirsch AT, Ringleb PA, Hacke W, Topol EJ. Amplified benefit of clopidogrel versus aspirin in patients with diabetes mellitus. *Am J Cardiol.* 2002;90(6):625–628.

Bousser MG, Eschwege E, Haguenau M, Lefauconnier JM, Thibult N, Touboul D, et al. "AICLA" controlled trial of aspirin and dipyridamole in the secondary prevention of athero-thrombotic cerebral ischemia. *Stroke.* 1983;14(1):5–14.

Brott TG, Hobson RW, 2nd, Howard G, Roubin GS, Clark WM, Brooks W, et al. Stenting versus endarterectomy for treatment of carotid-artery stenosis. *N Engl J Med.* 2010;363(1):11–23. Epub 2010/05/28.

Brown RD, Whisnant JP, Sicks JD, O'Fallon WM, Wiebers DO. Stroke incidence, prevalence, and survival: secular trends in Rochester, Minnesota, through 1989. *Stroke.* 1996;27(3):373–380.

Camm AJ, Kirchhof P, Lip GYH, et al. Guidelines for the management of atrial fibrillation: The Task Force for the Management of Atrial Fibrillation of the European Society of Cardiology (ESC). *European Heart Journal.* 2010;31:2369–2429. http://www.escardio.org/guidelines-surveys/esc-guidelines/GuidelinesDocuments/guidelines-afib-FT.pdf.

CAPRIE Steering Committee. A randomised, blinded, trial of clopidogrel versus aspirin in patients at risk of ischaemic events (CAPRIE). *Lancet.* 1996;348(9038):1329–1339.

Chambers BR, Norris JW. Outcome in patients with asymptomatic neck bruits. *N Engl J Med.* 1986;315(14):860–865.

Chimowitz MI, Lynn MJ, Derdeyn CP, Turan TN, Fiorella D, Lane BF, et al. Stenting versus aggressive medical therapy for intracranial arterial stenosis. *N Engl J Med.* 2011;365(11):993–1003. Epub 2011/09/09.

Chimowitz MI, Lynn MJ, Howlett-Smith H, Stern BJ, Hertzberg VS, Frankel MR, et al. Comparison of warfarin and aspirin for symptomatic intracranial arterial stenosis. *N Engl J Med.* 2005;352(13):1305–1316.

Chobanian AV, Bakris GL, Black HR, Cushman WC, Green LA, Izzo JL, Jr., et al. The Seventh Report of the Joint National Committee on Prevention, Detection, Evaluation, and Treatment of High Blood Pressure: the JNC 7 report. *JAMA.*2003;289(19):2560–2572.

Collins R, Armitage J, Parish S, Sleight P, Peto R. Effects of cholesterol-lowering with simvastatin on stroke and other major vascular events in 20536 people with cerebrovascular disease or other high-risk conditions. *Lancet.* 2004;363(9411):757–767.

Connolly et al. Guidelines for the management of aneurysmal subarachnoid hemorrhage : a guideline for healthcare professionals from the American Heart Association/American Stroke Association. *Stroke.* July 2013.

Connolly SJ, Ezekowitz MD, Yusuf S, Eikelboom J, Oldgren J, Parekh A, et al. Dabigatran versus warfarin in patients with atrial fibrillation. *N Engl J Med.* 2009;361(12):1139–1151. Epub 2009/09/01.

Dahlof B, Lindholm LH, Hansson L, Schersten B, Ekbom T, Wester PO. Morbidity and mortality in the Swedish Trial in Old Patients with Hypertension (STOP-Hypertension). *Lancet.* 1991;338(8778):1281–1285.

Dannenberg AL, Garrison RJ, Kannel WB. Incidence of hypertension in the Framingham Study. *Am J Public Health.* 1988;78(6):676–679.

Di Tullio M, Sacco RL, Gopal A, Mohr JP, Homma S. Patent foramen ovale as a risk factor for cryptogenic stroke. *Ann Intern Med.* 1992;117(6):461–465.

Diener HC, Bogousslavsky J, Brass LM, Cimminiello C, Csiba L, Kaste M, et al. Aspirin and clopidogrel compared with clopidogrel alone after recent ischaemic stroke or transient ischaemic attack in high-risk patients (MATCH): randomised, double-blind, placebo-controlled trial. *Lancet.* 2004;364(9431):331–337.

Diener HC, Darius H, Bertrand-Hardy JM, Humphreys M. Cardiac safety in the European Stroke Prevention Study 2 (ESPS2). *Int J Clin Pract.* 2001;55(3):162–163.

Djousse L, Ellison RC, Beiser A, Scaramucci A, D'Agostino RB, Wolf PA. Alcohol consumption and risk of ischemic stroke: The Framingham Study. *Stroke.* 2002;33(4):907–912.

Dutch TIA Study Group. The Dutch TIA trial: protective effects of low-dose aspirin and atenolol in patients with transient ischemic attacks or nondisabling stroke. *Stroke.* 1988;19(4):512–517.

EC/IC Bypass Study Group. Failure of extracranial-intracranial arterial bypass to reduce the risk of ischemic stroke. Results of an international randomized trial. *N Engl J Med.* 1985;313(19):1191–1200.

Elkind MS, Sciacca R, Boden-Albala B, Rundek T, Paik MC, Sacco RL. Moderate alcohol consumption reduces risk of ischemic stroke: the Northern Manhattan Study. *Stroke.* 2006;37(1):13–19. Epub 2005/11/25.

Endovascular versus surgical treatment in patients with carotid stenosis in the Carotid and Vertebral Artery Transluminal Angioplasty Study (CAVATAS): a randomised trial. *Lancet.* 2001;357(9270):1729–1737.

European Carotid Surgery Trialists' Collaborative Group. MRC European Carotid Surgery Trial: interim results for symptomatic patients with severe (70–99%) or with mild (0–29%) carotid stenosis. European

Carotid Surgery Trialists' Collaborative Group. *Lancet.* 1991;337(8752):1235–1243.

European Stroke Prevention Study (ESPS). Principal end-points. The ESPS Group. *Lancet.* 1987;2(8572):1351–1354.

Executive Summary of The Third Report of The National Cholesterol Education Program (NCEP) Expert Panel on Detection, Evaluation, and Treatment of High Blood Cholesterol in Adults (Adult Treatment Panel III). *JAMA.* 2001;285(19):2486–2497.

Farrell B, Godwin J, Richards S, Warlow C. The United Kingdom transient ischaemic attack (UK-TIA) aspirin trial: final results. *J Neurol Neurosur Ps.* 1991;54(12):1044–1054.

Feinberg WM, Blackshear JL, Laupacis A, Kronmal R, Hart RG. Prevalence, age distribution, and gender of patients with atrial fibrillation. Analysis and implications. *Arch Intern Med.* 1995;155(5):469–473.

Fiore M. US Tobacco Use and Dependence Guideline Panel. *Treating Tobacco Use and Dependence: Clinical Practice Guideline.* Rockville, MD: US Department of Health and Human Services, USPHS; 2000.

Fontaine KR, Redden DT, Wang C, Westfall AO, Allison DB. Years of life lost due to obesity. *JAMA.* 2003;289(2):187–193.

Furlan AJ, Reisman M, Massaro J, Mauri L, Adams H, Albers GW, et al. Closure or medical therapy for cryptogenic stroke with patent foramen ovale. *N Engl J Med.* 2012;366(11):991–999. Epub 2012/03/16.

Gent M, Blakely JA, Easton JD, Ellis DJ, Hachinski VC, Harbison JW, et al. The Canadian American Ticlopidine Study (CATS) in thromboembolic stroke. *Lancet.* 1989;1(8649):1215–1220.

Gaede P, Vedel P, Larsen N, Jensen GV, Parving HH, Pedersen O. Multifactorial intervention and cardiovascular disease in patients with type 2 diabetes. *N Engl J Med.* 2003;348(5):383–393.

Gage BF, Waterman AD, Shannon W, Boechler M, Rich MW, Radford MJ. Validation of clinical classification schemes for predicting stroke: results from the National Registry of Atrial Fibrillation. *JAMA.* 2001;285(22):2864–2870.

Gill JS, Shipley MJ, Tsementzis SA, Hornby RS, Gill SK, Hitchcock ER, et al. Alcohol consumption—a risk factor for hemorrhagic and non-hemorrhagic stroke. *Am J Med.* 1991;90(4):489–497.

Gillum RF. Risk factors for stroke in blacks: a critical review. *Am J Epidemiol.* 1999;150(12):1266–1274.

Goldstein LB, Adams R, Alberts MJ, Appel LJ, Brass LM, Bushnell CD, et al. Primary prevention of ischemic stroke: a guideline from the American Heart Association/American Stroke Association Stroke Council: cosponsored by the Atherosclerotic Peripheral Vascular Disease Interdisciplinary Working Group; Cardiovascular Nursing Council; Clinical Cardiology Council; Nutrition, Physical Activity, and Metabolism Council; and the Quality of Care and Outcomes Research Interdisciplinary Working Group: the American Academy of Neurology affirms the value of this guideline. *Stroke*. 2006;37(6):1583–1633.

Gorelick PB. Alcohol and stroke. *Stroke*. 1987;18(1):268–271.

Gorelick PB, Richardson D, Kelly M, Ruland S, Hung E, Harris Y, et al. Aspirin and ticlopidine for prevention of recurrent stroke in black patients: a randomized trial. *JAMA*. 2003;289(22):2947–2957.

Granger CB, Alexander JH, McMurray JJ, Lopes RD, Hylek EM, Hanna M, et al. Apixaban versus warfarin in patients with atrial fibrillation. *N Engl J Med*. 2011;365(11):981–992. Epub 2011/08/30.

Guiraud-Chaumeil B, Rascol A, David J, Boneu B, Clanet M, Bierme R. Prevention des recidives des accidents vasculaires cerebraux ischemiques par les anti-agregants plaquettaires. Resultats d'un essai therapeutique controle de 3 ans. [Prevention of recurrences of cerebral ischemic vascular accidents by platelet antiaggregants. Results of a 3-year controlled therapeutic trial]. *Rev Neurol (Paris)*. 1982;138(5):367–385.

Halkes PH, van Gijn J, Kappelle LJ, Koudstaal PJ, Algra A. Aspirin plus dipyridamole versus aspirin alone after cerebral ischaemia of arterial origin (ESPRIT): randomised controlled trial. *Lancet*. 2006;367(9523):1665–1673.

Hass WK, Easton JD, Adams HP, Jr., Pryse-Phillips W, Molony BA, Anderson S, et al. A randomized trial comparing ticlopidine hydrochloride with aspirin for the prevention of stroke in high-risk patients. Ticlopidine Aspirin Stroke Study Group. *N Engl J Med*. 1989;321(8):501–507.

He J, Klag MJ, Wu Z, Whelton PK. Stroke in the People's Republic of China. I. Geographic variations in incidence and risk factors. *Stroke*. 1995;26(12):2222–2227.

Heart Outcomes Prevention Evaluation Study Investigators. Effects of ramipril on cardiovascular and microvascular outcomes in people with diabetes mellitus: results of the HOPE study and MICRO-HOPE substudy. *Lancet*. 2000;355(9200):253–259.

Henderson RD, Eliasziw M, Fox AJ, Rothwell PM, Barnett HJ. Angiographically defined collateral circulation and risk of stroke in patients with severe carotid artery stenosis. North American Symptomatic Carotid Endarterectomy Trial (NASCET) Group. *Stroke*. 2000;31(1):128–132.

Hennerici M, Hulsbomer HB, Hefter H, Lammerts D, Rautenberg W. Natural history of asymptomatic extracranial arterial disease. Results of a long-term prospective study. *Brain*. 1987;110 (Pt 3):777–791.

Homma S, Sacco RL, Di Tullio MR, Sciacca RR, Mohr JP. Effect of medical treatment in stroke patients with patent foramen ovale: patent foramen ovale in Cryptogenic Stroke Study. *Circulation*. 2002;105(22):2625–2631.

Homma S, Thompson JLP, Pullicino PM, Levin B, Freudenberger RS, Teerlink JR, et al. Warfarin and aspirin in patients with heart failure and sinus rhythm. *N Engl J Med*. 2012;366:1859–1869.

Inzitari D, Eliasziw M, Gates P, Sharpe BL, Chan RK, Meldrum HE, et al. The causes and risk of stroke in patients with asymptomatic internal-carotid-artery stenosis. North American Symptomatic Carotid Endarterectomy Trial Collaborators. *N Engl J Med*. 2000;342(23):1693–1700.

Jauch EC, Saver JL, Adams HP, Jr., Bruno A, Connors JJ, Demaerschalk BM, et al. Guidelines for the early management of patients with acute ischemic stroke: a guideline for healthcare professionals from the American Heart Association/American Stroke Association. *Stroke*. January 31, 2013.

Julius S, Alderman MH, Beevers G, Dahlof B, Devereux RB, Douglas JG, et al. Cardiovascular risk reduction in hypertensive black patients with left ventricular hypertrophy: the LIFE study. *J Am Coll Cardiol*. 2004;43(6):1047–1055.

Kannel WB, McGee DL. Diabetes and cardiovascular disease: The Framingham study. *JAMA*. 1979;241(19):2035–2038.

Kappelle LJ, Eliasziw M, Fox AJ, Sharpe BL, Barnett HJ. Importance of intracranial atherosclerotic disease in patients with symptomatic stenosis of the internal carotid artery: The North American Symptomatic Carotid Endarterectomy Trial. *Stroke*. 1999;30(2):282–286.

Kiely DK, Wolf PA, Cupples LA, Beiser AS, Myers RH. Familial aggregation of stroke: The Framingham Study. *Stroke*. 1993;24(9):1366–1371.

Kittner SJ, Stern BJ, Feeser BR, Hebel R, Nagey DA, Buchholz DW, et al. Pregnancy and the risk of stroke. *N Engl J Med*. 1996;335(11):768–774.

Kurth T, Gaziano JM, Berger K, Kase CS, Rexrode KM, Cook NR, et al. Body mass index and the risk of stroke in men. *Arch Intern Med*. 2002;162(22):2557–2562.

Lee CD, Folsom AR, Blair SN. Physical activity and stroke risk: a meta-analysis. *Stroke*. 2003;34(10):2475–2481.

Liao D, Myers R, Hunt S, Shahar E, Paton C, Burke G, et al. Familial history of stroke and stroke risk: The Family Heart Study. *Stroke*. 1997;28(10):1908–1912.

Lightwood JM, Glantz SA. Short-term economic and health benefits of smoking cessation: myocardial infarction and stroke. *Circulation*. 1997;96(4):1089–1096.

Lin HJ, Wolf PA, Kelly-Hayes M, Beiser AS, Kase CS, Benjamin EJ, et al. Stroke severity in atrial fibrillation: The Framingham Study. *Stroke*. 1996;27(10):1760–1764.

Loh E, Sutton MS, Wun CC, Rouleau JL, Flaker GC, Gottlieb SS, et al. Ventricular dysfunction and the risk of stroke after myocardial infarction. *N Engl J Med.* 1997;336(4):251–257.

Lyrer P, Engelter S. Antithrombotic drugs for carotid artery dissection. *Cochrane Database Syst Rev.* 2003(3):CD000255.

Mackey AE, Abrahamowicz M, Langlois Y, Battista R, Simard D, Bourque F, et al. Outcome of asymptomatic patients with carotid disease. Asymptomatic Cervical Bruit Study Group. *Neurology.* 1997;48(4):896–903.

Mas JL, Chatellier G, Beyssen B, Branchereau A, Moulin T, Becquemin JP, et al. Endarterectomy versus stenting in patients with symptomatic severe carotid stenosis. *N Engl J Med.* 2006;355(16):1660–1671.

Mas JL, Zuber M. Recurrent cerebrovascular events in patients with patent foramen ovale, atrial septal aneurysm, or both and cryptogenic stroke or transient ischemic attack. French Study Group on Patent Foramen Ovale and Atrial Septal Aneurysm. *Am Heart J.* 1995;130(5):1083–1088.

Mayberg MR, Wilson SE, Yatsu F, Weiss DG, Messina L, Hershey LA, et al. Carotid endarterectomy and prevention of cerebral ischemia in symptomatic carotid stenosis. Veterans Affairs Cooperative Studies Program 309 Trialist Group. *JAMA.* 1991;266(23):3289–3294.

Mazzaglia G, Britton AR, Altmann DR, Chenet L. Exploring the relationship between alcohol consumption and non-fatal or fatal stroke: a systematic review. *Addiction.* 2001;96(12):1743–1756.

Mohr JP, Thompson JL, Lazar RM, Levin B, Sacco RL, Furie KL, et al. A comparison of warfarin and aspirin for the prevention of recurrent ischemic stroke. *N Engl J Med.* 2001;345(20):1444–1451.

MRC Working Party. Medical Research Council trial of treatment of hypertension in older adults: principal results. *BMJ.* 1992;304(6824):405–412.

MRC/BHF Heart Protection Study of cholesterol lowering with simvastatin in 20,536 high-risk individuals: a randomised placebo-controlled trial. *Lancet.* 2002;360(9326):7–22.

Mzimba ZS, Beevers DG, Lip GY. Antihypertensive therapy before, during, and after stroke. *Basic Res Cardiol.* 1998;93 Suppl 2:59–62.

North American Symptomatic Carotid Endarterectomy Trial Collaborators (NASCETC). Beneficial effect of carotid endarterectomy in symptomatic patients with high-grade carotid stenosis. *N Engl J Med.* 1991;325(7):445–453.

Patel MR, Mahaffey KW, Garg J, Pan G, Singer DE, Hacke W, et al. Rivaroxaban versus warfarin in nonvalvular atrial fibrillation. *N Engl J Med.* 2011;365(10):883–891. Epub 2011/08/13.

Pfeffer MA, Braunwald E, Moye LA, Basta L, Brown EJ, Jr., Cuddy TE, et al. Effect of captopril on mortality and morbidity in patients with left ventricular dysfunction after myocardial infarction. Results of the survival and ventricular enlargement trial. The SAVE Investigators. *N Engl J Med.* 1992;327(10):669–677.

Powers WJ, Clarke WR, Grubb RL, Jr., Videen TO, Adams HP, Jr., Derdeyn CP. Extracranial-intracranial bypass surgery for stroke prevention in hemodynamic cerebral ischemia: the Carotid Occlusion Surgery Study randomized trial. *JAMA.* 2011;306(18):1983–1992. Epub 2011/11/10.

PROGRESS Collaborative Group. Randomised trial of a perindopril-based blood-pressure-lowering regimen among 6,105 individuals with previous stroke or transient ischaemic attack. *Lancet.* 2001;358(9287):1033–1041.

Randomised trial of endarterectomy for recently symptomatic carotid stenosis: final results of the MRC European Carotid Surgery Trial (ECST). *Lancet.* 1998;351(9113):1379–1387.

Rashid P, Leonardi-Bee J, Bath P. Blood pressure reduction and secondary prevention of stroke and other vascular events: a systematic review. *Stroke.* 2003;34(11):2741–2748.

Reynolds K, Lewis B, Nolen JD, Kinney GL, Sathya B, He J. Alcohol consumption and risk of stroke: a meta-analysis. *JAMA.* 2003;289(5):579–588.

Ringleb PA, Allenberg J, Bruckmann H, Eckstein HH, Fraedrich G, Hartmann M, et al. 30 day results from the SPACE trial of stent-protected angioplasty versus carotid endarterectomy in symptomatic patients: a randomised non-inferiority trial. *Lancet.* 2006;368(9543):1239–1247.

Ringleb PA, Bhatt DL, Hirsch AT, Topol EJ, Hacke W. Benefit of clopidogrel over aspirin is amplified in patients with a history of ischemic events. *Stroke.* 2004;35(2):528–532.

Risk factors for stroke and efficacy of antithrombotic therapy in atrial fibrillation: Analysis of pooled data from five randomized controlled trials. *Arch Intern Med.* 1994;154(13):1449–1457.

Roger VL, Go AS, Lloyd-Jones DM, Adams RJ, Berry JD, Brown TM, et al. Heart disease and stroke statistics—2011 update: a report from the American Heart Association. *Circulation.* 2011;123(4):e18–e209. Epub 2010/12/17.

Rothwell PM, Eliasziw M, Gutnikov SA, Warlow CP, Barnett HJ. Endarterectomy for symptomatic carotid stenosis in relation to clinical subgroups and timing of surgery. *Lancet.* 2004;363(9413):915–924.

Sacco RL, Adams R, Albers G, Alberts MJ, Benavente O, Furie K, et al. Guidelines for prevention of stroke in patients with ischemic stroke or transient ischemic attack: a statement for healthcare professionals from the American Heart Association/American Stroke Association Council on Stroke: co-sponsored by the Council on Cardiovascular Radiology and Intervention: the American Academy of Neurology affirms the value of this guideline. *Stroke.* 2006;37(2):577–617.

Sacco RL, Boden-Albala B, Abel G, Lin IF, Elkind M, Hauser WA, et al. Race-ethnic disparities in the impact of stroke risk factors: the northern Manhattan stroke study. *Stroke*. 2001;32(8):1725–1731.

Sacco RL, Boden-Albala B, Gan R, Chen X, Kargman DE, Shea S, et al. Stroke incidence among white, black, and Hispanic residents of an urban community: the Northern Manhattan Stroke Study. *Am J Epidemiol*. 1998;147(3):259–268.

Sacco RL, Diener HC, Yusuf S, Cotton D, Ounpuu S, Lawton WA, et al. Aspirin and extended-release dipyridamole versus clopidogrel for recurrent stroke. *N Engl J Med*. 2008;359(12):1238–1251.

Sacco RL, Elkind M, Boden-Albala B, Lin IF, Kargman DE, Hauser WA, et al. The protective effect of moderate alcohol consumption on ischemic stroke. *JAMA*. 1999;281(1):53–60. Epub 1999/01/19.

Sacco RL, Shi T, Zamanillo MC, Kargman DE. Predictors of mortality and recurrence after hospitalized cerebral infarction in an urban community: the Northern Manhattan Stroke Study. *Neurology*. 1994;44(4):626–634.

Schievink WI, Mokri B, O'Fallon WM. Recurrent spontaneous cervical-artery dissection. *N Engl J Med*. 1994;330(6):393–397.

Schrader J, Luders S, Kulschewski A, Berger J, Zidek W, Treib J, et al. The ACCESS Study: evaluation of Acute Candesartan Cilexetil Therapy in Stroke Survivors. *Stroke*. 2003;34(7):1699–1703.

Shindler DM, Kostis JB, Yusuf S, Quinones MA, Pitt B, Stewart D, et al. Diabetes mellitus, a predictor of morbidity and mortality in the Studies of Left Ventricular Dysfunction (SOLVD) Trials and Registry. *Am J Cardiol*. 1996;77(11):1017–1020.

SSYLVIA Study Investigators. Stenting of Symptomatic Atherosclerotic Lesions in the Vertebral or Intracranial Arteries (SSYLVIA): study results. *Stroke*. 2004;35(6):1388–1392.

Staessen JA, Fagard R, Thijs L, Celis H, Arabidze GG, Birkenhager WH, et al. Randomised double-blind comparison of placebo and active treatment for older patients with isolated systolic hypertension. The Systolic Hypertension in Europe (Syst-Eur) Trial Investigators. *Lancet*. 1997;350(9080):757–764.

Suk SH, Sacco RL, Boden-Albala B, Cheun JF, Pittman JG, Elkind MS, et al. Abdominal obesity and risk of ischemic stroke: the Northern Manhattan Stroke Study. *Stroke*. 2003;34(7):1586–1592.

Turcato E, Bosello O, Di Francesco V, Harris TB, Zoico E, Bissoli L, et al. Waist circumference and abdominal sagittal diameter as surrogates of body fat distribution in the elderly: their relation with cardiovascular risk factors. *Int J Obes Relat Metab Disord*. 2000;24(8):1005–1010.

UK Prospective Diabetes Study Group (UKPDS). Efficacy of atenolol and captopril in reducing risk of macrovascular and microvascular complications in type 2 diabetes: UKPDS 39. *BMJ*. 1998b;317(7160):713–720.

UK Prospective Diabetes Study Group (UKPDS). Tight blood pressure control and risk of macrovascular and microvascular complications in type 2 diabetes: UKPDS 38. *BMJ*. 1998a;317(7160):703–713.

Visser CA, Kan G, Meltzer RS, Lie KI, Durrer D. Long-term follow-up of left ventricular thrombus after acute myocardial infarction. A two-dimensional echocardiographic study in 96 patients. *Chest*. 1984;86(4):532–536.

WATCHMAN left atrial appendage system for embolic protection in patients with atrial fibrillation. Ongoing. Available from: http://www.strokecenter.org/trials/TrialDetail.aspx?tid=716.

Weber MA, Julius S, Kjeldsen SE, Brunner HR, Ekman S, Hansson L, et al. Blood pressure dependent and independent effects of antihypertensive treatment on clinical events in the VALUE Trial. *Lancet*. 2004;363(9426):2049–2051.

Wolf PA, D'Agostino RB, Kannel WB, Bonita R, Belanger AJ. Cigarette smoking as a risk factor for stroke. The Framingham Study. *JAMA*. 1988;259(7):1025–1029.

Wolf PA, D'Agostino RB, O'Neal MA, Sytkowski P, Kase CS, Belanger AJ, et al. Secular trends in stroke incidence and mortality. The Framingham Study. *Stroke*. 1992;23(11):1551–1555.

Wolz M, Cutler J, Roccella EJ, Rohde F, Thom T, Burt V. Statement from the National High Blood Pressure Education Program: prevalence of hypertension. *Am J Hypertens*. 2000;13(1 Pt 1):103–104.

Yadav JS, Wholey MH, Kuntz RE, Fayad P, Katzen BT, Mishkel GJ, et al. Protected carotid-artery stenting versus endarterectomy in high-risk patients. *N Engl J Med*. 2004;351(15):1493–1501.

You RX, Thrift AG, McNeil JJ, Davis SM, Donnan GA. Ischemic stroke risk and passive exposure to spouses' cigarette smoking. Melbourne Stroke Risk Factor Study (MERFS) Group. *Am J Public Health*. 1999;89(4):572–575.

Yusuf S, Sleight P, Pogue J, Bosch J, Davies R, Dagenais G. Effects of an angiotensin-converting-enzyme inhibitor, ramipril, on cardiovascular events in high-risk patients. The Heart Outcomes Prevention Evaluation Study Investigators. *N Engl J Med*. 2000;342(3):145–153.

Zweifler RM, Silverboard G. Arterial Dissections. 4th ed., pp. 549–573. Mohr JP, Choi DW, Grotta JC, Weir B, Wolf PA, eds. Philadelphia: Churchill Livingstone; 2004.

7

Risk Reduction for Other Major Diseases of Adulthood

BARBARA P. YAWN

Risk reduction is aimed at decreasing the morbidity and premature mortality associated with the causes of death and disability in adults in the United States. In general, risk factors are due to the individual's genetic makeup, environment, lifestyle, or a combination of these factors. Risk reduction may affect the onset of a condition or disease (primary prevention), the early identification of a disease to prevent adverse events (secondary prevention), or the limitation of disability from a disease that has already led to a serious adverse event (tertiary prevention), as discussed throughout *Prevention Practice in Primary Care*. Immunizations can prevent death or disability from several conditions; influenza and pneumonia vaccines prevent deaths, and the shingles vaccine can prevent morbidity and disability (Oxman et al., 2005; Yawn et al., 2007; Ortqvist et al., 1998; Greci, Katz, & Jekel, 2005). Appropriate dietary intake can prevent rickets or scurvy. Osteoporosis screening does not prevent disease but may prevent a hip or other fracture thereby preventing fracture-associated morbidity and premature mortality (Rousseau, 1997; Borer, 2005). Exercise, nutritional advice and educational support (rehabilitation) may slow declines in quality of life and morbidity in patients who have had chronic obstructive pulmonary disease (COPD) adverse events such as exacerbation (Paz-Diaz et al., 2007). In this Chapter we will identify strategies that are appropriate for health professionals and institutions to use in addressing the risk factors related to the most common causes of morbidity and premature mortality in adults (other than cancer and cardiovascular disease, which have been covered in previous Chapters). Screening is not enough, however; when feasible, the need for a second stage of evaluation or follow-up will be addressed (Kroenke, 2001). While many of the

recommendations presented will be based on the work of the US Preventive Services Task Force (USPSTF) sponsored by the Agency for Health Care Research and Quality (http://www.uspreventiveservicestaskforce.org) and the Community Guide supported by the Centers for Disease and Prevention (http://www.thecommunityguide.org/about/default.htm), the Chapter also touches on recommendations related to basic nutritional requirements including vitamins and minerals, recommended levels of exercise, the need for balance of intake and exercise, and stress reduction. These recommendations for general health are often overlooked when physicians and health care organizations focus on specific conditions, procedures, testing, and "medical" interventions.

The USPSTF is a group of 15 experts in general medicine, nursing and mental health who review the evidence related to specific conditions and make recommendations supporting screening or counseling (A and B level recommendations; http://www.uspreventiveservicestaskforce.org/uspstf/uspsabrecs.htm), recommendations requiring clinical judgment for individual cases (C recommendations), recommendations against screening or counseling (D recommendations), and "I statements," which indicate that evidence is insufficient for recommendations (Sawaya et al., 2007; Barton et al., 2007). Their work is supported through the Agency for Health Care Research and Quality (AHRQ). The Task Force on community Preventive Services is a group of 12 experts on primary health care, epidemiology, and community health who develop the Community Guide (http://www.thecommunityguide.org/about/default.htm). Their work is supported by the Centers for Disease and Prevention (CDC). The work of these groups is based on specific evidence reviews developed for each topic. Once the topic of interest is determined, a series of questions are developed and fit into a logic model or framework (Sawaya et al., 2007). An evidence-based review is developed to answer the questions in the logic model and is synthesized by the Evidence Based Practice Centers (Sawaya et al., 2007) and the members of the Task Forces. Final recommendations include a specific screening or counseling recommendation with a strength of evidence labeled A through D as explained above. The recommendations include clinical considerations as well as suggestions for further research to fill in the evidence gaps (Barton et al., 2007).

Tables 7-1 and 7-2 are the 2012 summary of recommendations pertaining to adults from the USPSTF (www.ahrq.gov/clinic/uspstf/upstopics.htm). The separation between adult and children may seem artificial to health professionals caring for people across the age span. Topics such as infant car seat use and childhood immunizations must be discussed with parents. However, in this Chapter the primary focus will be on topics that relate to recommendations that pertain to adult health and prevention that is done with adults in primary care (Donaldson et al., 2001). The recommendations highlighted in the tables relate to issues of cancer or cardiovascular disease and have been discussed in previous Chapters.

GENERAL ISSUES WITH SCREENING/COUNSELING IN CONTINUITY CARE PRACTICES

Most primary care practices offer continuity care for adults of all ages. These practices need to deal with both the initiation and repetition of screening or counseling. Some of the basic evaluations for prevention begin at age 20 to 25 in both men and women and are repeated periodically for the rest of the person's life. The exact nature of the initial screening or counseling is usually specified. However, details on repetition may be less available. Repeated assessment may not always require the same intensity as the initial assessment. For example, the use of safety belts in motor vehicles should be reassessed, but if the initial answer is "I always use them," a simple "Are you still using seat belts?" may be adequate, with greater scrutiny at times such as during pregnancy, when a woman may not know how to adjust seat belt use to her changing shape. For many prevention recommendations, the frequency of the repeated assessment may not be specified; even if it is, the recommendations are seldom based on the same high

TABLE 7-1. RISK REDUCTION RECOMMENDATIONS FOR ADULT WOMEN FROM THE USPSTF

Pregnant–any age
Laboratory testing
Hepatitis B
Chlamydia
Syphilis
Gonorrhea
Anemia
Bacteruria
Rh incompatibility at first visit and 24 to 28 weeks
Recommendations
Breast feeding counseling
Nutrition (folic acid intake) assessment
Tobacco use counseling Influenza immunization
Non-pregnant–20–40
Laboratory testing
Cholesterol assessment beginning at 20 for women at high risk of CVD
Diabetes screening in those with sustained BP > 135/80
Pap smear—in sexually active women
Recommendations
Blood pressure assessment
Obesity assessment
Tobacco-yes/no and? ready to quit
Alcohol abuse assessment
Depression
Sexual history—onset and number of partners—consider screening chlamydia, gonorrhea, and HIV screening
Family CVD history Family breast/ovarian Ca history counseling regarding BRCA
Immunizations
Influenza immunizations yearly
TdaP once and then dT every 10 years
41–64–Add
Laboratory testing
Lipids (cholesterol) beginning at age 45 years
Recommendations
Daily aspirin at age 50
Immunizations
Zostravax once beginning at age 50 (non-immune compromised individuals)
Imaging studies
Mammogram beginning at age 50 years
Colonoscopy or stool occult blood beginning at age 50 years
> 65-Add:
Immunizations
-Pneumovax once
Imaging
-Bone density screening

Source: Adapted from http://www.uspreventiveservicestaskforce.org/uspstf/uspsabrecs.htm plus the ACIP.cv

TABLE 7-2. RISK REDUCTION
RECOMMENDATIONS FOR ADULT MEN
FROM THE USPSTF

20–35
Blood pressure assessment
Diabetes screening if sustained BP >135/80
Obesity assessment
Tobacco—yes/no and? ready to quit
Alcohol abuse assessment
Depression screening
Sexual history
HIV screening
Family CVD history
Influenza immunization yearly
DTaP once, then dT every 10 years

35–49–Add
Laboratory
Lipids (cholesterol)
Recommendations
Daily aspirin at age 40

50–65–Add
Zostavax immunization in those without immunocompromise
Imaging/testing
Colorectal cancer screening beginning at age 50 years

>65–Add
Immunizations
Pneumovax at least once
Imaging
If smoker, aortic aneurysm screening

Source: Aadapted from www.ahrq.gov/clinic/uspstf/upstopics.htm.

level of evidence as the recommendation for when and how to make the initial assessment. Clinical judgment and common sense are required when considering reassessments. For example, between the ages of 25 and 40 it is unlikely that height will change significantly in the average adult. While the initial assessment of height is important for obtaining a body mass index (BMI) and as a baseline for height loss in later life, staff time may be better spent on collecting other vital signs than yearly heights during this period. For some assessments such as weight, the risk and benefits should address where weights are obtained. The risk of weighing obese people in a public setting such as a high traffic hallway outside patient examination rooms may be significant in the eyes of the patient, suggesting the need and desirability of in-examination room weighing opportunities. Several studies have demonstrated

women's reluctance and delay in seeking medical care due to weight assessments, especially those done in more public settings (Olson, Schumaker, & Yawn, 1994). Repeat screening assessments are not intended to follow problems or abnormalities that are identified, but to identify new problems in those without previously identified conditions. Therefore, repeat screening frequency is different from repeated assessment and evaluation of treatment for identified issues such as obesity or osteoporosis.

Many of the screening and counseling procedures in younger adults are based on questions, questionnaires, or history taking. Unlike procedure-based screening such as a colonoscopy, question- or history-based screening processes may be initiated by patient-completed surveys distributed by the receptionists or medical assistants. However, simply asking is not sufficient. Screening must be linked to appropriate and available follow-up for abnormal results (www.ahrq.gov/clinic/uspstf/upstopics.htm). For example, every physician, nurse practitioner, or physician's assistant must be ready and able to do smoking cessation counseling and support including pharmacotherapy or referral. The 5 As (ask, advise to quit, assess willingness, assist to quit and arrange follow-up and support) (Prochaska & Velicer, 1997; Anatchkova, Velicer, & Prochaska, 2006) and the 5Rs (relevance, risks, rewards, roadblocks, and repetition) are useful frameworks for assessment and support but must be enhanced by specific knowledge of smoking cessation strategies, even when referral is anticipated. Like most other chronic diseases, tobacco use and addiction is a chronic relapsing condition requiring not only initial evaluation and therapy but ongoing monitoring and support (Rise et al., 2008; Fiore et al., 2004; Ritchie, Schulz, & Bryce, 2007). Smoking status should be reassessed regularly, but it can be frustrating to ask the same questions of those who have never smoked or who quit successfully 10 to 20 years ago. The simple question "Has your smoking status changed?" is usually sufficient for those who have never smoked. For those who have smoked, it is good to acknowledge the quit attempt or success. For anyone who continues to smoke or has relapsed, repeat of the full 5 As plus the 5 Rs is recommended (www.acponline.org/journals/news/apr02/smoking.htm, jeny.ipro.org/showthread.php?t=219) (see Table 7-3).

Alcohol misuse assessment is recommended to begin in early adolescence and continues throughout

TABLE 7-3. THE 5 AS AND 5RS OF SMOKING CESSATION

The 5As (Five Major Steps to Intervention) counseling framework can be used as an approach to engage patients in smoking cessation discussions.

1. Ask about tobacco use.
2. Advise to quit through clear personalized messages.
3. Assess willingness to quit.
4. Assist to quit.
5. Arrange follow-up and support.

Common complementary practices include using motivational interviewing and the 5Rs.

1. Relevance of smoking and cessation to current life and lifestyle.
2. Risks of continued smoking to the person and his or her family.
3. Rewards of smoking cessation may include money, family recognition.
4. Roadblocks to smoking cessation, including a partner that smokes.
5. Repetition is needed to successfully quit.

life (www.ahrq.gov/clinic/uspstf/upstopics.htm). At least three categories of alcohol misuse have been established: risky/hazardous, harmful, and dependence. The definitions of these terms can help determine what should be included in an assessment. Risky/hazardous is defined by more than 7 drinks per week for women, 14 per week for men, or more than 3 at one time for women or 6 for men. Harmful drinking is causing the drinker physical, social, or psycho-social harm (WHO, 2005). Several tools has been tested in primary care practices to identify problem drinking behaviors, including AUDIT (Fiellen, Reid, & O'Connor, 2000; Reinert & Allen, 2002; Bradley et al., 2003), and CAGE (Ewing, 1984; McCusker et al., 2002; Aertgeerts et al., 2000). Support for modifying drinking behaviors can be done in the primary care setting (Whitlock et al., 2002). However, treatment of alcohol dependency usually requires formal programs, which can be completed in many settings. Like smoking, alcohol misuse is a chronic relapsing condition that will require ongoing monitoring and support. Little information is available to determine exactly how and how often alcohol use should be reassessed following intensive therapy or cessation of use. The Community Guideline stresses the importance of recommending the use of a designated driver for

all who drink at sites other than their own home. The value of this recommendation by a health professional as a stand-alone program has not been assessed but fits well into multidimensional community programs (http://www.thecommunityguide.org/about/default.htm).

The high prevalence of depression and depressive symptoms among adults in the United States has led to recommendations for routine and repeated depression screening in all adults (Ohayon, 2007). The exact age when depression screening should begin is not clear, nor is the recommended frequency of repeated screening in those without previous depression (www.ahrq.gov/clinic/uspstf/upstopics.htm). However, the high prevalence and potentially devastating effects of postpartum depression suggest that routine screening might begin no later than the age of the first pregnancy for both men and women (Gjerdingen & Yawn, 2007; Burt & Stein, 2002). Several self-administered screening tools are available for depression screening. The PHQ-9 and PHQ-2 have been the most widely validated screening tools in primary care practice in the United States (Cameron et al, 2008; Li et al, 2007) and are available free for use by any practicing physician or other clinician (http://www.depression-primarycare.org/clinicians/toolkits/materials/forms/phq9/questionnaire/). The PHQ-9 includes a question related to suicidal ideation. Therefore, any practice doing this type of depression screening must have the resources and plans to deal with positive depression screening and reports of suicidal ideation. While in some communities this is as simple as referral to the easily accessible emergency department of an adjacent hospital, all practices need to develop an action plan for evaluation or referral for patients reporting suicidal thoughts (Yawn et al., 2008).

Other screening begins with history and may lead to simple affirmation of healthy choices or to further, more specific testing. Sexual history is important at any age and will guide the need for specific testing for HIV, chlamydia, and gonorrhea (www.ahrq.gov/clinic/uspstf/upstopics.htm), and counseling to prevent unwanted pregnancies (http://www.thecommunityguide.org/about/default.htm). Sexual history should include information regarding the onset of intercourse or oral "sex," the number of partners, whether partners are the same or different sex or both and history of previous pregnancies and sexually transmitted infections (STIs). The USPSTF recommends regular (yearly perhaps) screening for chlamydia in all women <25 years who have had intercourse. Screening for gonorrhea and HIV should be considered for pregnant women, men and women who have had multiple partners or sex given in exchange for money or drugs, and men who have sex with men (USPSTF, 2008). How to phrase the questions regarding sexual history may depend on the community in which the patient lives, but simply ignoring this important screening because a man or women is assumed to have no potential for risk is not appropriate (Wallis, 1998).

Osteoporosis screening for women 60 years and older is the only other A or B level recommendation of the USPSTF not related to cancer or cardiovascular disease USPSTF, 2008). This also begins with self-completed questions using tools such as the Osteoporosis Risk Assessment Instrument with more specific bone imaging for women found to be high risk. The two step process allows the more expensive and specific procedure to be done only in the higher risk women (Cadarette et al., 2001).

Some screening procedures are to be done in those at increased risk, but the first step of screening is not a questionnaire but the presence of another disease. For example, the USPSTF recommends screening for diabetes in adults with hypertension or hyperlipidemia, which is most adults over the age of 45 to 50. The Community Guide also addresses diabetes but focuses on secondary and tertiary prevention in those with known diabetes. These disease management suggestions include monitoring of glycosylated hemoglobin, lipids, retinal vessels, renal function, foot lesions, and signs of neuropathy (mono-filament testing) all of which have been shown to identify risk factors and complications to allow additional secondary and tertiary prevention strategies to be started and thereby improve outcomes (American Diabetes Association, 2001a, 2001b, 2001c, 2001d; Diabetes Control and Complications Trial Research Group, 1993; UKPDS, 1998a, 1998b; Fontbonne et al, 1989; Bild et al., 1989; Rith-Najarian, Stolusky, & Gohdes, 1992; ETDRS, 1991; Ravid et al., 1996; Bakris et al., 2000).

Not all possible screening is appropriate to undertake at the present time. Few would argue with the lack of evidence and potential risks of recommending routine screening with a full body CT scan at any age (Brenner & Elliston, 2004). Groups interested in a specific condition or those who have spent years treating the end stage of a disease often find it difficult to accept the lack of evidence as a reason to not screen. However, some types of screening have sufficient evidence to recommend *against* routine screening in *asymptomatic* adults. Types of screening not recommended (excluding cancer and cardiovascular disease which have been discussed previously) include screening for asymptomatic bacteriuria in non-pregnant adults, for genital herpes, hepatitis B, syphilis, and hemochromatosis (www.ahrq. gov/clinic/uspstf/upstopics.htm). Unfortunately, the USPSTF's list of "I" statements that have *insufficient evidence to recommend for or against screening* is even longer (see Table 7-4, adapted from http:// www.uspreventiveservicestaskforce.org/uspstf/ uspsabrecs.htm). Several of these screening and counseling procedures are recommended by specialty and advocacy groups who are willing to accept limited evidence and may rely heavily on subspecialty expert opinion (Leppäniemi, 2008). Such recommendations may not apply to the average patient in primary care practice who has a lower prior probability of disease than those who move on from primary care to subspecialty care due to concerns or unexplained symptoms.

Table 7-5 is a summary of the recommendations from the Community Guide. Some overlap with recommendations from the USPSTF, but others deal with less disease-specific assessments and counseling. Many of the recommendations from the Community Guide deal with community-based

---

TABLE 7-4. SUMMARY OF "I" STATEMENTS* BY USPSTF FOR ADULT RISK REDUCTION

Gonorrhea screening in adults not at increased risk.
Family violence screening in those without signs or symptoms.
Screening for dementia in asymptomatic older adults.
Screening for suicide risk in those without symptoms or depression.
Behavioral counseling for healthy diet in unselected general population.
Counseling to promote sustained weight loss in overweight and obese adults.
Counseling to promote physical activity.
Screening for thyroid disease in adults.
Counseling interventions for the prevention of low back pain.
Screening for glaucoma.

*Insufficient evidence found.
Source: Adapted from www.ahrq.gov/clinic/uspstf/upstopics.htm.

TABLE 7-5. RISK REDUCTION FOR ADULTS FROM THE COMMUNITY GUIDE

Alcohol—lower level acceptable for driving

Motor vehicle safety—driving after drinking alcohol, designated driver

Tobacco—prevention and cessation

Physical activity—encourage community programs

Obesity—community based programs

Diabetes—case management and self-care

Nutrition—community and school-based programs

Sexual behavior—school and community based programs

Oral health—community water fluoridation and community programs for face mask use

Violence—community-based programs

Mental health—follow through after screening

Vaccines—program to increase rates in vaccines recommended by the CDC

Source: Adapted from http://www.thecommunityguide.org/about/default.htm.

programs, which may or may not include screening and education given at health professional sites. For example, programs for lowering acceptable alcohol levels while driving are actually advocacy activities that can be joined by individual health professionals. Programs for obesity, diabetes, sexual behavior, mental health, vaccines, and tobacco are designed to include health professional sites such as primary care offices and emergency departments. Nutritional balance assessment (calorie intake and exercise) and behavioral counseling on nutrition is not recommended by the USPSTF (an "I "statement for insufficient evidence) (USPSTF, 2008), although obesity screening is. Exercise evaluation is recommended by the Community Task Force to be supported by community programs based in schools without specific recommendations for the office-based health professional. The balance of intake and exercise affects many chronic conditions that result in significant morbidity and mortality (Must et al, 1999; Mokdad et al., 2005). Both underweight and overweight adults require assessment, support, and often referral. Many commercial community-based programs are more intensive than those that many primary care offices can provide and have been shown to be effective (Fabricatore & Wadden, 2010). For people living in more rural and remote areas, Internet-based programs are being tested. So unless you are prepared to provide intensive long-term support in counseling in your office,

it is important to learn the strengths, weaknesses, costs, and outcomes of programs available in your community and to make referrals to those programs. Exercise assessment and advice should accompany nutritional assessment and is appropriate for the normal as well as over and underweight individuals (Petrella & Wright, 2000; Warburton, Nicol, & Bredin, 2006; Sorensen et al., 2007). Unfortunately, we have limited information on how this can be accomplished easily in the office setting.

For motor vehicle safety, two issues are stressed (Caswell, 2001): safety belts are 45–60% effective in reducing deaths and 50–65% effective in reducing moderate-to-critical injuries (NHTSA, 2000), and the risk for fatal crash involvement increases as blood alcohol levels increase (Zador, Krawchuk, & Voas, 2000).

Infectious disease prevention other than HIV prevention is based on adult immunization recommendations from the Advisory Committee on Immunization Practices (ACIP) and the CDC. Some immunization recommendations are unique to young adults attending college or joining the military (meningococcal vaccine), or for cancer prevention in young women and men (HPV vaccine)   (http://www.cdc.gov/mmwr/preview/mmwrhtml/mm6050a3.htm). Specific immunizations for all adults include the influenza vaccine yearly, tetanus and diphtheria every 10 years with the inclusion of pertussis once, pneumococcal vaccine once at age 65 years for healthy adults but beginning at age 20 years in smokers and others with chronic diseases; all of these deal with primary prevention. The pertussis immunization prevents some morbidity in adults but is primarily directed to the prevention of pertussis in infants by removing transmission from adults sources of pertussis (Coudeville, van Rie, & Andre, 2008). Herpes zoster vaccine for immuno-compotent adults aged 50   years   (http://www.cdc.gov/mmwr/preview/mmwrhtml/mm6044a5.htm) and older, whether or not they have had a previous episode of herpes zoster is a unique type of secondary prevention, preventing a reactivation years or decades after primary chickenpox (Oxman et al., 2005). Of these vaccines, the use of influenza vaccine in young adults and the herpes zoster vaccine are the newest recommendations. The benefits gained from the yearly influenza vaccine vary widely, depending on the particular strain of influenza, its virulence, and the spread of influenza across the country. While estimates are published for the cost effectiveness of influenza vaccine use in all age groups, the value of herd immunity is difficult to estimate since most cases of influenza are unrecognized, not associated with medical care, and unreported even among patients who are health professionals (Molinari et al., 2007). Estimates of the cost and personal burden of herpes zoster have been published and suggest that vaccine use is cost effective (Di Legami et al., 2007; Dworkin et al., 2007).

Counseling of individual "normal weight" patients in the health professional's office related to healthy diet, appropriate use of vitamin, mineral, and other food supplements, and exercise are not addressed in either the USPSTF or the Community Guide. Such counseling is often limited to those with identified health problems such as obesity. Perhaps the best currently available screening method is to evaluate the individual patient's use of supplements, including herbs and "natural" and alternative therapies, and to counsel those with use of multiple supplements, supplements in high doses and supplements that are known to interact with common drugs. Our limited knowledge about the interactions and impact of many supplements requires significant additional research and is likely to make the use of computers with powerful and intelligent search engines a must in primary care practices (van Binsbergen, Delaney, & van Weel, 2003; Brotons et al., 2003).

The public health basis for screening has been discussed in the early Chapters of this book. The suggestions that screening should be for common conditions, should provide a way to recognize disease in asymptomatic individuals, should provide better outcomes than diagnosis at a later stage of disease, and should have an adequately sensitive and specific screening method (http://www.medicine.ox.ac.uk/bandolier/band5/b5-1.html) are being challenged. We no longer do universal screening only for common conditions; for example, there is mandated routine screening of newborns for rare metabolic diseases. For adults we are screening for depression by helping people and health professionals identify existing symptoms that may have been ignored or that the patient is reluctant to bring to the health professional's attention. Currently we have no way to identify the asymptomatic person who will become depressed. Similar types of screening may become possible with conditions such as chronic obstructive pulmonary disease (COPD) or dementia (which are usually diagnosed in late stages) for which earlier recognition might prevent morbidity

or improve the person's and family's quality of life, even if progression remains inevitable (Schermer & Quanjer, 2007). This reassessment of the basic tenets for screening may result in widely expanded screening recommendations over the next few years, and it is likely that advances in genetics and proteomics will bring other screening recommendations in areas other than cancer during the next decades (Sogawa et al., 2007; Myers et al, 2004).

PRIORITIZING AND IMPLEMENTING RISK REDUCTION ACTIVITIES AND RECOMMENDATIONS

Yarnall et al. have published data suggesting that implementation of the USPSTF guidelines would be impossible in clinical practice (2003). This is undoubtedly true if all guidelines were to be implemented at one visit. Fortunately, primary care is also continuity care (Donaldson et al., 2001), which allows the provision of services, counseling, and education over several visits and perhaps even over several years. When not all risk reduction can be completed at a single visit, it is necessary to prioritize what is provided. In clinical practice, the prioritization should be consistent with the patient's needs, interests, and questions, but it should also reflect the diseases and conditions that are most likely to affect the health and mortality of people of the patient's age and gender. Figure 7-1 shows the most common sources of mortality by age in the United States in 2009. Figure 7-2 shows the most common causes of disability of US adults by age and gender, also from 2009.

In addition, priorities should include an assessment of the marginal benefit likely to accrue from each of the prevention strategies. Most health and social marketing efforts are based only on the population rates of morbidity or mortality, probably because it is easy to understand that cancer is the "number one killer" of Americans (Figure 7-2). It is less easy to explain that more women die every year of heart disease and lung disease than of breast cancer. It is even more difficult to explain that the marginal benefit of screening for and addressing tobacco use cessation and perhaps balance of intake and exercise is greater than the marginal benefit gained from yearly mammography after age 40 (Keen at al., 2007; Evidence-Based Radiology Working Group, 2001) or from screening for and treating hyperlipidemia with statin therapy (Chan et al., 2007; Newby et al., 2002). While in some cases explaining the marginal benefit

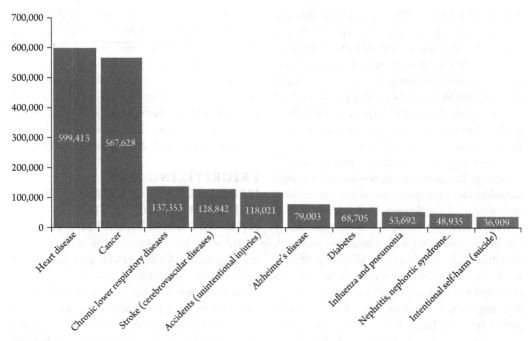

FIGURE 7-1: Most Common Causes of Death in US Adults, 2009.

Source: http://www.cdc.gov/nchs/fastats/Icod.htm.

or even finding data in a format to allow assessment of comparable numbers needed to screen or treat is difficult, in other cases it is impossible since the data has not been collected or analyzed. For example, the marginal benefit of eating two cups of fruit daily versus two cups of fruit a week is unknown. Similarly, the marginal benefit of yearly mammography versus bi-annual mammography often gets lost in gender politics, rhetoric, and health marketing (Keen et al., 2007). For the health professional seeing an individual patient, data based on the average US adult of that age and gender may not apply—no patient is truly "average." It is this view that often leads to the use of personal "expert" opinion not only for a specific individual but for all people within the practice—a group to which the average US data is likely to apply. Therefore, implementation of screening recommendations requires the health professional to develop priorities based on knowledge of the person, the evidence behind the recommendations, and whenever available, information on marginal benefit or number needed to screen or treat.

Mortality rates vary significantly by age, as do the causes of those deaths. Cancer, cardiovascular, stroke and lung disease deaths all increase with age. Conversely, as a percent of deaths, motor vehicle injuries, accidents, and homicides are more common in younger adults. Therefore, it may be of greater marginal benefit to discuss seat belt use and the importance of a designated driver with a young adult than to discuss future needs for mammography or colon cancer screening. For the middle-aged adult, the priority is less clear-cut, since by age 40–50 many prevention measures are recommended for early diagnosis as well as primary prevention. Dietary and exercise recommendations are important throughout the life span since both diet and exercise may be considered part of primary, secondary, and even tertiary prevention in most common chronic health conditions.

Priority 1 for All Ages

At any age, screening for tobacco use and offering smoking cessation is the highest priority. Smoking has been related to over 3 million premature deaths in the US and up to 40% of all chronic diseases in the United States (Mendez & Warner, 2004; Fiore et al., 2004). For 50–80% of patients, depending on the geographic locale (e.g., Kentucky versus Minnesota), screening requires only a single question—"Have you ever smoked more than 100 cigarettes?" A "no" can lead to an affirmation of the patient's healthy decision, and a notation in the medical record suggesting future screening can be limited to "Has your smoking status changed?"

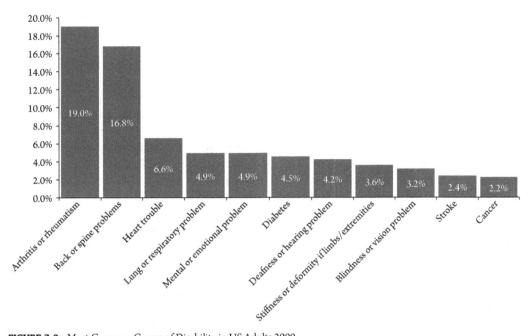

FIGURE 7-2: Most Common Causes of Disability in US Adults 2009.

Source: MMWR. May 1, 2009;58(16). U.S. Census Bureau, Survey of Income and Program Participation, 2004 Panel, Wave 5, June–September 2005.

Note: Based on responses from an estimated 45.1 million persons (94% of total) reporting disability (i.e., difficulty with activities of daily living, instrumental activities of daily living, specific functional limitations [except vision, hearing or speech], limitation in ability to do housework or work at a job or business) who also reported the main cause of their disability.

Weighted numbers in 1,000s.

Participants reporting disability were asked: "Which condition or conditions cause these difficulties?" and shown this list of conditions. Those who chose more than one condition were asked to identify the main cause of their disability.

Confidence interval.

*Weighted estimates less than 200,000 are based on a small sample, are likely unreliable and should be interpreted with caution (4).

Patients have come to expect tobacco use screening and usually do not object to having a nurse, medical assistant or even a receptionist ask about smoking status, including it as a vital sign (Ahluwalia et al., 1999) (see Table 7-5).

Priority 2 for All Ages

Immunizations are one of the few therapies we have to prevent morbidity and mortality with a single or recurrent series of prevention delivery. The patient has to agree to and receive the immunization, but no lifestyle changes or daily therapy is required. The side effects are minimal, and for almost all the evidence is strong and includes effectiveness data. Adult immunizations may be one of the simpler gaps in prevention to address with standing orders, use of immunization registries to assess individual patient's needs, and other practice system enhancements that require little clinician time for most patients.

Priority 3 for All Ages, Especially Younger Adults

The next priority may be an assessment of the balance of nutritional intake and exercise. Obesity and lack of exercise are associated with the onset of several chronic diseases such as diabetes, cancer and osteoarthritis (Must et al., 1999; Mokdal et al., 2005). For other diseases such as asthma, COPD, and many musculoskeletal conditions, obesity and inadequate exercise lead to greater morbidity and symptoms burden (WHO, 2005; Department of Health, 2005). Obesity is easy to asesss using the BMI. Unfortunately, we have few simple programs to address these issues that are appropriate for the average primary care. Until we do, screening and referral to intensive behavorial or commercial weight management programs and a commonsense approach to increasing physical activities are at least a beginning.

Priority 4 for All Ages

The World Health Organization (WHO) has identified mental health as the largest health problem in the world (WHO, 2005; http://www.who.int/mental_health/en/). In the United States, depression is common, affecting as many as 40% of adults over a lifetime (http://www.who.int/mental_health/en). Depression is often a chronic relapsing condition that requires long-term monitoring and care (Ohayon, 2007). While screening is easy, the depth of that screening and next steps for patients who screen positive must be considered before the first patient receives a PHQ-2 or PHQ-9 or CES-D. Is the office ready to deal with a patient unexpectedly reporting suicidal ideation? Are you or is someone else in the office comfortable making a clinical evaluation to diagnose depression? Who will be able to prescribe, monitor, and modify anti-depressant therapy? Are there local resources, in-person or telemedicine resources, to provide cognitive behavioral counseling (CBT), which has been shown to be effective in managing depression? Deciding to add two questions to a patient visit is easy compared to the preparation required to deal with the patients' answers, which may be positive in 12–20% of adults and higher in those with chronic disease such as substance abuse, diabetes, COPD, and arthritis (Davis et al., 2008; Norwood, 2007). Several programs have been designed to support depression screening in primary care and are feasible but require the same type of interest and office champions that make quality improvement programs doable in any condition (Nutting et al., 2008; Lee et al., 2007; Stinchfield, 2008).

Priority 5 for All Ages

Several of the screening activities suggested by the Community Task Force do not have validated surveys or questionnaires but are simply recommended to be part of a rapid review of systems and issues. Prevention and education related to most topics is intended to be supplemented by community health programs: consistent use of seat belts and car seats, yearly influenza immunizations, regular exercise, and use of a designated driver. Community programs and seasonal posters displayed in office waiting rooms may help shorten the time required to cover these issues (Stinchfield, 2008; Reynolds et al., 2008). During the primary care office visit, advice in these areas does not have to require an extended time. Selecting a single topic for education based on what you know about the patient's age, lifestyle, and season of the visit is a good way to cover a variety of topics over a period of years. Handing patients a group of printed pamphlets has been shown to be of little value. However, focusing on a single issue with a simple pamphlet or even a note hand written on a prescription pad emphasizes the importance that the physician or nursing staff placed on the topic. For example, the note may simply say, "Use a designated driver any time you are drinking more than 2 glasses of wine, more than 2 beers, or 2 or more mixed drinks in a period of 2 hours or less."

Priority 6 by Ages

The recommendations of the USPSTF can be divided into tasks by age, gender, and pregnancy status (Tables 7-1 and 7-2). It should be noted that not each of the activities is recommended to be completed yearly. For example, the list for women 50 and older looks long. But the only tests suggested yearly (other than mammography, which has been discussed earlier) are blood pressure, influenza immunization, perhaps depression screening, obesity screening, and tobacco use screening. Of these, the blood pressure, tobacco use status, and obesity assessment are all a part of routine vital signs. Influenza immunizations are seasonal and can be done using a standing order that does not require an office visit (Ahmed et al., 2004). Depression screening can be done with a two-question screener given to people before they come into the examination room (Li et al., 2007). However, it is important to determine that you are ready to deal with the results of the screening before you begin screening (Dietrich et al., 2004).

A factor that has begun to affect the prioritization of screening activities is financial reward systems such as "Pay for Performance" (Keen et al., 2007; Glickman et al., 2008). These programs will be discussed in later Chapters. It is not feasible for an individual physician or even a small- to moderate-sized practice to spend the time and money required to assess how and whether these "required or recommended" measures are appropriate or truly evidence- rather than expert opinion–based. It is reasonable, however, to demand that for the well-being of our patients and the populace that the evidence basis of "Pay for Performance" measures meet or exceed the standards used by other groups that make national health care recommendations, such as the USPSTF and the Community Guide (Sawaya et al., 2007).

Putting It All Together

Books, unlike patients, are divided into Chapters. This Chapter deals only with prevention activities other than those for cancer, stroke, and cardiovascular disease, which have been covered previously. Unfortunately, patients do not come as pieces of the whole or with clear labels helping us determine how and when to prioritize prevention. But we are in a much better position than we were 30 years ago when our patients had few educational resources and often relied upon us to be the sole source of prevention information. It is a rare person that has not heard about flu shots and diabetes or osteoporosis screening. The guidance that patients often need from the health professional is when to begin screening, what the purpose of screening really is (e.g., not to prevent diabetes but to recognize it earlier), and how often the screening should be repeated. In this time of stress on health care resources conservation, it is no longer acceptable to ignore the evidence and just do everything every year (Merenstein, Daumit, & Powe, 2006). Prioritization and selectivity requires time and familiarity with the evidence; it can be very frustrating when not all health care professionals and facilities implement that philosophy.

When discussing screening and prevention issues, at least three groups of health professionals can be identified: those who follow national guidelines very closely, those who are minimalists in regard to screening and counseling, and those who find it easier to perform everything all the time without prioritization or selecting specific times for repeat screening. For the first group, this Chapter is simply another confirmation of what is being done. For the group of minimalists, the book provides suggestions for what should be done. And finally, for the "everything" group, the view of a skeptic may be helpful. An ounce of prevention may be worth a pound of cure, but without high levels of supporting evidence, "prevention" can result in a ton of tests. According to Chris Knight, MD (http://sci.washington.edu/info/forums/reports/prevention_primarycare.asp), even the most vocal advocate of "prevention" should consider the potential harm done when evidence is ignored or manipulated to suit the opinions of an individual physician or other clinician. Principles to consider: "If it is not fixable, don't break it." Before screening for a condition that you cannot prevent, treat, improve, or cure, make sure you have a plan for dealing with the results and some evidence that knowing the results will benefit the patient or family.

Currently, this may relate to several types of genetic screening. However, the balance of harm and benefit must be reassessed as genomics moves forward and is linked to therapies that may change disease progression or outcomes. Second, remember that "what you know can hurt you." False positive results often lead to extensive and expensive workups to prove that they are false positives, while a false negative will be reassessed in the plan of repeated screenings. And third, don't burn the haystack to find the needle. "The rarer the disease, the safer and more specific the test needs to be" (http://sci.washington.edu/info/forums/reports/prevention_primarycare.asp) (Hogy et al., 2008).

CONCLUSIONS

Prevention must be a part of all primary care practices. However, it will take many years and many new discoveries and new innovative programs to identify ways to use our screening results to prevent many of the common causes of morbidity and mortality. This and the previous Chapters have outlined our current and limited knowledge of primary, secondary, and tertiary prevention activities that have the potential to improve our patients' and society's quality of life and longevity. The next Chapters will discuss the state of the art in implementing and integrating these activities into primary care practices.

REFERENCES

Aertgeerts B, Buntinx F, Bande-Knops J, Vandermeulen C, Roelants M, Ansoms S, et al. The value of CAGE, CUGE, and AUDIT in screening for alcohol abuse and dependence among college freshmen. *Alcohol Clin Exp Res.* 2000 Jan;24(1):53–57.

Ahluwalia JS, Gibson CA, Kenney RE, Wallace DD, Resnicow K. Smoking status as a vital sign. *J Gen Intern Med.* 1999 Jul;14(7):402–408.

Ahmed F, Friedman C, Franks A, Latts LM, Nugent EW, France EK,et al. Effect of the frequency of delivery of reminders and an influenza tool kit on increasing influenza vaccination rates among adults with high-risk conditions. *Am J Manag Care.* 2004 Oct;10(10):698–702.

American Diabetes Association. Standards of medical care for patients with diabetes mellitus. *Diabetes Care.* 2001a;24(Suppl 1):S33–S55.

American Diabetes Association. Preventive foot care in people with diabetes. *Diabetes Care.* 2001b;24(Suppl 1):S56–S57.

American Diabetes Association. Management of dyslipidemia in adults with diabetes. *Diabetes Care.* 2001c;24(Suppl 1):S58–S61.

American Diabetes Association. Diabetic retinopathy. *Diabetes Care.* 2001d;24(Suppl 1): S73–S76.

Anatchkova MD, Velicer WF, Prochaska JO. Replication of subtypes for smoking cessation within the pre-contemplation stage of change. *Addict Behav.* 2006 Jul;31(7):1101–1115.

Bakris GL, Williams M, Dworkin L, et al. Preserving renal function in adults with hypertension and diabetes: a consensus approach. *Am J Kidney Dis.* 2000;36:646–661.

Barton MB, Miller T, Wolff T, Petitti D, LeFevre M, Sawaya G, et al. How to read the new recommendation statement: methods update from the U.S. Preventive Services Task Force. *Ann Intern Med.* 2007 Jul 17;147(2):123–127.

Bild DE, Selby JV, Sinnock P, Browner WS, Braveman P, Showstack JA. Lower-extremity amputation in people with diabetes: epidemiology and prevention. *Diabetes Care.* 1989;12:24–30.

Borer KT. Physical activity in the prevention and amelioration of osteoporosis in women: interaction of mechanical, hormonal and dietary factors. *Sports Med.* 2005;35(9):779–830.

Bradley KA, Bush KR, Epler AJ, Dobie DJ, Davis TM, Sporleder JL, et al. Two brief alcohol-screening tests From the Alcohol Use Disorders Identification Test (AUDIT): validation in a female Veterans Affairs patient population. *Arch Intern Med.* 2003 Apr 14;163(7):821–829.

Brenner DJ, Elliston CD. Estimated radiation risks potentially associated with full-body CT screening. *Radiology.* 2004 Sep;232(3):735–738

Brotons C, Ciurana R, Pineiro R, Kloppe P, Godycki-Cwirko M, Sammut MR. Dietary advice in clinical practice: the views of general practitioners in Europe. *Am J Clin Nutr.* 2003 Apr;77(4 Suppl):1048S–1051S.

Burt VK, Stein K. Epidemiology of depression throughout the female life cycle. *J Clin Psychiatry.* 2002;63 Suppl 7:9–15.

Cadarette SM, Jaglal SB, Murray TM, McIsaac WJ, Joseph L, Brown JP. Evaluation of decision rules for referring women for bone densitometry by dual-energy x-ray absorptiometry. *JAMA.* 2001 Jul 4;286(1):57–63.

Cameron IM, Crawford JR, Lawton K, Reid IC. Psychometric comparison of PHQ-9 and HADS for measuring depression severity in primary care. *Br J Gen Pract.* 2008 Jan;58(546):32–36.

Caswell, EA. Recommendations of the Community Task Force on Motor Vehicle Safety. *MMWR.* 2001:50:1–13.

Chan P, Nallamothu B, Gurm H, Hayward R. Sandeep Vijan. Incremental benefit and cost-effectiveness of high-dose statin therapy in high-risk patients with coronary artery disease. *Circulation.* 2007;115:2398–2409.

Coudeville L, van Rie A, Andre P. Adult pertussis vaccination strategies and their impact on pertussis in the United States: evaluation of routine and targeted (cocoon)strategies. *Epidemiol Infect.* 2008 May;136(5):604–620.

Davis L, Uezato A, Newell JM, Frazier E. Major depression and comorbid substance use disorders. *Curr Opin Psychiatry.* 2008 Jan;21(1):14–18.

Department of Health. *Choosing Activity: A Physical Activity Action Plan.* London: DH; 2005.

Di Legami V, Gianino MM, Atti MC, Massari M, Migliardi A, Tomba GS, et al. Epidemiology and costs of herpes zoster: background data to estimate the impact of vaccination. *Vaccine.* 2007 Oct 23;25(43):7598–7604.

Diabetes Control and Complications Trial Research Group. Effect of intensive treatment of diabetes on the development and progression of long-term complications in insulin-dependent diabetes mellitus. *N Engl J Med.* 1993;329:977–986.

Dietrich AJ, Oxman TE, Williams JW, Schulberg HC, Bruce ML, Lee PW, et al. Re-engineering systems for the treatment of depression in primary care: cluster randomised controlled trial. *BMJ.* 2004 Sep 11;329(7466):602.

Donaldson M, Yordy K, Lohr K, Neal A. Vanselow, eds. Committee on the Future of Primary Care, Institute of Medicine. *Primary Care: America's Health in a New Era.* Washington, DC: Institute of Medicine; 2001; 1996.

Dworkin RH, White R, O'Connor AB, Baser O, Hawkins K. Healthcare costs of acute and chronic pain associated with a diagnosis of herpes zoster. *J Am Geriatr Soc.* 2007 Aug;55(8):1168–1175.

Early Treatment Diabetic Retinopathy Study Research Group (ETDRS). Early photocoagulation for diabetic retinopathy: ETDRS Report Number 9. *Ophthalmology.* 1991;98:766–785.

Evidence-Based Radiology Working Group. Evidence-based radiology: a new approach to the practice of radiology. *Radiology.* 2001;220:566–575.

Ewing JA. Detecting alcoholism. The CAGE questionnaire. *JAMA.* 1984 Oct 12;252(14):1905–1907.

Fabricatore AN, Wadden TA. Lifestyle modification in the treatment of obesity. In: Goldstein D, ed. *The Management of Eating Disorders and Obesity.* 2nd ed. Totowa, NJ: Humana Press; 2010.

Fiellin DA, Reid MC, O'Connor PG. Screening for alcohol problems in primary care: a systematic review. *Arch Intern Med.* 2000 Jul 10;160(13):1977–1989.

Fiore MC, Croyle RT, Curry SJ, Cutler CM, Davis RM, Gordon C, et al. Preventing 3 million premature deaths and helping 5 million smokers quit: a national action plan for tobacco cessation. *Am J Public Health.* 2004 Feb;94(2):205–210.

Fiore MC, McCarthy DE, Jackson TC, Zehner ME, Jorenby DE, Mielke M, et al. Integrating smoking cessation treatment into primary care: an effectiveness study. *Prev Med.* 2004 Apr;38(4):412–420.

Fontbonne A, Eschwege E, Cambien F, et al. Hypertriglyceridaemia as a risk factor of coronary heart disease mortality in subjects with impaired glucose tolerance or diabetes: results from the 11-year follow-up of the Paris Prospective Study. *Diabetologia.* 1989;32:300–304.

Gjerdingen DK, Yawn BP. Postpartum depression screening: importance, methods, barriers, and recommendations for practice. *J Am Board Fam Med.* 2007 May-Jun; 20(3):280–288.

Glickman SW, Schulman KA, Peterson ED, Hocker MB, Cairns CB. Evidence-based perspectives on pay for performance and quality of patient care and outcomes in emergency medicine. *Ann Emerg Med.* 2008 May;51(5):622–631.

Greci LS, Katz DL, Jekel J. Vaccinations in pneumonia (VIP): pneumococcal and influenza vaccination patterns among patients hospitalized for pneumonia. *Prev Med.* 2005 Apr;40(4):384–388.

Hogg J, Lemelin J, Graham I, Grimshaw J, Martin C, Moore L, et al. Improving prevention in primary care: evaluating the effectiveness of outreach facilitation. *Fam Pract.* 2008;25:40–48.

Keen JD, Keen JE, Ganott MA, Sumkin JH, Gur D. Does the Marginal Benefit Exceed the Marginal Cost? *Radiology.* 2007;243:299–300.

Kroenke K. Screening is not enough. *Ann Intern Med.* 2001 Mar 6;134(5):418–420.

Lee PW, Dietrich AJ, Oxman TE, Williams JW, Barry SL. Sustainable impact of a primary care depression intervention. *J Am Board Fam Med.* 2007 Sep-Oct;20(5):427–433.

Leppäniemi A. From eminence-based to error-based to evidence-based medicine and surgery. Scand J Surg 2008;97(1):2–3.

Li C, Friedman B, Conwell Y, Fiscella K. Validity of the Patient Health Questionnaire 2 (PHQ-2) in identifying major depression in older people. *J Am Geriatr Soc.* 2007 Apr;55(4):596–602.

McCusker MT, Basquille J, Khwaja M, Murray-Lyon IM, Catalan J. Hazardous and harmful drinking: a comparison of the AUDIT and CAGE screening questionnaires. *QJM.* 2002 Sep;95(9):591–595.

Mendez D, Warner KE. Adult cigarette smoking prevalence: declining as expected (not as desired). *Am J Public Health.* 2004 Feb;94(2):251–252.

Merenstein D, Daumit GL, Powe NR. Use and costs of non-recommended tests during routine preventive health exams. *Am J Prev Med.* 2006 Jun;30(6):521–527.

Mokdad AH, Marks JS, Stroup DF, Gerberding JL. Correction: actual causes of death in the United States, 2000. JAMA (2005 Jan 19) 293(3):293–294.

Molinari NA, Ortega-Sanchez IR, Messonnier ML, Thompson WW, Wortley PM, Weintraub E, et al. The annual impact of seasonal influenza in the US: measuring disease burden and costs. *Vaccine.* 2007 Jun 28;25(27):5086–5096.

Must A, Spadano J, Coakley E, Field A, Colditz G, Dietz W. The Disease Burden Associated With Overweight and Obesity. JAMA 1999;282:1523–1529.

Myers J, Macleod M, Reed B, Harris N, Mires G, Baker P. *Use of proteomic patterns as a novel screening tool in pre-eclampsia. J Obstet Gynaecol.* 2004 Nov;24(8):873–874.

National Highway Traffic Safety Administration (NHTSA). *Traffic Safety Facts 1999: Occupant Protection.* Washington, DC: US Department of Transportation, National Highway Traffic Safety Administration; 2000. Publication no. DOT HS 809 090.

Newby LK, Kristinsson A, Bhapkar MV, Aylward PE, Dimas AP, Klein WW, et al. Early statin initiation and outcomes in patients with acute coronary syndromes. *JAMA.* 2002 Jun 19;287(23):3087–3095.

Norwood RJ. A review of etiologies of depression in COPD. *Int J Chron Obstruct Pulmon Dis.* 2007;2(4):485–491.

Nutting PA, Gallagher K, Riley K, White S, Dickinson WP, Korsen N, et al. Care management for depression in primary care practice: findings from the RESPECT-Depression trial. *Ann Fam Med.* 2008 Jan-Feb;6(1):30–37.

Ohayon MM. Epidemiology of depression and its treatment in the general population. *J Psychiatr Res.* 2007 Apr-Jun;41(3–4):207–213.

Olson CL, Schumaker HD, Yawn BP. Overweight women delay medical care. *Arch Fam Med.* 1994 Oct;3(10):888–889.

Ortqvist A, Hedlund J, Burman LA, Elbel E, Hofer M, Leinonen M, et al. Randomised trial of 23-valent pneumococcal capsular polysaccharide vaccine in prevention of pneumonia in middle-aged and elderly people. Swedish Pneumococcal Vaccination Study Group. *Lancet.* 1998 Feb 7;351(9100):399–403.

Oxman MN, Levin MJ, Johnson GR, Schmader KE, Straus SE, Gelb LD, et al. A vaccine to prevent herpes zoster and postherpetic neuralgia in older adults. *N Engl J Med.* 2005 Jun 2;352(22):2271–2284.

Paz-Diaz H, Montes de Oca M, Lopez JM, Celli BR. Pulmonary rehabilitation improves depression, anxiety, dyspnea and health status in patients with COPD. *Am J Phys Med Rehabil.* 2007 Jan;86(1):30–36.

Petrella RJ, Wight D. An office-based instrument for exercise counseling and prescription in primary care. The Step Test Exercise Prescription (STEP). *Arch Fam Med.* 2000 Apr;9(4):339–344.

Pitta F, Troosters T, Probst VS, Langer D, Decramer M, Gosselink R. Are patients with COPD more active after pulmonary rehabilitation? *Chest.* 2008 Aug;134(2):273–280.

Prochaska JO, Velicer WF. The transtheoretical model of health behavior change. *Am J Health Promot* 1997 Sep-Oct;12(1):38–48.

Ravid M, Lang R, Rachmani R, Lishner M. Long-term renoprotective effect of angiotensin-converting enzyme inhibition in nonBinsulin-dependent diabetes mellitus: a 7-year follow-up study. *Arch Intern Med.* 1996;156:286–289.

Reinert DF, Allen JP. The Alcohol Use Disorders Identification Test (AUDIT): a review of recent research. Alcohol Clin Exp Res (2002 Feb) 26(2):272–279.

Reynolds CE, Snow V, Qaseem A, Verbonitz L. Improving immunization rates: initial results from a team-based, systems change approach. *Am J Med Qual.* 2008 May-Jun;23(3):176–183.

Rise J, Kovac V, Kraft P, Moan IS. Predicting the intention to quit smoking and quitting behaviour: extending the theory of planned behaviour. *Br J Health Psychol.* 2008 May;13(Pt 2):291–310.

Ritchie D, Schulz S, Bryce A. One size fits all? A process evaluation—the turn of the 'story' in smoking cessation. *Public Health.* 2007 May;121(5):341–348.

Rith-Najarian SJ, Stolusky T, Gohdes DM. Identifying diabetic patients at high risk for lower-extremity amputation in a primary health care setting: a prospective evaluation of simple screening criteria. *Diabetes Care.* 1992;15:1386–1389.

Rousseau ME. Dietary prevention of osteoporosis. *Lippincotts Prim Care Pract.* 1997 Jul-Aug;1(3): 307–319.

Sawaya GF, Guirguis-Blake J, LeFevre M, Harris R, Petitti D. Update on the methods of the U.S. Preventive Services Task Force: estimating certainty and magnitude of net benefit. *Ann Intern Med.* 2007 Dec 18;147(12):871–875.

Schermer TR, Quanjer PH. COPD screening in primary care: who is sick? *Prim Care Respir J.* 2007 Feb;16(1):49–53.

Sogawa K, Itoga S, Tomonaga T, Nomura F. Diagnostic values of surface-enhanced laser desorption/ionization technology for screening of habitual drinkers. *Alcohol Clin Exp Res.* 2007 Jan;31(1 Suppl):S22–S26.

Sorensen JB, Kragstrup J, Kjaer K, Puggaard L. Exercise on prescription: trial protocol and evaluation of outcomes. *BMC Health Serv Res.* 2007;7:36.

Stinchfield PK. Practice-proven interventions to increase vaccination rates and broaden the immunization season. *Am J Med.* 2008 Jul;121(7 Suppl 2):S11–S21.

Tinkelman DG, Price D, Nordyke RJ, Halbert RJ. COPD screening efforts in primary care: what is the yield? *Prim Care Respir J.* 2007 Feb;16(1):41–48.

UK Prospective Diabetes Study (UKPDS) Group. Intensive blood-glucose control with sulphonylureas or insulin compared with conventional treatment and risk of complications in patients with type 2 diabetes (UKPDS 33). *Lancet.* 1998a;352:837–853.

UK Prospective Diabetes Study Group (UKPDS). Tight blood pressure control and risk of macrovascular and microvascular complications in type 2 diabetes: UKPDS 38. *BMJ.* 1998b;317:703–713.

US Preventive Services Task Force (USPSTF). *The Guide to Clinic Preventive Services.* AGRQ Pub No. 08–05100. September 2008. Rockville, MD: USPSTF; 2008.

van Binsbergen JJ, Delaney BC, van Weel C. Nutrition in primary care: scope and relevance of output from the Cochrane Collaboration. *Am J Clin Nutr.* 2003 Apr;77(4 Suppl):1083S–1088S.

Wallis LA, ed. *Textbook of Women's Health.* Philadelphia : Lippincott-Raven; 1998.

Warburton DE, Nicol CW, Bredin SS. Prescribing exercise as preventive therapy. *CMAJ.* 2006 Mar 28;174(7):961–974.

Whitlock EP, Orleans CT, Pender N, Allan J. Evaluating primary care behavioral counseling interventions: an evidence-based approach. *Am J Prev Med.* 2002 May;22(4):267–284.

World Health Organization (2005). *Preventing Chronic Diseases: A Vital Investment.* Geneva: WHO.

Yarnall KSH, Pollak KI, Ostbye T, et al. Primary care: is there enough time for prevention? *Am J Public Hea lth.*2003;93:635–641.

Yawn B, Dietrich A, Wollan P, Bertram S, Kurland M, Graham D et al. The IAP: A simple tool to guide assessment and immediate action for suicidal ideation. *J Fam Pract Mgmt.* (2009) 16(5):17–20.

Yawn BP, Saddier P, Wollan PC, St Sauver JL, Kurland MJ, Sy LS. A population-based study of the incidence and complication rates of herpes zoster before zoster vaccine introduction. *Mayo Clin Proc.* 2007 Nov;82(11):1341–1349.

Zador PL, Krawchuk SA, Voas RB. Alcohol-related risk of driver fatalities and driver involvement in fatal crashes in relation to driver age and gender: an update using 1996 data. *J Stud Alcohol.* 2000;61:387–395.

8

Personalizing Prevention

MARC S. WILLIAMS

BACKGROUND

One of the many challenges facing primary care providers (PCPs) is the sheer volume of preventive messages to deliver. A study by Yarnall et al. (2003) estimated that 7.4 hours per working day are needed for the provision of the preventive services recommended by the US Preventive Services Task Force (USPSTF). They appropriately conclude that, "[t]ime constraints limit the ability of physicians to comply with preventive services recommendations." There is increasing pressure on PCPs to be compliant with an expanding suite of preventive services inconsistent with the coexisting economic pressure to see more patients in a given unit of time. The need to reconcile these issues has led to a variety of strategies, including moving some preventive services outside the physician visit (e.g., immunization clinics, computerized prevention messages [Sciamanna et al., 2002], use of allied health personnel [Palmer & Midgette, 2008]) and prioritization of preventive services (e.g. smoking cessation for active smokers; weight control for overweight/obese). A recent study by Pollak et al. (2008) demonstrated that PCPs' prioritization was reasonably consistent with the USPSTF's "A" rated (good evidence) recommendations, with the exception of smoking cessation and Pap smear. The authors also note that PCPs spent relatively more time on two interventions, prostate-specific antigen (PSA) and exercise counseling, despite an "I" rating (inconclusive evidence of effectiveness), indicating that prioritization was using principles other than evidence in some cases. These factors are not well understood. In one study almost no correlation was found between PCPs' perceptions of the importance of a preventive measure, their effectiveness at delivering the preventive service and the actual delivery of the preventive service to patients (Litaker et al., 2005). The authors concluded that "[p]hysicians' attitudes toward prevention are necessary, but not sufficient in ensuring the delivery of preventive services." Cornuz et al. (2000) identified three general categories of barriers to the delivery of preventive services: lack of time, lack of patient interest, and lack of training. They also noted that certain provider behaviors were associated with negative attitudes toward alcohol and smoking counseling. These included consumption of more than three alcoholic drinks per day, sedentary lifestyle, lack of national certification (study was from Switzerland), and lack of awareness of their own blood pressure.

Patient receptiveness to preventive messages influences not only patient compliance with recommendations, but the ongoing willingness of PCPs to take time to deliver preventive services. Many studies have identified a variety of patient-related factors impacting compliance with preventive health recommendations (which also differ based on other factors such as race, ethnicity, socioeconomic status, health literacy, and the type of intervention). As a first approximation, it is reasonable to say that these issues are centered on the communication of risk in a way that is understandable and meaningful to the patient, as effective communication accounts for most of the individual patient factors listed above, as also discussed in Chapters 1 and 11. This view is confirmed by recent initiatives to make sure that communication with patients, whether written or verbal, is done in the patient's native language, at an appropriate literacy level and with attention to cultural competency, although the impact of this approach on outcomes should be studied (Anderson et al., 2003). Personalizing communication is the first step to personalizing prevention, but are there ways to also personalize the preventive interventions so that they account for individual biological, environmental, and behavioral differences among patients? The Chapter will explore approaches to personalizing prevention; additional discussion of personalized medicine for prevention is found in Chapter 12. The primary focus will be on 3 of the 10 essential public health functions as described by the Association of State and Territorial Health Officials (ASTHO): monitor health (assessment); diagnose and investigate (assessment); and evaluate (assurance; see Figure 8-1). The reader will be aware of the fact that changes in services as described will either require or lead to changes in other essential functions.

PERSONALIZED VERSUS PRECISION

Is a "personalized" approach to prevention, diagnosis, and treatment a new idea? Most providers would say that they have always practiced personalized medicine. The history of medicine is replete with exhortations to personalize care. Hippocrates emphasized the observation of the individual patient, documentation of signs and symptoms, and tailoring treatment to the individual, based not only on the signs and symptoms, but the values of the patient. Indeed, this probably represents the first recorded reference to patient-centered care.

Another problem that is appearing in the discussion of personalized care is the tendency for some to equate personalized medicine with genomic medicine. Given the profusion of genetic and genomic discoveries in the past decade, it is hard to argue against the potential for this new information to transform

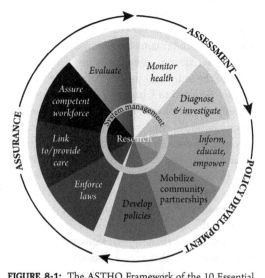

FIGURE 8-1: The ASTHO Framework of the 10 Essential Public Health Services.

medicine. There is a sense that this knowledge is so fundamental to our understanding of health and disease that it will relegate other information to a second-class status. The image of our genetic code on a credit card that will be inserted into a computer in the doctor's office so that our personal data can be used to direct care is compelling, although the complexity of the science suggests that this vision is unlikely to be realized in the near term. Part of the issue is the tendency to conflate medical science and medical practice. Medical science is essential for the practice of medicine, but practice is extraordinarily complex and involves many factors that are beyond the scope of the science. Still, it is important to recognize that the use of biomarkers—genes or other biological substances that indicate the presence of a particular condition or propensity—to personalize therapy is not new. In 1930 the discovery of ABO blood groups by Karl Landsteiner allowed safe transfusion of blood products for the first time. ABO groups are genetically determined, but no one is suggesting that we substitute genetic testing for our current blood-typing methods. This introduces an important concept—that is, genomic strategies must be compared to other non-genomic ways to characterize an individual's likelihood to benefit from a given intervention, with no a priori assumptions that the genomic approach will be superior.

It is for these reasons that the definition of personalized medicine proposed by Pauker and Kassirer in 1987 seems to be most appropriate to use: "Personalized medicine is the practice of clinical decision-making such that the decisions made maximize the outcomes that the patient most cares about and minimizes those that the patient fears the most, on the basis of as much knowledge about the individual's state as is available." There are three key points captured by this definition. First is the focus on the outcomes of care; second is the central role of the patient in defining what outcomes, positive or negative, are of most importance. Third, notice that the words "genetic" or "genomic" do not appear in the definition. The authors emphasize the importance of using "...as much knowledge about the individual's state as is available." There are no assumptions that genetic or genomic information is superior to other information in caring for the patient. Only if evidence demonstrates that genetic information is superior should it be treated as such.

Although the concept of personalized medicine is not new, it is clear that the practice of medicine is in the process of being transformed. The realization of personalized medicine to this point has been empiric and dependent on the individual provider's knowledge and experience. This has led to care that has high variability and less than optimal outcomes. Christensen et al. (2009) refer to this as "intuitive medicine" and define it as "…care for conditions that can be diagnosed only by their symptoms and only treated with therapies whose efficacy is uncertain." The focus in care is moving from the intuitive to the precise. The same authors define precision medicine as "…the provision of care for diseases that can be precisely diagnosed, whose causes are understood, and which consequently can be treated with rules-based therapies that are predictably effective." It is at the intersection of personalized and precision medicine where the opportunity exists to optimize patient care and prevention.

PERSONALIZING PREVENTION

While genetic and genomic information has the potential to radically alter the approach to prevention, as noted above, there are few examples of genomic information being effectively used for prevention, with a few exceptions in pharmacogenomics where genomic information can be used to inform dose and effectiveness and prevent adverse drug events (ADE). The principles of personalized prevention can be illustrated with three examples: prevention of an adverse drug event; the impact of systematic screening for a highly penetrant single gene cancer predisposition disorder; and the use of family history information.

Prevention of an Adverse Drug Event

ADEs have a significant impact on the cost and quality of care. According to the Agency for Healthcare Research and Quality (AHRQ 2001), over 770,000 people are injured or die each year in hospitals from adverse drug events (ADEs). National hospital expenses to treat patients who suffer ADEs during hospitalization are estimated at between $1.56 and $5.6 billion annually. The costs of ADEs in the outpatient setting in 2000 were estimated to exceed $177 billion dollars in the United States (Ernst and Grizzle, 2001). Any strategy that could be reasonably expected to reduce ADEs could have a significant impact on morbidity, mortality, and cost. Genetic factors are known to play a role in the susceptibility to ADEs, although the magnitude of the effect remains uncharacterized for the most part.

The use of genetic information could personalize the prevention of ADEs.

Abacavir is a synthetic drug with inhibitory activity against human immunodeficiency virus (HIV-1). It, in combination with other antiretroviral agents, is indicated for the treatment of HIV-1 infection. Serious and sometimes fatal hypersensitivity reactions (HSR) have been associated with the use of abacavir. Investigation has found that patients who carry the HLA-B*5701 allele are at high risk for experiencing an HSR to abacavir (Mallal et al., 2008). Only 0–0.5% of patients who are HLA-B*5701 negative will develop hypersensitivity, while more than 70% who are HLA-B*5701 positive will develop hypersensitivity. The FDA issued an alert in July 2008 (FDA, 2008) about this, and information was added to the boxed warning with the following recommendations:

- Screening for the HLA-B*5701 allele is recommended for all patients prior to starting abacavir therapy. This approach has been found to decrease the risk of a hypersensitivity reaction.
- Patients who previously took abacavir and tolerated it have developed abacavir HSR upon restarting abacavir-containing therapy. Screening is recommended prior to reinitiation of abacavir in patients of unknown HLA-B*5701 status who have previously tolerated abacavir.
- For HLA-B*5701-positive patients, treatment with an abacavir-containing regimen is not recommended and should be considered only under exceptional circumstances when the potential benefit outweighs the risk.

Similar predispositions have been seen with two other drugs: carbamazepine and risk for Stevens-Johnson syndrome (HLA-B*1502) and nevirapine hypersensitivity analysis (HLA-B*3505). The predisposing HLA type for Stevens-Johnson syndrome associated with carbamazepine use is present almost exclusively in Asian and Asian-Indian ethnicities (Lim et al., 2008). The FDA boxed warning (FDA, 2007) recommends testing for HLA-B*1502 in all patients of Asian ethnicity prior to initiation of treatment with carbamazepine. The situation with nevirapine is more complex in that the genetic variant appears to interact with other clinical factors such as the patient's sex and CD4 count.

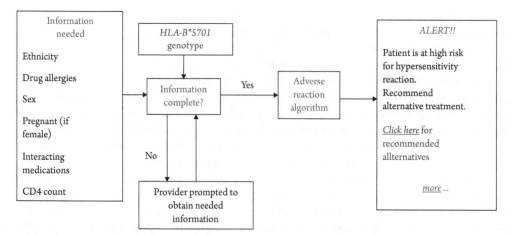

FIGURE 8-2: Example Use of the Electronic Health Record with Pharmacogenetic Findings Prior to the Use of Abacavir to Prevent ADEs.

Note: The left-hand box shows the information needed to populate the adverse drug event algorithm. Most of this information could be captured automatically from the EHR. The genotype could be automatically entered if known. The second box determines if all the information is available to allow the algorithm to run. If not, the provider is prompted to add the information, or to order the genetic test. When the information is complete, the algorithm runs. In this case an alert is triggered, represented in the box on the right. The alert allows the provider to choose from a list of acceptable alternative medications. This link allows seamless access to information about why the alert was received.

The HLA-B*3505 genotype is relatively infrequent except in patients of Thai ancestry (Chantarangsu et al., 2009). The evidence on this variant is still emerging and the FDA has not changed the boxed warning at this time, although some are recommending testing in patients of Thai ancestry.

How could pharmacogenetic testing prior to use of abacavir be used in clinical practice to prevent ADEs? In clinical situations such as this, the electronic health record (EHR) may have significant impact. If a practitioner is using an EHR that is enabled for computerized order entry (CPOE) for medications, the translation of this knowledge is straightforward, as illustrated in Figure 8-2. In this example, once the provider chooses to use abacavir, the ADE algorithm accumulates the necessary information from the EHR, eliminating the need for the provider to take time to hand-enter information. Only if information is missing is the provider prompted to add the information (or order a test). The output of the algorithm would either be low risk of ADE, in which case the order is filled, or high risk of ADE, in which case the provider receives an alert. This alert is functional in order to minimize disruption to the clinical workflow. When faced with an alert, providers may want to know what alternative medications would be available. In this alert, one click will take the provider to a list of acceptable alternatives, and the prescription can be ordered. Alternatively, if the

provider wants to know why the alert was triggered, a click on the "more" link directs the provider to other electronic information resources, such as the FDA black box warning or the primary medical literature. This eliminates the need to search for information and allows the provider to rapidly obtain the specific information needed to answer the clinical question. The basic framework, once constructed, can be used for other medications (such as carbamazepine) with minimal effort required to alter the required informational elements. This approach takes advantage of clinical decision support, which will be discussed in more detail in the family history section below.

LYNCH SYNDROME

Colorectal cancer (CRC) is one of the most common cancers worldwide, with more than a million cases detected and half a million who die from the disease annually (Center et al., 2009). Approximately 5–10% of CRC is familial, reflecting shared genetic and environmental predisposition (Burt, 1996). However, some CRC is due to genetic mutations that are highly likely to lead to disease. These are referred to as hereditary CRC to distinguish them as single gene disorders. An example of this is CRC due to mutations in DNA mismatch repair (MMR) genes (Lynch et al., 2008). When cells divide, genetic errors can occur. Mismatch repair proteins (coded for by the MMR genes) identify and repair these errors. If one of these proteins does not function normally, errors can accumulate that can lead to abnormal cell growth and ultimately cancer. Two to five percent of all CRC is due to genetic mutations in MMR genes collectively known as Lynch syndrome (LS), previously referred to as hereditary non-polyposis colorectal cancer (HNPCC) (Hampel et al., 2005). Individuals with LS have a lifetime risk of CRC as high as 70–80%, as well as higher risk of endometrial, ovarian, pancreatic, and urologic cancers. Importantly, risk for some of the cancers can be dramatically lowered by intensive surveillance of LS mutation carriers, principally colonoscopy beginning at an early age. If patients who have LS can be identified, testing of family members can rapidly identify those relatives who are at high risk and who would benefit from early surveillance and intervention. The challenge is how to identify the first case in a family. Family history was initially the recommended screening method but recent evidence has suggested substantial deficiencies in this approach (EGAPP, 2009). Not only is family history insensitive (estimated to detect only 50% of at-risk individuals under ideal circumstances), there is strong evidence that demonstrates that family histories obtained by health care providers who do not have specific training in genetics is insufficiently detailed, further lowering sensitivity (Grover et al., 2004).

These problems led investigators to study colorectal tumors for characteristics that indicated a high risk for LS. An Evaluation of Genomic Applications in Practice and Prevention (EGAPP) evidence review (EGAPP, 2009) supported a tumor-based screening approach to

identify patients for confirmatory genetic testing, followed by familial case finding. In other words, testing of a particular patient's tumor can lead to genetic testing in that individual to identify an MMR gene mutation, followed by identification of that patient's family members who are at increased risk and who could be tested. A recent modeling study by Mvundura et al. (2010) using conservative baseline estimates and modeling more contemporary screening protocols provided further evidence of the value of this screening, demonstrating an incremental cost effectiveness ratio of about $22,500 per life-year saved, compared to no LS screening, a very favorable result. This finding was confirmed by Ladabaum and colleagues (2011).

Based on this information, combined with internal analyses and consultation with clinical leaders, the decision was made to implement tumor-based Lynch syndrome screening at our institution. The full details of the implementation process are available to the interested reader (Gudgeon et al., 2011). The screening protocol is presented in Figure 8-3.

Making the diagnosis of LS has a significant impact on the patient and family members. For the patient, tumors that have microsatellite instability—a feature of LS—do not respond well to fluorouracil-based chemotherapeutic agents (Jover et al., 2011). Patients are at increased risk for developing other cancers, particularly women who are at increased risk for endometrial and ovarian cancer. These individuals can reduce the risk of developing a second cancer by using enhanced surveillance (e.g., annual colonoscopy, vaginal

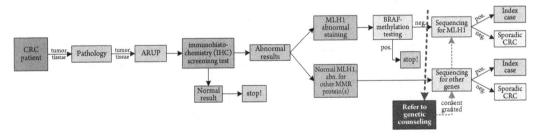

FIGURE 8-3: Example Lynch Syndrome Screening Protocol.

Note: CRC, colorectal cancer; ARUP, ARUP laboratories, the referral laboratory used for the tumor analysis; MMR, mismatch repair; methylation of the MLH1 promoter.

A patient who undergoes resection of a CRC has a portion of the tumor sent for immunohistochemical (IHC) analysis of the four MMR proteins (MLH1, MSH2, MSH6, PMS2). If the IHC is normal, LS is ruled out. If there is abnormal staining for MSH2, MSH6, or PMS2, the tumor is screen positive and the patient is referred for genetic counseling and specific gene sequencing. If there is abnormal staining for MLH1, additional testing is indicated. BRAF mutation analysis and methylation of the MLH1 promoter are done sequentially (i.e., MLH1 promoter is done only if BRAF is normal), as the presence of either of these changes identifies somatic changes, which when positive rule out the presence of LS. A patient with abnormal MLH1 staining and normal BRAF mutation analysis and methylation of the MLH1 promoter is screen positive and the patient is referred for genetic counseling and specific gene sequencing.

ultrasound) or prophylactic surgery (e.g., sub-total colectomy, total abdominal hysterectomy with bilateral salpingo-oophorectomy). Given the autosomal dominant inheritance of LS, the identification of a patient with LS offers the opportunity to identify other at-risk family members for familial mutation testing (relatively inexpensive). Family members with mutations are offered enhanced surveillance and prophylactic surgery as for the patient, while family members who do not carry the mutation are not at increased risk and can follow the general population recommendations for screening. The cost effectiveness as described by Mvundura et al. (2010) depends on the identification and prevention of cancer in unaffected mutation-positive family members.

FAMILY HISTORY

The first mention of the use of family history to prevent an adverse medical outcome may be found in the *Mishneh Torah* that dates from the second century. The law as recorded here stated that if two sons of the same mother die after circumcision, then future sons must not be circumcised. This is presumed to refer to excessive bleeding due to hemophilia, an X-linked disorder, although the law does not indicate that the deaths were due to bleeding.

Family history has been promoted as the first "genomic" tool for disease prevention and health promotion (Valdez et al., 2010). It has proven utility in the identification of rare, medically significant single gene disorders, as in the hemophilia example above, but has also been shown to have the ability to identify those at increased risk for common diseases of importance to public health, such as cancer, heart disease, and diabetes (Valdez et al., 2010). Advances in sequencing technology that enabled large-scale analysis of the genome were predicted by some to eliminate the need to know the family history, as all risk would be understood at the genomic level. Genome-wide association studies (GWAS) have identified many hundreds of variants associated with common, complex diseases such as diabetes and heart disease. However, in the vast majority of cases these variants, even if aggregated, explain only a small fraction of risk that is expected based on family studies. In complex disorders such as diabetes, it has been noted that adding validated genomic risk variants contributes little to improving risk prediction based on traditional factors such as family history, body mass index, age, sex, and so on (Imamura & Maeda, 2011). This leads to questions about the nature of

the so-called "missing heritability" (Manolio et al., 2009). Hypotheses about the nature of the missing heritability include larger numbers of variants of small effect that are unable to be detected using current approaches; rare variants of strong effect; structural variants that are not well-identified with current technology; gene-environment interactions (particularly shared environment among relatives); epistasis (gene-gene interactions); and imprecise phenotyping (Manolio et al., 2009). Manolio et al. (2009), in discussing new research strategies to discover the missing heritability, suggest that focusing on families with large sibships, particularly families that would allow recontact in order to gather additional information to refine the phenotype (what is called interative phenotyping) could be useful. Families that are highly penetrant for a given condition may represent ideal subjects for studies that address several of the hypotheses, including rare variants of high effect, structural variants, epistasis, and gene-environment interactions, given that families not only share genetic factors but share environmental exposures, particularly in first-degree relatives. Practically, it does not appear that genomic approaches will supplant the utility of family history in clinical care for some time. Indeed, family history may have increased importance as whole genome sequencing moves into the clinic in that novel variants that have characteristics suggesting they could be pathogenic could be contextualized by closely examining the family history for associated disorders. If these disorders were present, this would provide additional evidence that the novel variant could be pathogenic; absence of a family history does not exonerate the variant, however, given that it could have arisen for the first time in the patient.

Family history has been used to guide diagnosis in individuals presenting with signs and symptoms of a disease, to assist in reproductive decision making, to inform initiation and maintenance of therapies, and to inform the interpretation of genetic test results. It has also been shown to help build rapport with patients (Williams et al., 2011). Despite the extensive clinical use of family history, there has been inadequate study of its clinical utility for common, complex diseases, as exemplified by the 2009 *National Institutes of Health State of the Science Conference on Family History* (Berg et al., 2009). In contrast, the Centers for Disease Control and Prevention (CDC) have identified diseases where adequate evidence exists to stratify risk and modify care based on family history (Yoon et al., 2009). To formally address the *State of the Science*

Conference criticism, Qureshi and colleagues [2012] performed a pragmatic, matched-pair, cluster randomized, controlled trial to study the effect of adding systematic collection of family history to cardiovascular disease assessment. They found the mean increase in proportion of participants classified as having high cardiovascular risk was 4.8 percentage points in the intervention practices, compared with 0.3 percentage point in control practices when family history from patient records was incorporated. In addition, while not a formal part of the study, they found that significantly more patients in the intervention group stopped smoking compared to the control group.

Researchers have identified what family history is (or should be) collected by primary care physicians (specific diseases, age of onset, relation to patient, etc.) (Reid et al., 2009; Acheson et al., 2000; Summerton & Garrood, 1997) and have identified barriers to the collection of family history (time, perception that information from the patient isn't accurate or actionable, inadequate reimbursement, lack of training) (Rich et al., 2004). Other studies have indicated that many primary care physicians have concerns about their ability to use the family history they collect (Gramling et al., 2004; Every et al., 1999). These issues have led to highly variable use of family history in clinical practice, further reducing the utility of this information. While more research is needed on how family history can best be used to prevent common, chronic disease (Yoon et al., 2003), there is adequate information to implement family history in clinical care at present. The relevant questions relative to this implementation are: How can family history be collected in a systematic way to reduce inter-provider variability? Using the currently available evidence, how can family history information be analyzed to identify and counsel patients at risk for development of a chronic condition? How can information be obtained from the clinical setting to enhance the currently available evidence on the utility of family history in the identification and treatment of common, complex disease?

One of the major barriers to the use of family history is the time needed to collect the information within the constraints of the clinic visit (Rich et al., 2004). One solution to this is to collect the information outside the clinic visit. This has led to the creation of online family history collection tools such as the Surgeon General's "My Family Health Portrait Tool" and the CDC's "Family HealthWare," as well as institutional tools such as Intermountain

Healthcare's "Our Family Health.™" Usability testing has indicated a generally positive response to the use of these tools to enter information (Owens et al., 2011; Yoon et al., 2009; Intermountain Healthcare, unpublished data). The "Family Healthware" tool includes risk stratification algorithms for six diseases (coronary heart disease, stroke, diabetes, and colorectal, breast, and ovarian cancers) (Yoon et al., 2009). Patients reviewed their familial risk information with special attention to those diseases for which they had moderate or strong familial risk. They also reviewed information related to recommended changes in health behavior and requested linkage between their family health information and relevant aspects of their medical record such as blood pressure and lipid levels. "Family Healthware" has been used as the tool to answer research questions about the utility of family history information in the "Family Healthware Impact Trial (FHITr)." In one of the first studies to assess the impact of family history on patient outcomes, the FHITr demonstrated modest but significant improvement in health behaviors based on risk identified by the tool (Ruffin et al., 2011).

Another barrier identified by providers has been the concern about the accuracy of patient-provided information. While this may be a valid concern, it is important to note that most of the available family history relative risk information currently in use was derived from patient-reported data that were not validated by medical record review or consultation with relatives. As such, they are the basis for current recommendations about risk stratification and alterations in screening, and represent usual practice. A study by Facio et al. (2010) examined the validity of patient-entered information using the "My Family Health Portrait," using a genetic counselor obtained pedigree as a comparator. The sensitivity of the "My Family Health Portrait" was 67–100% and the specificity 92–100% compared to the counselor-generated pedigree with best concordance for diabetes and the cancers, and poorer agreement for coronary artery disease and stroke. Researchers are also beginning to assess the response of providers to patient-entered family history information. Kanetzke et al. (2011) studied pediatricians' perceptions about the "My Family Health Portrait" as a tool for health promotion and disease prevention in the pediatric setting. An assessment of future health care providers (specifically medical students and house officers) regarding the clinical use of the "My Family

Health Portrait" (MHFP) tool was generally posi-tive. Participants agreed or strongly agreed that the MFHP tool is understandable, easy to use, and suitable for general public use. Sixty-seven percent would encourage their patients to use the tool, although concerns were raised about the accessibil-ity of the tool for patients and the accuracy of the patient-entered information (Owens et al., 2011). Orlando et al. [2011] integrated a computerized family health history system within the context of a routine well-visit appointment and found that they were able to overcome many of the existing barriers to collection and use of family history information by primary care providers. The pilot was so suc-cessful that the providers requested that the system continue to fund the tool so it could continue to be used once the study ended.

Clinical decision support (CDS) "…refers broadly to providing clinicians and/or patients with clinical knowledge and patient-related informa-tion, intelligently filtered, or presented at appropri-ate times, to enhance patient care" (Osheroff et al., 2007). The use of CDS embedded within family history collection tools has the potential to enhance the use of family history and to mitigate issues of lack of training and interpretation of information needed to use family history effectively to improve care

(Hoffman and Williams, 2011). The Genetic Risk Assessment on the Internet with Decision Support (GRAIDS) trial is one such effort. GRAIDS is focused on improving the management of familial cancer risk in primary care (Emery et al., 2007). In comparing practices using the GRAIDS software, which incorporates the collection and assessment of family history specific to cancer, in practices provid-ing usual care, there was a significant increase in the number of referrals to the regional genetics clinic for familial cancer assessment and improved compli-ance with referral guidelines.

The previous discussion has identified patient or provider factors that can impact the use of family history. How might we take what has been learned from these and other studies to create a conceptual model of personalized prevention?

PERSONALIZED PREVENTION FOR CORONARY ARTERY DISEASE: A CASE EXAMPLE

In this section, a scenario that combines the com-ponents to personalize the risk for coronary artery disease (CAD) is presented in Figure 8-4. While this scenario is hypothetical at present, work con-tinues to implement this approach for CAD at Intermountain Healthcare.

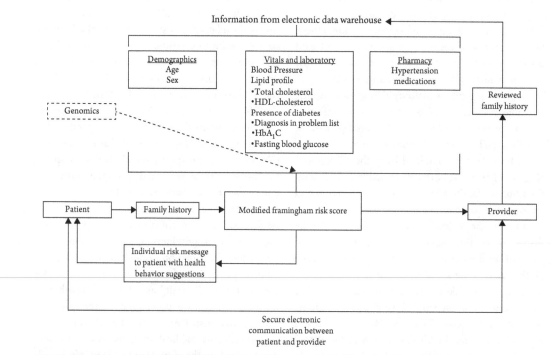

FIGURE 8-4: Example of Protocol for Adding Genomic Information to Risk Stratification.

A 50-year-old man logs into his patient portal account. He notices a new application to collect family history. He opens the program and creates a family history file. His demographic information is automatically populated from the electronic data warehouse (EDW) and he is asked to confirm that the information, including designation of race or ethnicity, is correct. He is prompted to enter his race or ethnicity and religion (Caucasian non-Hispanic, non-Jewish) and health behavior information regarding smoking and use of alcohol and drugs. He enters "no" to all these queries. He then proceeds to enter his family history information. Of relevance to this scenario are his father and one brother who had heart attacks before the age of 50 and his mother's sister who was diagnosed recently with colorectal cancer. When he clicks to exit the program, a message appears asking if he would like to have the family history reviewed for risk. He clicks "yes" and a number of risk algorithms utilized by his provider's health care system are run against the data provided in the family history form. Where needed, information such as vital signs or laboratory values is pulled from the EDW. The risk algorithm for CAD uses the Framingham Risk Score (FRS) modified to include family history information, as this has been shown to be an independent risk factor (Sivapalaratnam et al., 2010). Based on these factors, the patient is classified as intermediate risk for CAD. This information is presented to the patient and he is provided with the four health behaviors from the American Heart Association's "Life's Simple 7™":

1. Not smoking.
2. Achieving and maintaining a body mass index <25 kg/m².
3. Exercising at a moderate intensity ≥ 150 minutes (or 75 minutes at vigorous intensity) each week.
4. Eating a "healthy diet": adhering to four to five important dietary components
   - sodium intake <1.5 g/day;
   - sugar-sweetened beverage intake <36 oz. weekly;
   - ≥ 4.5 cups of fruits and vegetables/day;
   - ≥ three 1 oz. servings of fiber-rich whole grains/day;
   - ≥ two 3.5 oz. servings of oily fish/week.

He is also given the option of sending the information to his primary care provider (PCP). He clicks "yes" and the information from the family history tool and the risk algorithm result is sent via a secure electronic message to the PCP.

When the PCP opens the message from the patient, she is able to review the family history information and flag this as "reviewed" so it can be added to the electronic health record. The PCP is also notified that the patient is at intermediate risk for CAD; the provider is sent the specific family history, clinical information, and access to the algorithm and attendant literature that led to this determination. The PCP is also notified that the patient's most recent low density lipoprotein (LDL) level was 135 mg/dl and is informed that according to the health care system's evidence-based CAD primary prevention protocol, inflammatory marker testing (e.g., C-reactive protein) should be ordered to determine the LDL treatment target. As part of the notification, the PCP is given the option to order the marker test through an embedded link. She clicks "yes," and the system automatically creates a lab order and sends a secure electronic message to the patient indicating that the PCP has reviewed the family history and has ordered a test. The name of the test, the reason for the test, and the procedure for testing are provided to the patient in language appropriate for a lay person.

This case demonstrates how a primary prevention approach can be individualized based on information that exists or is provided in an electronic health record, using an automated process. Best evidence can be provided to optimize the preventive effort while not disrupting provider workflow. Figure 8-4 also illustrates that as genomic information emerges, it could be added to the algorithm to contribute to risk stratification. The findings could be accessed through a secure electronic connection either from the patient's electronic health record, or a central data repository, depending on the storage model utilized.

Bringing in the Patient's Perspective

If we are truly committed to capturing the patient's perspective in the preceding case, then one additional feature needs to be added. After entering the family history information, the patient should be asked, "Is there anything in your family history that you are concerned about, or you wish to talk with your doctor about?" In the example above, the patient could indicate "yes, I am concerned about my risk for colorectal cancer because of my aunt." If this message were also sent to the patient's PCP, she would recognize that the patient has a specific concern that should be addressed that was not related to the risk specified in the algorithm. Depending upon the patient's age, this could be an opportunity to reinforce colonoscopy for colorectal cancer prevention, for example. With the addition of the risk conferred by the aunt's diagnosis, the patient may move along the "stage of change" toward colorectal cancer screening (as discussed in Chapter 3), rather than preventing CAD (although many of the preventive behaviors in nutrition and exercise are similar) (Doherty et al., 1998). Preventive messages about exercise, weight, and healthy eating could be framed in the context of reducing risk for colorectal cancer (Lund et al., 2011), with the hope that the patient would be more likely to make these behavior changes based on his concern, recognizing that there would be attendant benefits for the CAD risk as well. This incorporates the admonition by Pauker and Kassirer (1987) that we "...maximize the outcomes that the patient most cares about and minimizes those that the patient fears the most..." and represents patient-centered care.

CONCLUSIONS

Personalizing prevention has the potential to optimize preventive care for individuals based on their risk and their health concerns. To make this a reality several things are required:

- Collection of all relevant information about an individual including but not limited to:
  - Demographics
  - Personal health history, health behaviors, and vital signs
  - Family history
  - Laboratory, imaging, and other studies
  - Genetic and genomic information as it becomes available and useful.
- Storage of information in a coded and computable format that can be used by electronic health record systems.
- Development of evidence-based risk algorithms that can accurately stratify risk and that are tied to specific preventive interventions.
- Evidence that the preventive interventions improve important health outcomes.
- Presentation of information and interventions to providers in the context of their clinical workflow to improve the efficiency and effectiveness of prevention.

- Capture of patient preferences and negotiation with the provider to prioritize the interventions most likely to benefit that specific patient.
- Improve communication of risk in a way that is understandable and meaningful to the patient.
- Measurement of defined health outcomes to insure that the intervention is resulting in the expected improvement in that specific patient.

The infrastructure needed to support personalized prevention is on the horizon. It will be important to invest in real world clinical research to rapidly target which diseases and interventions are best suited for personalization, to develop the evidence that outcomes are improved, and to promote dissemination and implementation.

REFERENCES

Acheson LS, Wiesner GL, Zyzanski SJ, Goodwin MA, Stange KC. Family history-taking in community family practice: implications for genetic screening. *Genet Med.* 2000;2:180–185.

AHRQ. 2001. Retrieved July 10, 2013, from http://www.ahrq.gov/qual/aderia/aderia.htm.

Anderson LM, Scrimshaw SC, Fullilove MT, Fielding JE, Normand J; Task Force on Community Preventive Services. Culturally competent healthcare systems: a systematic review. *Am J Prev Med.* 2003;24:68–79.

Berg AO, Baird MA, Botkin JR, Driscoll DA, Fishman PA, Guarino PD, Hiatt RA, Jarvik GP, Millon-Underwood S, Morgan TM, Mulvihill JJ, Pollin TI, Schimmel SR, Stefanek ME, Vollmer WM, Williams JK. National Institutes of Health State-of-the-Science Conference Statement: Family History and Improving Health. *Ann Intern Med.* 2009;151:872–877.

Burt RW. Cohorts with familial disposition for colon cancers in chemoprevention trials. *J Cell Biochem Suppl.* 1996;25:131–135.

Center MM, Jemal A, Ward E. International trends in colorectal cancer incidence rates. *Cancer Epidemiol Biomarkers Prev.* 2009;18:1688–1694.

Chantarangsu S, Mushiroda T, Mahasirimongkol S, Kiertiburanakul S, Sungkanuparph S, Manosuthi W, Tantisiriwat W, Charoenyingwattana A, Sura T, Chantratita W, Nakamura Y. HLA-B*3505 allele is a strong predictor for nevirapine-induced skin adverse drug reactions in HIV-infected Thai patients. *Pharmacogenet Genomics.* 2009;19:139–146.

Christensen CM, Grossman JH Hwang J. *The Innovator's Prescription a Disruptive Solution for Health Care.* New York: McGraw-Hill; 2009.

Cornuz J, Ghali WA, Di Carlantonio D, Pecoud A, Paccaud F. Physicians' attitudes towards prevention: importance of intervention-specific barriers and physicians' health habits. *Fam Pract.* 2000;17:535–540.

Doherty SC, Steptoe A, Rink E, Kendrick T, Hilton S. Readiness to change health behaviours among patients at high risk of cardiovascular disease. *J Cardiovasc Risk.* 1998;5:147–153.

EGAPP. Recommendations from the EGAPP Working Group: genetic testing strategies in newly diagnosed individuals with colorectal cancer aimed at reducing morbidity and mortality from Lynch syndrome in relatives. *Genet Med.* 2009;11:35–41.

Emery J, Morris H, Goodchild R, Fanshawe T, Prevost AT, Bobrow M, Kinmonth AL. The GRAIDS Trial: a cluster randomised controlled trial of computer decision support for the management of familial cancer risk in primary care. *Br J Cancer.* 2007;97:486–493.

Ernst FR, Grizzle AJ. Drug-related morbidity and mortality: updating the cost of-illness model. *J Am Pharm Assoc (Wash).* 2001;41:192–199.

Every J, Watson E, Rose P, Andermann A. A systematic review of the literature exploring the role of primary care in genetic services. *Fam Pract.* 1999;16:426–445.

Facio FM, Feero WG, Linn A, Oden N, Manickam K, Beisecker LG. Validation of My Family Health Portrait for six common heritable conditions. *Genet Med.* 2010;12:370–375.

FDA. 2007. Retrieved July 10, 2013, from http://www.fda.gov/ Drugs/DrugSafety/ Postmarket DrugSafety Informationfor Patientsand Providers /ucm124718.htm..

FDA. 2008. Retrieved July 10, 2013, from http://www.fda.gov/Drugs/ DrugSafety/PostmarketDrug Safety InformationforPatientsand Providers/ucm123927.htm

Gramling R, Nash J, Siren K, Eaton C, Culpepper L. Family physician self-efficacy with screening for inherited cancer risk. *Ann Fam Med.* 2004;2:130–132.

Grover S, Stoffel EM, Bussone L, Tschoegl E, Syngal S. Physician assessment of family cancer history and referral for genetic evaluation in colorectal cancer patients. *Clinical Gastroenterol Hepatol.* 2004;2:813–819.

Gudgeon JM, Williams JL, Burt RW, Samowitz WS, Snow GL, Williams MS. Lynch syndrome screening implementation: business analysis by a healthcare system. *Am J Manag Care.* 2011;17:e288–e300.

Hampel H, Frankel WL, Martin E, Arnold M, Khanduja K, Kuebler P, Nakagawa H, Sotamaa K, Prior TW, Westman J, Panescu J, Fix D, Lockman J, Comeras I, de la Chapelle A. Screening for the Lynch syndrome (hereditary nonpolyposis colorectal cancer). *N Engl J Med.* 2005;352:1851–1860.

Hoffman MA, Williams MS. Electronic medical records and personalized medicine. *Hum Genet.* 2011 130:33–39.

Imamura M, Maeda S. Genetics of type 2 diabetes: the GWAS era and future perspectives [Review]. *Endocr J.* 2011;58(9):723–739.

Jover R, Nguyen TP, Pérez-Carbonell L, Zapater P, Payá A, Alenda C, Rojas E, Cubiella J, Balaguer F, Morillas JD, Clofent J, Bujanda L, Reñé JM, Bessa X, Xicola RM, Nicolás-Pérez D, Castells A, Andreu M, Llor X, Boland CR, Goel A. 5-Fluorouracil adjuvant chemotherapy does not increase survival in patients with CpG island methylator phenotype colorectal cancer. *Gastroenterology.* 2011;140:1174–1181.

Kanetzke EE, Lynch J, Prows CA, Siegel RM, Myers MF. Perceived utility of parent-generated family health history as a health promotion tool in pediatric practice. *Clin Pediatr (Phila).* 2011;50:720–728.

Ladabaum U, Wang G, Terdiman J, Blanco A, Kuppermann M, Boland CR, Ford J, Elkin E, Phillips KA. Strategies to identify the Lynch syndrome among patients with colorectal cancer: a cost-effectiveness analysis. *Ann Intern Med.* 2011;155:69–79.

Lim KS, Kwan P, Tan CT. Association of HLA-B*1502 allele and carbamazepine-induced severe adverse cutaneous drug reaction among Asians, a review. *Neurol Asia.* 2008;13:15–21.

Litaker D, Flocke SA, Frolkis JP, Stange KC. Physicians' attitudes and preventive care delivery: insights from the DOPC study. *Prev Med.* 2005;40:556–563.

Lund EK, Belshaw NJ, Elliott GO, Johnson IT. Recent advances in understanding the role of diet and obesity in the development of colorectal cancer. *Proc Nutr Soc.* 2011;70:194–204.

Lynch HT, Lynch JF, Lynch PM, Attard T. Hereditary colorectal cancer syndromes: molecular genetics, genetic counseling, diagnosis and management. *Fam Cancer.* 2008;7:27–39.

Mallal, S, Phillips E, Carosi G, Molina JM, Workman C, Tomazic J, Jägel-Guedes E, Rugina S, Kozyrev O, Cid JF, Hay P, Nolan D, Hughes S, Hughes A, Ryan S, Fitch N, Thorborn D, Benbow A; PREDICT-1 Study Team. HLA-B*5701 screening for hypersensitivity to abacavir. *N Engl J Med.* 2008;358:568–579.

Manolio TA, Collins FS, Cox NJ, Goldstein DB, Hindorff LA, Hunter DJ, McCarthy MI, Ramos EM, Cardon LR, Chakravarti A, Cho JH, Guttmacher AE, Kong A, Kruglyak L, Mardis E, Rotimi CN, Slatkin M, Valle D, Whittemore AS, Boehnke M, Clark AG, Eichler EE, Gibson G, Haines JL, Mackay TF, McCarroll SA, Visscher PM. Finding the missing heritability of complex diseases. *Nature.* 2009;461:747–753.

Orlando LA, Hauser ER, Christianson C, Powell KP, Buchanan AH, Chesnut B, Agbaje AB, Henrich VC, Ginsburg G. Protocol for implementation of family health history collection and decision support into primary care using a computerized family health history system. *BMC Health Serv Res.* 2011;11:264.

Osheroff JA, Teich JM, Middleton BF, Steen EB, Wright A, Detmer DE. A roadmap for national action on clinical decision support. *J Am Med Inform Assoc.* 2007;14:141–145.

Owens KM, Marvin ML, Gelehrter TD, Ruffin MT 4th, Uhlmann WR. Clinical use of the Surgeon General's "My Family Health Portrait" (MFHP) Tool: opinions of future health care providers. *J Genet Couns.* 2011;20:510–525.

Palmer RC, Midgette LA. Preventive health patient education and counseling: a role for medical assistants? *J Allied Health.* 2008;37:137–143.

Pauker SG, Kassirer JP. Decision analysis. *New Eng J Med.* 1987;316:250–258.

Pollak KI, Krause KM, Yarnall KS, Gradison M, Michener JL, Østbye T. Estimated time spent on preventive services by primary care physicians. *BMC Health Serv Res.* 2008;8:245.

Qureshi N, Armstrong S, Dhiman P, Saukko P, Middlemass J, Evans PH, Kai J; ADDFAM (Added Value of Family History in CVD Risk Assessment) Study Group. Effect of adding systematic family history enquiry to cardiovascular disease risk assessment in primary care: a matched-pair, cluster randomized trial. *Ann Intern Med.* 2012;156:253–262.

Reid GT, Walter FM, Brisbane JM, Emery JD. Family history questionnaires designed for clinical use: a systematic review. *Public Health Genomics.* 2009;12:73–83.

Rich EC, Burke W, Heaton CJ, Haga S, Pinsky L, Short MP, Acheson L. Reconsidering the family history in primary care. *J Gen Intern Med.* 2004;19:273–280.

Ruffin MT 4th, Nease DE Jr, Sen A, Pace WD, Wang C, Acheson LS, Rubinstein WS, O'Neill S, Gramling R; Family History Impact Trial (FHITr) Group. Effect of preventive messages tailored to family history on health behaviors: the Family Healthware Impact Trial. *Ann Fam Med.* 2011;9:3–11.

Sciamanna CN, Diaz J, Myne P. Patient attitudes toward using computers to improve health services delivery. *BMC Health Serv Res.* 2002;2:19.

Sivapalaratnam S, Boekholdt SM, Trip MD, Sandhu MS, Luben R, Kastelein JJ, Wareham NJ, Khaw KT. Family history of premature coronary heart disease and risk prediction in the EPIC-Norfolk prospective population study. *Heart.* 2010;96:1985–1989.

Summerton N, Garrood PVA. The family history in family practice: a questionnaire study. *Fam Pract.* 1997;14:285–288.

Valdez R, Yoon PW, Qureshi N, Green RF, Khoury MJ. Family history in public health practice: a genomic tool for disease prevention and health promotion. *Annu Rev Public Health.* 2010;31:25.1–25.19.

Williams JL, Collingridge DS, Williams MS. Primary care physicians' experience with family history: an exploratory qualitative study. *Genet Med.* 2011;13:21–25.

Yarnall KS, Pollak KI, Østbye T, Krause KM, Michener JL. Primary care: is there enough time for prevention? *Am J Public Health.* 2003;93:635–641.

Yoon PW, Scheuner MT, Khoury MJ. Research priorities for evaluation family history in the prevention of common chronic diseases. *Am J Prev Med.* 2003;24:128–135.

Yoon PW, Scheuner MT, Jorgensen C, Khoury MJ. Developing Family Healthware, a family history screening tool to prevent common chronic diseases. *Prev Chronic Dis.* 2009;6:1–11.

9

Pay for Performance and Quality and Outcomes Frameworks for Prevention

FARUQUE AHMED AND STEVEN TEUTSCH

The findings and conclusions in this chapter are those of the authors and do not necessarily represent the official position of the Centers for Disease Control and Prevention.

This chapter is a US Government work and, as such, is in the public domain in the United States of America.

INTRODUCTION

The Institute of Medicine defines quality of care as "the degree to which health care services for individuals and populations increase the likelihood of desired health outcomes and are consistent with current professional knowledge" (Institute of Medicine, 1990). Quality of care encompasses the underuse, overuse, and misuse of health care services. The main cause of suboptimal quality of care is usually not deficiency in physician knowledge or motivation, but rather is attributable to system problems (Institute of Medicine, 2001). For an average adult primary care patient, there are 15.4 risk factors and 24.5 recommendations for preventive services (Medder, Kahn, Jr., & Susman, 1992). Urgent concerns tend to dominate visits to physicians (Szilagyi et al., 2005), as discussed in Chapter 1. In the United States, providers are not rewarded for providing higher quality under most of the existing payment mechanisms, and any financial benefits of increasing quality accrue mainly to payers and patients (Institute of Medicine, 2001; Robinson, 2001). The Institute of Medicine recommends better alignment of financial incentives for providers to promote higher quality of health care (Institute of Medicine, 2001; Institute of Medicine, 2006), as discussed in Chapter 12.

Pay for performance (P4P) is a relatively new policy initiative in which explicit financial incentives are offered by purchasers and health plans to primary care physicians, specialists, and hospital providers for achieving pre-defined quality targets. The interest in P4P programs can be attributed to several factors, including studies indicating that patients often do not receive recommended care, increased public awareness about patient safety as a result of publicity about Institute of Medicine reports, limited success of managed care activities to improve quality and control costs, and advances in the field of quality measurement (Institute of Medicine, 1999; Institute of Medicine, 2001; McGlynn et al., 2003; Young et al., 2005).

Economists have used the principal-agent theory to describe the relationship between payers of health care (principal) and providers (agent) in which the two parties have different abilities so it is desirable for payers to delegate responsibility for health care to providers. Further, there is asymmetric information between the two parties, as payers are unable to monitor all provider activities that can influence quality of care; the two parties have different goals in that quality is important to both parties, but payers may be more concerned with efficiency than providers' incomes, whereas providers may give precedence to income over cost control (Dudley et al., 2004; Frolich et al., 2007). Many economists therefore think that financial incentives should be used to ensure that providers focus on quality *and* efficiency.

In the United States, numerous health plans, employers, and the federal Centers for Medicare and Medicaid Services (CMS) have sponsored hundreds of P4P initiatives. In the United Kingdom, the National Health Service initiated a nationwide P4P program for general practitioners in 2004, known as the Quality and Outcomes Framework (QOF). P4P programs use national and/or locally developed quality measures to assess performance. A quality measure assesses the extent to which a health care process or outcome is attained, or the extent to which a structure to facilitate the delivery of health care is available (Donabedian, 1966; Hodgson, Simpson, & Lannon, 2008).

Examples of structure, process, and outcome measures include use of electronic health records, breast cancer screening, and stage of cancer at diagnosis, respectively. Process measures can be used to assess adherence to recommendations, while performance on outcome measures may be affected by several processes or factors. For example, diagnosis of cancer at an early stage depends not only on whether screening was done at recommended intervals but also on the quality of the screening procedure, the timeliness of follow-up of suspicious findings, and the aggressiveness of the tumor.

National quality measures are sponsored or endorsed by several organizations, including the National Quality Forum (NQF), the Ambulatory Care Quality Alliance (AQA), the American Medical Association Physician Consortium for Performance Improvement (PCPI), and the National Committee for Quality Assurance (NCQA) (Hodgson, Simpson, & Lannon, 2008). Clinical preventive services recommended by the US Preventive Services Task Force (USPSTF), the Advisory Committee on Immunization Practices (ACIP) of the US Centers for Disease Control and Prevention (CDC), and other organizations are commonly included in national performance measurement sets (CDC, 2013; AHRQ, 2012). Desirable attributes of performance measures include the importance of the measure (relevance to stakeholders, health importance, applicability to measuring disparities in care, potential for improving quality, susceptibility to being influenced by the health care system), scientific soundness (explicitness of evidence supporting the measure, strength of evidence, reliability, validity, allowance for patient factors as required, comprehensible), and feasibility (explicit specification of numerator and denominator, data availability, and accessibility) (AHRQ, 2013). Measures of clinical preventive services are particularly amenable to these attributes (Ahmed et al., 2001; Ahmed et al., 2002). Although a primary goal of P4P programs is improving the quality of care, some program sponsors expect to control costs by reducing variation in quality or inappropriate utilization (Trude, Au, & Christianson, 2006).

CONCEPTUAL MODEL

Figure 9-1 shows a conceptual model describing the response of providers to P4P programs. Characteristics of P4P programs play a key role in how providers perceive the need to respond to the incentive. The response may be influenced by contextual factors. Provider response may include

changes in the structure or process of care. Outcomes of interest include both desirable effects and undesirable consequences.

PROVIDER COMPENSATION MECHANISMS

An appreciation of the underlying provider compensation mechanisms is needed to understand how P4P initiatives may influence practice patterns. Payment mechanisms used by health plans include fee-for-service (FFS), capitation, or a combination of capitation with FFS for certain procedures. FFS payments are based on the number and types of services provided, whereas capitation denotes a fixed payment per patient per month to cover a defined set of services (e.g., primary care, specialty care) provided for patients.

Similarly, compensation methods for physicians include FFS, capitation, and salary. Salary denotes payment of a certain amount per month of work. Arrangements in which salary is tied to measures of individual productivity (e.g., insurance claims generated) can be considered to be a type of FFS payment. FFS is believed to provide an incentive to provide more care to increase income. Capitation is perceived to provide an incentive to provide less care, however (Berwick, 1996). When physicians are paid a salary, payment is independent of the level of care provided or the number of patients seen, but there is an incentive to minimize the time spent working (Dudley et al., 2004).

Physician organizations such as medical groups and independent practice associations (IPAs) may serve as financial intermediaries between physicians and health plans (Robinson et al., 2004). Individual physicians may participate in more than one physician organization and may also have direct contracts with health plans. Further, physician organizations may sometimes pay physicians using a mechanism that differs from that between the physician organization and the health plans (Dudley et al., 2004). For example, a physician organization may receive capitation payment but may pay physicians a salary.

FACTORS THAT MAY INFLUENCE EFFECTIVENESS OF P4P INITIATIVES

Factors that may influence the effectiveness of P4P initiatives in improving quality pertain to characteristics of the incentive program as well as contextual factors (Dudley et al., 2004). The same program

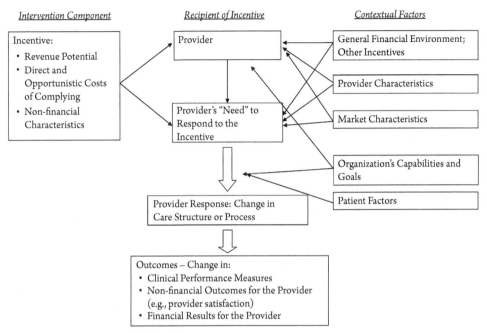

FIGURE 9-1: Model of a Provider's Response to Incentives.

Source: Adapted from Dudley, RA, Frolich A, Robinowitz DL, Talavera JA, Broadhead P, and Luft HS. Strategies to support quality-based purchasing: a review of the evidence summary, Technical Review 10. AHRQ Pub. No. 04-0057. Rockville, MD: Agency for Healthcare Research and Quality; 2004.

implemented in different contexts may produce different results.

Characteristics of the Incentive Program

Characteristics include the target and nature of the incentive, certainty and costs of achieving targets, performance measures, the scale of performance targets, and the publicity of performance scores.

Target of the Incentive

Incentive payments can be targeted to individual physicians, physician organizations, or both individual physicians and physician organizations. Targeting individual physicians provides more actionable information than aggregate data, enhances accountability, and allows greater control by physicians in receiving a bonus (Dudley & Rosenthal, 2006). Targeting physician organizations may enhance institutional cooperation and make it more feasible to invest in information systems and other infrastructures, which may not only lead to improvement in the areas measured but also have secondary benefits. Investments in decision

support systems or electronic health records can lead to greater adherence to guideline-based care, particularly preventive care, and may enhance monitoring activities; other potential benefits of such investments include enhancing patient safety through reducing medication errors and lowering the utilization of redundant or unnecessary care (Chaudhry et al., 2006). Targeting measurements to the physician group level, compared to the individual physician level, could lead to greater statistical precision for evaluating programs because of larger sample sizes.

Nature of the Incentive and Costs of Improving Performance

The attractiveness of performance incentives to providers will be influenced by the size of the incentive per patient, the proportion of a provider's panel that is covered by the incentive program(s), and costs to improve performance. The costs include both direct and opportunity, by not doing something else (Dudley et al., 2004). Costs may include investments in information technology, personnel, or the value of a provider's time (Rosenthal & Frank, 2006). Costs can be both fixed and variable, and may involve substantial start-up costs associated with changes in processes (Dudley et al., 2004). If up-front costs are involved, they may also be influenced by the perceived likelihood that the incentive program will be continued in the future. Investment costs may be relatively lower for larger practices, compared to solo or small practices, because of economies of scale.

Constructs of Performance Measures

Providers will give more importance to the incentive program if they believe that the performance measures are aligned with their perceptions of quality care and that they are based on accurate and valid data. Incentive programs can target measures pertaining to clinical quality, information technology, patient satisfaction, and cost efficiency. However, inclusion of cost-efficiency measures may undermine the credibility of P4P programs to providers (Dudley & Rosenthal, 2006). Providers may be more inclined to act in response to measures over which they have greater control than measures that may be influenced by a variety of factors (Dudley et al., 2004). The clinical validity of measures and the cost of data collection must be balanced (Rosenthal & Dudley, 2007). Administrative claims data are more readily accessible than medical records data but may be less accurate and may contain fewer clinical details. Adjusting for differences in patient populations across providers may increase the burden of data collection because claims data may not contain the required information and more costly chart abstractions may be necessary.

Scale of Performance Targets

Incentives can be based on absolute performance targets (e.g., mammography rate of 85% or higher), on relative performance (e.g., bonuses paid to the top 10% of providers), or on a percentage improvement (Dudley & Rosenthal, 2006). Absolute targets reward high-quality providers and have the advantage of simplicity. Providers with low performance may feel discouraged, however, as there are no rewards if improvements fall short of the threshold, and high-quality providers may receive bonuses with little or no improvement. Such payments to high-quality providers may be viewed as a reward for a job already well done, but it may not fully mesh with the concept of using financial incentives to improve quality of care. The relative performance strategy can create competition, but may limit collaboration and sharing of best practices (Rosenthal & Dudley, 2007). It also introduces uncertainty because a physician's bonus

depends not only on her or his performance but also on that of the peers. The percentage improvement strategy can result in the distribution of more bonus dollars toward providers with lower initial performance, but may be fairer to providers who serve a larger proportion of vulnerable populations. Providers with high initial performance may be at a disadvantage because there is less room for improvement (ceiling effect), however. Concerns regarding fairness in comparing performance across providers may be ameliorated by appropriate risk adjustment. Risk adjustment may be less of an issue for the improvement approach, in which providers are compared against their own baseline, than if only the top-ranked providers are rewarded (Dudley & Rosenthal, 2006).

Other ways that incentives can be structured include differentially rewarding providers for achievements along a continuum of performance thresholds (graduated bonuses), for example, offering a full bonus to providers whose performance is above the prior year's 85th percentile level and 50% of that amount to providers whose performance is between the prior year's 75th and 85th percentiles. Providers can also be rewarded in a continuous manner in proportion to their achievement (Dudley et al., 2004; Dudley & Rosenthal, 2006).

Provider Feedback and Public Reporting of Performance

P4P program sponsors may provide feedback to providers on their performance and that of their peers, and may also publicly report performance information. Feedback and public reporting may complement the effect of financial incentives through its effect on provider competitiveness, self-esteem, and reputation (Frolich et al., 2007), as also described in Chapter 10. Public reporting may have an indirect financial impact if patients seek out or are steered to higher-performing providers, or if better quality can be reflected in higher charges.

Contextual Factors

Contextual mediators include the financial environment, provider, market, organizational, and patient characteristics.

Financial Characteristics of the Environment

The proportion of income from FFS, capitation, and salary may influence the response to financial incentives. The potential for opportunity costs is greatest for providers who predominantly receive FFS payments (Dudley et al., 2004). For example, giving more immunizations may detract from performing activities that generate more fees per unit time or from seeing new patients. For providers receiving capitation payments, each extra activity is an added cost, and activities that may attract sicker patients or lead to additional follow-up activities (e.g., tests, prescriptions) will tend to be avoided, unless the additional income from the incentive offsets the added costs. Preventive services, such as influenza immunizations for the elderly, that prevent near-term complications may be more readily accepted by a capitated provider, compared to a screening procedure that generates the need for additional services to evaluate positive or false-positive results. For salaried physicians, there is no financial opportunity cost, as income is not related to what is done, but there is likely to be increased workload associated with performing additional activities. The extent of competing incentives may also influence the response of providers; for example, providers may give less attention to P4P programs with smaller payouts.

Market Characteristics

Factors include the extent of competition faced by a provider, the degree to which payers adopt similar P4P programs, and local professional initiatives to improve quality (Frolich et al., 2007).

Provider Characteristics

Factors that may influence response to P4P initiatives include provider demographics (e.g., years since the completion of training), specialty, workload, and proportion of patients where the incentive is relevant (Dudley et al., 2004; Frolich et al., 2007). Other factors influencing provider acceptance of pay for performance include intrinsic motivation, professionalism, altruism, assumptions about patient preferences, and whether a physician has already achieved her or his target income.

Organizational Characteristics

Organizational determinants of P4P adoption include practice size, electronic information systems capabilities, supportive medical leadership, organizational culture, and whether incentives that target physician groups are passed down to individuals (Dudley et al., 2004; Frolich et al., 2007). If there are no mechanisms to share incentives with group members, it may weaken the effect of the incentive on motivating change in individual behavior (Eijkenaar, 2011).

Patient Characteristics

Factors modulating P4P include socioeconomic characteristics and education level of patients, health insurance status, and structure of insurance benefits (e.g., co-pay amounts) (Dudley et al., 2004; Frolich et al., 2007). Patients who are low income or have low health literacy may have poorer health behaviors than others. There may also be varying norms across cultures. For example, Hispanics tend to have a more fatalistic attitude toward cancer than non-Hispanics (Perez-Stable et al., 1992).

POTENTIAL EFFECT ON DISPARITIES

Concern has been expressed that P4P programs may have an unintended effect of increasing disparities. Disparities may widen if quality improvement initiatives do not take into account cultural, linguistic, and educational needs of minority patients; if providers drop or avoid vulnerable populations; or if resource gaps are widened because of the greater difficulty of providers that predominantly serve vulnerable populations to qualify for bonuses (Casalino et al., 2007b; Chien et al., 2007; Chien et al., 2012; Friedberg et al., 2010). Vulnerable populations obtain medical care from a relatively small number of providers; these providers tend to have lower baseline performance scores and therefore would need to improve more to achieve absolute performance targets (Bach et al., 2004). Adjusting or stratifying performance scores based on race or socioeconomic status and rewarding improvement may increase fairness (Casalino et al., 2007b). However, adjusting performance scores may imply that a lower standard of care is acceptable for vulnerable populations. Several strategies have been suggested to reduce the likelihood of increasing disparities: collecting race and ethnicity data at the individual or community level; emphasizing quality measures on conditions that are more prevalent in minority populations; establishing guidelines and/or measures on disparity (e.g., the provision of culturally, literacy, and linguistically appropriate services); and rewarding improvement in addition to rewarding absolute performance (Chien et al., 2007).

PHYSICIAN CONCERNS ABOUT P4P PROGRAMS

Buy-in of physicians is important for the success of P4P programs. Professional medical societies generally support incentive programs to improve the quality of care (ACP, 2005; AAFP, 2010; Brush, Jr., et al., 2006; Bufalino et al., 2006; Hodgson, Simpson, &

Lannon, 2008). However, concerns regarding P4P initiatives include the choice and validity of performance measures, increased administrative burdens, physician autonomy, patient actions and preferences, and possible unintended adverse consequences. The unintended consequences could include dropping or not accepting difficult patients, neglecting aspects of care that are not measured, undermining trust of patients in their physicians, and providing unnecessary or inappropriate care to patients with terminal or severe comorbid illnesses (Casalino, 1999; Casalino et al., 2007a; Snyder & Neubauer, 2007; Werner & Asch, 2007).

SOURCES OF FUNDS FOR P4P PROGRAMS

Sources of funds for P4P incentives include new money, expected savings from cost reductions (through improved quality or through cost-saving measures such as generic prescribing), reallocation of funds from previous incentive programs, redirection of all or a portion of annual payment increases to incentive pay, and the redistribution of funds from lower performing providers to higher performing providers (Baker & Delbanco, 2008; Dudley & Rosenthal, 2006). Health plans may not be able to offset costs because most of the health and financial gains of improving quality are long term and because of substantial membership turnover. Purchasers who believe that health care costs are already high may be reluctant to provide substantial additional funds (Christianson, Leatherman, & Sutherland, 2008). Providers may favor funding incentive payments through mechanisms that do not threaten their income but offer the potential for rewards (Maynard, 2012).

CASE STUDY OF A MAJOR P4P PROGRAM

The Rewarding Results demonstration projects serves as a case study for illustrating issues in designing and implementing P4P programs (Young et al., 2005; Young, Burgess, Jr., & White, 2007). The demonstration projects were jointly sponsored by the Robert Wood Johnson Foundation, California HealthCare Foundation, and the Commonwealth Fund. The reward payers were health plans in six projects and employers in one project. Projects were located in California, Kentucky, Massachusetts, Michigan, New York, and Ohio. The focus was mainly on primary care physicians; in two projects,

the unit of accountability was physician organizations (i.e., group practices and independent practice associations); in two projects, the unit was individual physicians; and both individual physicians and physician organizations were accountable in two projects. Hospitals were the unit of accountability in one project. Most of the quality measures were based on NCQA's Healthcare Effectiveness Data and Information Set (HEDIS) performance measures.

Dimensions that were considered in designing and implementing the projects included provider awareness of financial incentives, size and structure of financial incentives, clinical relevance of performance targets, accountability for performance targets, and the fairness of the programs (Young et al., 2005; Young, Burgess, Jr., & White, 2007).

Provider Awareness of Financial Incentives

Because providers are inundated with clinical and reimbursement information from payers and professional organizations, it may be difficult for payers to create awareness of the quality targets, the measurement systems, and payout formulas. Multiple types of P4P programs in a geographic area may also create confusion among providers. Payers in the seven projects used local and regional meetings, hard-copy and electronic mailings, and websites to raise awareness. In two of the projects, efforts were made to standardize performance measures among payers. Physicians in these demonstration projects generally had inadequate understanding of the details of the P4P programs in which they were participating, however, regardless of the unit of accountability.

Size and Structure of Financial Incentives

The size of the incentive needed to motivate providers is likely to be larger if substantial investments are needed to attain the performance targets, such as the development of disease registries, the use of support staff, and the adoption of information technology. In these projects, all but one site structured the incentive as a bonus; one site used a combination of bonus and withhold for primary care physicians (i.e., a 10% withhold from all claims, and payout of between 50% and 150% of the withhold amount, depending on performance). Although the incentive amount was perceived by physicians to be inadequate, many providers gave greater attention to quality targets that were linked to incentives.

Clinical Relevance of Quality Targets

Providers' perceived clinical relevance of the performance measures may be an important factor in the success of the program. Program sponsors preferred well-established standardized measurement sets such as HEDIS because they were readily available, were familiar to providers, and did not generally require substantial additional data collection efforts. Providers participated in selecting or adapting particular measures from the measurement sets. However, providers were concerned about the accuracy of determining patient eligibility for a given performance measure and the validity of reports based on electronic claims data.

Accountability for Performance Targets

The demonstration projects differed in whether provider organizations or individual physicians were the units of accountability. Investment in quality improvement infrastructure appeared to be substantially greater in project sites where the unit of accountability was provider organizations rather than individual physicians. Physicians felt that better infrastructure would facilitate their ability to meet performance targets. Some provider organizations were reported to retain all of the incentive amounts for investing in infrastructure, which may, however, reduce the willingness of physicians to engage in the program. Some physicians were offended by the external oversight of performance associated with financial incentives and performance measurement that is counter to the traditional notions of clinical accountability, professionalism, and patients' trust in physicians.

Fairness of P4P Programs

Providers have concerns regarding how performance targets are defined (e.g., provider ranking, threshold values, percentage improvement). Most of the sites used threshold values, such as mammography rates of 80%. Providers who are already performing well have an advantage when threshold values are used, however. Further, providers may have concerns about fairness if sociodemographic characteristics and health status of patients could affect the achievement of performance targets.

EVALUATION OF P4P PROGRAMS IN THE UNITED STATES

A study of 27 early adopters of P4P programs reveals that payers increased the size of financial incentives and the number of performance measures over time (Rosenthal et al., 2007). Measures of clinical processes (e.g., mammography rates) and patient satisfaction were the most common types used initially; inclusion of measures of outcomes (e.g., glycosylated hemoglobin level control, low-density lipoprotein cholesterol level control, and blood pressure control), information technology, and cost efficiency (e.g., generic prescribing, formulary compliance) increased over time. Some payers subsequently eliminated measures on which performance was consistently very high (e.g., smoking cessation counseling; well-baby and well-child visits; measles, mumps, and rubella vaccination; mammography; cervical cancer screening; colorectal cancer screening). The most common provider type targeted was primary care physicians; the inclusion of specialists and hospital providers increased over time. The incentives were initially based on absolute performance targets, which were subsequently expanded to include incentives based on improvement. Despite increases in the size of the incentives, the amount represented a very small portion of providers' incomes; the average bonus amount was approximately 2.3% of reimbursement. Major challenges that were identified included overcoming physician resistance, determining the incentive size that is meaningful to providers, and finding funds to sustain the programs. The lessons learned included the importance of involving providers early in the development process, maintaining communication and transparency, starting small, and developing trust and building measurement and quality improvement capabilities over time.

Healthplan Activities

A national survey of health maintenance organizations (HMOs) reported that P4P is commonly used (Rosenthal et al., 2006). Most HMOs targeted medical groups or both medical groups and individual physicians; very few targeted only individual physicians. Types of performance measures used, in order of frequency, were; clinical quality, information technology, patients' satisfaction, and cost. The clinical measures most commonly included; diabetes care, mammography, and asthma medication. Bonuses based on absolute targets were more common than bonuses based on relative performance or on improvement. Certain HMO characteristics were associated with having P4P programs: paying primary care physicians by capitation; requiring that enrollees select their own primary care physicians; and having contracts between HMOs and purchasers that included bonuses or penalties for performance. Having a designated primary care physician and payment by capitation make it easier to identify accountable physicians. HMOs in the South were less likely to have P4P programs than those in the Northeast, the Midwest, or the West.

Provider Responses

A 2006 study assessed the attitudes and reactions of executives of physician organizations in Massachusetts, a state where health plans have widely implemented P4P programs (Bokhour et al., 2006). The executives felt that rewarding quality was more acceptable to physicians than previous financial incentives for decreasing utilization. However, the multiple measurement systems, differences in performance targets, and frequent changes in the targets were reported to be confusing and difficult to monitor. Many executives believed that physicians are inherently motivated to provide good quality care and that the bonus was a well-deserved reward for a job already well done. However, some executives believed that physicians were much more likely to pay attention to report cards that were tied to financial incentives and that financial incentives could result in system-level changes. Many physicians felt that they were unfairly penalized when patients did not adhere to their recommendations, and that non-compliant patients should be excluded from the performance measurement. A major concern was that the recording and reporting of data were not accurate and that what was measured did not truly constitute quality. The way the performance measures were defined was not consistent with their definitions of quality. Some physicians believed that the measurement system failed to reflect the good quality care they were giving, and so they had little control over receiving the incentive payments. Therefore, provider input in identifying quality goals and measures was considered to be important to ensure

that performance targets are aligned with clinical goals and relevant to clinical practice.

The way the financial incentives were distributed varied within the provider organizations: (1) money was distributed based on the performance of individual physicians on the performance measures; (2) money was distributed based on performance on an internal rating system; (3) money was distributed equally to all providers; (4) money was retained by the organization; and (5) money was divided between the organization and individual physicians. Problems in distributing the money included; more than one physician provided care to a patient, but only the physician identified as the primary provider would receive the financial incentive; non-availability of physician-specific data from each health plan; and physicians with small numbers of eligible patients. The rationale for retaining all money by the organization was that the involvement of both physicians and support staff was needed to provide quality care; money needed to be invested for system-level changes such as electronic medical records or hiring additional staff; and the avoidance of conflict as to which physician was actually responsible for providing the service.

Effect on Quality Improvement Activities

A survey of leaders of physician groups in Massachusetts found an association between P4P incentives and the use of quality improvement initiatives (Mehrotra et al., 2007). Most physician groups had P4P incentives with at least one health plan. Performance domains commonly included quality measures, followed by measures on utilization (e.g., use of formulary medications, emergency department visits) and information technology (e.g., use of electronic medical records, use of electronic prescribing); patient satisfaction measures were least commonly used. The most common type of quality improvement activity was development of a registry and a system for giving feedback to providers about their performance. Quality improvement initiatives commonly targeted mammography screening, glycosylated hemoglobin measurement, and asthma controller medication use. Few medical groups had quality improvement initiatives targeting low-density lipoprotein cholesterol level control and hypertension control.

An initiative to improve asthma care in 13,000 children across 44 pediatric practices (165 physicians) that coupled P4P with building improvement capability and promoting system changes reported substantive and sustainable improvement (Mandel & Kotagal, 2007). The financial incentive of a 7% fee schedule increase was structured into three levels: a first-level reward of 2% fee schedule increase for participation, regardless of practice-specific performance; a second-level reward of an additional 2% fee schedule increase for overall network performance, regardless of practice-specific performance (receipt of influenza vaccination by at least 30% of asthma patients, receipt of controller medications by at least 70% of patients with persistent asthma); and a third-level reward of 3% fee schedule increase for improvement capability (development of asthma registries by practices and collection of concurrent data on key processes and outcomes) and practice performance (influenza vaccination of at least 50%, controller medication at least 75%, and written self-management plan at least 80%). The first-level reward provided compensation for time and effort of physicians, nurses, office managers, and other staff; the second-level reward was geared toward enhancing communication and collaboration among practices to promote the sharing of successful interventions; and the third level rewarded improved infrastructure and the performance of individual practices. The percentage of asthma patients receiving perfect care (written self-management plan; controller medications for patients with persistent asthma) increased from 4% at baseline to 88% during the third year. The percentage receiving influenza vaccine increased from 22% to 62%.

Impact on Quality of Care

A systematic review of 15 studies assessing the effect of financial incentives at the provider group or individual physician level showed mixed results (Petersen et al., 2006). Thirteen of these 15 studies assessed process measures, mostly for preventive services. Of the nine studies at the provider group level, two studies showed an increase across all the measures of quality, five studies reported improvement in some measures but not others, and two studies found no effect. Most of the improvements were small. Of the six studies on incentives at the physician level, five reported an increase in some or all of the performance measures. Among the 15 studies, three showed that financial incentives improved documentation rather than increased the use of preventive services.

A Cochrane review of the effect of financial incentives on the quality of health care provided by primary care physicians included seven studies published from 2000 to 2009 (Scott et al., 2011). The outcomes examined included smoking cessation, cervical cancer screening, mammography screening, diabetes management (HbA1C testing, lipoprotein density level, urinalysis, eye examination), childhood immunization, chlamydia screening, and appropriate asthma medication. Six studies showed modest effects in improving the quality of care for some, but not all, outcome measures. One study showed no improvement.

EVALUATION OF THE UK QUALITY AND OUTCOMES FRAMEWORK

The Quality and Outcomes Framework (QOF) is a government program introduced by the UK National Health Service (NHS) in 2004 to provide financial incentives to general practitioners (GPs) for improving quality of care (Roland, 2004). Every NHS patient must select a GP, who is paid primarily by capitation and who serves as a gatekeeper to specialist care. The nationwide quality initiative was supported by an increase of about £1.8 billion (US $3.4 billion) in the NHS budget over 3 years.

Performance indicators were developed in close collaboration with physicians and are reviewed every 2 years. A total of 146 quality indicators were established in 2004 that covered clinical care for 10 chronic diseases, the organization of care, and patient experiences with care. The performance of each physician's practice, which typically has two to six physicians, is measured using data extracted from electronic medical records maintained by the practices. Performance levels are publicly reported based on points assigned to each quality indicator, which can range from 1 to 56 points. For each indicator, there is a minimum threshold performance that a practice must meet to begin accruing points, and an upper performance target at which a practice earns all available points; points are allocated on a sliding scale for performance scores that are between the minimum and maximum thresholds. For example, a practice receives one point if blood pressure is controlled for at least 25% of patients with coronary heart disease, and the maximum 19 points are earned if blood pressure is controlled for at least 70% of such patients. Practices are allowed to exclude inappropriate patients from the performance calculations, for example, patients who fail to attend an office visit despite at least three reminders, who have terminal illness or are extremely frail, who are taking the maximum tolerated dose of medication but whose levels remain suboptimal, or who do not agree to the investigation or treatment. The number of points earned, taking into consideration practice size and disease prevalence, determines the incentive award. GPs can increase their income by up to 30% based on performance on the quality indicators.

In response to the program, practices have employed more nurses and administrative staff, have set up chronic-disease clinics, and have increased the use of information technology (Doran et al., 2006). Information technology systems are designed for clinicians to respond to the performance incentives and to monitor their own performance on an ongoing basis (McDonald, White, & Marmor, 2009). For example, computer pop-up boxes prompt clinicians for needed action, and the software provides a running total of points achieved. Nurses have become the primary source of care for managing chronic conditions (Campbell, McDonald, & Lester, 2008). For example, a nurse may manage all asthma patients visiting a practice. By 2006, nurses managed a third of all patient consultations (Doran & Roland, 2010).

Practices attained a median of 95.5% of the available points during the first year of the program (Doran et al., 2006). No baseline information on performance scores of practices was collected prior to the implementation of the QOF program, and the attained score was much higher than the 75% predicted by the Department of Health for developing budget estimates. The overall proportion of eligible patients for whom indicated care was provided was 83.4%. The attainment score is higher than the proportion obtaining indicated care because a practice can obtain all available points for a quality indicator if the maximum threshold is met. A median 6% of patients were excluded from the performance calculations by the practices, with 1.1% of practices excluded more than 15% of their patients. It is unclear whether the exclusion of large numbers of patients by the few practices was done for appropriate reasons. Concern has also been expressed that the performance thresholds may have been set too low (Timmins, 2005). Although additional nursing and administrative costs were borne by the practices, the incentive payments generally also increased the personal earnings of GPs who owned the practices (Doran et al., 2006).

Another study assessed the effect of the QOF program on the quality of care for patients with diabetes, asthma, or coronary heart disease (Campbell et al., 2009). The percentage of eligible patients obtaining indicated care for diabetes, asthma, and coronary heart disease improved an average rate of 1.8%, 2.0%, and 3.5% per year, respectively, in the pre-introduction period from 1998 through 2003. From 2003–2005, there was a significant increase in the percentage obtaining indicated care over and above the preexisting trend for diabetes (7.5 percentage points increase beyond the pre-introduction trend) and asthma (9.4 percentage points increase), but not coronary heart disease (non-significant increase of 2.8 percentage points). However, the percentage plateaued between 2005 and 2007 for all three conditions. There may be little financial incentive to further improve after maximum thresholds for scoring points have been reached, or clinicians may become exhausted (Doran & Roland, 2010). A study has reported a reduction in health equalities across populations classified into five categories based on the level of area deprivation (Doran et al., 2008). In year 1 of the QOF program (2004–2005), the percentage of eligible patients for whom indicated care was provided by 7,637 practices for 48 clinical indicators ranged from a median of 86.8% for the least deprived area to 82.8% for the most deprived area. The difference in median achievement between the least deprived and most deprived areas decreased from 4.0% in year 1 to 0.8% in year 3.

Some questions raised about manipulation or gaming to increase performance scores include inappropriate use of exceptions or the removal of difficult patients from disease registers, checking off indicators without fully meeting all requirements, and inaccurate recording (e.g., blood pressure recording bias) (Doran & Roland, 2010; McDonald, White, & Marmor, 2009). However, audits are performed on randomly selected practices, and there are severe penalties for fraud. Unintended consequences include; less attention to some aspects of care not linked to incentives, and reduced continuity of care (Campbell et al., 2009). It may have been more difficult for patients to see their usual doctor after the introduction of the QOF program because access to a doctor within 48 hours (not necessarily the usual doctor) was linked to incentives, or because many practices delegated the management of chronic diseases to nurses. It is also reported that physicians had less time to focus on the doctor-patient relationship and the patient's agenda because of competing demands for meeting performance targets (e.g., large number of pop-up boxes, increased time spent on collecting and entering data into electronic medical records) (McDonald & Roland, 2009).

The UK program differs from those that have been implemented in the United States on several aspects: a single payer; a single nationally agreed-upon set of performance measures; a larger number of performance measures; a single method for assessing performance scores; the close involvement of physicians in selecting performance measures and developing methods for scoring performance; the discretion of physicians to exclude non-compliant patients or patients for whom an indicator is judged to be inappropriate; the magnitude of the incentive; use of data extracted from the practices' own electronic medical records (almost all practices now have electronic medical records); the ability of physicians to monitor performance on an ongoing basis; and the greater consciousness by physicians of the performance targets (McDonald, White, & Marmor, 2009).

CONCLUSIONS

There is little rigorous evidence for the effect of design and contextual factors on the effectiveness of P4P that could guide the implementation of P4P programs (Chassin, 2006; Christianson, Leatherman, & Sutherland, 2008; Eijkenaar, 2011; Frolich et al., 2007; Galvin, 2006; Van et al., 2010). In the United States, physicians may be affiliated with one or more physician organizations, and individual physicians and physician organizations may contract with a variety of health plans and insurers, including preferred provider organizations (PPOs), health maintenance organizations (HMOs), traditional indemnity insurers, and government Medicare and Medicaid plans. Collaboration and coordination between program sponsors in a geographic area can facilitate the adoption of a common set of performance measures, reduce confusion faced by providers, and make the program more manageable for physician practices. The engagement of physicians in program design and the selection of performance measures from an early stage can increase physician buy-in. P4P may have a sustained effect in improving the quality of care if it can serve as a catalyst for changing systems of care (e.g., the use of information technology, care provided by multidisciplinary teams). However, P4P should not be viewed as a panacea. Multipronged approaches are needed to improve the quality of care.

ADDITIONAL RESOURCES

The Leapfrog Group. Incentive and reward compendium. Available at http://www.leapfroggroup.org/compendium2.

UK Quality and Outcomes Framework. Available at http://www.qof.ic.nhs.uk/.

National Quality Measures Clearinghouse. Available at http://www.qualitymeasures.ahrq.gov/.

REFERENCES

AAFP. *Pay-for-Performance*. 2010. Available from http://www.aafp.org/about/policies/all/pay-performance.html.

ACP. *Linking Physician Payments to Quality Care*. 2005. Available from http://www.acponline.org/acp_policy/policies/linking_physician_payments_quality_care_2005.pdf.

AHRQ. *U.S. Preventive Services Task Force (USPSTF)*. 2012. Available from http://www.ahrq.gov/professionals/clinicians-providers/guidelines-recommendations/uspstf/index.html.

AHRQ. *Desirable Attributes of a Quality Measure*. 2013. Available from http://www.qualitymeasures.ahrq.gov/tutorial/attributes.aspx.

Ahmed F, Elbasha EE, Thompson BL, Harris JR, Sneller VP. Cost-benefit analysis of a new HEDIS performance measure for pneumococcal vaccination. *Med Decis Making*. 2002;22(5 Suppl):S58–S66.

Ahmed F, Harris JR, Shih S, Pawlson LG. New HEDIS performance measure on influenza immunization for 50- to 64-year-old adults. *Prev Med Manag Care*. 2001;2(5):215–221.

Bach PB, Pham HH, Schrag D, Tate RC, Hargraves JL. Primary care physicians who treat blacks and whites. *N Engl J Med*. 2004;351(6):575–584.

Baker G, Delbanco S. *Provider Pay-For-Performance Incentive Programs: 2006–2007 National Study Results*. 2008. Available from http://www.medvantage.com/resources.htm.

Berwick DM. Quality of health care. Part 5: Payment by capitation and the quality of care. *N Engl J Med*. 1996;335(16):1227–1231.

Bokhour BG, Burgess JF, Jr, Hook JM, White B, Berlowitz D, Guldin MR, Meterko M, Young GJ. Incentive implementation in physician practices: A qualitative study of practice executive perspectives on pay for performance. *Med Care Res Rev*. 2006;63(1 Suppl):73S–95S.

Brush JE, Jr, Krumholz HM, Wright JS, Brindis RG, Cacchione JG, Drozda JP, Jr, Fasules JW, Flood KB, Garson A, Jr, Masoudi FA, McBride T, McKay CR, Messer JV, Mirro MJ, O'Toole MF, Peterson ED, Schaeffer JW, Valentine CM. American College of Cardiology 2006 principles to guide physician pay-for-performance programs: a report of the American College of Cardiology Work Group on Pay for Performance (A Joint Working Group of the ACC Quality Strategic Direction Committee and the ACC Advocacy Committee). *J Am Coll Cardiol.* 2006;48(12):2603–2609.

Bufalino V, Peterson ED, Burke GL, LaBresh KA, Jones DW, Faxon DP, Valadez AM, Brass LM, Fulwider VB, Smith R, Krumholz HM, Schwartz JS. Payment for quality: guiding principles and recommendations: principles and recommendations from the American Heart Association's Reimbursement, Coverage, and Access Policy Development Workgroup. *Circulation* 2006;113(8):1151–1154.

Campbell SM, McDonald R, Lester H. The experience of pay for performance in English family practice: a qualitative study. *Ann.Fam.Med.* 2008;6(3):228–234.

Campbell SM, Reeves D, Kontopantelis E, Sibbald B, Roland M. Effects of pay for performance on the quality of primary care in England. *N Engl J Med.* 2009;361(4):368–378.

Casalino LP. The unintended consequences of measuring quality on the quality of medical care. *N Engl J Med.* 1999;341(15):1147–1150.

Casalino LP, Alexander GC, Jin L, Konetzka RT. General internists' views on pay-for-performance and public reporting of quality scores: a national survey. *Health Aff. (Millwood).* 2007a;26(2):492–499.

Casalino LP, Elster A, Eisenberg A, Lewis E, Montgomery J, Ramos D. Will pay-for-performance and quality reporting affect health care disparities? *Health Aff. (Millwood).* 2007b;26(3):w405–w414.

Centers for Disease Control (CDC). 2013. *Advisory Committee on Immunization Practices (ACIP).* Available from http://www.cdc.gov/vaccines/acip/.

Chassin MR. Does paying for performance improve the quality of health care? *Med Care Res Rev.* 2006;63(1 Suppl):122S–125S.

Chaudhry B, Wang J, Wu S, Maglione M, Mojica W, Roth E, Morton SC, Shekelle PG. Systematic review: impact of health information technology on quality, efficiency, and costs of medical care. *Ann Intern Med.* 2006;144(10):742–752.

Chien AT, Chin MH, Davis AM, Casalino LP. Pay for performance, public reporting, and racial disparities in health care: how are programs being designed? *Med Care Res Rev.* 2007;64(5 Suppl):283S–304S.

Chien AT, Wroblewski K, Damberg C, Williams TR, Yanagihara D, Yakunina Y, Casalino LP. Do physician organizations located in lower socioeconomic status areas score lower on pay-for-performance measures? *J Gen Intern Med.* 2012;27(5):548–554.

Christianson JB, Leatherman S, Sutherland K. Lessons from evaluations of purchaser pay-for-performance programs: a review of the evidence. *Med.Care Res.Rev.* 2008;65(6 Suppl):5S–35S.

Donabedian A. Evaluating the quality of medical care. *Milbank Mem Fund Q.* 1966;44(3 Suppl):206.

Doran T, Fullwood C, Gravelle H, Reeves D, Kontopantelis E, Hiroeh U, Roland M. Pay-for-performance programs in family practices in the United Kingdom. *N Engl J Med.* 2006;355(4):375–384.

Doran T, Fullwood C, Kontopantelis E, Reeves D. Effect of financial incentives on inequalities in the delivery of primary clinical care in England: analysis of clinical activity indicators for the quality and outcomes framework. *Lancet* 2008;372(9640):728–736.

Doran T, Roland M. Lessons from major initiatives to improve primary care in the United kingdom. *Health Aff. (Millwood).* 2010;29(5):1023–1029.

Dudley RA, Frolich A, Robinowitz DL, Talavera JA, Broadhead P, Luft HS. *Strategies to Support Quality-Based Purchasing: A Review of the Evidence Summary, Technical Review 10.* (Prepared by the Stanford-University of California San Francisco Evidence-based Practice Center under Contract No. 290-02-0017). AHRQ Pub. No. 04-0057. Rockville, MD: Agency for Healthcare Research and Quality; 2004.

Dudley RA, Rosenthal MB. *Pay for Performance: A Decision Guide for Purchasers.* AHRQ Pub. No. 06-0047. Rockville, MD: Agency for Healthcare Research and Quality; 2006.

Eijkenaar F. Key issues in the design of pay for performance programs. *Eur J Health Econ.* 2013;14(1):117–131.

Friedberg MW, Safran DG, Coltin K, Dresser M, Schneider EC. Paying for performance in primary care: potential impact on practices and disparities. *Health Aff. (Millwood).* 2010;29(5):926–932.

Frolich A, Talavera JA, Broadhead P, Dudley RA. A behavioral model of clinician responses to incentives to improve quality. *Health Policy* 2007;80(1):179–193.

Galvin RS. Evaluating the performance of pay for performance. *Med Care Res Rev.* 2006;63(1) Suppl:126S–130S.

Hodgson ES, Simpson L, Lannon CM. Principles for the development and use of quality measures. *Pediatrics* 2008;121(2):411–418.

Institute of Medicine. *Medicare, A Strategy for Quality Assurance.* Volume 1. Washington, DC: National Academies Press; 1990.

Institute of Medicine. *To Err is Human: Building a Safer Health System.* Washington, DC: National Academies Press; 1999.

Institute of Medicine. *Crossing the Quality Chasm: A New Health System for the 21st Century.* Washington, DC: National Academies Press; 2001.

Institute of Medicine. *Rewarding Provider Performance: Aligning Incentives in Medicare.* Washington, DC: National Academies Press; 2006.

Mandel KE, Kotagal UR. Pay for performance alone cannot drive quality. *Arch Pediatr Adolesc Med.* 2007;161(7):650–655.

Maynard A. The powers and pitfalls of payment for performance. *Health Econ.* 2012;21(1):3–12.

McDonald R, Roland M. Pay for performance in primary care in England and California: comparison of unintended consequences. *Ann Fam Med.* 2009;7(2):121–127.

McDonald R, White J, Marmor TR. Paying for performance in primary medical care: learning about and learning from "success" and "failure" in England and California. *J Health Polit Policy Law.* 2009;34(5):747–776.

McGlynn EA, Asch SM, Adams J, Keesey J, Hicks J, DeCristofaro A, Kerr EA. The quality of health care delivered to adults in the United States. *N Engl J Med.* 2003;348(26):2635–2645.

Medder JD, Kahn NB Jr, Susman JL. Risk factors and recommendations for 230 adult primary care patients, based on U.S. Preventive Services Task Force guidelines. *Am J Prev Med.* 1992;8(3):150–153.

Mehrotra A, Pearson SD, Coltin KL, Kleinman KP, Singer JA, Rabson B, Schneider EC. The response of physician groups to P4P incentives. *Am J Manag Care.* 2007;13(5):249–255.

Perez-Stable EJ, Sabogal F, Otero-Sabogal R, Hiatt RA, McPhee SJ. Misconceptions about cancer among Latinos and Anglos. *JAMA.* 1992;268(22):3219–3223.

Petersen LA, Woodard LD, Urech T, Daw C, Sookanan S. Does pay-for-performance improve the quality of health care? *Ann Intern Med.* 2006;145(4):265–272.

Robinson JC. Theory and practice in the design of physician payment incentives. *Milbank Q.* 2001;79(2):149–177, III.

Robinson JC, Shortell SM, Li R, Casalino LP, Rundall T. The alignment and blending of payment incentives within physician organizations. *Health Serv Res.* 2004;39(5):1589–1606.

Roland M. Linking physicians' pay to the quality of care—a major experiment in the United Kingdom. *N Engl J Med.* 2004;351(14):1448–1454.

Rosenthal MB, Dudley RA. Pay-for-performance: will the latest payment trend improve care? *JAMA.* 2007;297(7):740–744.

Rosenthal MB, Frank RG. What is the empirical basis for paying for quality in health care? *Med Care Res Rev.* 2006;63(2):135–157.

Rosenthal MB, Landon BE, Howitt K, Song HR, Epstein AM. Climbing up the pay-for-performance learning curve: where are the early adopters now? *Health Aff. (Millwood).* 2007;26(6):1674–1682.

Rosenthal MB, Landon BE, Normand SL, Frank RG, Epstein AM. Pay for performance in commercial HMOs. *N Engl J Med.* 2006;355(18):1895–1902.

Scott A, Sivey P, Ait OD, Willenberg L, Naccarella L, Furler J, Young D. The effect of financial incentives on the quality of health care provided by primary care physicians. 2011. *Cochrane Database Syst Rev.,* no. 9:CD008451.

Snyder L, Neubauer RL. Pay-for-performance principles that promote patient-centered care: an ethics manifesto. *Ann Intern Med.* 2007;147(11):792–794.

Szilagyi PG, Shone LP, Barth R, Kouides RW, Long C, Humiston SG, Jennings J, Bennett NM. Physician practices and attitudes regarding adult immunizations. *Prev Med.* 2005;40(2):152–161.

Timmins N. Do GPs deserve their recent pay rise? *BMJ* 2005;331(7520):800.

Trude S, Au M, Christianson JB. Health plan pay-for-performance strategies. *Am J Manag Care* 2006;12(9):537–542.

Van Herck P, De Smedt D, Annemans L, Remmen R, Rosenthal MB, Sermeus W. Systematic review: Effects, design choices, and context of pay-for-performance in health care. *BMC Health Serv Res.* 2010;10:247.

Werner RM, Asch DA. Clinical concerns about clinical performance measurement. *Ann Fam Med* 2007;5(2):159–163.

Young GJ, Burgess JF, Jr, White B. Pioneering pay-for-quality: lessons from the rewarding results demonstrations. *Health Care Financ.Rev.* 2007;29(1):59–70.

Young GJ, White B, Burgess JF, Jr, Berlowitz D, Meterko M, Guldin MR, Bokhour BG. Conceptual issues in the design and implementation of pay-for-quality programs. *Am J Med Qual.* 2005;20(3):144–150.

10

Provider and Office-Based Approaches to Prevention in Primary Care

SHERRI N. SHEINFELD GORIN

This Chapter explores a potentially transformative model of primary care practice, the Patient Centered Medical Home (PCMH), and the coordination of care, which is one of its core principles. In this Chapter, two approaches that facilitate the sharing of evidence to support the aims of the PCMH—practice facilitation and academic detailing—are examined, alongside provider assessment and feedback, learning collaboratives, and medical informatics to improve prevention practice in primary care.

THE PATIENT-CENTERED MEDICAL HOME (PCMH)

The patient-centered medical home (PCMH) is a model of primary care transformation that seeks to organize and deliver primary health care that is patient- and family-centered, comprehensive, coordinated, accessible, and structured to continuously improve quality and safety (AHRQ, 2011; Agency for Healthcare Research and Quality, 2011; Scholle, Torda, Peikes, Han, Genevro, 2010; Moreno, Peikes, Krilla, 2010; Stange et al., 2010).

The term "medical home" was first used by the American Academy of Pediatrics in 1967 to describe the concept of a single centralized source of care and medical record for children with special health care needs (Sia, Tonniges, Osterhus, & Taba, 2004). In 2004, the "Future of Family Medicine" report (Martin, Avant, Bowman, et al., 2004) detailed the "New Model of Family Medicine" (Green, Graham, Bagley, et al., 2004; Nutting, Miller, Crabtree, Jaen, Stewart, & Stange, 2009), helping to initiate the national conversations leading to the PCMH. The National Demonstration Project (NDP) was launched in June 2006 by the American Academy of Family Physicians (TransforMED, 2009) to test this new model; the NDP was subsequently updated to be consistent with the emerging consensus principles of the PCMH, as described later in this Chapter (Patient-Centered Primary Care Collaborative, 2009). The 40 years of efforts since the late 1960s to redesign primary care to improve quality, along with the concepts of the chronic care model (CCM; Wagner et al., 2001), have greatly enlarged the concept of the PCMH (Kilo, Wasson, 2010; Carrier, Gourevitch, & Shah, 2009).

As described in Chapter 3, the Chronic Care Model (CCM; Wagner, Austin, & Von Korff, 1996; Wagner, Glasgow, Davis, et al., 2001; Wagner, Austin, David, Hindmarsh, Shaefer, & Bonomi, 2001) is a conceptual model for organizing systems of health care for quality improvement in chronic illnesses; the CCM is associated with improved health outcomes and is the cornerstone of PCMH (McDonald, Sundaram, Bravata, et al., 2007). The CCM rests on the following assumption: high-quality chronic illness care is characterized by productive interactions between the practice team and patients that consistently provide the assessments, support for self-management, optimization of therapy, and follow-up associated with good outcomes. The CCM includes six elements: (1) self-management support; (2) delivery system design; (3) decision support; (4) clinical information systems; (5) organized health care system; and (6) community resources and policies (Wagner, Austin, & Von Korff, 1996; Wagner, Glasgow, Davis, et al., 2001). The CCM has been used by more than 100 health organizations in collaborative quality improvement activities (Wagner, Austin, Davis, Hindmarsh, Schaefer, & Bonomi, 2001). Interventions based on the chronic care model (CCM) and focused on single conditions such as diabetes mellitus, asthma, chronic obstructive pulmonary disease, or depression have been shown to improve patient outcomes and/or quality of care (Adams, Smith, Allan et al., 2007; Bodenheimer, Wagner, & Grumbach, 2002; Coleman, Austin, Brach, et al., 2009; Tsai, Morton, Mangione, et al., 2005). The PCMH builds on the CCM model and is intended to address the full range of patient-focused health care needs (Agency for Healthcare Research and Quality, Patient Centered Medical Home Resource Center, 2011; http://effectivehealthcare.ahrq.gov/index.cfm/search-for-guides-reviews-and-reports/?produ ctid=1177&pageaction=displayproduct).

The core principles of the PCMH are the following: wide-ranging, team-based care; patient-centered orientation toward the whole person; care that is coordinated across all elements of the health care system and the patient's community; enhanced access to care that uses alternative methods of communication; and a systems-based approach to quality and safety (Scholle, Torda, Peikes, Han, & Genevro, 2010). In February 2007, the four major primary care physician associations, representing over 300,000 physicians, endorsed the Joint Principles of the Patient-Centered Medical Home, including the American Academy of Family Physicians (AAFP), the American Academy of Pediatrics (AAP), the American College of Physicians (ACP), and the American Osteopathic Association (AOA).

The Joint Principles (http://www.pcpcc.net/content/joint-principles-patient-centered-medical-home) include:

- Each patient has an ongoing relationship with a personal physician trained to provide first contact, continuous and comprehensive care.
- The personal physician leads a team of individuals who collectively take responsibility for the ongoing care of each patient.
- The personal physician is responsible for providing all the patient's health care needs or taking responsibility for appropriately arranging care with other qualified professionals. This includes care for all stages of life, acute care, chronic care, preventive services, and end-of-life care.
- Care is coordinated and/or integrated: care is coordinated across all elements of the complex health care system (e.g., subspecialty care, hospitals, home health agencies, nursing homes) and the patient's community (e.g., family, public and private community-based

services). Care is facilitated by registries, information technology, health information exchange, and other means to assure that patients get the indicated care when and where they need and want it in a culturally and linguistically appropriate manner.

Quality and safety are ensured through the following:

- Practices advocate for their patients to support the attainment of optimal, patient-centered outcomes that are defined by a care-planning process driven by a compassionate, robust partnership between physicians, patients, and the patient's family.
- Evidence-based medicine and clinical decision-support tools guide decision making.
- Physicians are accountable for continuous quality improvement through voluntary engagement in performance measurement and improvement.
- Patients actively participate in decision making, and feedback is sought to ensure that patients' expectations are being met.
- Information technology is utilized appropriately to support optimal patient care, performance measurement, patient education, and enhanced communication.
- Practices go through a voluntary recognition process by an appropriate non-governmental entity to demonstrate that they have the capabilities to provide patient-centered services consistent with the medical home model.
- Patients and families participate in quality improvement activities at the practice level.
- Enhanced access to care is available through systems such as open scheduling, expanded hours, and new options for communication between patients, their personal physician, and practice staff.

Payment recognizes the added value provided to patients who have a patient-centered medical home, and should be based on the following framework:

- Reflect the value of physician and non-physician staff patient-centered care management work that falls outside the face-to-face visit.

- Pay for services associated with coordination of care both within a given practice and between consultants, ancillary providers, and community resources.
- Support the adoption and use of health information technology for quality improvement.
- Support the provision of enhanced communication access, such as secure e-mail and telephone consultation (review in: Car, Gurol-Urganci, de Jongh, Vodopivec-Jamsek, & Atun, 2012).
- Recognize the value of physician work associated with remote monitoring of clinical data using technology.
- Allow for separate fee-for-service payments for face-to-face visits. (Payments for care management services that fall outside the face-to-face visit, as described above, should not result in a reduction in the payments for face-to-face visits.)
- Recognize case mix differences in the patient population that is being treated within the practice.
- Allow physicians to share in savings from reduced hospitalizations associated with physician-guided care management in the office setting.
- Allow for additional payments for achieving measurable and continuous quality improvements.
- Focus evaluations on quality, cost, and experience.

In 2010, to advance the adoption of the PCMH under the Affordable Care Act, the Centers for Medicare and Medicaid (CMS) launched the Multi-Payer Advanced Primary Care Practice Demonstration initiative. Under this demonstration, CMS participates in multi-payer reform initiatives (including both Medicaid and private health plans) that are currently being conducted by states to make advanced primary care (APC) practices more broadly available (including Federally Qualified Health Centers serving Medicare beneficiaries). In accord with the PCMH principles outlined previously, practices that are participating in the demonstration use a team approach to care, with the patient at the center. APC practices emphasize prevention, health information technology, care coordination, and shared decision making among patients and their providers. The goal is to improve the quality and coordination of health care services. The demonstration program pays a monthly care management fee for beneficiaries receiving primary care from APC practices. The care management fee is intended to cover care coordination, improved access, patient education, and other services to support chronically ill patients. Additionally, each participating state has mechanisms to offer APC practices community support and linkages to state health promotion and disease prevention initiatives.

The following states were selected to participate in this demonstration: Maine, Vermont, Rhode Island, New York, Pennsylvania, North Carolina, Michigan, and Minnesota. Medicare participation in three of the state's programs (Vermont, New York, and Rhode Island) started on July 1, 2011. Two additional states (North Carolina and Michigan) were effective on October 1, 2011, and the three remaining states became operational on January 1, 2012. Each state's program will be operational for 3 years. By the end of the 3-year demonstration, approximately 1,200 medical homes serving over 900,000 Medicare beneficiaries are expected to be participating (http://www.cms.gov/Medicare/ DemonstrationProjects/DemoProjectsEvalRpts/ downloads/mapcpdemo_Factsheet.pdf; Agency for Healthcare Research and Quality, 2012).

PCMH Certification

National Committee on Quality Assurance (NCQA, discussed in Chapter 2), an organization that helps to establish standards by which insurance companies monitor the quality of care, has established a PCMH certification program for practices. The NCQA's Physician Practice Connections—Patient Centered Medical Home® (PPC-PCMH) applies a scoring method to rate the level of medical home that a practice provides, alongside different levels of qualification (www.ncqa.org;). NCQA has already established physician recognition certification for a number of specific areas, including back pain, diabetes, cardiovascular disease and stroke, and physician practice connections (use of information technology). Enhanced recognition can lead to performance improvement and enhanced payment or referrals from insurance companies (www.ncqa.org; http:// www.coloradoafp.org/medical6.html#topic2).

The PPC-PCMH includes nine standards for medical practices to meet, with a total potential score of 100 (see Figures 10-1 and 10-2). Ten elements are listed as "Must Pass Elements;"

PPC-PCMH Content and Scoring

Standard 1: Access and Communication	Pts
A. **Has written standards for patient access and patient communication****	4
B. **Uses data to show it meets its standards for patient access and communication****	5
	9

Standard 2: Patient Tracking and Registry Functions	Pts
A. Uses data system for basic patient information (mostly non-clinical data)	2
B. Has clinical data system with clinical data in searchable data fields	3
C. Uses the clinical data system	3
D. **Uses paper or electronic-based charting tools to organize clinical information****	6
E. **Uses data to identify important diagnoses and conditions in practice****	4
F. Generates lists of patients and reminds patients and clinicians of services needed (population management)	3
	21

Standard 3: Care Management	Pts
A. **Adopts and implements evidence-based guidelines for three conditions ****	3
B. Generates reminders about preventive services for clinicians	4
C. Uses non-physician staff to manage patient care	3
D. Conducts care management, including care plans, assessing progress, addressing barriers	5
E. Coordinates care//follow-up for patients who receive care in inpatient and outpatient facilities	5
	20

Standard 4: Patient Self-Management Support	Pts
A. Assesses language preference and other communication barriers	2
B. **Actively supports patient self-management****	4
	6

Standard 5: Electronic Prescribing	Pts
A. Uses electronic system to write prescriptions	3
B. Has electronic prescription writer with safety checks	3
C. Has electronic prescription writer with cost checks	2
	8

Standard 6: Test Tracking	Pts
A. **Tracks tests and identifies abnormal results systematically****	7
B. Uses electronic systems to order and retrieve tests and flag duplicate tests	6
	13

Standard 7: Referral Tracking	PT
A. **Tracks referrals using paper-based or electronic system****	4
	4

Standard 8: Performance Reporting and Improvement	Pts
A. **Measures clinical and/or service performance by physician or across the practice****	3
B. Survey of patients' care experience	3
C. **Reports performance across the practice or by physician ****	3
D. Sets goals and takes action to improve performance	3
E. Produces reports using standardized measures	2
F. Transmits reports with standardized measures electronically to external entities	1
	15

Standard 9: Advanced Electronic Communications	Pts
A. Availability of Interactive Website	1
B. Electronic Patient Identification	2
C. Electronic Care Management Support	1
	4

**Must Pass Elements

FIGURE 10-1: The National Committee on Quality Assurance's (NCQA's) Physician Practice Connections—Patient Centered Medical Home® (PPC-PCMH) Content and Scoring.

PPC-PCMH Scoring

Level of Qualifying	Points	Must Pass Elements at 50% Performance Level
Level 3	75 - 100	10 of 10
Level 2	50 – 74	10 of 10
Level 1	25 – 49	5 of 10
Not Recognized	0 – 24	< 5

Levels: If there is a difference in Level achieved between the number of points and "Must Pass", the practice will be awarded the lesser level; for example, if a practice has 65 points but passes only 7 "Must Pass" Elements, the practice will achieve at Level 1.

Practices with a numeric score of 0 to 24 points or less than 5 "Must Pass" Elements do not Qualify.

FIGURE 10-2: The National Committee on Quality Assurance's (NCQA's) Physician Practice Connections—Patient Centered Medical Home® (PPC-PCMH) Scoring and Certification Levels.

practices must pass at least five of these elements. The qualification levels include: Not Recognized, Level 1, Level 2, and Level 3. To achieve Level 1 a minimum score of 25 out of 100 must be achieved. It is not clear what level will be required to qualify for additional reimbursement from insurance companies.

Four national primary care societies also provide PCMH accreditation, certification, achievement, and recognition. These include the American Academy of Family Physicians, the American Academy of Pediatrics, the American College of Physicians, and the American Osteopathic Association.

Evaluations of the PCMH

Implementation of the principles of the PCMH varies widely (Vest et al., 2010). A recent review that was conducted as part of the Agency for Healthcare Quality and Research's (AHRQ's) "Closing the Quality Gap: Revisiting the State of the Science" series (Agency for Healthcare Research and Quality, 2011) revealed that across 19 comparative studies, PCMH interventions had a small positive effect on patient experiences and small to moderate positive effects on the delivery of preventive care services (moderate strength of evidence). Staff experiences were also improved by a small to moderate degree (low strength of evidence). Evidence suggested a reduction in emergency department visits (risk ratio [RR], 0.81 [95% CI, 0.67–0.98]) but not in hospital admissions (RR, 0.96 [95% CI, 0.84–1.10]) in older adults (low strength of evidence). There was no evidence for overall cost savings. They concluded that current evidence is insufficient to determine the effects on clinical and most economic outcomes (Jackson et al., 2013).

Coordination of Care

One of the Joint Principles of the PCMH is to provide coordinated care; integrated care is complex and depends upon careful coordination among multiple treatments and providers and upon technical information exchange and regular communication flow among all of those involved in treatment, including patients, family members, specialist physicians, other specialty disciplines, primary care physicians, and support services (Fennell et al., 2010; Patient-Centered Primary Care Collaborative, http://www.pcpcc.net/node/14.). Many diseases, including cancer, in particular, involve multimodality

therapies that require the engagement of multiple primary and subspecialty physicians, other health care professionals, family, and even community organizations, which often provide support during and after treatment and deliver hospice care at end of life (Ballard-Barbash, 2010; Han & Rayson, 2010).

The challenges to the health care system of coordinating patient care across multiple organizational levels and the full range of tasks, conditions, services, providers, and sites of care over time require changes in the design, dissemination, implementation, and maintenance of care processes, policies, and payment systems (IOM, 2001). Yet, evidence for the effectiveness of care coordination models at the interfaces of public and private health care systems and between primary and specialty care is limited (Ballard-Barbash, 2010; Taplin & Rodgers, 2010; Fennell et al., 2010; Hesse et al., 2010).

Definitions of Care Coordination

A recent systematic review identified more than 40 definitions of coordination of care (Care Coordination Atlas (*Atlas*; McDonald et al., 2007, 2010). The authors concluded with the following general definition:

> Care coordination is the deliberate organization of patient care activities between two or more participants (including the patient) involved in a patient's care to facilitate the appropriate delivery of health care services. Organizing care involves the marshalling of personnel and other resources needed to carry out all required patient care activities and is often managed by the exchange of information among participants responsible for different aspects of care.

Best Practices in Care Coordination

In 2000, Mathematica assessed the best practices of coordinated care among the Medicare Fee For Service (FFS) programs nationally. They restricted their search to programs with evidence of reductions in hospital admissions (the costliest Medicare-covered service) or in total medical costs, and to programs serving adults with chronic, systemic illness or providing true care coordination (not, for example, medical devices or programs for wound care). They interviewed a selected subset to assess the reasons for their program's success (http://www.mathematica mpr.com/publications/pdfs/bestpractices.pdf;http://www.ahrq.gov/downloads/pub/evidence/pdf/caregap/caregap.pdf).

According to their findings, best practices in care coordination include:

1. Programs that follow three steps (Assess and Plan, Implement and Deliver, Reassess and Adjust) for all enrolled patients.
   - Step one concludes with a written plan of care.
   - Step two includes the establishment of an ongoing care coordinator-patient relationship, and the provision of excellent patient education.
   - Step three includes a periodic reassessment of patients' progress.
2. Programs have expressed goals of the prevention of health problems and crises, and of early problem detection and intervention (a proactive approach, in other words).
3. Disease-specific programs incorporate national evidence-based or consensus-based guidelines into their interventions.
4. Care coordinators are nurses with at least a bachelor's degree in nursing.
5. Programs have significant experience in care coordination and demonstrate evidence of having reduced hospital use or total medical costs.

As discussed later in this Chapter, Health Information Technology (HIT) can play an important role in the coordination of care among patients and providers, as well as among providers.

Measures of Care Coordination

As discussed previously, the Atlas was developed to help evaluators identify appropriate measures for assessing care coordination interventions in research studies and demonstration projects, particularly those measures focusing on care coordination in ambulatory care. The Atlas includes measures of patient and caregiver experiences with care coordination, as well as experiences of health care professionals and health system managers. In the *Atlas*, measures were mapped to domains, or mechanisms for achieving coordination, including coordination activities (e.g., establish accountability or negotiate responsibility, communicate, facilitate transitions, assess needs and goals) and broad approaches (e.g., teamwork focused on coordination and medication management). Measurement perspectives included those of the patient/family (e.g., reports of satisfaction with coordination of care), the health care professional (e.g., nurses' reports of confusion or hassle in time spent coordinating referrals), and system representatives (e.g., developing a system to post reminders to patients and providers when a follow-up examination is due). While measurement characteristics vary considerably, as do findings on their implementation in US clinical settings, many of the measures are robust and are relevant to advancing preventive care.

Evaluations of Care Coordination

To determine whether varied care coordination programs reduced hospitalizations and Medicare expenditures and improved quality of care for chronically ill Medicare beneficiaries, Peikes et al. (2009) conducted a two-arm randomized contolled trial. Participants were eligible, volunteer Medicare FFS patients diagnosed, in the main, with congestive heart failure, coronary artery disease, and diabetes. Their usual health care sites were among the 15 that were participating in a national care coordination demonstration project (i.e., under the Medicare Coordinated Care Demonstration ([MCCD]). Each participant was assigned at random to a treatment or control care coordination program using a variety of models.

Although patients in the treatment group reported more help arranging care than those in the comparison condition, vaccinations and routine preventive services did not differ between the two groups. Thirteen of 15 sites implementing care coordination programs failed to show differences in hospitalizations. Elements of the two more successful programs included more frequent in-person contact with the care coordinator, a patient mix with neither too low risk nor too seriously ill patients, ability to teach patients how to take their medications, ability of the care coordinators to work closely with local hospitals and interact frequently (and informally) with treating physicians (Peikes, 2009). This study concluded that these 15 programs had favorable effects on none of the outcomes measured, and few of the included quality of care indicators. The findings of this trial across several chronic diseases highlight the importance of substantial in-person contact, and programs that target moderate to severe patients for both cost neutrality and benefit.

By contrast, initial findings from a systematic review and meta-analysis of cancer care coordination in the United States and Canada that includes studies published between 1980 and 2013 reveal that cancer care coordination interventions led to improvements in over two-thirds of outcomes including screening, patient experiences with care, and quality of end-of-life care. In a meta-analysis of a subset of these studies, cancer care coordination interventions were almost twice as efficacious in promoting desired outcomes as comparable interventions. The literature on cancer care coordination is heterogeneous, but available studies suggest a strong and robust effect of cancer care coordination on improving health outcomes in varied settings across the cancer care continuum (Sheinfeld Gorin et al., 2013a, 2013b).

ACADEMIC DETAILING

One promising physician-directed intervention, academic detailing (AD), focuses primarily on disseminating information to providers to enable them to improve the care that they provide to their patients (Avorn & Soumerai, 1983; Soumerai & Avorn, 1990). Traditionally employed by pharmaceutical companies to promote prescription drug uptake among physicians, academic detailing programs began by providing patient-oriented materials to help patients understand why their doctor was not recommending an antibiotic for common cold symptoms (Fischer, 2012).

Academic detailing rests on three major understandings of primary care practice:

- Better medical care is given when physicians follow the best available evidence.
- There are more data available than physicians have time to keep up with on their own.
- Delivering useful and reliable information via one-on-one customized encounters offers the best opportunity for physicians to be able to apply key evidence directly into their practices.

At its core, AD is about basing medical decisions on the best available (impartial) evidence (Fischer, 2012). In practice, academic detailing starts with evidence derived from clinical research, evidence reviews, published guidelines, or other credible and unbiased sources. The evidence is distilled into compact and practical messages that can be delivered to front-line clinicians in a usable format. Academic detailers (often physicians or nurses) tailor the messages to the providers' needs.

The multicomponent AD intervention also includes techniques and tools that address office-based barriers to screening (Dickey, Gemson, & Carney, 1999; Hulscher, Wensing, van der Weijden, & Grol, 2002). These include physician reminders (e.g., chart flags, manual or computerized reminder systems; Austin & Balas, 1994; Curry & Emmons, 1994) and multilingual, low-literacy patient education materials (Pignone, Harris, 2000; Chan & Kaufman, 2011) to change prevention practices in the office.

From the perspective of behavioral science, this timely (Hensley, 2006) intervention approach is uniquely suited to identifying and moderating the pragmatic barriers to change identified in primary care practices. In particular, outreach visits and the provision of evidence (rather than opinion) are critical to change through AD. The provision of information in response to specific physician queries, a critical aspect of academic detailing, is consonant with general understandings of the clinical problem-solving approaches used by physicians (Burke, 1982).

To encourage the practice of prevention, academic detailing seeks to change physicians' attitudes and beliefs toward the behavior (e.g., screening) through persuasive communications, and to alter their cognitions though tailored feedback and reinforcement. Concomitantly, a prevention-oriented office context (e.g., through trained staff) and cues in office procedures (e.g., flagged medical charts) enrich the physician's memory for new information and reinforce behavioral patterns (Bouton, 2000; see Figure 10-3 and Table 10-1).

Digital Detailing

Of late, academic detailing with face-to-face contact has been supplemented with digital detailing. Digital detailing has been tested via the Internet and CD-ROMs. In a study of digital detailing components, we developed a set of four standardized patient cases that were delivered to primary care providers via a web-accessible CD-ROM. Each patient case contained one or more of the structural, testing, or normative barriers to CRC screening, alongside physician response choices. The CD-ROM was designed to provide feedback to the PCP around

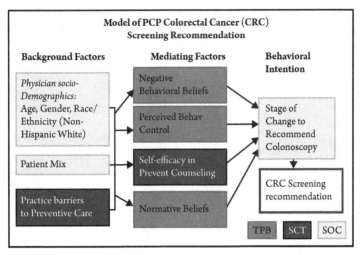

FIGURE 10-3: Model of Primary Care Provider Colorectal Cancer Screening Recommendations.

Note: TPB: Theory of Planned Behavior; SCT: Social Cognitive Theory; SOC: Stages of Change (Trans-theoretical Model)

Source: Honda K, Sheinfeld Gorin S. A model of stage of change to recommend colonoscopy among urban primary care physicians. *Health Psychology.* 2006;25:65–73. Reproduced with permission

---

TABLE 10-1. SUMMARY OF THEORETICAL CONSTRUCTS AND ACADEMIC DETAILING INTERVENTION COMPONENTS

Reinforcement and improvement of behavioral capacities (knowledge & skills), outcome expectancies, self-efficacy	Multiple approaches, skills training and mastery, specific changes in small steps, model positive outcomes
Pros and cons of screening, social norms, perceived behavioral control in patient care	Stage-tailored feedback: barriers, screening performance, goal-setting
Reinforcement, cues to action	Office-based, patient-oriented tools, procedures

---

how to address these barriers to change, using scientific evidence, clinical advice from our physician advisory board, and relevant theory (Chapter 3; see Figures 10-4 to 10-10; Honda & Sheinfeld Gorin, 2006). As detailed in Figure 10-4, each case began with archetypal patients who expressed their presenting problems, structural (e.g., financial), testing (e.g., embarrassment), or normative barriers (e.g., limited support from family) to colorectal cancer screening. The primary care physician was presented with several response choices to each patient. In Figure 10-5, at a brief "decision point," the physician was asked to select an answer that reflected his or her realistic response to the archetypal patient. In Figure 10-6, at the "response evaluation," the physician's response to the archetypal patient was rated on how informative, responsive, and appropriate it is. The "expansion of the decision point" is illustrated in Figure 10-7. With a "click," the physician could expand the decision point to obtain additional information on the patient, to assist with his or her decision making; for example, the patient's pedigree is presented in Figure 10-7. Access to numerous online (and printable) resources (for the physician, the team, and patients and families) was provided to assist with decision making. The home page for the study of informed decision making for prostate cancer screening that is illustrated in Figure 10-8 used web-based digital detailing only, without any face-to-face contacts. Each of these cases varied along the unique barriers to prostate cancer screening (including cultural competence). Figure 10-10 shows the front page of a web-based program (password-accessible) for primary care physicians to explore HPV inoculation with adolescents and young adults.

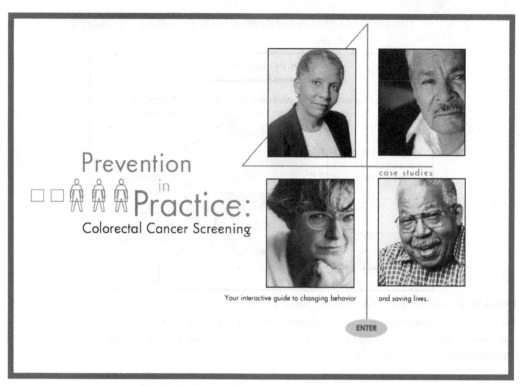

FIGURE 10-4: Digital Detailing for Colorectal Cancer Screening via a Web-Accessible CD-ROM.

Note: Each of four archetypal patient cases contained one or more of the structural, testing, or normative barriers to screening, alongside physician response choices.

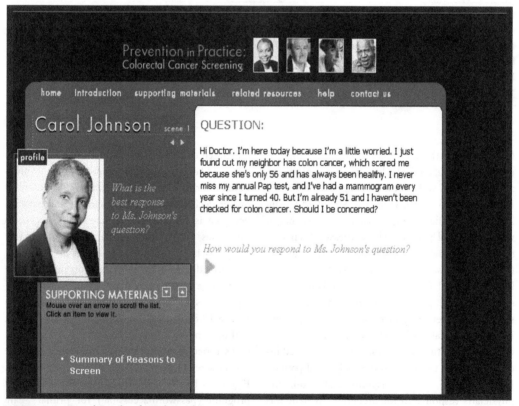

FIGURE 10-5: Digital Detailing for Colorectal Cancer Screening: Decision Point.

Note: At a brief "decision point," the physician is asked to select an answer that reflects his or her realistic response to the archetypal patient.

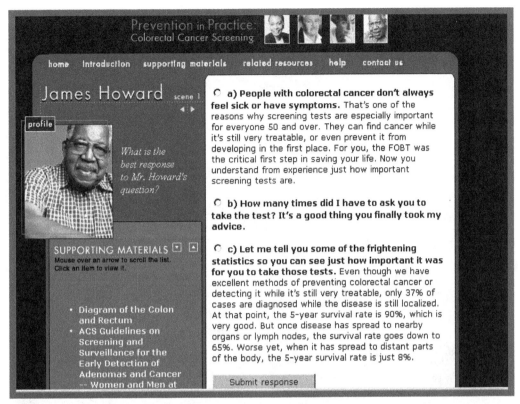

FIGURE 10-6: Digital Detailing for Colorectal Cancer Screening: Response Evaluation.

Note: The physician's response to the archetypal patient is also rated on how informative, responsive, and appropriate it is.

Evaluation of Academic Detailing

We evaluated the four cases in Figures 10-4 to 10-9 for face validity with a series of patient focus groups, then physician focus groups. We looked at the impact of the multi-component AD program for primary care physicians to evaluate colorectal cancer screening with patients at 12-months post-randomization. More than one-half (58%) of the intervention primary care physicians (PCPs) reported that the CD-ROM assisted them in counseling for colorectal cancer screening with patients, (Shankaran, Bennett, Graff Zivin, Scoppettone, & Sheinfeld Gorin, 2009).

Usability testing of the web-based program for primary care physicians to explore shared/informed decision making for prostate cancer screening (see Figures 10-8 and 10-9) revealed favorable usability for this interactive educational program among PCPs. The program was used as intended, read from the introduction to the cases, then resource materials. Overall, the program was used quite rapidly, with limited and rapid downloading of optional resource pages. Two scientific articles were downloaded most frequently. The most often accessed resource was the page on cultural competence (see Figure 10-9), suggesting the overall importance of providing easily accessible full-text high-impact publications, culturally relevant materials and approaches for prostate cancer screening, particularly to primary care physicians working in low resource communities (Sheinfeld Gorin, Franco, Hajiani, & Senathirajah, 2007).

More generally, Academic Detailing has consistently demonstrated physician breast, cervical, and colorectal cancer screening of patients in inceased accord with professional guidelines, as well as change in vaccination practices across a number of systematic reviews (Briss, Rodewald, Hinman, Shefer, Stirkas, Bernier, Carande-Kulis, Yusuf, Ndiaye, Williams, & the Task Force on Community Preventive Services, 2000; Hulscher, Wensing, van der Weijden, & Grol, 2002; Walsh & McPhee, 1992). These findings have

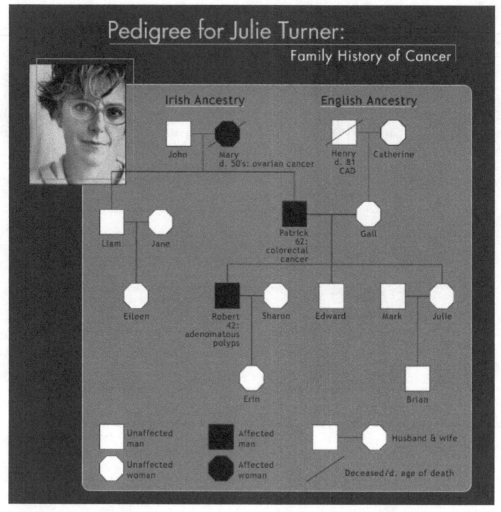

FIGURE 10-7: Digital Detailing for Colorectal Cancer Screening: Expansion of the Decision Point.

Note: With a "click," the physician may expand the decision point to obtain additional information on the patient, for example, a family pedigree, to assist with his or her decision making. Access to online (and printable) resources (for physician or patient and families) is provided to assist with decision making.

been reported in our own rigorous randomized clinical trials as well (Ashford, Gemson, Sheinfeld Gorin, et al., 2000; Sheinfeld Gorin, Gemson, Ashford, et al., 2000; Sheinfeld Gorin, Ashford, Lantigua, et al., 2007; Sheinfeld Gorin, Ashford, Lantigua, et al., 2007; Sheinfeld Gorin et al., 2002; Sheinfeld Gorin, Graff Zivin, & NYPAC Study Group, 2003; Sheinfeld Gorin, Glenn, & Perkins, 2011; Shankaran, Bennett, Graff Zivin, Scoppettone, & Sheinfeld Gorin, 2009; Sheinfeld Gorin, Ashford, Lantigua, Hossain, et al., 2006; Sheinfeld Gorin, Franco, Westhoff, & NYPAC Study Group, 2006;

Sheinfeld Gorin, Wang, Raich, Bowen, Hay, 2006). The effects of multicomponent AD on increasing cancer screening have also been sustained over time (Dietrich et al., 1994).

While some findings on AD for quality improvement purposes have been mixed (Hulscher, Wensing, van der Weijden, & Grol, 2002) due to under-resourced approaches (Ganz et al., 2005), Academic Detailing, alongside patient intervention, has demonstrated modest (but statistically non-significant) effects on increased colorectal cancer screening among health plan members in

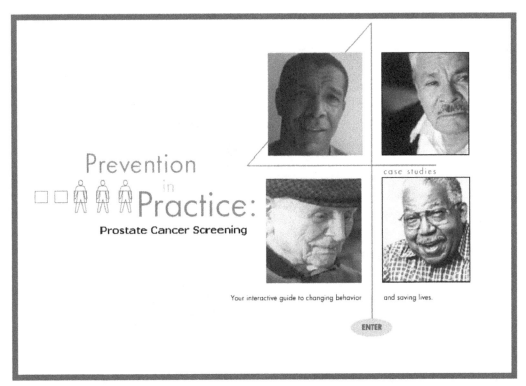

FIGURE 10-8: Digital Detailing for Prostate Cancer Shared/Informed Decision Making and Screening.

Note: This program was delivered via a password-accessible website.

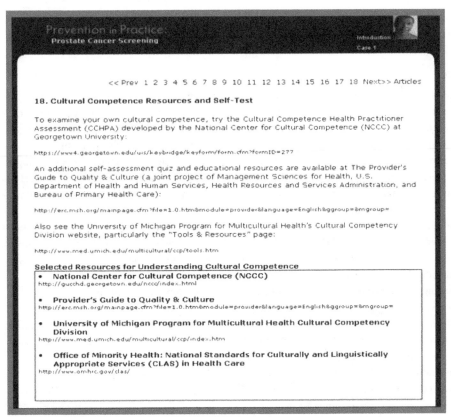

FIGURE 10-9: Digital Detailing for Prostate Cancer Shared/Informed Decision Making and Screening, Page on Cultural Competence.

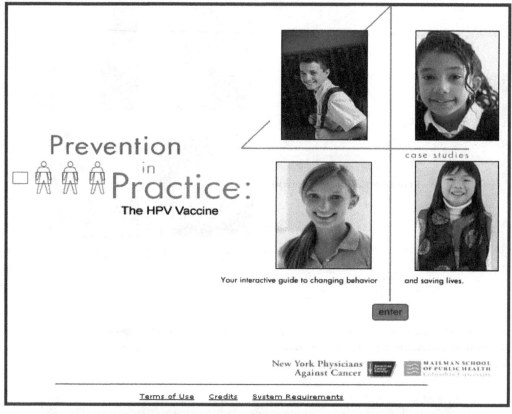

FIGURE 10-10: Digital Detailing for Inoculation with the Human Papillomavirus (HPV) Vaccine.

Note: This program is delivered via a password-accessible website.

two states (Pignone, Winquist, Schild, et al., 2011). The most recent study results on AD changing formulary ordering practices have been uniformly positive, however (Simon et al., 2005; Solomon et al., 2001; Simon et al., 2006; Van der Elst et al., 2006).

At present, there are several large US, Canadian, and Australian nationwide programs relying on academic detailing designed to change formulary ordering practices (State of Pennsylvania; New York State Medicaid Prescriber Education Program; Canadian Academic Detailing Collaboration; NPSMedicineWise), preventive behaviors such as smoking cessation (City of New York), and country-wide to increase shared decision making for prostate cancer screening among PCPs (Australia), as well as to increase evidence-based treatments (particularly pharmacologic) within the Veterans Administration San Diego Health Care System (VA Academic Detailing Service; Lehmann, 2012). While some findings are still emerging, based on the findings to date, the evidence is strong enough to recommend multicomponent academic detailing for

breast and colorectal cancer screening, particularly in medically underserved areas. Further, the effectiveness of multicomponent academic detailing on physician behavior change compares favorably with other physician-directed intervention approaches in health care such as Continuing Medical Education (Bloom et al., 2005) and reducing clinical inertia (Sperl-Hillen, et al., 2000; O'Connor, 2005).

To further advance the dissemination of academic detailing, partnerships with the following entities are promising:

- Departments of Health;
- Quality Improvement Organizations (QIOs);
- Area Health Education Centers (AHECs);
- HITECH Regional Extension Centers (RECs);
- Practice-based research networks (PBRNs);
- Primary care associations (PCAs);
- Accountable care organizations (ACOs);
- Chartered value exchanges (CVEs);
- Large health care systems;

- Medicare (pay-for-performance);
- Malpractice insurance providers;
- Union-based benefit plans (e.g., 1199SEIU Funds).

These partners, alongside emerging new systems of primary care practice, can provide a number of organizational opportunities for the establishment of academic detailing programs to help physicians and other health care professionals deploy the best possible evidence in day-to-day practice (Avorn, 2012).

PRACTICE FACILITATION

Facilitators, also known as quality improvement coaches, assist practices with coordinating their quality improvement activities and help to build capacity for those activities, potentially enhancing system-wide quality, safety, and the implementation of evidence-based practices. Coaches also enhance direct patient care by coordinating care and helping patients navigate the system, improving access for patients, and communicating across the care team. These important, complementary roles aim to help primary care practices deliver coordinated, accessible, comprehensive, and patient-centered care (Taylor, 2012, 2013).

Specifically, practice facilitators are specially trained individuals who work with primary care practices "to make meaningful changes designed to improve patients' outcomes. [Practice Facilitators] help physicians and improvement teams develop the skills they need to adapt clinical evidence to the specific circumstance of their practice environment" (DeWalt, Powell, Mainwaring, et al., 2010; Nagykaldi Z, Mold JW, & Aspy CB. 2005).

Practice facilitation models have been widely implemented, notably in North Carolina's Statewide Quality Improvement Program, through an AHEC (http://www.ncahec.net/pubs/newsletters/2012_Winter/duke_endowment.html), and in the Oklahoma Health Care Authority and Practice-Based Research Networks: Oklahoma (http://www.okhca.org/research.aspx?id=88&parts=7447 and http://www.okhca.org/WorkArea/linkit.aspx?LinkIdentifier=id&ItemID=13379).

Emerging best practices in practice facilitation include:

- Creating key-driver models to identify activities and strategies to reach desired outcomes. These help to maintain a focus on high-yield activities.

- Using a variety of Quality Improvement approaches. James Mold, University of Oklahoma (2012), suggests that "[p]ractice facilitation should occur in the context of other efforts and strategies such as payment reform, benchmarking, and academic detailing."
- Determining the stages of practice facilitation intervention.
- Deciding on dose and delivery.
- Selecting onsite versus distance practice facilitation delivery.

Regarding the recruitment and hiring of practice facilitators, best practices have emerged around:

- Looking for core competencies in practice facilitators.
- Facilitating interpersonal and project management skills.
- Seeking competencies in acquiring and using data to drive improvement and transformation, quality improvement methods, and those needed for specific interventions.
- Selecting a staffing model that includes hiring facilitators as program employees; internal employees of the practice; contracting with consultants; or even using volunteers as facilitators.
- Assessing the different roles in redesigning and improving care delivery provided by practice facilitators and care managers.

Evaluations of Practice Facilitation

Several rigorous evaluations have been conducted of practice facilitation, notably in the context of implementing and assessing PCMHs. A recent meta-analysis of studies of practice facilitation within primary care settings concluded that primary care practices are almost three times as likely to adopt evidence-based guidelines through practice facilitation compared with no-intervention control group practices, however (Baskerville, Liddy, Hogg, 2012).

According to a recent systematic review, practice facilitation has a moderately robust effect of 0.56 (95% CI, 0.43–0.68); primary care practices are 2.76 (95% CI, 2.18–3.43) times more likely to adopt evidence-based guidelines through practice facilitation relative to control group practices. Evidence-based guideline adoption within primary care was influenced by tailoring, the number of practices per facilitator, and the intensity of the intervention; these modifications of practice facilitation have resource implications (Baskerville, Liddy, & Hogg, 2012).

In a qualitative analysis, the National Demonstration Project (NDP) of practices' transition to PCMHs looked at the impact of practice facilitation on practice redesign among early adopter practices and found that facilitation increased the practices' capability to make and sustain change and increased organizational capacity to adopt new methods and service models, compared to non-facilitated practices (Nutting et al., 2010). This study was followed by a systematic comparative analysis of patient outcomes in the NDP. In 2006, a total of 36 family practices were randomized to facilitated or self-directed intervention groups. Progress toward the PCMH was measured by independent assessments of how many of 39 NDP model components the practices adopted. Two types of patient outcomes were assessed: (1) patient-rated (patient empowerment, general health status, and satisfaction with the service relationship); (2) condition-specific, using measures of the quality of care from the Ambulatory Care Quality Alliance (ACQA) Starter Set (for example, tobacco use, drug therapy for lowering LDL cholesterol, drug therapy for lowering LDL cholesterol; http://www.ahrq.gov/qual/aqastart.htm) and other measures of delivery of clinical preventive services and chronic disease care. While all practices adopted substantial numbers of NDP components over 26 months, facilitated practices adopted significantly more new components on average than self-directed practices. Ambulatory Care Quality

Alliance (ACQA) scores improved significantly over time in both groups, as did chronic care scores, with no significant differences between groups. There were no improvements in patient-rated outcomes. In sum, after slightly more than 2 years, implementation of PCMH components, whether by facilitation or practice self-direction, was associated with small improvements in condition-specific quality of care but not patient experience. Thus, PCMH models that call for practice change without altering the broader delivery system may not achieve their intended results, at least in the short term (Nutting, Crabtree, Miller, Stewart, Stange, & Jaén, 2010).

Model of Practice Change

The practice facilitation approach, although generally atheoretical, shares many of its components with the chronic care model as discussed earlier and in Chapter 3 (Glasgow, Orleans, & Wagner, 2001; Epping-Jordan, Pruitt, Bengoa, & Wagner, 2004). The practice facilitation approach is also informed by the findings from regional and national collaboratives focused on service improvements (Berwick, 1998; Langley, Nolan, Nolan, Norman, & Provost, 1996; Solberg, 2005).

The Solberg framework for change, too, has undergirded much of the work on practice facilitation. The framework is based on practice experience with "insightful implementers" (Solberg, 2007). The model proposes that priority, change process, and care process content are necessary for measurable improvements in quality of care and patient outcomes, although internal and external barriers must also be attended to and addressed (see Figure 10-11; Solberg, 2007).

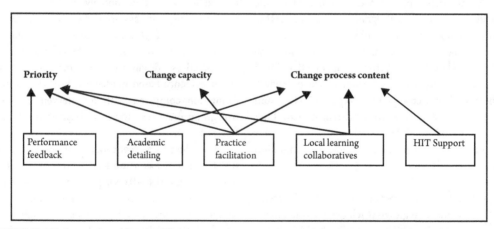

FIGURE 10-11: Approaches to Practice Change.

Source: Solberg L. Improving medical practice: a conceptual framework. *Ann Fam Med.* 2007;5:251–256.

Priority

Unless there is a strong desire and resource allocations for the specific organizational change as well as freedom from competing or more important priorities, major change is unlikely to happen. The leader's priority must be shared by other personnel at all levels and must be reinforced by focused actions and commitment of resources. The equivalent of a "burning platform" is the best metaphor for this change factor.

Change Process Capability

A qualitative study of Health Partners Medical Group's change efforts suggests that at least the following factors are important in the capacity of an organization to change (Hroscikoski, Solberg, Sperl-Hillen, Harper, & Crabtree, 2006):

1. Strong effective leadership, both centrally and locally;
2. A commonly understood framework and infrastructure for managing the change process;
3. People at all levels with change management skills;
4. Adequate resources and time devoted to the change process;
5. A mature and capable clinical information system;
6. Good communication and measurement skills;
7. A high degree of trust and teamwork;
8. Individual accountability;
9. A high degree of involvement and engagement by personnel at all levels.

Care Process Content

Care process content emphasizes systems-level changes in the practice environment rather than asking individuals to simply do better or to do things that are unlikely for human beings (such as having perfect memory or completely consistent actions). Many care process examples fit within four of the six CCM elements: delivery system redesign, self-management support, decision support, and clinical information system.

To improve care, each of the above-listed factors must be addressed in an overall environment that minimizes barriers (e.g., a poor financial situation, reimbursement that does not reward quality, inadequate information technology, physician resistance, and physicians that are too busy; Bodenheimer, Wang, Rundall, et al., 2004). Similarly, the environment must maximize facilitators (e.g., strong. leadership and an organizational culture that values quality). To apply the framework to change, each CCM factor must be focused on a clear goal. Then, by considering which of the barriers are most amenable to changes, external or internal change agents may be able to target the specific factor that is impeding movement toward the selected goal.

As shown in Figure 10-11 (a schematic), priorities for change may be affected by: academic detailing and practice facilitation, as well as practice feedback and local learning collaboratives, by encouraging, motivating, and facilitating local champions of change. Change processes may be affected only by practice facilitation, as practice facilitators are generally based within a practice, rather than consulting to it (as academic detailers often are), or external to the practice (as in learning collaboratives). Generally, change process content may be affected by all approaches but performance feedback, unless that feedback is continuous, and accompanied by tactics for overcoming barriers to change. Provider assessment and feedback, learning collaboratives, and medical informatics (health information technology, or Health IT) are discussed briefly forthwith.

Provider Assessment and Feedback

Provider assessment and feedback approaches may both evaluate provider performance in delivering or offering preventive services including screening to clients (assessment) and present providers with information about their performance in providing screening services (feedback; http://www.thecommunityguide.org/cancer/screening/provider-oriented/assessment.html). Feedback may describe the performance of a group of providers (e.g., mean performance for a practice) or an individual provider, and may be compared with a goal or standard. Several reviews cited by the *Guide to Community Preventive Services* have associated provider performance assessment and feedback with increased cancer screening (Sabatino et al., 2012; Community Preventive Services Task Force, 2012). Multicomponent academic detailing may also incorporate provider assessment and feedback.

LEARNING COLLABORATIVES

The "learning collaborative" approach, in which clinical staff work together to redesign their systems to become more patient-focused and efficient, holds promise for many health care settings. Perhaps the best-known "breakthrough" collaboratives are led by the Institute for Healthcare Improvement (IHI); these bring together groups of health care organizations that share a commitment to making major, rapid system changes (Wagner et al., 2001). Through shared learning, teams from a variety of organizations work with each other and IHI faculty to test and implement rapid-cycle quality improvement approaches, using the Plan-Do-Study-Act (PDSA) cycle (http://www.ihi.org). In practice, the collaborative becomes a temporary and powerful learning organization that can motivate; it provides knowledge, skills, and support, and develops its own culture. The collaborative can equip and empower teams to address quality problems, if the home organization's senior management and its culture are supportive, as described further forthwith.

A published description of multi-organizational collaborative improvement projects in health care across North America, the United Kingdom, and Sweden has reported changed processes and outcomes (Øvretveit, Bate, Cleary, et al., 2002). For example, a UK primary health care collaborative focused on improving access and reducing delays between primary and specialty care reduced the risk of coronary heart disease by 34% in the involved practices (Oldham et al., 2002). Similar results were also reported for "spread practices," that is, those to which the ideas were spread beyond the collaboratives in the United Kingdom. While there are still marked variations among both collaboratives and teams (to be discussed later in this Chapter) the following *team* factors may influence the success or failure of quality-focused collaboratives (Øvretveit, Bate, Cleary, et al., 2002):

1. Their ability to work as a team;
2. Their ability to learn and apply quality methods;
3. The strategic importance of their work to their home organization;
4. The culture of their home organization; and
5. The type and degree of support from management.

In the United States, the Agency for Healthcare Research and Quality (AHRQ) sponsored a learning collaborative to reduce health care disparities among minority populations in nine national or regional health care firms, including Aetna, Cigna, Kaiser Permanente, United Healthcare, WellPoint–Kaiser Permanente, Harvard Pilgrim Healthcare of Massachusetts, HealthPartners of Minnesota, Highmark Blue Cross-Blue Shield Organization in Pennsylvania, and Molina Healthcare, Inc., headquartered in California (http://www.ahrq.gov/about/evaluations/learning/learning2.htm). The collaborative reported changed processes, but the outcomes are not yet reported.

The Commonwealth Fund used a learning collaborative among four under-resourced community health centers in New York to make improvements in key operations: getting patients in and out of centers quickly; offering appointments with the patient's primary care provider on demand; enhancing revenue collections; and attracting and retaining patients (http://www.commonwealthfund.org/Innovations/Tools/2005/Jun/Improving-Health-Care-Delivery-The-Learning-Collaborative-Approach.aspx).

Learning collaboratives informed the original development of the CCM and, as discussed previously in this Chapter, have been used by a large number of health care systems across the United States (Berwick, 1998; Langley, Nolan, Nolan, Norman, Provost, 1996; Solberg, 2005).

MEDICAL INFORMATICS

Medical informatics[1] has been defined as "the field that concerns itself with the cognitive, information processing, and communication tasks of medical practice, education, and research." (Greenes & Shortliffe, 1990). Medical informatics has been used to develop information systems to support the infrastructure of medicine for education, decision making, communication, and many other aspects of professional activity (Greenes & Shortliffe, 1990; Eysenbach, 2000). More recent applications of medical informatics include consumer health informatics, as described more fully in Chapters 11 and 12.

Health Information Technology (HIT; see Figure 10-11) is an umbrella term for information processing and services in the health care field. The role of Health Information Technology (HIT) as a change technique is illustrated in Figure 10-11. The application of medical informatics in primary

---

1 The section on "Medical Informatics" was drafted by Yalini Senathirajah, Ph.D.

care—particularly for prevention—has grown considerably. In this Chapter, provider-directed uses of medical informatics, electronic health records, personal health records, security and privacy are discussed. Additional discussion of the burgeoning role of medical informatics in prevention for patients is found in Chapter 11 and its role in the future in Chapter 12.

Provider-Directed Use of Medical Informatics

Providers most often use medical informatics for e-mail, electronic and personal health records, and for care coordination. Security and privacy remain key concerns throughout their use.

The asynchronous communication afforded by e-mail, for example, offers some benefits to both providers and patients, including convenience and efficient use of time, with the potential to reduce costs. Costs include less direct communication, so potentially less dialogue, although alternative technologies, such as telehealth, could mitigate this potential problem (Haggstrom, 2013).

Electronic Health Records

Electronic health records (EHRs) are electronic versions of patients' medical records, including their medical history, diagnoses, treatments, medication regiments, imaging reports, and other clinical documents. Electronic health records can provide many benefits for providers and their patients, but they depend on how the EHRs are used.

As of May 2013, over 50% of physicians' (and other health care providers') offices and 80% of US hospitals had adopted electronic medical records in some form (http://www.hhs.gov/news/press/2013pres/05/20130522a.html). There are 6 companies responsible for about three-quarters of the electronic medical records installations around the country that are not in-house systems (HIMSS Analytics Database; h/t Modern Healthcare).

A rapid growth in EHRs over the past year reflects the advent of incentives from the Centers for Medicare & Medicaid Services (CMS) Incentive Programs and the Meaningful Use portion of the Health Information Technology for Economic and Clinical Health (HITECH) Act. This Act mandated electronic health records for all US health care providers (http://www.healthit.gov/policy-researchers-implementers/hitech-act-0; Health IT Policy Council Recommendations to the National Coordinator for Defining Meaningful Use). Meaningful use (MU) is the set of standards defined by CMS Incentive Programs that govern the use of electronic health records and allow eligible providers and hospitals to earn incentive payments by meeting specific criteria that progress through stages 1–3 (http://www.healthit.gov/policy-researchers-implementers/meaningful-use; Blumenthal & Tavenner, 2010). Stage 1 is focused on data capture and sharing; stage 2 criteria seek to advance clinical processes; and stage 3 criteria are designed to improve outcomes. Throughout, meaningful use requirements mandate the reporting of specific sets of prevention measures, such as smoking cessation counseling and diabetes HbA1c monitoring, as well as depression, alcohol, substance use disorder, and suicide screening (http://www.healthit.gov/policy-researchers-implementers/behavioral-health-expert-panel). Meaningful use implementation began in 2011 with stage 1; stage 2 is planned for 2014, and stage 3 is proposed for 2016. At present, the criteria for implementing stage 3 criteria are still in formation (http://www.cdc.gov/ehrmeaningfuluse/).

Stage 1 criteria include the collection and sharing of a common (core) MU dataset (see Figure 10-12). Further, providers and eligible hospitals must report on clinical quality measures (e.g., in diabetes, asthma, and vaccinations, including those

---

FIGURE 10-12: COMMON MEANINGFUL USE (MU) DATA SET

---

(1) Patient name
(2) Sex
(3) Date of birth
(4) Race
(5) Ethnicity
(6) Preferred language
(7) Smoking status
(8) Problems
(9) Medications
(10) Medication allergies
(11) Laboratory test(s)
(12) Laboratory value(s)/result(s)
(13) Vital signs—height, weight, blood pressure, BMI (Body Mass Index, or weight/height × height)
(14) Care plan field(s), including goals and instructions
(15) Procedures
(16) Care team member(s)

Note: Data should be expressed according to the specified standard[s]), e.g., § 170.207(a-c)(2-4) *From:* ONC, 2012

with National Quality Forum [NQF)] endorsement) in order to successfully attest to meaningful use and receive an incentive payment.

Particularly important provisions for patients are included in the stage 2 criteria of the MU initiative, as patients are able to obtain copies of their medical records, as well as a customizable clinical summary of their records (ONC, 2012). Access by third parties to the patient's medical record must be logged and the patient must be provided with information on (1) the type of action (view, download, transmission) that occurred; (2) the date and time that each action occurred; and (3) the user who took the action (ONC, 2012). The initiative also mandates that the electronic health records maintained by practices provide patients with secure log-on access to a portal, commonly termed a Personal Health Record (PHR). The PHR must provide the patient with the following capabilities:

- View the common MU data set in English, provider's name and contact information, admission and discharge dates if the patient was an inpatient;
- Download a summary in human-readable format; and
- Transmit this to a third party electronically (with the information on parties and transmission made available to the patient).

Personal Health Records

Personal health records (PHRs) are electronic records (often accessible online) that are designed primarily for the patient's use. They have been the focus of much recent innovative efforts, for example, *PatientsLikeMe, Dossia, IndivoHealth*, and *My Health Manager*. For example, in *PatientsLikeMe*, people connect with others who have the same disease; they track and share their own experiences on-line; can regularly discuss their treatment histories and side effects, symptoms, disease-specific functional scores, moods, and quality of life. In *PatientslikeMe*, individuals can share a detailed record over time; and organize their personal data into charts and graphs. Aggregated patient data, that are deidentified are sold (Haggstrom, 2013). Nonetheless, the major Internet companies, *GoogleHealth* and *Microsoft HealthVault*, have abandoned this field, due to limited adoption of their products.

PHRs can enable patients to gain insights into patterns of their own health; and to place their experiences in context. In particular, PHRs can enhance chronic disease management by facilitating the tracking of behaviors, medications, visits, laboratory results, and other patient data. They provide a "one-stop" shop for patients, and can facilitate their recall of important dates or other relevant information about their health, particularly if a disease is complex or long-standing. Many PHRs allow the patient to assign permissions for sharing with others such as caregivers, family members, or other health care providers, facilitating wider communication and coordination of care. PHRs may be populated by information from the regular provider's electronic health record, known as a "tethered" PHR. They can allow the patient to correct errors in the record, to record patient preferences to facilitate shared decision making, provide decision support tools, and assist with informed consent. Practical tools such as appointment schedulers and refill requests, as well as direct communication with providers via messaging platforms, can ease patients' communication between appointments and provide continuous access to their medical data. PHRs can also be "untethered" to the electronic medical record, as discussed in Chapter 11, via mobile apps, self-tracking of health (for example, symptoms such as pain), and patient-directed decision support (using self-management tools).

There are several considerations in the design of effective PHRs. These include the use of medical terms that are comprehensible to the average layperson, preferably at an eighth-grade or lower reading level. As some medical information in the PHR (e.g., laboratory findings) may not be understood by the patient, the PHR may include supplemental explanatory resources. Or, the patient may be restricted from viewing the record until the provider can inform the patient, for example, of the findings from an HIV-AIDS test or a cancer diagnosis. Parts of the EHR may not be included in the PHR, for example, psychiatric notes which in the opinion of the provider would not be appropriate for viewing by patients or their relatives. Data visualization can be an important component of the PHR, allowing patients to better understand the significance of trends in their medical data over time, for example, in smoking cessation or weight reduction.

Use of PHRs may vary widely, based on the patient's health status, and his or her affinity for technology. Patients with chronic disease conditions that require careful recordkeeping, monitoring, and communication with multiple providers may find this more useful than those with minimal health problems. Prevention of adverse events, tracking of medication adherence and exercise regimens, aggregation of information from multiple providers, labs, and institutions are potential benefits of PHRs. Some commercial PHRs allow the patient to give permission for data to be imported from multiple sources. In fact, Schnipper et al. found that patient insertion of medication information into a PHR medication review tool, coordinated with EHR information, resulted in a decrease in unexplained potentially harmful medication discrepancies. (Schnipper et al., 2012).

Patients' objections to PHRs include; concerns about their ability to accurately record information, assumptions about whether providers may view (or trust) the information, possible errors in the record, and concerns about privacy. Physicians may express concerns about the time needed to review the record with the patient.

Medical Informatics and Care Coordination

Generally, health Information Technology has been shown to improve healthcare quality more generally by: increasing adherence to guidelines; enhancing disease surveillance: and decreasing medication errors. The major benefits result from decreased utilization of medical care; the effects on time use are mixed, however (Basit & Shekelle, 2006; Haggstrom, 2013).

In cancer, health IT has been found to efficiently link patients, primary and specialty care teams, and technical service providers to coordinative cancer care (Hesse et al., 2010). "Meaningful use" of health IT for coordination of cancer care also has great promise, but has not yet been fully addressed in legislation or implemented in practice (Health IT Policy Council Recommendations to the National Coordinator for Defining Meaningful Use; Hesse et al., 2010)

For example, the use of health IT at the point of care—in the home or community via mobile technology, such as tablet computers and personal digital assistants (PDAs)—holds considerable promise (Blumenthal, 2010). Having the capability to view test results at the point of care enables providers to use these findings to make timely decisions about treatment, as well as to order medications. Further, if the office or medical center also has an electronic

medical record with the same functionalities, information from the mobile technology could be rapidly integrated across provider locations, facilitating coordinated patient care.

Security and Privacy

Major concerns in the adoption of EHRs, PHRs, and other medical informatics tools are privacy and security. Public concerns about breaches in the security of data about health exceed worries about financial data insecurity (https://www.cdt.org/about). Technologies and policies, as well as commercial practices, are changing rapidly; many commercial entities regard *eHealth* and *mHealth* as "the next big thing" and a potential gold mine (review in: Free, Phillips, Felix, Galli, Patel, & Edwards, 2010; Silberg, Lundberg, & Musacchio, 1997). Yet, a recent report from the Office of Inspector General reported a lack of Health Information Technology security in government-funded programs (including Medicare and Medicaid) and the audited hospitals. The security provisions in the Health Insurance Portability and Accountability Act (HIPAA) have not kept pace with technology (Office of Inspector General, 2011). Thus the patient, in order to be protected, must be aware of the many potential concerns that a loss of privacy or security bring, as not all are dues to a technical breach of informatics systems.

Concerns include:

a. Breaching information systems due to malicious or profit intent;

b. Breaching information systems accidents with a loss of privacy;

c. Forming agreements with third party businesses to the health care provider or institution

d. Selling of patient data by commercial entities with acceptable privacy policies that merge or go out of business;

e. Obtaining health information using implied or express consent of the user with entities not covered by HIPAA, such as health websites.

f. Re-identifying de-identified research data to which consent has been given. For example, a study by Gymrek et al. demonstrated that de-identified genetic information used for research could be re-identified when combined with public databases (Gymrek et al., 2013; see Chapter 12).

g. Disclosing health information, either by accident or deliberately, via social networking sites. For example, *Facebook* privacy policies may be inadequate, and information conveyed among friends or relatives may be viewable by others.

h. Requiring consent and a full explanation for genetic data, as these data have particularly far-ranging implications for privacy. For example, consent obtained from a patient for disclosure does not include consent by his or her relatives or descendants, who must be informed of the risks and benefits of disclosure (see Chapter 12).

CONCLUSIONS

Over the past 20 years, considerable evidence has emerged about effective approaches to primary care practice change. As discussed in Chapter 3, implementation of the practice change approaches that are discussed in this Chapter—PCMH, academic detailing, practice facilitation, learning collaboratives, and medical informatics—depend on senior management support and a receptive culture, among other features of the site, the change agent or "champion," and the idea itself. The PCMH has the potential to transform health care; studies conducted to date suggest that the PCMH interventions have had a small positive effect on patient experiences and small to moderate positive effects on the delivery of preventive care services. There is moderately robust evidence for increasing primary care effectiveness toward prevention via academic detailing and practice facilitation. Enhanced engagement with individual sites, networks of practices, public health agencies, and health care systems will be necessary to increase the use and cost-effectiveness of both academic detailing and practice facilitation. Provider assessment and feedback have increased cancer screening among providers, but there are limited studies in preventing other diseases. Learning "breakthrough" collaboratives across health care systems, like those led by the IHI, have increased the adoption of quality-directed innovations. There is limited evidence about the cost-effectiveness and the long-term outcomes of collaboratives compared with other approaches,

however. Medical informatics has had a strong impact on the conduct of prevention in primary care practices, through the meteoric rise in the use of the Internet and social media. Within the primary care practice, the Electronic Medical Record and Personal Health Records have been widely implemented. Security and privacy of these increasingly interconnected records are prime concerns.

MEDICAL INFORMATICS RESOURCES

Informatics methods for prevention will change rapidly as innovations and testing increase; therefore providers should consult the latest online information for up-to-date applications and advice. Below are some curated resources that aim to provide healthcare providers with useful and/or tested tools. *Happtique*, for example, is a list of mobile health tools curated by doctors and nurses, and evaluated for usability by patients.

http://www.happtique.com. Curated list of mobile health applications.

http://www.mhealthsummit.org/. Major yearly conference with online recordings, covering new developments in mHealth.

http://search.proquest.com/docview/199954 6113/13BB52F4BE325D04D80/10?accoun tid=35803. Tailored interventions for multiple risk behaviors.

http://www.ncbi.nlm.nih.gov/pmc/articles/ PMC1127483/. Definitions and concepts of consumer health informatics.

http://www.ncbi.nlm.nih.gov/pubmed/ 22519523. Internet methods for HIV assistance.

REFERENCES

Adams SG, Smith PK, Allan PF, et al. Systematic review of the chronic care model in chronic obstructive pulmonary disease prevention and management. *Arch Intern Med.* 2007;167(6):551–561.

Agency for Healthcare Research and Quality. Patient Centered Medical Home Resource Center. Retrieved January 24, 2012, from http://pcmh.ahrq.gov/.

Agency for Healthcare Research and Quality. *Closing the Quality Gap: Revisiting the State of the Science—Series Overview.* June 23, 2011. Retrieved March 13, 2012, from www.effectivehealthcare.ahrq.gov/index.cfm/ search-for-guides-reviews-and-reports/?pageaction=

displayproduct&productid=715. AHRQ Publication No. AHRQ 11-0091September 2011.

Ashford A, Gemson D, Sheinfeld Gorin S, Bloch S, Lantigua R, Ahsan H, Neugut AI. Cancer screening and prevention practices of inner city physicians. *Am J Prev Med*. 2000;19:59–62.

Austin SM, Balas EA, Mitchell JA, Ewigman BG. Effect of physician reminders on preventive care: meta-analysis of randomized clinical trials. In *Proceedings: Symposium on Computer Applic Med Care*. 1994:121–124.

Avorn J, Soumerai SB. Improving drug-therapy decisions through educational outreach: a randomized controlled trial of academically based "detailing." *N Engl J Med*. Jun 16 1983;308(24):1457–1463.

Avorn J. AD History Part III: the future of academic detailing. *Academic Detailing Today* newsletter, Fall/Winter 2012. Ballard-Barbash R. Foreword. *J Natl Cancer Inst Monogr*. 2010;40(theme issue):1–2.

Basit C, Shekelle P. Systematic Review: Impact of Health Information Technology on Quality, Efficiency, and Costs of Medical Care, Annals of Internal Medicine, 2006.

Baskerville NB, Liddy C, Hogg W. Systematic review and meta-analysis of practice facilitation within primary care settings. *Ann Fam Med*. 2012;10(1):63–74.

Bercovitz AR, Park-Lee E, Jamoom E. *Adoption and Use of Electronic Health Records and Mobile Technology by Home Health and Hospice Care Agencies*. National Health Statistics Reports Number 66, May 20, 2013. http://www.cdc.gov/nchs/data/nhsr/nhsr066.pdf.

Berwick DM. Developing and testing changes in delivery of care. *Ann Intern Med*. 1998;128(8):651–656.

Blumenthal D. Launching HITECH. *N Engl J Med*. 2010;362(5):382–385.

Blumenthal D, Tavenner M. The "meaningful use" regulation for electronic health records. *New Engl J Med*. 2010;363 (6):501–504.

Briss PA, Rodewald LE, Hinman AR, Shefer AM, Stirkas RA, Bernier RR, Carande-Kulis VG, Yusuf HR, Ndiaye SM, Williams SM, the Task Force on Community Preventive Services. Reviews of evidence regarding interventions to improve vaccination coverage in children, adolescents, and adults. *Am J Prev Med*. 2000;18(1S):97–140.

Bodenheimer T, Wang MC, Rundall TG, et al. What are the facilitators and barriers in physician organizations' use of care management processes? *Jt Comm J Qual Saf*. 2004;30(9):505–514.

Bodenheimer T, Wagner EH, Grumbach K. Improving primary care for patients with chronic illness: the chronic care model, Part 2. *JAMA*. 2002;288(15):1909–1914.

Bouton ME. A learning theory perspective on lapse, relapse, and the maintenance of behavior change. *Health Psychol*. Jan 2000;19(1 Suppl):57–63.

Car J, Gurol-Urganci I, de Jongh T, Vodopivec-Jamsek V, Atun R. Mobile phone messaging reminders for attendance at healthcare appointments. *Cochrane Database of Systematic Reviews*. 2012;7:CD007458.

Carrier E, Gourevitch MN, Shah NR. Medical homes: challenges in translating theory into practice. *Med Care*. 2009;47:714–722.

Chan CV, Kaufman DR. A framework for characterizing eHealth literacy demands and barriers. *J Med Internet Res*. 2011;13:e94.

Coleman K, Austin BT, Brach C, et al. Evidence on the Chronic Care Model in the new millennium. *Health Aff (Millwood)*. 2009;28(1):75–85.

Community Preventive Services Task Force. Updated recommendations for client- and provider-oriented interventions to increase breast, cervical, and colorectal cancer screening. *Am J Prev Med*. 2012;43(1):760–764.

Curry SJ, Emmons KM. Theoretical models for predicting and improving compliance with breast cancer screening. *Ann Behav Med*. 1994;16:302–316.

Deborah Peikes, PhD; Arnold Chen, MD, MSc; Jennifer Schore, MS, MSW; Randall Brown, PhD Effects of Care Coordination on Hospitalization, Quality of Care, and Health Care Expenditures Among Medicare Beneficiaries15 Randomized Trials. JAMA. 2009;301(6):603–618. doi:10.1001/jama. 2009.126.

Dickey LL, Gemson DH, Carney P. Office system interventions supporting primary care-based health behavior change counseling. *Am J Prev Med*. 1999;17:299–308.

Dietrich AJ, Sox CH, Tosteson TD, Woodruff CB. Durability of improved physician early detection of cancer after conclusion of intervention support. *Cancer Epidemiol Biomarkers Prev*. 1994;3:335–340.

Epping-Jordan JE, Pruitt SD, Bengoa R, Wagner EH. Improving the quality of health care for chronic conditions. *Qual Saf Health Care*. 2004;13(4):299–305.

Eysenbach G. Consumer health informatics. *BMJ*. 2000;320:1713.http://dx.doi.org/10.1136/bmj.320. 7251.1713.

Fennell ML, Prabhu Das I, Clauser S, Petrelli N, Salner A. The organization of multidisciplinary care teams: modeling internal and external influences on cancer care quality. *J Natl Cancer Inst Monogr*. 2010;40(theme issue):72–80.

Fischer, Michael. *Patient-Centered Outcomes Research and Academic Detailing*. http://www.narcad.org/newsletter/fall2012adtoday/.

Free C, Phillips G, Felix L, Galli L, Patel V, & Edwards P. The effectiveness of M-health technologies for improving health and health services: a systematic review protocol. *BMC Research Notes*. 2010;3:250.

Glasgow RE, Orleans CT, Wagner EH. Does the chronic care model serve also as a template for improving prevention? *Milbank Q*. 2001;79(4):579–612, iv–v.

Green LA, Graham R, Bagley B, et al. Task Force 1. Report of the task force on patient expectations, core values, reintegration, and the new model of family medicine. *Ann Fam Med.* 2004;2(Suppl 1):S33–S50.

Greenes RA, Shortliffe EH. Medical informatics. An emerging academic discipline and institutional priority. *JAMA.* 1990;263:1114–1120.

Gymrek G, McGuire A, Golan D, Halperin E, Erlich Y. Identifying Personal Genomes by Surname Inference. *Science.* 2013;33:321–324.

Haggstrom, DA. *Cancer care coordination: health information technology.* Presentation to the Society of Beahvioral Medicine. San Francisco, CA, 2013.

Han PJK, Rayson D. The coordination of primary and oncology specialty care at the end of life. *J Natl Cancer Inst Monogr.* 2010;40(theme issue):31–37.

Health IT Policy Committee. *Recommendations to the National Coordinator for Health IT.* Accessed July 2013 from: http://www.healthit. gov/policy- researchers- implementers/health-it-policy-committee- recommendations- national-coordinator-heal.

Hensley S. As drug bill soars, some doctors get an "unsales" pitch. *Wall Street Journal,* March 13, 2006.

Hesse BW, Hanna C, Massett HA, Hesse NK. Outside the box: will information technology be a viable intervention to improve the quality of cancer care? *J Natl Cancer Inst Monogr.* 2010;40(theme issue):81–89.

Honda K, Sheinfeld Gorin, S. A model of stage of change to recommend colonoscopy among urban primary care physicians. *Health Psychology.* 2006;25(1):65–73.

Hroscikoski MC, Solberg LI, Sperl-Hillen JM, Harper P, Crabtree BF. The challenges of change: a qualitative study of Chronic Care Model implementation. *Ann Fam Med.* 2006;4(4)317–326.

Hulscher MEJL, Wensing M, van der Weijden T, Grol R. Interventions to implement prevention in primary care. *Cochrane Database of Systematic Reviews.* 2002; 2.

Institute of Medicine. *Crossing the Quality Chasm: A New Health System for the 21st Century.* Washington, DC: National Academies Press; 2001, 24.

Jackson GL, Powers BJ, Chatterjee R, Prvu Bettger J, Kemper AR, Hasselblad V, Dolor RJ, Irvine RJ, Heidenfelder BL, Kendrick AS, Gray R, Williams JW. The patient-centered medical home: a systematic review. *Ann Intern Med.* 2013;158(3):169–178.

Kilo CM, Wasson JH. Practice redesign and the patient-centered medical home: history, promises, and challenges. *Health Aff (Millwood).* 2010;29: 773–778. [PMID: 20439860]

Langley GJ, Nolan KM, Nolan TW, Norman CL, Provost LP. *Improvement Guide: A Practical Approach to Enhancing Organizational Performance.* San Francisco, CA: Jossey-Bass; 1996.

Lehmann D. Role of academic detailing in healthcare improvement. National Resource Center for Academic Detailing's (NaRCAD) annual conference, November 12–13, 2012, Boston, MA.

Martin JC, Avant RF, Bowman MA, et al. The future of family medicine: a collaborative project of the family medicine community. *Ann Fam Med.* 2004;2-(Suppl 1):S3–S32.

McDonald KM, Sundaram V, Bravata DM, et al. Care Coordination. Vol. 7 of: Shojania KG, McDonald KM, Wachter RM, Owens, DK, editors. *Closing the Quality Gap: A Critical Analysis of Quality Improvement Strategies. Technical Review 9* (Prepared by the Stanford University-UCSF Evidence-based Practice Center under contract 290-02-0017). AHRQ Publication No. 04(07)-0051-7. Rockville, MD: Agency for Healthcare Research and Quality; June 2007.

McDonald KM, Schultz E, Albin L, Pineda N, Lonhart J, Sundaram V, Smith-Spangler C, Brustrom J, and Malcolm E. *Care Coordination Atlas Version 3* (Prepared by Stanford University under subcontract to Battelle on Contract No. 290-04-0020). AHRQ Publication No. 11-0023-EF. Rockville, MD: Agency for Healthcare Research and Quality; November 2010.

Mold JW. *Academic Detailing and Renal Disease.* Comparative Effectiveness Summit, Washington, DC, November, 2012.

Moreno L, Peikes D, Krilla A. *Necessary But Not Sufficient: The HITECH Act and Health Information Technology's Potential to Build Medical Homes.* (Prepared by Mathematica Policy Research under Contract No. HHSA290200900019ITO2.) AHRQ Publication No. 10-0080-EF. Rockville, MD: Agency for Healthcare Research and Quality; June 2010.

Nagykaldi Z, Mold JW, & Aspy CB. Practice facilitators: A review of the literature. *Fam Med.* 2005; 37(8):581–585).

Nutting PA, Miller WL, Crabtree BF, Jaen CR, Stewart EE, Stange KC. Initial lessons from the first national demonstration project on practice transformation to a patient-centered medical home. *Ann Fam Med.* 2009; 7 (3): 254–260

Nutting PA, Crabtree BF, Miller WL, Stewart EE, Stange KC, Jaén CR. Journey to the patient-centered medical home: a qualitative analysis of the experiences of practices in the National Demonstration Project. *Ann Fam Med.* 2010;8(Suppl 1):s45–s56.

Nutting et al. 2010. Effects of facilitation on practice outcomes in the National Demonstration Project Model of the Patient-Centered Medical Home. *Ann Fam Med.* 8(supplement 1):S33–S44.

O'Connor PJ. Commentary: improving diabetes care by combating clinical inertia. *Health Serv Res* 2005; 40:1854–1861.

Office of Inspector General. *Audit of Information Technology Security Included in Health Information Technology Standards 05-16-2011.* Accessed June 2013 from: http://oig.hhs.gov/oas/reports/other/180930160.asp

Oldham R, et al. How to spread good practice to 7 million patients. Presentation at the 7th European Quality Forum, Edinburgh, March 2002.

Øvretveit J, Bate P, Cleary P, et al. Quality collaboratives: Lessons from research. *Qual Safe Health Care.*
2002;11:345–351.

Patient-Centered Primary Care Collaborative (PCPCC).
Joint Principles of the Patient Centered Medical Home.
Accessed January 16, 2013, from http://www.pcpcc.
net/node/14.

Pignone M, Harris R, Kinsinger L. Videotape-based decision aid for colon cancer screening. *Ann Int Med.*
2000; 133(10):761–769.

Pignone M, Winquist A, Schild L, Lewis C, Scott T,
Hawley J, Rimer BK, Glanz K. Effectiveness of a
patient and practice-level colorectal cancer screening
intervention in health plan members: The CHOICE
Trial. *Cancer.* 2011 117(15): 3352–3362.

Sabatino SA, Lawrence B, Elder R, Mercer SL, Wilson
KM, DeVinney B, Melillo S, Carvalho M, Taplin S,
Bastani R, Rimer BK, Vernon SW, Melvin CL, Taylor
V, Fernandez M, Glanz K, Community Preventive
Services Task Force. Effectiveness of interventions
to increase screening for breast, cervical, and colorec-
tal cancers: nine updated systematic reviews for The
Guide to Community Preventive Services. *Am J Prev
Med.* 2012;43(1):765–786.

Schnipper JL, Gandhi TK, Wald JS, Grant RW, Poon
EG, Volk LA, et al. Effects of an online personal health record on medication accuracy and
safety: a cluster-randomized trial. *JAMA.* 2012;19:
728–734.

Scholle S, Torda P, Peikes D, Han E, Genevro J. *Engaging
Patients and Families in the Medical Home* (Prepared
by Mathematica Policy Research under Contract No.
HHSA290200900019ITO2.) AHRQ Publication
No. 10-0083-EF. Rockville, MD: Agency for
Healthcare Research and Quality; June 2010.

Scholle S, Torda P, Peikes D, Han E, Genevro J. *Engaging
Patients and Families in the Medical Home* (Prepared
by Mathematica Policy Research under Contract No.
HHSA290200900019ITO2.) AHRQ Publication
No. 10-0083-EF. Rockville, MD: Agency for
Healthcare Research and Quality; June 2010.

Shankaran V, Bennett C, Graff Zivin J, Scoppettone M,
Sheinfeld Gorin S. Costs and cost-effectiveness of a
health care provider-directed intervention to promote colorectal cancer screening among underserved
populations. *J Clin Oncol.* 2009; 27: 5370–5375.

Sheinfeld Gorin S, Ashford A, Lantigua R, Hossain A,
Desai M, Troxel A, Gemson D. Effectiveness of academic detailing on breast cancer screening among
primary care physicians in an underserved community. *J Am Board Fam Med* 2006; 19: 110–121.

Sheinfeld Gorin S, Ashford A, Lantigua R, Hossain
A, Desai M, Troxel A, Gemson D (deceased).
Disseminating breast cancer screening to primary care
physicians in an underserved community. *Implement
Sci.* 2007;2:43. http://www.implementationscience.
com/content/2/1/43.

Sheinfeld Gorin S, Ashford A, Lantigua R, Hajiani F,
Franco R, Heck J, Gemson D (deceased). Intraurban
influences on physician colorectal cancer screening
practices. *JAMA.* 2007;99(12):1371–1380.

Sheinfeld Gorin S, et al. Outcomes of a trial to increase
physician breast cancer detection practices in underserved communities. *Cancer Epidemiol Biomarkers
Prev.* 2002;11:222.

Sheinfeld Gorin S, Franco R, Hajiani F, Senathirajah, Y.
Systematic development and usability testing of a
physician-based prostate cancer education program
in an African American community. *Proceedings of the
AMIA Annual Meeting* 2007; AMIA-0372-S2007.

Sheinfeld Gorin S, Franco R, Westhoff C, NYPAC. HPV
knowledge among physicians and their low-income
patients: survey findings and approaches for change.
Program/Proceedings of the Eurogen Conference
2006: Human papillomavirus infection and global
prevention of cervical cancer: priorities, practices and
new directions 2006;G423C0165:57–62.

Sheinfeld Gorin S, Gemson D, Ashford A, Bloch S,
Lantigua R, Ahsan H, Neugut AI. Cancer education
among primary care physicians in an underserved
community. *Am J Prev Med.* 2000;19:53–58.

Sheinfeld Gorin S, Glenn BA, Perkins RB. The human
papillomavirus (HPV) vaccine and cervical cancer: uptake and next steps. *Advances in Therapy,*
2011;28(8):615–639.

Sheinfeld Gorin S, Graff Zivin J, NYPAC Study Group.
Effects of academic detailing for colorectal cancer
screening among primary care physicians: self report
and cost effectiveness findings. *Cancer Epidemiol
Biomarkers Prev.* 2003;12:1276s–1279s.

Sheinfeld Gorin S, Haggstrom D, Fairfield K, Han P,
Krebs P, Clauser SB, QCCC CCI Working Group.
Cancer care coordination systematic review and
meta-analysis: twenty-two years of empirical studies.
2013 Annual Meeting, Abstract #115962, June 2013b.

Sheinfeld Gorin S, McDonald K, Haggstrom D, Han
P, Clauser S. Coordinating cancer care: what have
we learned from twenty years of empirical studies?
Symposium presented to the Society of Behavioral
Medicine, March 2013a.

Sheinfeld Gorin S, Wang C, Raich P, Bowen DJ, Hay J.
Decision-making in cancer prevention and chemoprevention. *Ann Behav Med.* 2006;32:179–187.

Sia C, Tonniges TF, Osterhus E, Taba S. History of
the medical home concept. *Pediatrics.* 2004;113:
1473–1478.

Silberg WM, Lundberg GD, Musacchio RA. Assessing, controlling, and assuring the quality of medical information
on the Internet: Caveant lector et viewor – let the reader
and viewer beware. *JAMA.* 1997;277:1244–1245.

Simon SR, Majumdar SR, Prosser LA, Salem-Schatz
S, Warner C, Kleinman K, Miroshnik I, Soumerai
SB. Group versus individual academic detailing to
improve the use of antihypertensive medications in

primary care: a cluster-randomized controlled trial. *Am J Med*. May 2005;118(5):521–528.

Simon SR, Smith DH, Feldstein AC, Perrin N, Yang X, Zhou Y, Platt R, Soumerai SB. Computerized prescribing alerts and group academic detailing to reduce the use of potentially inappropriate medications in older people. *J Am Geriatr Soc*. Jun 2006;54(6):963–968.

Solberg L. Improving medical practice: a conceptual framework. *Ann Fam Med*. 2007;5:251–256.

Solberg LI. If you've seen one quality improvement collaborative. *Ann Fam Med*. 2005;3(3):198–199.

Soumerai SB, Avorn J. Principles of educational outreach ("academic detailing") to improve clinical decision making. *JAMA*. Jan 26 1990;263(4):549–556.

Sperl-Hillen JM, O'Connor PJ, Carlson R, et al. Improving diabetes care in a large health care system: an enhanced primary care approach. *Jt Comm J Qual Improv*. 2000; 26:615-22.

Stange KC, Nutting PA, Miller WL, Jaen CR, Crabtree BF, Flocke SA, et al. Defining and measuring the patient-centered medical home. *J Gen Intern Med*. 2010;25:601–612.

Taplin SH, Rodgers AB. Toward improving the quality of cancer care: addressing the interfaces of primary and oncology-related subspecialty care. *J Natl Cancer Inst Monogr*. 2010;40(theme issue):3–10.

Taylor EF and Agency for Healthcare Research & Quality and Mathematica Policy Research. *Enhancing the Primary Care Team to Provide Redesigned Care: The Roles of Practice Facilitators and Care Managers*, webinar presentation to the PCMH, 2012.

Taylor EF, Machtal RM, Meyers DS, Genevro J, Peikes DN. Enhancing the primary care team to provide redesigned care: the roles of practice facilitators and care managers. *Annals of Family Medicine* 2013;11(1):80–83.

The Office of the National Coordinator for Health IT (ONC). *Meaningful Use Stage II requirements*. Accessed May 12, 2012, from: http://www.healthit.gov/policy-researchers-implementers/meaningful-use

TransforMED. *National Demonstration Project*. Accessed January 16, 2009, from http://www.trans-formed.com/ndp.cfm.

Tsai AC, Morton SC, Mangione CM, et al. A meta-analysis of interventions to improve care for chronic illnesses. *Am J Manag Care*. 2005;11(8):478–488. PMID: 16095434.

Vest JR, Bolin JN, Miller TR, Gamm LD, Siegrist TE, Martinez LE. Medical homes: "where you stand on definitions depends on where you sit." *Med Care Res Rev*. 2010;67:393–411.

Wagner EH, Austin BT, David C, Hindmarsh M, Shaefer J, & Bonomi A. Improving chronic illness care: translating evidence into action. *Health Affairs*. 2001;20(6):64–78.

Wagner EH, Austin BT, Von Korff M. Organizing care for patients with chronic illness. *Milbank Q*. 1996;74(4):511–544.

Wagner EH, Glasgow RE, Davis C, Bonomi AE, Provost L, McCulloch D, et al. Quality improvement in chronic illness care: a collaborative approach. *Joint Comm J Qual Im*. 2001;27:63–80.

Walsh JM, McPhee SJ. A systems model of clinical preventive care: an analysis of factors influencing patient and physician. *Health Educ Q*. 1992;19(2):157–175.

Walsh JM, McPhee SJ. A systems model of clinical preventive care: an analysis of factors influencing patient and physician. *Health Educ Q*. 1992;19(2):157–175.

11

Patient-Directed Approaches to Prevention

SHERRI N. SHEINFELD GORIN

Patient-directed—in fact, patient-centered—approaches are at the core of the clinical practice of prevention. In this Chapter, several well-established approaches to patient behavioral change that emphasize patient self-management and clinical collaboration are examined, including goal-setting, shared decision making, the 5 As, and motivational interviewing. (Some of these approaches are also described in Chapter 3.) This Chapter then describes tailored telephone interviewing and computer-assisted counseling. Risk assessment is key to prevention. Risk is the probability that a disease will develop in an individual during a specified time period. At the population level, with changes in health behaviors, the *risk* of disease is either reduced (as in the case of many infectious diseases today) or postponed until later in life (as in heart disease and various cancers; http://www.diseaseriskindex.harvard.edu/update/). Given the centrality of the concept of risk to prevention, the Chapter discusses in some detail risk assessment approaches using office-based tools. Finally, the Chapter introduces some emerging screening tools for primary care.

BEHAVIOR CHANGE AND THE PROVIDER/PATIENT ENCOUNTER

Patient-centered approaches that promote patient activation and self-management skills are key to desirable health outcomes among patients with many of the illnesses that are explored in Chapters 4 through 7 (Glasgow & Goldstein, 2007; Bodenheim, Lorig et al., 2002; Glasgow, Kaplan, Ockene, Fisher, Emmons, 2012). A patient-centered approach emphasizes collaboration, understanding, and empathizing with the patients' experience, negotiating goals, and helping patients to identify and overcome barriers to adherence and behavior change.

Lessons learned from the Chronic Illness Care Breakthrough Series and other efforts to integrate self-management support into health care settings (such as the Chronic Care Model; Wagner et al., 2001; discussed in Chapters 3 and 10) suggest that the following elements are critical to success: (a) assessment of patient beliefs, behavior, and knowledge; (b) collaborative goal setting; (c) identification of personal barriers and supports; (d) problem solving to overcome barriers; and (e) developing a personal action plan that is based on the previous four steps (Glasgow, Funnell, Bonomi, et al., 2002; Rorer & Kinmouth, 2002; see Table 11-1). These approaches may be used to address health behavior change issues across a variety of medical conditions and patient populations (Lorig & Holman, 2003).

PATIENT DECISION MAKING FOR PREVENTION

Prevention decisions within the clinical encounter include whether to take a chemopreventive agent, to quit smoking, to increase fruit and vegetable consumption, or to begin a program of physical activity. These decisions also involve *which* prevention strategy

---

TABLE 11-1. PRINCIPLES OF EFFECTIVE COMMUNICATION THAT ENCOURAGE PATIENT SELF-MANAGEMENT

- Explore and hear the patient's perspective
- Provide emotional support and express empathy
- Share information that is useful and relevant
- Negotiate a plan
- Anticipate problems and barriers and identify potential solutions

Modified from Rorer D. Kinmonth AI. What is the evidence that increasing participation of individuals in self-management improves the processes and outcomes of care? In: Williams R, Kinmonth A, Warchain N, et al. eds., *The Evidence Base for Diabetes Care.* Hoboken, NJ: John Wiley and Sons, 2002.

to employ, that is, whether to quit smoking cold tur-key or to use nicotine replacement therapy, and deci-sions about *whether* to exercise on one specific day or another. A rational decision-making process begins with a choice that must be made; in prevention, the choice involves actions that one would undertake to reduce morbidity and mortality. Generally, a rational decision is time-delimited; would involve options, each linked to potential benefits and harms; and *may* reflect (at least in part) the decision maker's own pref-erences. Many of those decisions are also made out-side the medical encounter (Sheinfeld Gorin, Wang, Raich, Bowen, Hay, 2006).

Yet we know very little about how individuals decide to undertake, maintain, or discontinue pre-ventive behaviors. People may decide to eat more fruits and vegetables in a store when they see the dif-ferent varieties of greens. This decision tends to inte-grate into the fabric of daily life, so it may seem "ad hoc." Alternatively, the decision may be conscious and designed to change a lifestyle. The individual then decides how best to implement the change and how to adhere to the developed action plan (Sheinfeld Gorin, Wang, Raich, Bowen, Hay, 2006).

And there is little theoretical guidance either for acquiring new healthy behaviors, or for main-taining health behavior change over time. We know that the acquisition of behaviors is influenced by favorable expectations regarding future outcomes, whereas behavioral maintenance is likely influenced by satisfaction with the outcomes of behavior change (Rothman, 2000; Bouton, 2000). For example, the decision to quit smoking may entail a set of facilitators and barriers that would be quite different from the facilitators and barriers to maintaining cessation over time. Similarly, self-regulation theory (Leventhal, 1970), as described in Chapter 3, proposes that peo-ple concurrently develop two action plans to cope with illness (or potential illness): one for managing the objective demands of the illness (or potential ill-ness) itself, and a second for managing affect associ-ated with the illness threat. The development of these action plans may change over time, however, based on characteristics of the potential illness as well as facili-tators and barriers of the coping (and proactive cop-ing) process (Aspinwell & Taylor, 1997; Sheinfeld Gorin, Wang, Raich, Bowen, Hay, 2006).

Further, some (e.g., the use of tamoxifen or statins), not all, prevention decisions rest on evi-dence. Yet evidence must always be translated both into practice by the clinician and compliance by the patient, so it seems that *all* prevention and chemo-prevention decisions that engage action are fun-damentally preference sensitive (Sheinfeld Gorin, Wang, Raich, Bowen, Hay, 2006).

In addition to developing and implementing evidence for prevention decisions and identifying patient preferences, the challenge in prevention is to identify the useful decision points, and to find ways of actually measuring them (Sheinfeld Gorin, Wang, Raich, Bowen, Hay, 2006).

APPROACHES TO PATIENT BEHAVIOR CHANGE IN PRIMARY CARE

In most cases, the physician serves as a motiva-tor who can briefly emphasize the importance of behavioral goals to the patient and can collaborate on their formation; the subsequent intervention and follow-up are often conducted by a nurse, case man-ager, or other interventionist. In some practices, the physician both motivates and intervenes, with rein-forcement from other team members.

Goal Setting

After an assessment period, often using an auto-mated or rapidly scored instrument as discussed later in this Chapter, goal setting begins the change process. SMART (specific, measureable, attainable, realistic, and timely) goals can begin the clinical col-laboration on patient behavioral change, particularly when goals are reinforced by other team members (see Table 11-2 for an example) (Glasgow, 2005).

Shared Decision Making (SDM)

Given the more recent view of primary care deci-sion making as a partnership between providers and patients, there is growing interest in shared decision making. In fact, the Patient Protection and Affordable Care Act of 2010 (Affordable Care Act, P.L. 111-148) includes eight provisions to facilitate and encourage the use of the shared decision-making process (http://www.ama-assn.org/resources/doc/cms/a10-cms-rpt-7.pdf). In SDM, the provider and patient go through all phases of the decision-making process together, share treatment preferences, and reach an agreement on treatment choice. The Foundation for Informed Medical Decision-Making, a non-profit organization based in Boston, Massachusetts, defines shared decision making as "the process by which a health care [provider] com-municates to the patient personalized information

TABLE 11-2. SMART GOALS

Specific: I will increase my running mileage by 10% each week.

Measureable: I will keep track of my running distance each day so that I can track my progress toward my goal.

Attainable: Is the goal attainable for me? Yes, given my current schedule and my desire to accomplish this goal. I feel that this is attainable.

Realistic: Is the goal realistic for me? Yes, I have everything I need to make this goal a reality. I have the support and resources in place.

Timely: I will sign up to run a half-marathon in 3 months and a full marathon in 6 months.

Example to increase adherence with medication and psychotherapy use for a depressed patient: I will take my fluoxetine (Prozac) each morning before I go to work, and will go to Dr. Tappler's office every Tuesday at 4 pm, as scheduled, for the next month.

Example to increase intake of low-fat foods: Using the list that I received from my doctor's office, I will choose low-fat foods over high-fat foods at one meal each day over the next 4 weeks.

Example for smoking cessation: I will substitute a walk for my morning cigarette, chew 4 mg nicotine replacement gum every time that I feel like smoking, and wear a nicotine patch on my left arm for the next 3 months.

Another Example to increase physical activity: I will jog outside or use the elliptical machine at the gym at a moderate intensity for 30 minutes 4 times per week and stop eating potato chips every day to lose 1-2 lbs per week over the next 3 weeks.

Adapted from: Croteau J, Ryan D. Achieving your SMART health goals. BeWell@Stanford. 2013; http://bewell.stanford.edu/smart-goals. Accessed Jan, 2013. O'Neil J. SMART Goals, SMART Schools. *Educational Leadership*. 2000;Feb:46–50.
Examples from: Sheinfeld Gorin S, Krist A. Using MOHR for Behavior Change: A Webinar for Providers. http://healthpolicy.ucla.edu/mohr.

about the options, outcomes, probabilities, and scientific uncertainties of available treatment options and the patient communicates his or her values and the relative importance he or she places on benefits and harms" (http://informedmedicaldecisions.org/). Although patients always have the right to participate in decisions about their medical treatment, using formal shared decision-making processes can be especially useful in cases where more than one treatment option is available, and no treatment is considered "best" according to clinical evidence.

"Shared decision making (SDM) is defined as decisions that are shared by doctors and patients, informed by the best evidence available and weighted according to the specific characteristics and values of the patient." SDM is reflected in four of the ten "simple rules" for the redesign of health care: (1) customization based on patients' needs and values; (2) patient as source of control; (3) shared knowledge and free flow of information; and (4) evidence-based decision making (IOM, 2001; http://geiselmed.dartmouth.edu/ocer/pdf/shared_decision_making.pdf). SDM is key to a patient-centered decision, defined as the extent to which it reflects the considered needs, values and expressed preferences of a well-informed patient (Sepucha, Fowler, & Mulley, 2004).

As to patient autonomy and responsibility for medical decisions, the SDM concept stands midway between the paternalistic approach and the informed choice concept (Charles, Gafni, Whelan, 1997; Charles, Gafni, Whelan, 1999; Elwyn, Edwards, Kinnersley, Grol, 2000; Elwyn, Edwards, Kinnersley, 1999). According to Elwyn et al. (2000), SDM is most feasible in situations of professional equipoise where several legitimate choices exist and the provider does not have a clear preference about the treatment choice to make. One important prerequisite for SDM (Charles, Gafni, Whelan, 1997) is the mutual exchange of information between physician and patient, because the knowledge of both is needed to manage an illness successfully. The doctor contributes medical expert knowledge on causes of disease, symptoms, treatment options, and prognosis, whereas the patient discloses expectations, preferences, fears, attitudes to risk, values, experience of illness, and social circumstances (Coulter, 1999). After a process of negotiation with a final agreement, doctor and patient plan steps to put their shared decision into action. In SDM, more than one treatment option exists, as discussed previously.

If the options are limited, however, informed decision making (IDM) provides tools to support patient information about the benefits and harms of treatment choices, expecting the patient to make the final decision (Bieber, Müller, Blumenstiel, Schneider, Richter, Wilke, Hartmann, Eich, 2006).

The Ottawa Decision Support Framework emphasizes core elements that are essential to helping
individuals work through decisions (O'Connor,
Tugwell, Wells, et al., 1998). Informed decisions
occur when an individual (a) understands the
disease or condition being addressed and comprehends what the intervention involves, including its benefits, risks, limitations, alternatives, and
uncertainties; (b) has considered his or her own
preferences, as appropriate; (c) believes that he or
she has participated in decision making at a desired
level; and (d) makes a decision consistent with
those preferences (Sheridan, Harris, Woolf, 2004).
Informed decision making is a conscious process
that culminates in an action plan and may be supported by tools that supply patient information
about the benefits and harms of treatment choices
(Greenfield, Kaplan, Ware, 1985) and values clarification (Llewellyn-Thomas, 1995).

The decision to screen for prostate cancer is an
example that is amenable to shared decision making.
As discussed in Chapter 4, because the evidence of
benefits is not clearer than the risks for prostate cancer
screening using the PSA (Prostate-Specific Antigen)
test, all of the major professional groups—the
American Cancer Society, the American Urological
Association, the American Academy of Family
Practitioners, and the US Preventive Services Task
Force (that also does not recommend prostate cancer
screening)—recommend informed or shared decision
making between the primary care provider and each
age-eligible man (Smith, vonEschenbach, Wender,
Levin, Byers et al., 2001). Table 11-3 provides a provider guide to SDM with prostate cancer screening.

Evaluation of SDM

Despite the considerable interest in applying SDM
clinically, little research regarding its effectiveness has
been done to date (Joostena, DeFuentes-Merillasa,
de Weertc, Senskye, van der Staakd, de Jonga,
2008). A recent Cochrane Collaboration review systematically examined 11 randomized controlled trials (RCTs) on the effectiveness of SDM for patient
satisfaction, treatment adherence, and health status.
Five RCTs showed no difference between SDM and
control, one RCT showed no short-term effects but
positive longer-term effects, and five RCTs reported
a positive effect of SDM on outcome measures.
Two of these studies included individuals diagnosed with mental illness. The findings suggest that
SDM is particularly suitable for reaching treatment

agreement regarding long-term decisions, notably in
the context of a chronic illness, and when the intervention contains more than one session. Evidence
for the effectiveness of SDM in the context of other
types of decisions, or in general, is still inconclusive.

Decision Support Aids: Definitions, Frameworks, and Evaluations

Formal shared decision-making processes are generally facilitated through the use of electronic or
paper-based patient decision support aids; these are
often developed by third parties and licensed for use
by health plans, hospitals, or physicians. Through
tools such as booklets, videos, interactive computer
programs, and structured personal coaching, patients
receive evidence-based information about treatment
options and outcomes that are specifically designed
to help them evaluate trade-offs in the context of their
own feelings and preferences. Decision support aids
supplement direct communication between the physician and patient by offering patients an opportunity
to process complex—and possibly frightening—
information at their own pace, using information
that addresses the emotional as well as the clinical
aspects of medical care (http://www.ama-assn.org/
resources/doc/cms/a10-cms-rpt-7.pdf).

Patient decision aids have three core elements: clinical information, "values clarification,"
and guidance to help patients make and communicate their treatment decisions (O'Connor,
Llewellyn-Thomas, Flood, 2004). The clinical information component represents a synthesis of relevant evidence-based information about the patient's
medical condition, available treatment options, and
the potential risks, benefits, and outcomes associated with each option. The "values clarification"
component of patient decision aids helps patients
quantify the more subjective elements of addressing their medical condition and pursuing a course
of treatment. The decision aids (patient testimoni-
als, anecdotes, and questionnaires) are designed
to help patients learn about and identify with the
physical, emotional, and social aspects of each treatment option, so that they can visualize how their life
might be affected by various treatments. The guidance and communication elements of patient decision aids help lead patients through the process of
synthesizing the clinical and values information that
they have obtained and making decisions that they
are comfortable with. Entities that develop patient

TABLE 11-3. APPROACH TO SHARED DECISION MAKING (SDM)

A Sample Approach to Shared Decision Making (SDM) for Prostate Cancer Early Detection

1. Inform your patient about the following issues (decision aids can help in this process):
   - Types of prostate cancer
   - Risk of dying from the disease among men of the same age, family history, and race/ethnicity
   - Risk relative to other men's health issues such as heart disease
   - Ability of PSA to detect prostate cancer early
   - Uncertainty about whether treatment would extend his life
   - Issue of over-diagnosis
   - Side effects of treatment
2. Discuss his questions and concerns.
   Once your patient has considered key information about prostate cancer, the next step is to answer questions and address concerns. Many men have misconceptions about prostate cancer that you can help correct:
   - Cancer may sound more important than any other health concern; while it is an important issue for men's health, there are many others.
   - Help him understand that issues regarding prostate cancer and its detection and treatment may be different than he thinks.
   - Many men with prostate cancer do not die from it, even without treatment. But prostate cancer can kill, so it is important to be well informed.
3. Make it clear that he should help decide what is best for him because his values and preferences are key. He may be surprised that you're not telling him what to do.
   - Tell him there is no rush to make a decision. Give him time to think or learn more. Tell him that you can discuss it again and decide at a later visit.
   - Offer him a decision aid to take home.
   - Suggest that he may want to discuss it with family members.
   - Discuss why different men choose different options. Ask which man sounds the most like your patient feels:
     - One man may be more worried about dying of prostate cancer than about treatment side effects. He thinks early detection and treatment may save his life. He wants any prostate cancer to be detected despite the uncertainty.
     - Another man may be more worried about the harms associated with screening, such as over-diagnosis and treatment side effects. He thinks those harms outweigh the uncertainty about benefits. He would not want treatment so he wouldn't want to know whether he had cancer.
   - Tell him you will support any choice he makes.
4. Listen and make a joint decision.
   - A man may be ready to decide but still want your reassurance that either option is reasonable. Listen to whether the patient is leaning one way or the other, then tell him the choice is okay.
   - You can also tell him, if he is not ready to decide, that you will be available to discuss it when he is ready.
   - If he asks what you would choose, tell him you know men who have chosen both options.
   - In a few rare cases, a patient won't be able to make his own decision. If you must choose for him, try to think about which patient scenario best fits your patient.

---

decision aids often market them similarly to disease management programs. They may include personalized coaching by a nurse or other health care professional to help guide patients through the whole process. In some cases, especially in very sensitive areas such as decisions about end-of-life care, decision support aids have been designed to help structure and improve patient-physician conversations per se, with the physician taking the explicit role of professional guide (http://www.ama-assn.org/resources/doc/cms/a10-cms-rpt-7.pdf).

Many decision aids have been routinized using computer-based applications, particularly to help health care professionals integrate a patient's preferences (values) with scientific evidence, the patient's history, and local constraints. These decision aids are especially desirable when the optimal management strategy depends on the strength of the patient's preferences for the different health outcomes that may result from the decision (Gilhooly & McGhee, 1991). For example, a decision system for contraceptives choice would not only take into account personal risk factors (such as smoking) to determine the best choice but would also determine the values the patient places on different outcomes, such as unwanted pregnancy or venous thrombosis.

Decision support interventions could support choices in cancer prevention and chemoprevention by clarifying the decision (e.g., by providing details on the condition, evidence-based recommendations, benefits and harms of the option), elucidating the values underlying the choice (e.g., individuals' perception of benefits relative to harms), screening for implementation problems (e.g., self-efficacy), and providing referrals for additional support (e.g., evidence-based interventions).

For some prevention decisions, such as undertaking physical activity or eating more fruits and vegetables each day, there may be no readily measurable decision points, so intervening artificially imposes a structure or a "stopping rule" on a seemingly continuous process. The imposition of a structure may be useful in mapping the complexity of the decision, however.

For example, one may make the decision to make dietary change; second, one may develop an action plan to accomplish this; and third, one may make decisions day by day as the process is implemented. Because decisions are neither right nor wrong, individuals may encounter considerable difficulties or conflict in making these types of decisions. Sometimes these decisions may involve doing nothing as a reasonable option. Decision support in this context would focus on clarifying the decision, including the benefits, harms, and scientific uncertainties, as well as the importance and value that an individual may place on them (Sheinfeld Gorin, Wang, Raich, Bowen, Hay, 2006).

Evaluation of Decision Aids

Standards evaluating the quality of patient decision aids have been developed by the International Patient Decision Aids Standards (IPDAS) Collaboration, a multidisciplinary effort, led by researchers from Canada and the United Kingdom. Researchers, practitioners, patients, and policy makers from 14 countries have used online tools to establish a consensus on criteria that could be used to measure the reliability of a decision aid in three broad areas: content, development process, and effectiveness (Elwyn et al., 2006).

The IPDAS instrument (IPDASi) identifies 10 specific elements that should be evaluated to determine the comprehensiveness and integrity of the tool (information, probabilities, values, guidance, development, evidence, disclosure, plain language, evaluation, and test; http://www.ipdasi.org/; Ekwyn, O'Connor, Stacey, Volk, Edwards, et al., 2006). For example, evaluation elements include whether the tool adequately describes the health condition and all treatment options (including no treatment); what methods are used to help patients clarify values; whether a systematic development process followed; how developer credentials are documented and scientific evidence verified; and how conflicts of interest are identified and handled. The National Committee for Quality Assurance (NCQA, described in Chapter 2) has communicated with the IPDAS Collaboration steering committee about the possibility of developing accreditation standards for decision aids or the process of using them.

When compared to controls, decision aids help uncertain patients at baseline to increase their knowledge, reduce decisional conflict, and increase their desire to participate in decision making, without increasing anxiety (O'Connor, Fiset, DeGrasse, et al., 1999; O'Connor, Rostom, Fiset, et al., 1999; Molenaar, Sprangers, Postma-Schuit, et al. 2000; Sheinfeld Gorin, Wang, Raich, Bowen, Hay, 2006). A recent Cochrane Review systematically assessed 86 studies (Stacey, Bennett, Barry, Col, & Eden, 2011); the findings revealed that decision aids with explicit values clarification exercises improved informed values-based choices; decision aids appeared to have a positive effect on patient-practitioner communication; and decision aids had a variable effect on the length of consultation and choices. Decision aids increased the involvement in decision making and improved knowledge and a realistic perception of outcomes; however, the size of the effect varied across studies. Decision aids reduced the choice of discretionary surgery and had no apparent adverse effects on health outcomes or satisfaction with the decision. The effects on adherence with the chosen option, patient-practitioner communication, cost-effectiveness, and use with lower literacy populations needed further evaluation. Little is known about the degree of detail that decision aids need in order to have positive effects on attributes of the decision or the decision-making process itself.

THE FIVE As

The 5 As framework (ask, advise, assess, assist, and arrange; http://www.ahrq.gov/clinic/tobacco/5steps.htm) was first developed for smoking-cessation counseling (Glynn & Manley, 1989), as described previously in Chapters 4 through 7. The 5 As were first published in the influential *Treating Tobacco Use and Dependence* (Fiore et al., 2000), alongside the 5 Rs to enhance motivation for cessation (relevance, risk, rewards, roadblocks, and repetition; see Figure 11-1). In 2002, The Counseling and Behavioral Interventions Work Group of the US Preventive Services Task Force (USPSTF) recommended adoption of the "5 As" as a unifying framework for evaluating and describing health behavior counseling interventions in clinical settings (Whitlock, Orleans, & Pender, 2002).

Application of the 5 As to Tobacco Cessation

Tobacco-related disease is one of the leading preventable causes of death in the United States, as discussed throughout Chapters 4 through 7. Given the proportion of American adults who currently smoke cigarettes (19%; Adams, Kirzinger, Martinez,, 2012), even if health professionals have only a small effect on quit rates, the public health impact of this change could potentially be enormous.

Cessation Counseling among Health Care Providers

Application of the 5 As for smoking cessation in clinical practice vary, as discussed in Sheinfeld Gorin and Heck (2004). A survey of 1,400 smokers found that over one-half welcomed physician advice and stated that it would have a strong influence on their decision to quit (Ossip Klein, McIntosh, Utman, Burton, Spada, Guido, 2000). The majority of health care providers report inquiring about patients' smoking status and recording smoking status on the medical chart, although these practices vary by the patient's age (McIlvain, Crabtree, Backer, Turner, 2000). From 21–74% of patients (Jamal et al., 2012; Eckert, Junker, 2001; Rogers, Johnson, Young, & Graney, 1997) have reported receiving cessation advice from their providers. Depending on the setting, 45–81% of physicians (Easton, Husten, Elon, Pederson, Frank, 2001; O'Loughlin, Makni, Tremblay, et al.,

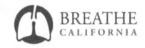

THE 5 A's OF INTERVENTION

ASK - 1 minute
Ask patient to describe their smoking status.
A. I NEVER smoked or smoked LESS THAN 100 cigarettes.
B. I stopped smoking more than 2 weeks ago but less than 1 year ago.
C. I stopped smoking more than 1 year ago.
D. I smoke regularly/not thinking of quitting in the next 30 days.

If B or C, reinforce their decision to quit, congratulate and encourage.

If D, document smoking status on their chart. Begin steps below.

ADVISE - 1 minute
Provide clear, strong advice to quit with personalized messages about the impact of smoking on health; urge every tobacco user to quit.

ASSESS - 1 minute
Assess the willingness to make a quit attempt within 30 days.
• Patient is willing to make a quit attempt in the next 14-30 days
• Patient is not willing to make a quit attempt (review the 5 R's below)

ASSIST - 3 minutes
Recommend the use of approved pharmacotherapy.
Refer to community cessation services or Internet when appropriate.
AND/OR
Help the patient develop a quit plan.
Provide problem-solving methods and skills for cessation.
Provide social support as a part of the treatment.
Help patient obtain extra treatment/social support for quitting in the smoker's environment.
Recommend the use of approved pharmacotherapy.
Provide self-help smoking cessation materials.

ARRANGE - 1 minute +
Assess smoking status every visit, reinforce/encourage cessation.

THE 5 R's OF MOTIVATION

RELEVANCE - 1 minute
Ask patient about how quitting may be personally relevant.
• Longer and better quality of life   • Extra money
• People you live with will be healthier
• Decrease chance of heart attack, stroke or cancer
• If pregnant, improves chance of healthy baby

RISKS - 1 minute
Ask the patient about their perception of short-term, long-term and environmental risks of continued use.
• Acute (breathing, asthma, pregnancy) • Long-term (heart, lungs, health)

REWARDS - 1 minute
Ask the patient about perceived benefits/rewards for quitting tobacco use.
• Health (self & others)   • Food taste
• Sense of smell   • Feel better
• Example to others   • Additional years of life

ROADBLOCKS - 3 minutes +
Ask patient about perceived roadblocks to quitting.
• Withdrawal symptoms   • Fear of failure
• Weight gain   • Lack of support
• Depression   • Enjoyment of tobacco

REPETITION - 1 minute +
Respectfully repeat 5 R's each visit, providing motivation and information.
Refer non-pregnant patient to 1-866-PITCH-EM and pregnant patient to 1-866-66START, community cessation services or Internet as appropriate.

FIGURE 11-1: Five As and Five Rs of Smoking Cessation.

Source: http://www.sccgov.org/sites/sccphd/en-us/HealthProviders/TobaccoPreventionDocumentsForm%20C_5A's%20and%205R's%20 of%20cessation.pdf.

2001; Gottlieb, Guo, Blozis, Huang, 2001), 36–71% of nurses (Sarna, Brown, Lillington, Rose, Wewers, Brecht, 2000; McEwen, West, 2001), and 51–61% of dentists (Lodi, Bez, Rimondini, Zuppiroli, Sardella, Carrassi, 1997; John, Yudkin, Murphy, Ziebland, Fowler, 1997) report having advised patients to quit, although fewer report assisting patients in cessation or arranging follow-up (Goldstein, DePue, Monroe, et al., 1998; Grimley, Bellis, Raczynski, Henning, 2001). Factors associated with receiving counseling include white race, male gender, being healthier, younger, and having insurance (Doescher & Saver, 2000; Borum, 2000). Primary care physicians and obstetricians-gynecologists report higher rates of counseling than do pediatricians (Easton, Husten, Malarcher, et al., 2001). Research has found that counseling is done most often during new patient visits, with younger patients, and by physicians who have been in practice for fewer years (Fiore et al., 2000).

Surveys of medical professionals have evaluated their receptivity to providing tobacco cessation counseling (among nurses, McCarty, Hennrikus, Lando, Vessey, 2001; among dentists, Fried & Cohen, 1992; Allard, 2000). Some of the common barriers cited by health care professionals were time (Pollak, Arredondo, Yarnall, et al., 2001), greater perceived complexity of a smoking cessation protocol (Bolman, de Vries, Mesters, 2002), and confidence in ability to counsel in this area (Sheinfeld Gorin, 2001). Other factors related to the provision of counseling include educational level (e.g., year of residency; Gottlieb, Guo, Blozis, Huang, 2001), having received training in cessation counseling (Hepburn, Johnson, Ward, Longfield, 2000), whether the provider smoked (Sheinfeld Gorin, 2001), the provider's race/ethnicity (Sheinfeld Gorin, 2001), and the strength of the provider-patient relationship (Coleman, Murphy, Cheater, 2000). Providing feedback to physicians may improve their motivation to counsel patients in cessation (Andrews, Tingen, Waller, Harper, 2001).

Several meta-analyses and literature reviews have assessed the efficacy of smoking cessation advice from varied health care professionals; they report a relationship between in-person advice, support from the medical team, the number and duration of sessions and patient quit rates (among physicians, Kottke et al., 1988; Ockene and Zapka, 1997; among nurses; Rice, 1999). Although the literature is sparse, advice from dentists may be effective in symptomatic populations (e.g., those with

pre-malignant oral lesions (Newton, Palmer, 1997; Gordon, Severson, 2001; Joseph, 2002; Hirshberg, Calderon, Kaplan, 2002).

A 2008 Cohrane review of randomized clinical trials on smoking cessation among physicians concluded that simple advice had a small effect on cessation rates. Assuming an unassisted quit rate of 2–3%, a brief advice intervention can increase quitting by a further 1–3% at least 6 months post-counseling. Additional components appear to have only a small effect, though there is a small additional benefit of more intensive interventions compared to very brief interventions. Providing follow-up support after offering the advice may increase the quit rates slightly (Stead, Bergson, & Lancaster, 2008).

Training programs have been designed to improve medical professionals' effectiveness, skills, and self-efficacy in this area. In the short term, they have been effective in improving providers' (particularly physicians') confidence and perceived effectiveness, and increasing rates of asking, advising, and providing self-help materials for cessation (Cornuz, Zellweger, Mounoud, Decrey, Pecoud, Burnand, 1997; Kawakami, Nakamura, Fumimoto, Takizawa, Baba, 1997).

The USPHS Guideline summarized the effects of physicians' counseling on tobacco cessation, finding them more effective than any other professional group alone (Fiore et al., 2008). In 2004, we reported that various health care professionals have critical influences on smoking cessation among their patients, yet they differ in their cessation efficacy. Using a meta-analysis of 37 randomized clinical trials or quasi-experiments (with control groups) of health care provider–delivered smoking cessation interventions, our findings revealed that physicians were the most effective at cessation. They were followed by multiprovider teams, dentists, and nurses. These findings suggest that contact with a health care professional will increase cessation; however, additional training in tobacco control for nurses is warranted. Longer-term studies of smoking cessation, particularly among dentists, are necessary (Sheinfeld Gorin & Heck, 2004).

THE 5 As APPLIED TO OTHER CHRONIC ILLNESSES: TWO SUBSTITUTE As

The 5 As have been expanded to include elements of relationship formation (with the substitution of "assess" for the first A, "ask" and "agree" for the third *A*) and have been applied to other health behaviors to enhance patient self-management in chronic illness care (Whitlock, Orleans, & Pender, 2002; Glasgow, Davis, Funnell et al, 2003; Glasgow, Funnell, Bonomi, et al., 2002; see Table 11-4). This 5 As framework is closely linked to the Principles of Effective Communication (Table 11-1), as relationship skills (e.g,. open-ended inquiry, reflective listening, and empathy) are essential elements of effective counseling interventions. Unlike the 5 As for smoking cessation, however, these 5 As include a specific relationship-building component. Both 5 As frameworks have advantages as tools for learning and the dissemination of prevention behaviors (Whitlock, Orleans, Pender et al., 2002; Goldstein, Whitlock, DePue, 2004; Glasgow & Goldstein, 2007).

Toward Routine Use of the 5 As in Clinical Practice

Given these findings, as well as those cited throughout Chapters 4 through 7, the primary care provider should ask about smoking at each visit, using a well-tested, brief model of the 5 As (ask/assess, advise, assess/agree, assist, and arrange; http://www. ahrq.gov/clinic/tobacco/5steps.htm). The Agency for Healthcare Research and Quality (AHRQ) recommends that smoking be considered a "vital sign," like blood pressure and weight, and thus should be queried and recorded at each visit (see Figure 11-2 for an example). A worksheet can integrate the 5As in clinical practices, although proposed routine (and often automated) patient assessment and screening tools (as described later in this Chapter) and many electronic health records also include cues for

smoking cessation (see Figure 11-3 for an example; http://healthpolicy.ucla.edu/mohr).

MOTIVATIONAL INTERVIEWING

The widely disseminated clinical method of motivational interviewing (MI) arose through a convergence of science and practice (Miller & Rose, 2009). Motivational interviewing focuses on exploring and resolving ambivalence and centers on motivational processes within the individual that facilitate change. MI supports change in a manner congruent with the person's own values and concerns, rather than coercing or imposing change. A current definition of motivational interviewing (2009) is: "A collaborative, person-centered form of guiding to elicit and strengthen motivation for change" (Miller & Rose, 2009). Components of MI may be applied by the physician in primary care, as discussed in Chapter 5, but it is generally applied in full by a trained therapist, wherein the patient is considered the counselor's client.

The definition of MI includes three core elements:

1. MI is a particular kind of conversation about change that is *collaborative* between the provider and the client.
2. MI is a *person-centered* counseling method that is *goal-oriented*, emphasizing the autonomy of the client.
3. MI is *evocative*, that is, it seeks to call forth the person's *own* motivation for and movement toward a specific goal by eliciting and exploring the person's own arguments for change (http://www.motivationalinterview. org/Documents/1%20A%20MI%20 Definition%20Principles%20&%20 Approach%20V4%20012911.pdf).

The Motivational Interviewing Approach

Motivational Interviewing focuses on building rapport in the initial stages of the counseling relationship. A central concept of MI is the identification, examination, and resolution of ambivalence about changing behavior.

As stated previously, central to change through MI is the client relationship. The clinician expresses empathy, develops discrepancy, avoids

---

Blood pressure: _____

Pulse: _____ Weight: _____

Temperature: _____

Respiratory rate: _____

Smoking: Current   Former   Never
                        (*circle one*)

FIGURE 11-2: Vital Signs Stamp with Smoking Status.

Source: Fiore MC. The new vital sign: assessing and documenting smoking status. *JAMA.* 1991;266:3183–3184.

> **OFFICE PRACTICE PLANNING**
> **MATRIX FOR IMPLEMENTING 5 A's**
>
> | Component | Who | What | When | Where | Resources needed | Notes |
> |---|---|---|---|---|---|---|
> | *ASSESS* | | | | | | |
> | *ADVISE* | | | | | | |
> | *AGREE* | | | | | | |
> | *ASSIST* | | | | | | |
> | *ARRANGE* | | | | | | |

FIGURE 11-3: Example of Worksheet to Integrate the Five As into Primary Care Practice.

Source: Glasgow RE, Goldstein MG. Introduction to the principles of health behavior change. In: Woolf S, ed. *Health Promotion and Disease Prevention in Clinical Practice,* 2nd ed., pp. 129–147. Philadelphia: Williams and Wilkins; 2007.

argumentation, rolls with resistance, and supports self-efficacy (http://www.motivationalinterview.org/Documents/METDrugAbuse.PDF).

Ambivalence, that is, feeling two ways about behavior change, is seen as a natural part of the change process. By contrast, provider exhortations or arguments for change tend to build resistance. Thus, when "change talk," which is discussed later in this Chapter, is elicited or spontaneously expressed by the patient, the clinician provides affirmation and support to help build and deepen commitment (Rollnick, Mason, & Butler, 1999; Miller & Rollnick, 1998). *Rolling with resistance* involves backing off when the patient expresses it, by acknowledging that change is difficult while also inviting the patient to consider new information or perspectives. The provider *supports self-efficacy* by helping the patient to build on past successes, take achievable small steps toward change, and problem solve to overcome barriers (Miller & Rollnick, 2002).

To address client ambivalence and "roll with resistance," the provider thoughtfully uses techniques and strategies that are responsive to the client. These MI strategies are built on three components of the counseling interchange: collaboration, evocation, and autonomy.

Collaboration (versus Confrontation)

Collaboration is a partnership between the clinician and the client, grounded in the point of view and experiences of the client. The therapeutic process is focused on mutual understanding, not the therapist being right.

Evocation (Drawing Out, Rather Than Imposing Ideas)

In the MI approach, the clinician draws out the individual's own thoughts and ideas, rather than imposing an opinion to motivate a commitment to change.

Autonomy (versus Authority)

Ultimately, it is up to the individual to follow through with making change happen. Clinicians reinforce that there is no single best way to change. In addition to deciding whether they will make a change, clients are encouraged to take the lead in developing a menu of options as to how to achieve the desired change.

THE PRINCIPLES OF MOTIVATIONAL INTERVIEWING

The clinician employing MI will seek to abide by these four principles throughout treatment (express empathy, support self-efficacy, roll with resistance, and develop discrepancy).

Express Empathy

The process of expressing empathy relies on the client's experiencing the provider as able to see the world as the client sees it.

Support Self-Efficacy

As discussed previously, self-efficacy concerns the individual's confidence in successfully accomplishing the task of change (e.g., smoking cessation; Bandura, 1986, 1998; as discussed in Chapter 3). MI is a strengths-based approach that believes that clients have within themselves the capabilities to change successfully. In motivational interviewing, clinicians support self-efficacy by focusing on previous successes and highlighting skills and strengths that the client already has.

Roll with Resistance

From an MI perspective, resistance in treatment occurs when the client experiences a conflict between his or her view of the problem or the solution and that of the provider, or when the client experiences infringement on his or her autonomy. These experiences are often based in the client's ambivalence about change. As stated previously, in MI, clinicians avoid eliciting resistance by not confronting the client; when resistance occurs, they "roll with it," working to de-escalate and avoid a negative interaction. Actions and statements that demonstrate resistance remain unchallenged, especially early in the counseling relationship. When the provider rolls with resistance, the session does not resemble an argument. When the MI provider values the client defining his or her problem and developing his or her own solutions, little is left for the client to resist. A frequently used metaphor is "dancing" rather than "wrestling" with the client. In exploring client concerns, clinicians invite clients to examine new points of view, and are careful not to impose their own ways of thinking. A key concept is that a clinician avoid the "righting reflex," a tendency to ensure that the client understands and agrees with the need to change and solves problems for the client.

Develop Discrepancy

Motivation for change occurs when people perceive a mismatch between where they are and where they want to be; a provider practicing motivational interviewing works to develop this by helping clients examine the discrepancies between their current circumstances or behaviors and their values and future goals. When clients recognize that their current behaviors place them in conflict with their values or interfere with the accomplishment of self-identified goals, they are more likely to experience increased motivation to make important life changes. It is important that the provider using MI does not use strategies to develop discrepancy at the expense of the other principles, yet gradually helps clients to become aware of how their current behaviors may lead them away from, rather than toward, their important goals.

Motivational Interviewing Strategies

The practice of motivational interviewing involves the skillful use of certain counseling techniques, including non-verbal communications, to establish a therapeutic alliance (or a "beneficial client-therapist attachment"; Horvath & Luborsky, 1993) and to capitalize on the client's potential for change. These are known by the acronym OARS, which describes open-ended questions, affirmations, reflections, and summaries.

- Open-ended questions, that is, those that are not easily answered by yes/no, or by a short, specific, limited response, are posed by the clinician. Open-ended questions invite elaboration and thinking more deeply about an issue. Closed-ended questions are used for assessment, however.
- Affirmations are statements that recognize client strengths and support client self-efficacy. They also assist in building rapport and in helping the client to see that change is possible. Affirmations include reframing behaviors or concerns as evidence of positive client qualities.
- Reflections, or reflective listening, are perhaps the most crucial skill in MI. Through the use of these skills, the client comes to feel that the provider understands the issues from his or her perspective and is empathic. With the use of reflections (i.e., repeating or rephrasing what the client has said, paraphrasing the client, or reflecting the client's feelings), the clinician guides the client toward resolving ambivalence by a focus on the negative aspects of the status quo and the positive aspects of making change.
- Summaries are a special type of reflection in which the clinician recaps what has occurred in all or part of a counseling session(s).

Summaries communicate interest and understanding and call attention to important elements of the discussion. They may be used to shift attention or direction and to prepare the client to move on. Summaries can highlight both sides of a client's ambivalence about change and can promote the development of discrepancy by strategically selecting what information should be included and what can be minimized or excluded.

Change Talk

OARS is implemented alongside the client's change talk. Change talk contains statements by the client revealing the consideration of, motivation for, or commitment to change, known as *DARNCAT*:

Desire (I want to change);

Ability (I can change);

Reason (It's important to change);

Need (I should change);

Commitment (I will make changes);

Activation (I am ready, prepared, and willing to change);

Taking steps (I am taking specific actions to change).

Strategies for Evoking Change Talk

Some specific therapeutic strategies are likely to elicit and support change talk in motivational interviewing:

1. Ask evocative questions: Ask an open question, the answer to which is likely to be change talk.
2. Explore decisional balance: Ask for the pros and cons of both changing and staying the same.
3. Good things/Not so good things: Ask about the positives and negatives of the target behavior.
4. Ask for elaboration/examples: When a change talk theme emerges, ask for more details. In what ways? Tell me more? What does that look like? When was the last time that happened?
5. Look back: Ask about a time before the target behavior emerged. How were things better or different?
6. Look forward: Ask what may happen if things continue as they are (status quo).

For example, If you were 100% successful in making the changes you want, what would be different? How would you like your life to be 5 years from now?

7. Query extremes: What are the worst things that might happen if you don't make this change? What are the best things that might happen if you do make this change?
8. Use "change rulers": Ask: On a scale from 1 to 10, how important is it to you to change [the specific target behavior], where 1 is not at all important, and 10 is extremely important? Follow up: And why are you at ____ and not ____ [a lower number than stated]? What might happen that could move you from ____ to [a higher number]? Alternatively, you could also ask: How confident are you that you could make the change if you decided to do it?
9. Explore goals and values: Ask what the client's guiding values are. What does he or she want in life? Ask how the continuation of target behavior fits in with the person's goals or values. Does it help realize an important goal or value, interfere with it, or is it irrelevant?
10. Come alongside: Explicitly side with the negative (status quo) side of ambivalence. Perhaps _____ is so important to you that you won't give it up, no matter what the cost.

Example of the Use of MI with a Diabetic Patient

A brief (scripted) example of the use of MI with a diabetic patient to encourage eating less high-fat foods follows:

- *Provider*: You know, we've discussed this many times before; perhaps eating high-fat foods is so important to you that you won't give it up, no matter what the cost. (*Come alongside*)
- *Patient response*: I really should change; my health and staying around for my family are more important than eating burgers at McD's. (*Change talk*)
- *Provider*: That's great to hear you say; in what (specific) ways could you reduce the high-fat foods in your diet? (*Ask for elaboration/examples*)

Shortened Form of MI for Primary Care Practices

Brief versions of MI have been developed for use by providers in primary care and other health care settings (Rollnick, Mason, & Butler, 1999; Goldstein, 2002; Goldstein, 2002; Rollnick & Butler, 2005; Rollnick, Mason, & Butler, 1999) These versions emphasize the MI strategies described earlier and the assessment of two specific dimensions of motivation: (1) conviction or importance regarding the need for change, and (2) confidence or self-efficacy about taking action. Assessment is followed by the tailoring of counseling to address the patient's level of conviction and confidence, agreeing on a realistic and achievable goal, and assisting the patient in developing a behavior change plan.

As a general rule, if both conviction and confidence are low, it is most efficient to first focus on enhancing conviction. For patients with low conviction levels, effective counseling strategies include providing information and feedback (after asking the patient's permission), exploring ambivalence, and providing a menu of options for treatment and follow-up. Patients not ready to commit to action may agree to simply think about the possibilities for change or to seek assistance when they are ready to take action. For patients with low confidence, strategies include reviewing past experience, especially successes; teaching problem-solving and coping skills; and encouraging small steps that are likely to lead to initial success. For all patients, a follow-up plan is essential, as evidence suggests that follow-up is an important ingredient of all successful health behavior change counseling interventions (Goldstein, Whitlock, & DePue, 2004; Fiore et al., 2000; Norris, Nichols, Caspersen, et al., 2002; Glasgow & Goldstein, 2007; see Table 11-4 for a summary of these strategies within the 5 As).

Evaluation of Motivational Interviewing

MI has been found effective in decreasing substance abuse in a number of multisite clinical trials. The first multisite trial of motivational enhancement therapy (MET) provided a "check-up," or a 4-session intervention with a personal assessment, in addition to MI (Project MATCH, a 9-site psychotherapy trial with 1,726 clients; http://www.motivationalinterview.org/Documents/METDrugAbuse.PDF; Miller, Zweben, DiClemente, & Rychtarik, 1992); Project MATCH Research Group, 1993).

Outcomes through 3 years of follow-up were similar for a 4-session MET and the two 12-session treatment methods with which it was compared, yielding a cost-effectiveness advantage for MET (Babor & Del Boca, 2003; Holder et al., 2000; Project MATCH Research Group, 1997, 1998a). Similar positive findings emerged from the 3-site United Kingdom Alcohol Treatment Trial comparing MET with an 8-session family-involved behavior therapy (Copello et al., 2001; UKATT Research Team, 2005a, 2005b; Miller & Rose, 2009).

The Clinical Trials Network of the US National Institute on Drug Abuse has undertaken six multisite trials of MI and MET as compared with treatment-as-usual for drug problems and dependence (Carroll et al., 2002). MI-based interventions promote sustained reductions in alcohol use (Ball et al., 2007) and increased treatment retention (Carroll et al., 2006). MET exerted a significant beneficial effect at some sites but not others, however (Ball et al., 2007; Winhusen et al., 2008; Miller & Rose, 2009).

Not all trials have been positive. Null findings for MI have been reported, for example, among those with eating disorders (Treasure et al., 1998), drug abuse and dependence (Miller, Yahne, & Tonigan, 2003; Winhusen et al., 2008), in smoking cessation (Baker et al., 2006; Colby et al., 1998), and problem drinking (Kuchipudi, Hobein, Fleckinger, & Iber, 1990). Even within well-controlled multisite trials, MI has worked at some sites but not others, as mentioned previously (Ball et al., 2007; Winhusen et al., 2008). It is apparent that some providers are significantly more effective than others in delivering the same MI-based treatment (Project MATCH Research Group, 1998b); even in positive trials, a certain proportion of clients do not respond to MI (Miller & Rose, 2009).

The efficacy of MI also can vary across populations. A meta-analysis found that the effect size of MI was doubled when the recipients were predominantly from minority populations, as compared with white non-Hispanic Americans (Hettema, Steele, & Miller, 2005). A retrospective analysis of Project MATCH data found that Native Americans responded better to MET, as compared with other treatments (Villanueva, Tonigan, & Miller, 2007). Similarly, Clinical Trials Network studies found some evidence for differential benefit from MET among pregnant drug users from minority backgrounds relative to other women (Winhusen et al., 2008; Miller & Rose, 2009).

TABLE 11-4. THE 5 As FOR BEHAVIORAL COUNSELING AND HEALTH BEHAVIOR CHANGE

Assess:
- Ask about and assess behavioral health risks and factors that affect choice of behavior change goals and methods
- Assess beliefs, behaviors, knowledge, motivation, and past experience (some recommend performing this step as part of "Agree")
- Assessing behavioral risk factors identifies patients in need of intervention and provides a basis for tailoring brief interventions for maximum benefit

Advise:
- Give clear, specific, well-timed, and personalized behavior change advice, including information about personal health harms and benefits
- Provider advice establishes behavioral issues as an important part of health care
- Advise in a non-coercive, non-judgmental manner that respects readiness for change and patient autonomy
- Advice is most powerful when linked to the patient's own health concerns, past experiences, family/social situations, and level of health literacy

Agree:
- Collaboratively select appropriate goals and methods based on the patient's interest in and willingness to change the behavior
- Collaborate to find common ground and to define behavior change goals and methods
- Shared decision making (see above) is especially recommended for interventions that involve significant risk-benefit trade-offs
- Shared decision making about behavior change results in a greater sense of personal control, choices based in realistic expectations and patient values, improved patient adherence, and time saved in the examination room.

Assist:
- Using self-help resources and/or counseling, help the patient to achieve goals by acquiring skills, confidence, and social and environmental supports for behavior change
- Health care staff provide motivational interventions, address barriers to change, and/or secure support needed for successful change
- Effective interventions teach self-management and problem-solving or coping skills that enable patients to take the next immediate steps toward targeted behavior change

Arrange:
- An action plan is developed that lists goals, barriers, and strategies, and specifies follow-up plans
- Schedule follow-up (in person or by telephone) to provide ongoing assistance and support and to adjust the plan as needed, including referral to non-specialized interventions
- Consider behavioral risk factors as chronic problems that change over time
- Routine follow-up assessment and support through some kind of contact is usually necessary to promote and maintain behavior change

Goldstein M, Whitlock EP, DePue J. Multiple health risk behavior interventions in primary care: summary of research evidence. *Am J Prev Med.* 2004;27(2 Suppl):61–79.

While MI has been found effective across many rigorous trials, variability in outcomes across and within studies suggests the need to understand when and how a treatment works and the conditions of delivery that may affect its efficacy. These include the characteristics of the provider. Future research is needed to examine linkages between the processes of delivery and client outcomes, a form of research pioneered by Carl Rogers and his students (Truax & Carkhuff, 1967; Miller & Rose, 2009).

TAILORED TELEPHONE COUNSELING

Tailored telephone counseling (TTC) is a structured form of counseling, often supported by a counseling script that includes three components: (1) gathering information from the individual; (2) selecting messages from a message collection directly related to the individual's concerns or barriers; and (3) delivering the "tailored" messages (Luckmann, 2007). Generally, these interventions are led by trained counselors or health educators, rather than physicians;

some elements of TTC have been incorporated into routine primary care practice using computer aided telephone interviewing (CATI), for example.

The following section describes the application of TTC to promote the receipt of colorectal cancer (CRC) screening tests (developed by Randi Wolfe and Sherri Sheinfeld Gorin; unpublished manuscript; see Figure 11-4). The tailored telephone approach integrates a computer-assisted tailored interview (CATI) for assessment with a pre-defined set of questions (e.g., How likely are you to get an FOBT over the next 6 months?) and standardized health educator responses from a pre-tested message bank. The health educator tailors these messages to the patient's risk perceptions, knowledge, barriers and supports to change, and stage of change, as found in the patient's questionnaire that is completed during the assessment period (see the example later in this Chapter).

As described in Chapter 4, colorectal cancer screening tests include fecal occult blood test (FOBT), fecal immunochemical test (FIT), flexible sigmoidoscopy, colonoscopy, double-contrast barium enema (DCBE), CT (computed tomography), and colonography (or virtual colonoscopy). The stool DNA test has been tested for the early detection of colorectal cancer, but is not yet approved for clinical use by the Food and Drug Administration (http://www.fda.gov/MedicalDevices/default.htm).

Tailored Telephone Counseling (TTC) Intervention Process

The outcome of the TTC is that the patient obtains a CRC screening test within one year of the intervention. Health educators (including nurses, counselors, as well as other trained members of the medical team) tailor messages to the patient for this purpose. Health educators rely upon a web-accessible set of tailored messages (~97) and a branching structure for their messages to patients, as outlined on Figure 11-4. The three primary goals of the telephone contacts are to: (1) establish a positive and trusting rapport between the health educator and the participant; (2) provide information about screening guidelines, as well as the importance of early detection and treatment for colorectal cancer; and (3) encourage and prepare participants to receive a colorectal cancer screening test with consideration for the perceived risk (of disease), stage of change, and supports to and barriers to change. Emphasis is placed on positive reinforcement for learning about the risks for colorectal cancer (CRC), stressing the asymptomatic nature of the disease, the importance of early detection and treatment, and enhancing perceived self-efficacy

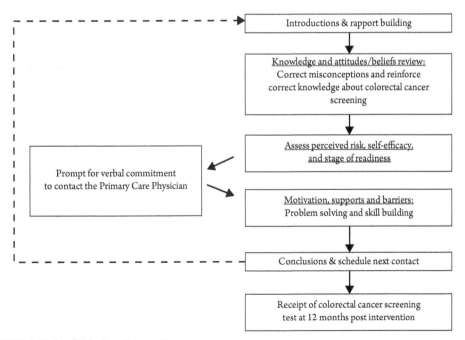

FIGURE 11-4: Tailored Telephone Intervention.

Source: Randi Wolfe and Sherri Sheinfeld Gorin (unpublished manuscript)

to overcome barriers to screening. As listed previously, the counseling is tailored to the following variables: level of knowledge and misconceptions; stage of change; motivation and barriers (e.g., ability to communicate with a primary care provider about a colorectal cancer screening test, ability to obtain and complete a CRC test). Patients are encouraged to contact their primary care providers (PCPs) directly for a CRC screening test. Improving implementation of cancer screening guidelines must involve not only acceptance of the procedures by PCPs but also compliance by their patients with completing the recommended tests or examinations.

Tailored telephone interviewing includes the following components:

Introductions and rapport building: The health educator explains that he or she is calling to discuss early detection and treatment of colorectal cancer and the study procedures. Established techniques are used for building rapport, as described previously.

Review of knowledge and attitudes/beliefs related to colorectal cancer screening tests: During the initial contact, the health educator highlights select factual information pertaining to the magnitude of colorectal cancer, risk factors, the often asymptomatic nature of disease, and the importance of early detection and treatment. In addition, the health educator discusses current professional guidelines (e.g., American Cancer Society) for colorectal cancer. Responses to questions from an initial assessment (e.g., via a questionnaire) are used to tailor the initial call with the goal of reinforcing accurate information and correcting misconceptions. Some of these questions are derived from the Core CRC Screening Questions (Vernon et al., 2004) and include: (1) When did you do your most recent [name the] test? (2) Why did you do your most recent [name the] test? (3) When did you do the [name the] test before your most recent one? (4) Why did you have that [name the] test?

Information about screening guidelines and the importance of early detection and treatment for CRC are reinforced at each subsequent telephone contact.

Prompt for verbal commitment and assessment of stage of readiness to talk to physician: The health educator attempts to elicit a verbal commitment from the participant to contact the PCP to obtain a CRC screening test. The health educator tailors the discussion based on the participant's stage of change, as it may vary over time. Obtaining (or striving to obtain) a verbal commitment is key to the behavior change process, and it justifies subsequent contacts with the participant. For example, if participants respond "Yes" when asked if they intend to contact their PCPs for a colorectal cancer screening test within the next 12 months, the health educator considers them to be in the "preparation" phase (of the stages of change, as described in Chapter 3). The health educator offers participants the necessary tools to assist with the behavior change (e.g., assistance with making an appointment). In this stage, the focus is on increasing the participant's confidence (self-efficacy) so that he or she can attempt this change and succeed.

Assessment of motivation and addressing barriers: Once a stage of change is determined, the health educator probes about both higher (e.g., action) and lower (e.g., contemplation) stages of change. For example, if a participant is only thinking about having a colorectal cancer screening test within the next 12 months, the health educator probes: "You are thinking about a colorectal cancer screening test. Can you tell me why you are thinking about a colorectal cancer screening test in the next 12 months, and not now? What would it take to get you to have a colorectal cancer screening test now?" During this segment of the discussion, the health educator identifies the supports and barriers to change, which are addressed through a series of standardized approaches, such as role playing to build skills and joint problem solving. The health educator seeks to overcome resistance to obtaining a CRC screening test now.

Conclusion and scheduling next contact: At the end of each call, the health educator does, if necessary, continue to prompt for a verbal commitment from the participant to contact his or her PCP for a colorectal cancer screening test, and schedules a follow-up telephone contact. Notes taken during and after the discussion guide subsequent communications.

Follow-up contacts: The subsequent contacts, *within 1 to 2 months after the previous contact,* vary (*up to 6 maximum*), depending, for example, on whether the participant has scheduled an appointment, or has reported a colorectal cancer screening test. These contacts also are tailored based on information gleaned from the first contact, including the participant's level of understanding about colorectal cancer screening testing, as well as his or her stage of readiness to talk to a PCP about these tests, motivation and barriers. Generally, a follow-up contact begins by reviewing the prior conversation. For example, after reestablishing rapport, the health educator will say: "When we spoke last, you said you were going to contact your PCP about completing a colorectal cancer screening test. Were you able to complete the colorectal cancer screening test? For example, if participants state "Yes," then they are considered in the "action" stage. Here, he or she needs positive reinforcement for the changes attained and support for moving on to the "maintenance" stage. Participants are reminded of the periodicity of the American Cancer Society CRC screening recommendations, for example, unless screening is recommended more frequently by their PCPs or a gastroenterologist. On the other hand, if participants express that they are not ready now, the health educator probes for reasons, engaging in reflective listening and paraphrasing to maintain rapport, as in motivational interviewing. The health educator is prompted with a set of messages from the (computer-based) message bank in response to the participant's expressed supports and barriers to CRC screening. For example, if patients report that they are no longer thinking about having a colorectal cancer screening test now, the health educator will ask: "What would it take for you to obtain a CRC screening test now?" The health educator notes how the stages of change might change from session to session and uses the appropriate messages for each stage. For example: "Last week you were ready to obtain a CRC screening test, but this week you are not. Can you tell me a why that might be?" At the conclusion of each follow-up contact, the participant is asked to make a commitment to schedule an appointment with his or her PCP, if he or she has not already done so. If the participant has made an appointment,

he or she will be asked for a verbal commitment to keep the appointment. The next contact is also scheduled.

Evaluation of Tailored Telephone Counseling

There is a growing body of evidence linking tailored interventions to increased cancer screening compliance (Vernon, 1999), compliance with retinopathy for diabetes (Jones, Walker, Schechter, & Blanco, 2010), and that tailoring interventions can affect preventive health behavior (Owen, Klapow, Hicken & Tucker, 2001; McPhereson, Higginson, & Heaarn, 2001), including reducing sedentary lifestyles, less eating of red meat, more eating of fruits and vegetables (Speck & Looney, 2001; Dubbert, 2002; Marcus, Bock, Pinto, Forsyth, Roberts, & Traficante, 1998; Brug, Campbell, & Van Assema, 1999). TTC has improved compliance with colposcopy (Lerman, Hanjani, Caputo, Miller, Delmoor, Nolte, et al., 1992) and improved follow-ups of abnormal Pap smears (Yabroff, Mangan, Mandelblatt, 2003; Miller, Siejak, Schroeder, Lerman, Hernandez, & Helm, 1997). TTC has demonstrated effectiveness in smoking cessation (Britt, Curry, McBride, Grothaus, & Louie, 1994; Lando, Rommens, Klevan, Roski, Cherney, Lauger, 1997; Leed-Kelly, Russel, Bobo, McIlvain, 1996; Zhu, Stretch, Balabanis, Rosbrook, Sadler, Pierce, 1996; Strecher, 1999; Lipkus, Lyna, & Rimer, 1999). TTC can increase mammography utilization over a mailed reminder, alongside physician recommendation and the opportunity to schedule the test (Yabroff, Mandelblatt, 1999; Stoddard, Fox, Costanza, et al., 2002). Research on TTC to increase colorectal cancer screening is limited, although a modified TTC intervention delivered annually was found significantly more effective than a control in increasing rates of FOBT (OR=1.46, 95% Cl 1.1–2.0; Tilley, Vernon, Myers, & Hanz, et al., 1999). In a recent TTC outreach intervention for CRC screening that was loosely tied to patients' PCPs, but not to an opportunity for scheduling an appointment, 80% of eligible patients accepted a TTC call (White, Stark, Luckmann, Rosal, Clemow, & Costanza, 2006). It therefore demonstrates considerable promise.

Figure 11-5 illustrates a CATI system for counseling that has been used across a large health care system for breast cancer screening counseling. In this approach, a provider (not a computer) interacts with a client via telephone. The provider is supported by the computer program (Luckmann, 2007).

COUNSELING WITH RELATIONAL AGENTS

Prevention counseling has also been conducted entirely by computer, using "relational agents" (computational artifacts designed to build and maintain long-term, social-emotional relationships with their users, often looking like homunculi; http://www. ccs.neu.edu/home/bickmore/agents/). They use a computerized message bank and artificial intelligence approaches to tailor the relational agent's response to the human (see Figure 11-6). Since face-to-face conversation is the primary context of relationship building for humans, relational agents are considered a specialized kind of embodied

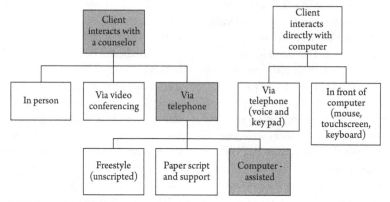

FIGURE 11-5: CATI Counseling for Cancer Screening. This diagram shows where CATI systems for counseling fit in a classification of counseling options. In this model, a counselor (not a computer) interacts with a client via telephone. The counselor is supported by the computer program.

Source: Luckmann R. *Applying Computer Assisted Telephone Interviewing (CATI) Methodology to Tailored Telephone Counseling (TTC) on Cancer Behavior.* Presentation to the Society of Behavioral Medicine, 2007.

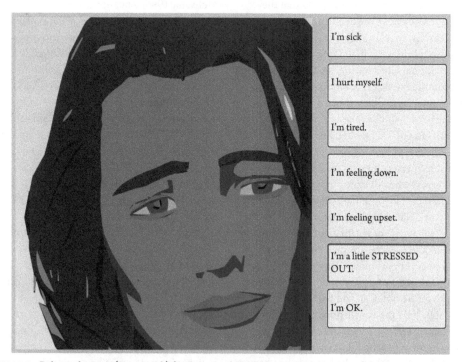

FIGURE 11-6: Relational Agents (Homunculi) for Automated Health Communication Systems.

Source: Bickmore T. *Relational Agents for Health Behavior Change.* Presentation to the Society of Behavioral Medicine, 2007.

conversational agent, with animated humanoid software agents that use speech, gaze, gesture, intonation, and other nonverbal modalities to emulate the experience of human face-to-face conversation. Relational agents are explicitly designed to remember past history and manage future expectations in their interactions with users (http://www.ccs.neu.edu/home/bickmore/agents/).

Evaluation of Relational Agents

One recent qualitative (focus group) and usability study of the use of a relational agent among a small sample of women from a safety net hospital and university increased the reporting of pre-conception health risks. Differences were noted in the effectiveness of the relational agent based on initial stage of change (Gardiner, Hempstead, Ring, et al., 2013). One study has suggested that counseling approaches using computerized relational agents could integrate best practices from provider-patient communication into automated health communication systems, thus enhancing possible wider dissemination (Vinson, Bickmore, Farrell, et al., 2011). Relational agents could provide an intuitive, engaging, and effective medium for behavioral interventions; they may be especially effective for individuals with low health, reading, or computer literacy (Bickmore, 2007; Gardiner, Hempstead, Ring, et al., 2013).

Recent work has demonstrated the ability of relational agents to establish and maintain relationships with people over a series of interactions. In this effort, the agent played the role of an advisor designed to motivate users to exercise more. One hundred subjects participated in a six-week longitudinal study (four week intervention and two week follow up) to determine the efficacy of this agent. Results indicate that the agent was successful at creating and maintaining a trusting, caring relationship with users and increasing their desire to continue interacting with it (http://www.ccs.neu.edu/home/bickmore/agents/). The evaluation of relational agents has been too limited thus far to assess its promise longer-term.

RISK ASSESSMENT APPROACHES IN PRIMARY CARE PRACTICE

Providers are increasingly urged—even mandated—to help patients make informed medical decisions by paying more attention to risk counseling. For some, the role of risk counseling is new and unfamiliar.

Schwartz, Woloshin, and Welch (1999) have suggested a three-pronged approach to risk communication (notably in cancer), including (1) developing a comprehensive population database about disease risk and treatment benefit to be created and maintained by the federal government; (2) helping health communicators (e.g., journalists) present data to the public clearly and objectively; and (3) educating patients via office-based visual aids and tutorials (Schwartz, Woloshin, & Welch, 1999). All three of these approaches are explored fully in a paper by Schwartz, Woloshin, and Welch (1999). Only the third element, educating the patient, primarily in cancer, will now be examined further.

Office-Based Visuals: Approaches to Educating Patients on Risk Assessment

A fundamental goal of health risk communication is to help people better understand the important health risks they face. This goal, a basic concept of contemporary medical ethics (Emanuel & Emanuel, 1992), also has practical implications. Patients who received more information from their physician were more satisfied and had higher compliance with medical regimens than those who received less (Hall, Roter, & Katz, 1988). At a minimum, understanding the magnitude of a risk (e.g., How big of a threat is breast cancer to me?) entails having some idea of what the risk is (What does it mean to have breast cancer?) and the chances of developing or dying of the condition. One reason that physicians may not engage in risk communication with patients is that they lack easy access to the relevant data. Simple office-based tools may help overcome this barrier (Schwartz, Woloshin, & Welch, 1999).

Office-based tools may stimulate and facilitate discussions about disease risks. Patients may want to know the answer to questions such as, What is the chance that a person my age will die of heart disease or breast cancer in the next 10 years? Similarly, patients may also find information about the benefit of various risk-reducing strategies valuable; for example, How does my chance of dying of breast cancer change if I have annual mammograms? To be useful, such office-based tools need to be up to date, immediately available, and easy for both providers and patients to use and to understand (Schwartz, Woloshin, & Welch, 1999).

Disease-Specific Tools

A number of tools that generate disease-specific risk estimates for an individual patient are now available. For example, the American Heart Association (Wilson, D'Agostino, Levy, Belanger, Silbershatz, Kannel, et al., 1998) has a website where an individual's risk of myocardial infarction can be calculated with the use of a model generated from the Framingham data, as discussed in Chapter 5. The Northern New England Cardiovascular Group (O'Connor, Plume, Olmstead, Coffin, Morton, Maloney, et al., 1992) uses a preprogrammed handheld computer to provide patients considering coronary artery bypass graft surgery with an estimate of the mortality risk they face from surgery. The National Cancer Institute (http://www.cancer.gov/bcrisktool/) has issued the Breast Cancer Risk Assessment Tool, which provides women with their risk of developing breast cancer to help women contemplating tamoxifen for the primary prevention of breast cancer (see Figure 11-7; Schwartz, Woloshin, & Welch, 1999). One of the most widely used tools, the *Disease Risk Index,* provides individuals the opportunity to find the risk of developing five major diseases in the United States and to obtain personalized approaches to preventing them (http://www.diseaseriskindex.harvard.edu/update/).

Implementing these tools in clinical practice entails collecting the necessary risk factor information from patients, preferably before a clinic visit, and generating a risk report (e.g., the breast cancer risk factors required for the Breast Cancer Risk Assessment Tool, reflected in Figure 11-7; Gail, Brinton, Byar, Corle, Green, Schairer, et al., 1989). Such risk reports (or the findings from assessment and screening tools as discussed later in this Chapter) could then be included in patients' medical records at the time of a scheduled clinic appointment with their providers to maximize the chance of discussion. Some evidence (Kalichman & Coley, 1995; Skinner, Strecher, & Hospers, 1994; Rimer & Glassman, 1998) suggests that such personalized—or tailored—messages may be more effective than generic messages. Whether the extra time, cost, and technical difficulty of these personalized reports outweigh this potential advantage is unknown, however (Schwartz, Woloshin, & Welch, 1999)

Although such tools are appealing because the disease-specific estimate is tailored to the patient, the inherent focus on a single disease taken out

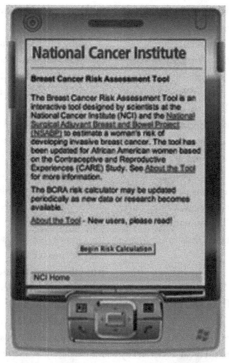

FIGURE 11-7: Breast Cancer Risk Assessment Screen. Reproduced with permission.

of context may overweigh its importance. When making a decision, a patient may find it helpful to understand where this particular disease fits into the important health threats that he or she faces. Patients may find it particularly helpful to know: How does my chance of dying of this particular disease compare with other diseases? What is my overall chance of dying? How does the overall mortality benefit of one intervention (e.g., mammography) compare with the benefit of another (e.g., giving up cigarettes)? (Schwartz, Woloshin, & Welch, 1999).

Comprehensive Visual Tools: Disease Risk and Benefit

To provide this context, charts with age- and sex-specific data about disease risks and treatment benefits are proposed. Figures 11-8 and 11-9 present examples of such simple office tools. Such low-tech tools can also be available online and can be downloaded either prior to, during, or after an office visit, for example, on an office-based kiosk. Simple paper-based tools are inexpensive and could be used anywhere (e.g., posted in any clinic office), require no special hardware and no additional personnel or maintenance (Schwartz, Woloshin, & Welch, 1999).

Disease Risk Chart

The disease risk chart shown in Table 11-5 displays 10-year disease-specific mortality data for five major diseases—in this case, coronary artery disease, breast cancer, lung cancer, colorectal cancer, and ovarian cancer—for women within 5-year age categories (Ries, Kosary, Hankey, Miller, Edwards, eds., 1999; National Center for Health Statistics, 1999). Moving across the table allows the user to compare the magnitude of each disease risk. Because many people may be even more concerned about their overall chance of dying than of diagnosis with a disease, the final column displays all-cause mortality to display how much each disease contributes to the overall chance of dying. Mortality data can be represented as counts, proportions, or rates; in this example, counts are presented with a stable denominator (e.g., 100,000 women) because there is some evidence suggesting that people find counts easiest to understand (Gigerenzer, 1996; Hoffrage & Gigerenzer, 1998; Schwartz, Woloshin, & Welch, 1999).

Benefit Chart

Table 11-6 presents an example of a benefit chart (for women). The goal of this chart is to help female patients compare the relative effect of a change

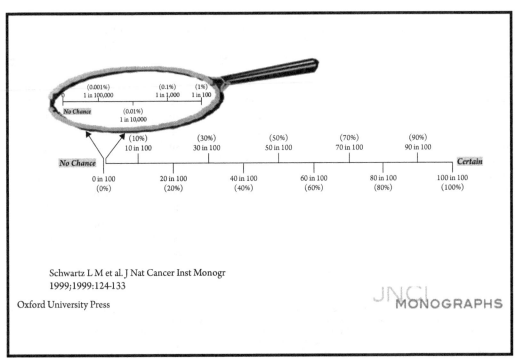

Schwartz L M et al. J Nat Cancer Inst Monogr 1999;1999:124-133

Oxford University Press

JNCI MONOGRAPHS

FIGURE 11-8: Visual Scale for Representing Event Probability. Reproduced with permission

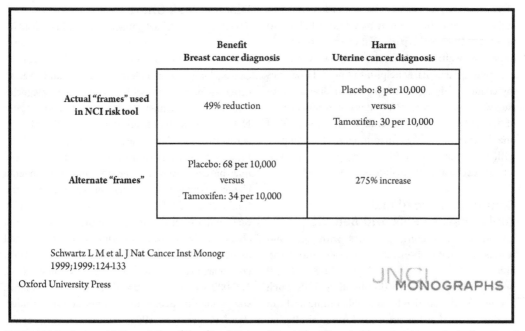

	Benefit Breast cancer diagnosis	Harm Uterine cancer diagnosis
Actual "frames" used in NCI risk tool	49% reduction	Placebo: 8 per 10,000 versus Tamoxifen: 30 per 10,000
Alternate "frames"	Placebo: 68 per 10,000 versus Tamoxifen: 34 per 10,000	275% increase

Schwartz L M et al. J Nat Cancer Inst Monogr
1999;1999:124-133
Oxford University Press

JNCI
MONOGRAPHS

FIGURE 11-9: Asymmetric Presentation of Benefit and Harms of Tamoxifen. The actual frames tend to emphasize benefit and minimize harm, whereas the alternate frames have the opposite effect. The numbers shown are the average annual event rates. Reproduced with permission

TABLE 11-5. DISEASE RISK CHART FOR WOMEN*: ESTIMATED 10-YEAR DISEASE-SPECIFIC AND ALL-CAUSE MORTALITY

Imagine 100,000 women your age.
> Over the next 10 years, how many will die of:

	Coronary Disease†	Lung Cancer	Breast Cancer	Colorectal Cancer	Ovarian Cancer	All Causes
For women age (y)						
20–24	8	1	6	2	2	600
25–29	30	5	30	6	5	700
30–34	70	20	70	10	10	1,000
35–39	140	50	150	30	20	1,500
40–44	300	130	270	50	50	2,100
45–49	630	310	420	100	90	3,300
50–54	1,200	600	550	180	150	5,100
55–59	2,200	1,000	680	300	210	8,100
60–64	3,900	1,500	830	440	280	12,000
65–69	6,500	1,800	970	640	350	18,000
70–74	11,000	2,000	1,100	880	400	27,000
75–79	18,000	1,900	1,200	1,200	440	41,000
80–84	34,000	1,500	1,200	1,500	400	67,000
85+	42,000	940	1,100	1,500	300	79,000

* We obtained 1996 mortality rates for 5-year age groups from Surveillance, Epidemiology, and End Results Program (cancer rates) and National Center for Health Statistics (coronary disease, all-cause mortality). We converted these annual rates into 10-year probabilities by applying the age-specific, disease-specific, and all-cause mortality rate for adjacent 5-year intervals. Numbers have been rounded to facilitate interpretation and represent rough estimates that should be accurate in terms of order of magnitude.
For example, about 8 of 100,000 women age 20–24 will die from coronary artery disease in the next 10 years compared with 3,900 out of 100,000 women age 60–64.
† Coronary artery disease includes deaths attributed to acute myocardial infarction, old myocardial infarction, angina, ischemic heart disease, and subacute/acute forms of ischemic heart disease. Schwartz L M et al. J Nat Cancer Inst Monogr1999;1999:124–133. Reproduced with permission

TABLE 11-6. PROTOTYPE BENEFIT CHART FOR WOMEN: 10-YEAR ALL-CAUSE MORTALITY WITH AND WITHOUT INTERVENTION AND DEATHS PREVENTED (95% CONFIDENCE INTERVAL)

Imagine 100,000 women your age.
Over the next 10 years, how many will die if they:

Age (y)	Quit Smoking			Start Annual Screening with Mammography			Start Annual Screening for Colon Cancer*		
	No	Yes	Deaths Prevented	No	Yes	Deaths Prevented*	No	Yes	Deaths Prevented*
55–59	13,000	6,500	6,500 (5,000–8,000)	8,100	7,900	200 (100–300)	8,100	8,000	100 (90–110)

*These numbers assume that the reduction in disease-specific mortality observed in trials is extended to all-cause mortality. Reductions in all-cause mortality have not been consistently observed in these screening trials. These estimates, therefore, represent best-case scenarios.
Schwartz L M et al. J Nat Cancer Inst Monogr 1999;1999:124–133. Reproduced with permission

in behavior or specific intervention on all-cause mortality. This example displays age- and female sex-specific 10-year all-cause mortality with or without a given intervention. The numbers shown in the chart are crude estimates that are accurate in their order of magnitude. The first scenario in the chart considers 100,000 smokers and displays their chance of dying in the next 10 years if they all continue to smoke or if they all quit smoking and the net effect—about 6,500 deaths prevented among 55–59-year-old smokers. Another scenario considers 100,000 women who do not have an annual screening mammography and those who do; it shows the net effect of 200 deaths prevented for 55–59-year-old women. These examples show that, for a 55-year-old female smoker, giving up cigarettes has a substantially greater effect on all-cause mortality than annual mammography (Schwartz, Woloshin, & Welch, 1999).

Ideally, a benefit chart would be created for an intervention only if the efficacy of screening or behavioral changes has been demonstrated in randomized clinical trials (e.g., mammography for women in their fifties) or when rigorous observational studies have convincingly demonstrated benefit and the interventions are routinely recommended (e.g., Pap screening for cervical cancer, smoking cessation counseling). Age and comorbidity present competing risks of disability or death that patients face in addition to the risk under consideration. These factors will influence the benefit of any intervention (behavioral changes or screening tests). The benefit charts may encourage explicit discussion between the patient and primary care physician about these issues. Because interventions can also have harms, an important challenge remains in how to convey data about side effects and poor outcomes. Studies comparing the effectiveness of these proposed comprehensive tools, disease-specific tools, and usual care are needed to learn which tools better help patients make important medical decisions (Schwartz, Woloshin, & Welch, 1999).

Teaching Patients to Be Better Consumers of Data

Efforts to promote informed patient decision making have become increasingly common, as discussed earlier in this Chapter. In general, these efforts have focused on providing disease-specific facts (Schwartz, Woloshin, & Welch, 1999). Unfortunately, there are reasons to question the likely effect of this commonsense approach to patient education. First, patients may not be ready for the data; problems with numeracy (i.e., low quantitative literacy) are common. For example, in the 2003 National Assessment of Adult Literacy (National Center for Education Statistics, 2003), 22% of the US population had only basic quantitative literacy, significantly less than in the 1992 survey; 11 million adults were non-literate in English so could not take the test. Low levels of numeracy strongly relate to difficulty in making use of quantitative data about the risk reduction of screening mammography (Schwartz, Woloshin, Black, & Welch, 1997). Second, patients may not know how to interpret the information they are given. Educators have long understood that presenting facts without first preparing the audience to receive them (i.e., integrating them into some organizing structure) is ineffective and probably counterproductive. In such a case, the members of the audience will absorb little information, it will be quickly forgotten; they will not understand how the information fits into their own experience, and may misinterpret what it means. With little experience in using data, for example, patients may be especially susceptible to the framing effects discussed in Chapter 3 (that is, how simple changes in the format of otherwise identical numerical information can profoundly influence its interpretation; Malenka, Baron, Johansen, Wahrenberger, & Ross, 1993; Forrow, Taylor, & Arnold, 1992; Naylor, Chen, & Strauss, 1992; Hux & Naylor, 1995; O'Connor, 1989; Tversky & Kahneman, 1981; McNeil, Pauker, Sox, & Tversky, 1982; Schwartz, Woloshin, & Welch, 1999).

Both written and verbal information regarding treatment is important to patients (Grime et al., 2007; Sleath et al., 2009; Elwyn et al., 2004). Elwyn and colleagues (2004) found that providers used written information more often to explain treatment risks to patients after they received training in shared decision making.

Personalizing the written information (e.g., using the word "you"), providing risk–benefit information in different formats, and giving patients a reflective task to work on when reading the information may improve patient perceptions of risk (Berry et al., 2002, 2003; Natter et al., 2004; O'Connor et al., 2009; Elwyn et al., 2011). This is particularly important as the information provided to patients in pharmacies is often not adequate to enable them to understand the risks and benefits of medications (Svarstad et al., 2004; Raynor et al., 2007; Winterstein et al., 2010). Yet, Svarstad and colleagues found that patients who received prescriptions in states with more stringent regulation of pharmacist counseling (e.g., states that require face-to-face counseling by a pharmacist) were more likely to receive medication risk information than patients in states with less regulatory intensity (Svarstad et al., 2004). As discussed in Chapter 2, the legislative context too is important to risk communication.

Understanding Numbers in Health: Best Practices

Best practices for office-based tutorials and online resources for risk assessment are summarized below

(e.g., from http://www.yourdiseaserisk.wustl.edu/ or http://www.diseaseriskindex.harvard.edu/update/):

1. *What is risk?* Attempts to discuss medical risk are easily undermined by confusing and imprecise use of language, so the program should begin with the multiple meanings of the word "risk," how to use words (and the limits of words) in describing risk, and ways to quantify risk (probability, percents, proportions, and rates). An example scale used to quantify and communicate small risks is found in Figure 11-8 (Schwartz, Woloshin, & Welch, 1999; as discussed in Chapter 3).

2. *What to look for in a statement about risk.* Patients are sensitized to ask questions, such as: What is the risk under discussion (e.g., is it the risk of being diagnosed or of dying)? What is the time frame under consideration (e.g., next 5 years or lifetime—and what does "lifetime" mean)? Who is at risk (i.e., does the statement refer to all women? women of a certain age? women with specific characteristics such as a family history of breast cancer)? (Schwartz, Woloshin, & Welch, 1999).

3. *Putting risk in context.* A salient but rare outcome, such as a celebrity dying of a rare cancer, may give undue weight to certain health risks, as discussed in Chapter 12. Patients are encouraged to ask questions, such as: How does the chance of this disease compare with other diseases or other familiar events? How dangerous is the disease (i.e., appreciating the difference between developing a condition and dying of it)? To illustrate competing risks, one may use the disease risk charts discussed previously and illlustrated in Figure 11-9 (Schwartz, Woloshin, & Welch, 1999).

4. *Changing risk.* This focuses on how to interpret statements that measure changes in risk given some exposure or intervention (e.g., relative and absolute risk reduction or number needed to treat). *Absolute risk* of a disease is the risk of developing the disease over a time period; for example, a 1 in 10 risk of developing a certain disease in over a lifetime can be expressed as a 10% risk. *Relative risk* is used to compare

the risk in two different groups of people, for example, smokers and non-smokers, as addressed in Chapter 3. This section can introduce the concept of framing (e.g., dying versus not dying). Benefit charts are used to highlight that not all risk factors and interventions are equally important (Schwartz, Woloshin, & Welch, 1999).

5. *Evidence.* Finally, there is uncertainty in what we know; this introduces the idea of grading evidence by highlighting the basic concepts of study design (e.g., observational study versus randomized clinical trial). Patients are encouraged to have a healthy skepticism and ask themselves, "Can I believe what I am being told? Could it be wrong?" (Schwartz, Woloshin, & Welch, 1999).

A recent summary of the evidence and a previous systematic review on patient education materials for risk communication suggested that these interventions had variable effects and, in general, left substantial room for improvement (Fischhoff, Brewer, Downs, 2011; review in: Schwartz, Woloshin, & Welch, 1999; Schwartz, Woloshin, & Black, 1997; O'Connor, Tugwell, Wells, Elmslie, Jolly, Hollingworth, et al., 1998; Lerman, Lustbader, Rimer, Daly, Miller, Sands, et al., 1995; Flood, Wennberg, Nease, Fowler, Ding, Hynes, 1996; Inglis & Farnill, 1993; Krueter & Strecher, 1995; Halpern, Blackman, & Salzman, 1989).

Evidence-based Risk Communication Approaches for Providers to Patients

While both this Chapter and Chapter 3 examine evidence-based approaches to communicating risk to patients, a recent review (Sleath & Goldstein, 2011) recommends that health care professionals receive specific training on how to communicate with patients about the risks and benefits of treatments. Two randomized controlled trials successfully demonstrated that physicians and pharmacists can be trained to communicate more effectively about medication risks (antidepressant medication) and benefits, however. Additional trials are needed to identify the most efficient and effective strategies for improving professionals' skills and promoting their use in actual encounters with patients (Rickles et al., 2006, Elwyn et al., 2004; Edwards et al., 2006). Existing models of

patient-centered communication (DiMatteo et al., 1995; Makoul et al., 2001; Stewart et al., 1995) and shared decision making (Frosch et al., 1999; Makoul & Clayman, 2006), as discussed in this Chapter, can be incorporated into this training.

As discussed throughout this book, patients who are more knowledgeable about their conditions, participate more actively in medical visits, and feel more confident about managing their conditions are more likely to follow through with treatment and achieve better outcomes (Anderson et al., 1995; Greenfield et al., 1988; Hibbard et al., 2005, 2007). Thus, strategies that focus on increasing patient participation in care may increase the likelihood that patients will ask for and receive needed information about the risks and benefits of medical treatments. Controlled trials of self-management support interventions that focus on increasing patients' confidence to self-manage have produced improvements in clinical outcomes across a number of other chronic conditions (Bodenheimer et al., 2003; Lorig et al., 2003; Warsi et al., 2004; Fisher et al., 2005; Glasgow et al., 2002).

Medical Informatics and Patient Health

After decades of development of information systems designed primarily for physicians and other health care managers and professionals, there is an increasing interest in reaching consumers and patients directly through computers and telecommunications systems.[1] Consumer health informatics is the branch of medical informatics that analyses consumers' needs for information; studies and implements methods of making information accessible to consumers; and models and integrates consumers' preferences into medical information systems (Eysenbach, 2000).

As discussed in Chapter 10, medical informatics has been defined as the study of the proper use of information in health care (http://www.amia.org/about/faqs/f7.html, 2012). Use of the Internet for health care information is widespread among the general population; Harris interactive 2011 found that 74% of all adults have looked online for health information (the same percentage as in Harlem; Cohall et al., 2011), with 60% having done so within

---

1 The section on "Medical Informatics" was drafted by Yalini Senathirajah, Ph.D.

the last month, and 39% saying they do so "often." Ninety percent said they were successful in their search, and 90% also said they found the information reliable. Information technologies are developing rapidly. In this Chapter, the applications of medical informatics to patient change, particularly among underserved populations, and online health interest communities are discussed. Additional explorations of the burgeoning role of medical informatics in prevention are found in Chapters 10 and 12.

Applications of Medical Informatics to Patient Change

Patient-directed informatics applications have been increasing over the past 10 years. This increase is due to enhanced awareness of the effect of behaviors on health, shifts in financial and management risks, and duties from payers to consumers, increased time pressures on providers, with an attendant change in the provider-patient relationship, as discussed in Chapter 1. At the national level, the Office of the National Coordinator for Health Information Technology (ONC) in the Department of Health and Human Services leads the strategy to increase electronic access to health information, to support the development of tools that enable people to take action with that information, and to shift attitudes related to the traditional roles of patients and providers, as discussed further below (Ricciardi, Mostashart, Murphy, Daniel, & Siminerio, 2013).

Informatics tools in health care practice have several advantages. They may provide information at times when health care providers are not available and in locations more comfortable to the patient, such as at home or while traveling. They may be scalable to larger populations in ways that individual provider attention may not be, and may include practical advice from fellow patients facing the same key issues; they allow for rapid feedback, and for different points of view regarding treatment and decision making. They may provide information that can be read or viewed at leisure, and that can be repeated for clarification (Ricciardi, Mostashart, Murphy, Daniel, & Siminerio, 2013). Mobile devices, carried by the patient, can be used to monitor physiological conditions at all times of day, with less intrusion than a human monitor. As with assessment and feedback to providers, tracking and displaying patient behavior can be used to motivate and change behavior patterns (Speck et al., 2010; Car et al., 2012). Common examples are the many self-tracking fitness "apps" that allow users to keep track of their running or walking program, distance and time, calories burned, that contribute to the "quantified self." Computer-based surveys (Speck et al., 2010; Cohall et al., 2007) that let the user answer questions privately can facilitate the examination of sensitive topics such as sexual behavior or substance abuse. Social networking technologies can assist patients with motivation and goal-setting alongside their peers. Text messaging is perhaps one of the most widely used means of giving patients reminders about health-related behaviors and appointments (e.g., *Txt4baby* supports expectant mothers during their pregnancies).

Medical Informatics among Underserved Populations

Access to information technology is a barrier to full participation in health care within low income communities. While access is gradually improving in these communities—a 2006 study of Harlem residents found that more than 90% of residents had access to cell phones—access to computers at work or school is more limited (Cohall, Nye, Moon-Howard, Kukafka, Dye, Vaughan, et al., 2011; Senathirajah, Kukafka, Guptarak, Cohall, 2006). Factors reducing access in poor communities like Harlem include limited health and *ehealth* literacy (Chan, Matthews, Kaufman, 2009; Chan, Kaufman, 2011), knowledge of the health care system and how to navigate it; unfamiliarity with medical vocabulary; an inability to navigate websites to find relevant information; limited and trust in the health care system (Senathirajah, Kukafka, Guptarak, Cohall, 2006).

Among residents of the diverse Harlem community, there were age-related differences in health information needs. Adolescents were more interested in information about a narrow range of conditions than adults, including sexually transmitted diseases (STDs) and their prevention, asthma, and their ability to handle situations that involved bullying. Adolescents were also more confident in their ability to find information online than adults. Adults had a wider range of disease concerns than adolescents, including diabetes, fitness, cancers, STDs, and psychosocial stresses (Cohall, Nye, Moon-Howard, Kukafka, Dye, Vaughan, et al., 2011; Senathirajah, Kukafka, Guptarak, Cohall, 2006).

For older patients, barriers to the use of medical informatics included a lack of computer experience and literacy or numeracy; difficulties with access (e.g., difficulty of getting to computer locations such as the library due to reduced mobility); and physical factors such as diminished eyesight for reading, poor eye-hand coordination limiting the use of a computer mouse, and limited memory (Cohall, Nye, Moon-Howard, Kukafka, Dye, Vaughan, et al., 2011; Senathirajah, Kukafka, Guptarak, Cohall, 2006).

Although there are more barriers to computer use among older adults than among adolescents, the computer can also be seen an enabling technology, providing companionship with distant relatives and friends via *Skype* (online video chat), connection with communities of interest for hobbies and specific diseases, self-paced learning, and, for immigrant groups, access to films, websites, and correspondence in other languages. Specific applications can facilitate the improvement of executive function in the elderly, within a relatively short time (15 minutes per day, 5 days per week, over 4 weeks; Nouchi, Takeuchi, Hashizume, et al., 2012).

Online Health Interest Communities

As an outgrowth of the active participation of individuals in their own health, a growing number of sites have enabled online support communities. The oldest of these is the Center for Health Enhancement Systems Studies (CHESS; http://chess.wisc.edu/chess/projects/current_studies_and_projects.aspx), which has developed and tested online disease management programs, for example, among breast cancer survivors (Shaw et al., 2000). Their mobile chronic disease management programs for breast cancer, as well as asthma, alcohol dependence, and lung cancer, allow intervention more frequently than with traditional care, reducing acute care episodes (Gustafson et al., 2011).

A recent trial using two types of online information networks, *podcasts* ("broadcast" + "(i) pod") only and *podcasts* and *Twitter* (including *tweets*, 140-character-long bursts of information), for weight loss. The randomized clinical trial was conducted among 96 overweight and obese men and women; the participants achieved a 2.7 percent weight loss at 6 months. Those who who engaged with *Twitter* were most successful at losing weight, such that every 10 posts to Twitter corresponded with approximately -0.5 percent weight loss. As opposed to traditional behavioral weight loss interventions that generally provide social support through weekly, face-to-face group meetings, this approach can be less costly and less burdensome to participants. The findings suggest that providing group support through online social networks can reach a large number of people who are interested in achieving a healthy weight. In the future, additional studies could be conducted to find ways (including *Facebook*) to provide social support for participants in remotely delivered weight loss programs in ways that are engaging, rewarding, and useful for a wide variety of participants (Turner-McGrievy & Tate, 2013).

ASSESSMENT AND SCREENING TOOLS

As discussed previously, there is significant interest in transforming health information technology to be more patient-centered (Krist, Woolf, 2011; Finkelstein, Knight, Marinopoulos, Gibbons, Berger, et al., 2012; Krist, Glenn, Glasgow, Balasubramanian, Chambers, et al., 2013). Further, there is a pressing need for greater attention to patient-centered health behavior and psychosocial issues in primary care, and for practical tools, study designs, and results of clinical and policy relevance (DHHS, 2011). To further integrate these several movements, one key element that has been missing is a set of brief, practical patient-reported items that are relevant to and actionable by patients and their health care teams (Glasgow, Kaplan, Ockene, Fisher, Emmons, 2012; Rabin, Purcell, Naveed, Moser, Henton, et al., 2012) and that are feasible to collect and act upon in the flow of general practice (Glasgow et al., 2012, Rabin et al., 2012). These tools can automate components of the 5 As (especially "ask" and "advise"), prompt "agree," shared decision making, and the crafting of SMART goals (Sheinfeld Gorin & Krist, http://healthpolicy.ucla.edu/mohr).

Practices may consider implementing health assessment for a variety of reasons. Some are looking for a way to systemically identify health issues of concern to their patients. Some wish to take advantage of incentives provided by insurers or accrediting agencies. Some want to implement the Medicare Annual Wellness Visit (AWV), an annual primary care visit that includes a medical history, a health risk assessment, an evaluation of physical condition, a screening for cognitive impairment, and a personalized prevention plan, as introduced in Chapter 2 (http://www.cms.gov/Outreach-and-Education/Medicare-Learning-Network-MLN/MLNProducts/

downloads/AWV_chart_ICN905706.pdf). Some practices want to implement a health assessment because of national initiatives like the National Committee for Quality Assurance (NCQA) Patient Centered Medical Home (PCMH) Recognition Program and the Centers for Medicare & Medicaid Services meaningful use standards (Office of the National Coordinator for Health IT (ONC). Meaningful Use Stage II Requirements. 2012), as discussed previously in Chapters 2 and 10. Automated assessment and screening tools can be adapted to append the electronic medical record, or to extend its use.

Particularly among older individuals, health care professionals can use these automated assessment and screening tools to monitor health status to detect early signs of health problems that would threaten independence and can ensure accurate distinctions in diagnosis. Increased use of screening tools in primary care for the assessment of depression and early cognitive deficits, such as the deterioration of memory, orientation, general intellect, specific cognitive capacities, and social functioning—the clinical precursors to dementia and Alzheimer's disease—as well as genetic risk factors (such as APOE), will become more important.

One example of a patient-reported tool for assessment and screening is My Own Health Report (MOHR), led by the National Cancer Institute. Begun in 2011, 93 national primary care, public health, health behavior, and psychosocial experts as well as patients engaged in a rigorous three-phase process to identify evidence-based, patient reported measures that if routinely collected could be used to improve health and monitor health status (DHHS, 2011). Seventeen brief, feasible screening questions evaluating 10 domains of health behaviors and psychosocial problems were identified (Estabrooks, Boyle, Emmons, Glasgow, Hesse, et al., 2012). The implementation of this patient-reported screening tool is currently being evaluated in 9 matched primary care practices across the United States (http://healthpolicy.ucla.edu/mohr).

Another example of a background Health Assessment in primary care, created for patients by the Colorado Research Network's Patient Advisory Council, is found in Figure 11-10.

CONCLUSIONS

Health providers should place a higher premium on fully involving patients in their own health care

FIGURE 11-10: A BACKGROUND HEALTH ASSESSMENT IN PRIMARY CARE, CREATED BY THE COLORADO RESEARCH NETWORK'S PATIENT ADVISORY COUNCIL

What is a health assessment?
A health assessment is a set of questions, answered by patients, that asks about personal behaviors, risks, life-changing events, health goals and priorities, and overall health.

Health assessments are usually structured screening and assessment tools used in primary care practices to help the health care team and patient develop a plan of care. Health assessment information can also help the health care team understand the needs of its overall population of patients. Health assessments can vary in length and scope. They can be completed during office visits or between office visits, either on paper or computers. Health assessment questions may be asked about patients of all ages, including children and adolescents.

Some common health assessment questions ask about:
- Tobacco use
- Stress
- Healthy eating
- Physical activity
- Sexual practices
- Sedentary behaviors such as sitting and watching TV or playing computer games
- Alcohol usage
- Addictive behaviors such as gambling or drug use
- Violence, bullying or physical abuse
- Depression or anxiety
- Emotional and social support
- Safety issues such as wearing a seat belt while driving
- Overall health or well-being.

From: CaReNet Patient Advisory Council © 2012

to the extent that patients choose. Providers should employ high-quality, reliable tools and skills for sharing decision making with patients, tailored to clinical needs, patient goals, social circumstances, and the degree of control that patients prefer. This Chapter has explored major approaches to patient behavioral change in primary care practice that encourage patient self-management and clinical collaboration. These approaches include the 5As, which have been recommended by the USPSTF across all health behavior counseling in primary care. Similarly, shared decision making has been recommended by the USPSTF and supported in the Affordable Care Act as an effective way of providing information when there is uncertainty about the evidence or when patient preferences are not clear, as in prostate cancer screening. SMART goals guide behavioral change toward measurable outcomes. Motivational interviewing fundamentals assist the primary care provider to "roll with resistance," helping patients to resolve their ambivalence about change. Tailored telephone interviewing, alongside other health care providers with computer assistance, can advance patients along the stages of change toward new behaviors. The application of relational agents to guide counseling shows some promise in disseminating counseling beyond the clinic. Office-based approaches to risk assessment and best practices for patient risk education address the barriers to understanding and applying data to prevention in practice. Medical informatics has propelled overwhelming changes in the routine practice of primary care through the electronic health record, particularly in underserved communities. Routine assessment and screening tools, such as the MOHR tool, could automate the use of the 5 As in practice (http://healthpolicy.ucla.edu/mohr).

In addition to health care providers and patients, health care delivery organizations should monitor and assess patients' perspectives and use those insights to improve care. They should establish patient portals to facilitate data sharing among providers, patients, and families; and make high-quality tools available for shared decision making with patients (IOM, 2012).

REFERENCES

Adams PF, Kirzinger WK, Martinez ME. Summary health statistics for the U.S. population: National Health Interview Survey, 2011. National Center for Health Statistics. Vital Health Stat 10(255). 2012.

Agency for Healthcare Research and Quality. *Five Major Steps to Intervention (The "5A's")*. US Public Health Service. Rockville, MD. Retrieved January 3, 2013, from: http://www.ahrq.gov/clinic/tobacco/5steps.htm.

Albert D, Ward A, Ahluwalia K, Sadowsky D. Addressing tobacco in managed care: a survey of dentists' knowledge, attitudes, and behaviors. *Am J Public Health.* 2002;92:997–1001.

Allard RH. Tobacco and oral health: attitudes and opinions of European dentists; a report of the EU working group on tobacco and oral health. *Int Dental J.* 2000;50:99–102.

Anderson, R., Funnell, M., Butler, P., Arnold, M., Fitzgerald, J., and Feste, C. (1995). Patient empowerment: Results of a randomized controlled trial. Diabetes Care, 18(7), 943-949.

Anderson, R., Funnell, M., Butler, P., Arnold, M., Fitzgerald, J., and Feste, C. (1995). Patient empowerment: Results of a randomized controlled trial. Diabetes Care, 18(7), 943-949.

Andrews JO, Tingen MS, Waller JL, Harper RJ. Provider feedback improves adherence with AHCPR Smoking Cessation Guideline. *Prev Med.* 2001;33:415–421.

Aspinwell LG, Taylor SE: A stitch in time: Self-regulation and proactive coping. *Psychol Bull.* 1997;121:417–436.

Babor, TF, Del Boca FK, eds. *Treatment Matching in Alcoholism.* Cambridge, UK: Cambridge University Press; 2003.

Baker A, Richmond R, Haile M, Lewin TJ, Carr VJ, Taylor RL, Jansons S, Wilhelm K. A randomized controlled trial of a smoking cessation intervention among people with a psychotic disorder. *Am J Psychiat.* 2006;163:1934–1942.

Ball SA, Martino S, Nich C, Frankforter TL, Van Horn D, Crits-Christoph P, Woody GE, Obert JE, Farentinos C, Carroll KM. Site matters: Multisite randomized trial of motivational enhancement therapy in community drug abuse clinics. *J Consult Clin Psychol.* 2007;75:556–567.

Bandura A. Health promotion from the perspective of social cognitive theory. *Psychol Health.* 1998;13:623–649.

Bandura A. *Social Foundations of Thought and Action.* Upper Saddle River, NJ: Prentice Hall; 1986.

Berry DC, Michas IC, Bersellin E. Communicating information about medication side effects: effects on satisfaction, perceived risk to health, and intention to comply. *Psychology and Health.* 2002;17:247–267.

Berry DC, Michas IC, Bersellini E. Communicating information about medication: the benefits of making it personal. *Psychology and Health.* 2003;18:127–139.

Bickmore T. *Relational Agents for Health Behavior Change.* Presentation to the Society of Behavioral Medicine, Washington, DC: 2007.

Bieber C, Müller KG, Blumenstiel K, Schneider A, Richter A, Wilke S, Hartmann M, Eich W. Long-term effects of a shared decision-making intervention on physician–patient interaction and outcome in fibromyalgia A qualitative and quantitative 1 year follow-up of a randomized controlled trial. *Patient Educ Couns.* 2006;63:357–366

Block DE, Block LE, Hutton SJ, Johnson KM. Tobacco counseling practices of dentists compared to other health care providers in a midwestern region. *J Dental Educ.* 1999;63:821–827.

Bodenheimer T, Lorig K, Holman H, Grumbach K. Patient self-management of chronic disease in primary care. *JAMA.* 2002;288(19):2469–2475.

Bolman C, de Vries H, Mesters I. Factors determining cardiac nurses' intentions to continue using a smoking cessation protocol. *Heart Lung.* 2002;31:15–24.

Borum ML. A comparison of smoking cessation efforts in African Americans by resident physicians in a traditional and primary care internal medicine residency. *J Natl Med Assoc.* 2000;92:131–135.

Bouton ME. A learning theory perspective on lapse, relapse, and the maintenance of behavior change. *Health Psychol.* 2000;19:57–63.

Brink SG, Gottlieb NH, McLeroy KR, Wisotzky M, Burdine JN. A community view of smoking cessation counseling in the practices of physicians and dentists. *Public Health Rep.* 1994;109:135–142.

Britt J, Curry SJ, McBride C, Grothaus L, Louie D. Implementation and acceptance of outreach telephone counseling for smoking cessation with nonvolunteer smokers. *Health Edu Q.* 1994;21:55–68.

Brug J, Campbell M, Van Assema P. The application and impact of computer-generated personalized nutrition education: a review of the literature. *Patient Educ Couns.* 1999;36:145–156.

Car J, Gurol-Urganci I, de Jongh T, Vodopivec-Jamsek V, Atun R. Mobile phone messaging reminders for attendance at healthcare appointments. Cochrane Database of Systematic Reviews. 2012;7:CD007458.

Car J, Gurol-Urganci I, de Jongh T, Vodopivec-Jamsek V, Atun R. Mobile phone messaging reminders for attendance at healthcare appointments. *Cochrane Database of Systematic Reviews.* 2012;7:CD007458.

Carroll KM, Ball SA, Nich C, Martino S, Frankforter TL, Farentinos C, Kunkel LE, Mikulich- Gilbertson SK, Morgenstern J, Obert JL, Polcin DL, Snead N, Woody GE. Motivational interviewing to improve treatment engagement and outcome in individuals seeking treatment for substance abuse: A multisite effectiveness study. *Drug and Alcohol Dependence.* 2006;81:301–312.

Carroll KM, Farentinos C, Ball SA, Crits-Cristoph P, Libby B, Morgenstern J, Obert JL, Polcin DL, Woody GE. MET meets the real world: Design issues and clinical strategies in the Clinical Trials Network. *J Subst Abuse Treat* 2002;23:73–80.

Carson KV, Verbiest MEA, Crone MR, Brinn MP, Esterman AJ, Assendelft WJJ, Smith BJ. Training health professionals in smoking cessation. Cochrane Database of Systematic Reviews 2012, Issue 5. Art. No.: CD000214. DOI: 10.1002/14651858.CD000214.pub2.

Chan CV, Kaufman DR. A framework for characterizing eHealth literacy demands and barriers. *J Med Internet Res.* 2011;13:e94.

Chan CV, Matthews LA, Kaufman DR. A taxonomy characterizing complexity of consumer eHealth Literacy. *AMIA Annual Symposium Proceedings.* 2009;2009:86–90.

Charles C, Gafni A, Whelan T. Decision-making in the physician– patient encounter: revisiting the shared treatment decision-making model. *Soc Sci Med.* 1999;49:561–651.

Charles C, Gafni A, Whelan T. Shared decision-making in the medical encounter: what does it mean? (or it takes at least two to tango). *Soc Sci Med.* 1997;44:681–692.

Cohall AT, Nye A, Moon-Howard J, Kukafka R, Dye B, Vaughan RD, et al. Computer use, internet access, and online health searching among Harlem adults. *Am J Health Promot.* 2011;25:325–333.

Cohall AT, Senathirajah Y, Dini S, Nye A, Powell D, Powell B. An online audio computer-assisted self-interview for pre-screening prior to rapid HIV testing in a vulnerable population. *AMIA Annual Symposium Proceedings.* 2007:915.

Colby SM, Monti PM, Barnett NP, Rohsenow DJ, Weissman K, Spirito A, Woolard RH, Lewander WJ. Brief motivational interviewing in a hospital setting for adolescent smoking: A preliminary study. *J Consult Clin Psychol.* 1998;66:574–578.

Coleman T, Murphy E, Cheater F. Factors influencing discussion of smoking between general practitioners and patients who smoke: a qualitative study. *Br J Gen Pract.* 2000;50:207–210.

Copello A, Godfrey C, Heather N, Hodgson R, Orford J, Raistrick D, et al. United Kingdom Alcohol Treatment Trial (UKATT): Hypotheses, design and methods. *Alcohol Alcoholism.* 2001;36:11–21.

Cornuz J, Zellweger JP, Mounoud C, Decrey H, Pecoud A, Burnand B. Smoking cessation counseling by residents in an outpatient clinic. *Prev Med.* 1997;26:292–296.

Coulter A. Paternalism or partnership. *BMJ.* 1999;319:719–720.

Croteau J, Ryan D. *Achieving your SMART health goals.* BeWell@Stanford. 2013. Accessed December 15, 2012, from: http://bewell.stanford.edu/smart-goals.

Department of Health and Human Services, National Institute of Health, Office of Behavioral and Social Sciences Research, National Cancer Institute. Identifying core behavioral and psychosocial data elements for the electronic health record. 2011. Accessed January 2013 from http://conferences.thehillgroup.com/OBSSR/EHR2011/index.html.

DiMatteo MR. Patient adherence to pharmacotherapy: the importance of effective communication. Formulary, 1995;30(10):596–598, 601–592, 605.

Doescher MP, Saver BG. Physicians' advice to quit smoking. The glass remains half empty. *J Fam Pract.* 2000;49:543–547.

Dubbert PM. Physical activity and exercise: Recent advances and current challenges. *J Consult Clin Psychol.* 2002;70(3):526–536.

Easton A, Husten C, Elon L, Pederson L, Frank E. Non-primary care physicians and smoking cessation counseling: Women Physicians' Health Study. *Women Health.* 2001;34:15–29.

Easton A, Husten C, Malarcher A, et al. Smoking cessation counseling by primary care women physicians: Women Physicians' Health Study. *Women Health.* 2001;32:77–91.

Eckert T, Junker C. Motivation for smoking cessation: what role do doctors play? *Swiss Med Wkly.* 2001;131:521–526.

Edwards A, Elwyn G, Hood K, Atwell C, Robling M, Houston H, et al. Patient-based outcome results from a cluster randomized trial of shared decision making skill development and use of risk communication aids in general practice. Fam Pract. 2004;21(4):347–354.

Elwyn G, O'Connor A, Stacey D, Volk R, Edwards A, Coulter A, Thomson R, Barratt A, Barry M, Bernstein S, Butow P, Clarke A, Entwistle V, Feldman-Stewart D, Holmes-Rovner M, Llewellyn-Thomas H, Moumjid N, Mulley AI, Ruland C, Sepucha K, Sykes A, Whelan T, on behalf of the International Patient Decision Aids Standards (IPDAS) Collaboration Developing a quality criteria framework for patient decision aids: online international Delphi consensus process. BMJ. 2006; 333:41721.

Elwyn G, Edwards A, Hood K, Robling M, Atwell C, Russell I, et al. Achieving involvement: process outcomes from a cluster randomized trial of shared decision making skill development and use of risk communication aids in general practice. *Fam Pract.* 2004;21(4):337–346.

Elwyn GJ, Edwards A, Kinnersley P. Shared decision-making in primary care: the neglected second half of the consultation. *Br J Gen Pract.* 1999;49:477–482.

Elwyn GJ, Edwards A, Kinnersley P, Grol R. Shared decision making and the concept of equipoise: the competences of involving patients in healthcare choices. *Br J Gen Pract.* 2000;50:892–899.

Emanuel EJ, Emanuel LL. Four models of the physician–patient relationship. *JAMA.* 1992;267:2221–2226.

Estabrooks PA, Boyle M, Emmons KM, Glasgow RE, Hesse BW, Kaplan RM, Krist AH, Moser RP, Taylor MV. Harmonized patient-reported data elements in the electronic health record: supporting meaningful use by primary care action on health behaviors and key psychosocial factors. *J Am Med Inform Assoc.* Jul 1 2012;19(4):575–582.

Eysenbach G. Consumer health informatics. *BMJ.* 2000 June 24; 320(7251): 1713–1716.

Finkelstein J, Knight A, Marinopoulos S, Gibbons C, Berger Z, Aboumatar H, Wilson R, Lau B, Sharma R, Bass E. Enabling patient-centered care through health information technology: Agency for Healthcare Research and Quality (US); 2012 Jun. (Evidence Reports/Technology Assessments, No. 206). Accessed February 2013 from http://www.ncbi.nlm.nih.gov/books/NBK99854/.

Fiore M. *US Tobacco use and dependence guideline panel.* Treating Tobacco Use and Dependence: Clinical Practice Guideline. Rockville, MD: US Department of Health and Human Services, USPHS; 2000.

Fiore MC, Jaén CR, Baker TB, et al. *Treating Tobacco Use and Dependence: 2008 Update. Clinical Practice Guideline.* Rockville, MD: US Department of Health and Human Services. Public Health Service. May 2008.

Fischhoff B, Brewer NT, Downs JS, eds. *Communicating Risks and Benefits: An Evidence-Based User's Guide.* Washington, DC: Food and Drug Administration (FDA), US Department of Health and Human Services, August 2011. Accessed April 13, 2013, from http://www.fda.gov/downloads/AboutFDA/ReportsManualsForms/Reports/UCM268069.pdf.

Fisher EB, Brownson CA, CO'Toole ML, Shetty G, Anwuri VV, Glasgow RE. Ecological approaches to self-management: the case of diabetes. *Am J Public Health.* 2005;95: 1523–1535.

Flood AB, Wennberg JE, Nease RF Jr, Fowler FJ Jr, Ding J, Hynes LM. The importance of patient preference in the decision to screen for prostate cancer. *J Gen Intern Med.* 1996;11:342–349.

Forrow L, Taylor WC, Arnold RM. Absolutely relative: how research results are summarized can affect treatment decisions. *Am J Med.* 1992;92:121–124.

Fried JL, Cohen LA. Maryland dentists' attitudes regarding tobacco issues. *Clin Preven Dentistry.* 1992;14:10–16.

Frosch DL, Kaplan RM. Shared decision making in clinical medicine: Past research and future directions. *Am J Prev Med.* 1999;17(4):285–294.

Gail MH, Brinton LA, Byar DP, Corle DK, Green SB, Schairer C, et al. Projecting individualized probabilities of developing breast cancer for white females who are being examined annually. *J Natl Cancer I.* 1989;24:1879–1886.

Gardiner P, Hempstead MB, Ring L, Bickmore T, Nyahkoon LY, Tran H, Paasche-Orlow M, Damus K, Jack B. Reaching women through health information technology: The Gabby Preconception Care System. *Am J Health Promot.* January/February 2013;27(3):eS11–eS20.

Gigerenzer G. The psychology of good judgment: frequency formats and simple algorithms. *Med Decision Making.* 1996;16:273–280.

Gilhooly ML, McGhee SM. Medical records: practicalities and principles of patient possession. *J Med Ethics.* 1991;17:138–143.

Glasgow RE. Medical office-based interventions. In: Frank Snoek F, Skinner TC, eds. Psychology in Diabetes Care. 2nd ed., pp. 109–133. Hoboken, NJ: John Wiley & Sons; 2005.

Glasgow RE, Davis CL, MM, et al. Implementing practical interventions to support chronic illness self-management. *Jt Comm J Qual.* 2003;29(11):563–574.

Glasgow RE, Funnell MM, Bonomi AE, Davis C, Beckham V, Wagner EH. Self-management aspects of the improving chronic illness care breakthrough series: implementation with diabetes and heart failure teams. *Ann Behav Med.* 2002 Spring;24(2):80–87.

Glasgow RE, Goldstein MG. Introduction to the principles of health behavior change. In: Woolf S, ed., *Health Promotion and Disease Prevention in Clinical Practice*. 2nd ed., pp. 129–147. Philadelphia: Williams and Wilkins; 2007.

Glasgow RE, Kaplan RM, Ockene JK, Fisher EB, Emmons KM. Patient-reported measures of psychosocial issues and health behavior should be added to electronic health records. *Health Aff (Millwood)*. 2012;31(3):497–504.

Glynn TM, Manley MW. *Flow to Help Your Patients Stop Smoking: A Manual for Physicians*. Report No.: NIH Publication #89-3064. Bethesda, MD: Smoking, Tobacco and Cancer Program, Division of Cancer Prevention and Control, National Cancer Institute; 1989.

Goldstein MC, Whitlock EP, DePue J. Multiple health risk behavior interventions in primary care: summary of research evidence. *Am J Prev Med*. 2004;27(2 Suppl):61–79.

Goldstein MG, DePue JD, Monroe AD, et al. A population-based survey of physician smoking cessation counseling practices. *Prev Med*. 1998;27:720–729.

Gordon JS, Severson HH. Tobacco cessation through dental office settings. *J Dental Educ*. 2001;65:354–363.

Gottlieb NH, Guo JL, Blozis SA, Huang PP. Individual and contextual factors related to family practice residents' assessment and counseling for tobacco cessation. *J Am Board Fam Pract*. 2001;14:343–351.

Greenfield S, Kaplan S, Ware JE, Jr. Expanding patient involvement in care. *Ann Intern Med*. 1985, 102:520–528.

Greenfield S, Kaplan SH, Ware JE Jr, Yano EM, Frank HJ. Patients' participation in medical care: Effects on blood sugar control and quality of life in diabetes. *J Gen Intern Med*. 1988;3(5):448–457.

Grime J, Blenkinsopp A, Raynor DK, Pollock K, Knapp P. The role and value of written information for patients about individual medicines: a systematic review. *Health Expect*. 2007;10(3):286–298.

Grimley DM, Bellis JM, Raczynski JM, Henning K. Smoking cessation counseling practices: a survey of Alabama obstetrician-gynecologists. *South Med J*. 2001;94:297–303.

Gustafson DH, Shaw BR, Isham A, Baker T, Boyle MG, Levy M. Explicating an evidence-based, theoretically informed, mobile technology-based system to improve outcomes for people in recovery for alcohol dependence. *Subst Use Misuse*. 2011;46:96–111.

Hall JA, Roter DL, Katz NR. Meta-analysis of correlates of provider behavior in medical encounters. *Med Care*. 1988;26:657–675.

Halpern DF, Blackman S, Salzman B. Using statistical risk information to assess oral contraceptive safety. *App Cogn Psychol*. 1989;3:251–260

Hepburn MJ, Johnson JM, Ward JA, Longfield JN. A survey of smoking cessation knowledge, training, and practice among U.S. Army general medical officers. *Am J Prev Med*. 2000;18:300–304.

Hettema J, Steele J, Miller WR. Motivational interviewing. *Ann Rev Clin Psychol*. 2005;1:91–111.

Hibbard JH, Mahoney ER, Stockard J, Tusler M. Development and testing of a short form of the patient activation measure. *Health Serv Res*. 2005;40(6 Pt 1):1918–1930.

Hibbard JH, Tusler M. Assessing activation stage and employing a "next steps" approach to supporting patient self-management. *J Ambul Care Manage*. 2007;30(1):2–8.

Hirshberg A, Calderon S, Kaplan I. Update review on prevention and early diagnosis in oral cancer. *Refuat Hapeh Vehashinayim*. 2002;19:38–48.

Hoffrage U, Gigerenzer G. Using natural frequencies to improve diagnostic inferences. *Acad Med*. 1998;73:538–540.

Holder HD, Cisler RA, Longabaugh R, Stout RL, Treno AJ, Zweben A. Alcoholism treatment and medical care costs from Project MATCH. *Addiction*. 2000;95:999–1013.

Horvath AO, Luborsky L. The role of the therapeutic alliance in psychotherapy. *J Consult Clin Psychol*. 1993;61(4):561–573.

Hux JE, Naylor CD. Communicating the benefits of chronic preventive therapy: does the format of efficacy data determine patients' acceptance of treatment? *Med Decis Making*. 1995;15:152–157.

Inglis S, Farnill D. The effects of providing preoperative statistical anaesthetic-risk information. *Anaesth Intens Care*. 1993;21:799–805.

Institute of Medicine. *Crossing the Quality Chasm*. Washington, DC: National Academies Press; 2001.

Jamal A, Dube SR, Malarcher AM, Shaw L, Engstrom MC. Tobacco use screening and counseling during physician office visits among adults–National Ambulatory Medical Care Survey and National Health Interview Survey, United States, 2005–2009. MMWR Morb Mortal Wkly Rep. 2012 Jun 15;61 Suppl:38–45.

John JH, Yudkin P, Murphy M, Ziebland S, Fowler GH. Smoking cessation interventions for dental patients-attitudes and reported practices of dentists in the Oxford region. *Br Dental J*. 1997;183:359–364.

Jones HL, Walker EA, Schechter CB, Blanco E. Vision is precious: a successful behavioral intervention to increase the rate of screening for diabetic retinopathy for inner-city adults. *Diabetes Educator*. 2010;36:118–126.

Joostena EAG, DeFuentes-Merillasa L,, de Weertc GH, Senskye T, van der Staakd PF, de Jonga CAJ. Systematic review of the effects of shared decision-making on patient satisfaction, treatment adherence and health status. *Psychother Psychosom*. 2008;77:219–226.

Joseph BK. Oral cancer: prevention and detection. *Med Prin Pract*. 2002;11:32–35.

Kalet A, Roberts JC, Fletcher R. How do physicians talk with their patients about risks? *J Gen Intern Med.* 1994;9:402–404.

Kalichman SC, Coley B. Context framing to enhance HIV-antibody-testing messages targeted to African American women. *Health Psychol.* 1995;14:247–254.

Kawakami M, Nakamura S, Fumimoto H, Takizawa J, Baba M. Relation between smoking status of physicians and their enthusiasm to offer smoking cessation advice. *Intern Med J.* 1997;36:162–165.

Kirsch IS, Jungeblut A, Jenkins L, Kolstad A. *Adult Literacy in America.* Washington, DC: Office of Education Research and Improvement, US Department of Education; 1993.

Kottke TE, Battista RN, DeFriese GH, Brekke ML. Attributes of successful smoking cessation interventions in medical practice: a meta-analysis of 39 controlled trials. *JAMA.* 1988;259:2883–2889.

Krist AH, Glenn AB, Glasgow RE, Balasubramanian B, Chambers DA, Fernandez M, Heurtin-Roberts S, Kessler R, Ory MG, Phillips SM, Ritzwoller DP, Roby DH, Rodriguez HP, Sabo RT, Sheinfeld Gorin S, Stange KC. Designing a valid randomized pragmatic primary care implementation trial: the my own health report (MOHR) project. *Implementation Science.* 2013;8:73. http://www.implementationscience.com/content/8/1/73.

Krist AH, Woolf SH. A vision for patient-centered health information systems. *JAMA.* 2011;305(3):300–301.

Krueter MW, Strecher VJ. Changing inaccurate perceptions of health risk: results from a randomized trial. *Health Psychol.* 1995;14:56–63.

Kuchipudi V, Hobein K, Fleckinger A, Iber FL. Failure of a 2-hour motivational intervention to alter recurrent drinking behavior in alcoholics with gastrointestinal disease. *J Stud Alcohol.* 1990;51:356–360.

Kviz FJ, Clark MA, Prohaska TR, et al. Attitudes and practices for smoking cessation counseling by provider type and patient age. *Preve Med.* 1995;24:201–212.

Lando HA, Rommens S, Klevan J, Roski J, Cherney L, Lauger G. Telephone support as an adjunct to transdermal nicotine in smoking cessation. *Am J Public Health.* 1997;87:1670–1674.

Leed-Kelly A, Russel KS, Bobo JK, Mcllvain H. Feasibility of smoking cessation counseling by phone with alcohol treatment center graduates. *J Subst Abuse Treat.* 1996;13(3):203–210.

Leventhal H. Findings and theory in the study of fear communications. In: Berkowitz L, ed. *Advances in Experimental Social Psychology,* pp. 120–186. New York: Academic; 1970.

Lipkus I, Lyna P, Rimer B. Using tailored interventions to enhance smoking cessation among African-Americans at a community health center. *Nicotine Tob Res.* 1999;1(1):77–85.

Llewellyn-Thomas H: Patients' health-care decision making: A framework for descriptive and experimental investigations. *Med Decis Making.* 1995, 15:101–106.

Lodi G, Bez C, Rimondini L, Zuppiroli A, Sardella A, Carrassi A. Attitude towards smoking and oral cancer prevention among northern Italian dentists. *Oral Oncol.* 1997;33:100–104.

Lorig KR, Holman HR. Self-management: education, history, definition, outcomes, and mechanisms. *Ann Behav Med.* 2003; 26: 1–7.

Luckmann R. *Applying Computer Assisted Telephone Interviewing (CATI) Methodology to Tailored Telephone Counseling (TTC) on Cancer Behavior.* Presentation to the Society of Behavioral Medicine, Washington, DC: 2007.

Makoul, G. Essential elements of communication in medical encounters: the Kalamazoo consensus statement. *Acad Med.* 2001;76(4):390–393.

Makoul G, Clayman ML. An integrative model of shared decision making in medical encounters. *Patient Educ Couns.* 2006;60(3):301–312.

Malenka DJ, Baron JA, Johansen S, Wahrenberger JW, Ross JM. The framing effect of relative and absolute risk. *J Gen Intern Med.* 1993;8:543–548.

Marcus B, Bock B, Pinto B, Forsyth L, Roberts M, Traficante R. Efficacy of an individualized, motivationally-tailored physical activity intervention. *Ann Behav Med.* 1998;20(3): 174–180.

McCarty MC, Hennrikus DJ, Lando HA, Vessey JT. Nurses' attitudes concerning the delivery of brief cessation advice to hospitalized smokers. *Preve Med.* 2001;33:674–681.

McEwen A, West R. Smoking cessation activities by general practitioners and practice nurses. *Tob Control.* 2001;10:27–32.

McIlvain HE, Crabtree BF, Backer EL, Turner PD. Use of office-based smoking cessation activities in family practices. *J Fam Pract.* 2000;49:1025–1029.

McNeil BJ, Pauker SG, Sox HC Jr, Tversky A. On the elicitation of preferences for alternative therapies. *New Engl J Med.* 1982;306:1259–1262.

McPherson CJ, Higginson I, Heaarn J. Effective methods of giving information in cancer: a systematic literature review of randomized controlled trials. *J Public Health Med.* 2001;23:227–234.

Miller SM, Siejak KK, Schroeder CM, Lerman C, Hernandez E, Helm CW. Enhancing adherence following abnormal Pap smears among lower income minority women: a preventive telephone counseling strategy. *J Natl Cancer I.* 1997;89:703–708.

Miller WB, Rose GS. Toward a theory of motivational interviewing. *Am Psychol.* 2009;64(6): 527–537

Miller WR. Motivational interviewing with problem drinkers. *Behav Psychoth.* 1983;11:147–172

Miller WR, Muñoz RF. *Controlling Your Drinking.* New York: Guilford Press; 2005.

Miller WR, Rollnick S, Moyers TB. *Motivational Interviewing* (7 videotape series). Albuquerque: University of New Mexico; 1998.

Miller WR, Rollnick S. *Motivational Interviewing: Preparing People for Change.* 2nd ed. New York: Guilford Press; 2002.

Miller WR, Rollnick S. Ten things that Motivational Interviewing is not. *Behav Cogn Psychoth.* 2009;37:129–140.

Miller WR, Rollnick S. *What Makes It Motivational Interviewing?* Presentation at the International Conference on Motivational Interviewing (ICMI). Stockholm, June 7, 2010. Accessed December 12, 2012, from http://www.fhi.se/Documents/ICMI/Dokumentation/June7/Plenary/Miller.

Miller WR, Rollnick S. *What's New since MI-2?* Presentation at the International Conference on Motivational Interviewing (ICMI). Stockholm, June 6, 2010. Accessed at http://www.fhi.se/Documents/ICMI/Dokumentation/June 6/Miller and Rollnick june6 pre conference workshop.pdf.

Miller WR, Rose GS. Toward a theory of motivational interviewing. *Am Psycholt.* 2009 September;64(6):527–537.

Miller WR, Sovereign RG. The check-up: a model for early intervention in addictive behaviors. In: Løberg T, Miller WR, Nathan PE, Marlatt GA, eds. *Addictive Behaviors: Prevention and Early Intervention,* pp. 219–231. Amsterdam: Swets & Zeitlinger; 1989.

Miller WR, Villanueva M, Tonigan JS, Cuzmar I. Are special treatments needed for special populations? *Alcohol Treat Q.* 2007;25(4):63–78.

Miller WR, Yahne CE, Moyers TB, Martinez J, Pirritano M. A randomized trial of methods to help clinicians learn motivational interviewing. *J Consult Clin Psychol.* 2004;72:1050–1062.

Miller WR, Yahne CE, Tonigan JS. Motivational interviewing in drug abuse services: A randomized trial. *J Consult Clin Psychol.* 2003;71:754–763.

Miller WR, Zweben A, DiClemente CC, Rychtarik RG. *Motivational Enhancement Therapy manual: A Clinical Research Guide for Therapists Treating Individuals with Alcohol Abuse and Dependence.* Rockville, MD: National Institute on Alcohol Abuse and Alcoholism; 1992.

Molenaar SM, Sprangers MA, Postma-Schuit FC, et al. Feasibility and effects of decision aids. *Med Decis Making.* 2000, 20:112–127.

Mullen PD, Holcomb JD. Selected predictors of health promotion counseling by three groups of allied health professionals. *Am J Prev Med.* 1990;6:153–160.

National Cancer Institute. *Breast Cancer Risk Tool: An Interactive Patient Education Tool* [software]. Bethesda (MD): National Cancer Institute; 1998.

National Cancer Institute. Grid-enabled measures database. 2011. Accessed January 2013 from https://www.gem-beta.org.

National Center for Health Statistics. *Mortality Data* [online]. 1999. Available from http://www.cdc.gov/nchswww/datawh/statab/upubd/mortabs.htm.

National Center for Health Statistics. *National Ambulatory Medical Care Survey: 1996.* Hyattsville, MD: US Department of Health and Human Services; 1997. Available online from: http://www.cdc.gov/nchswwv/data/ad295.pdf.

National Center for Health Statistics. *Summary Health Statistics for U.S. Adults: National Health Interview Survey,* 2011. Retrieved December 15, 2012, from http://www.cdc.gov/nchs/fastats/smoking.htm

Natter HM, Berry DC. Effects of active information processing on the understanding of risk information. *Applied Cognitive Psychology.* 2004;(19):123–135.

Naylor CD, Chen E, Strauss B. Measured enthusiasm: does the method of reporting trial results alter perceptions of therapeutic effectiveness? *Ann Intern Med.* 1992;117:916–921.

Newton JT, Palmer RM. The role of the dental team in the promotion of smoking cessation. *Br Dental J.* 1997;182:353–355.

Norris SL, Nichols PJ, Caspersen CJ, et al. The effectiveness of disease and case management for people with diabetes: a systematic review. *Am J Prev Med.* 2002;22 (4 Suppl):15–38.

Nouchi R, Taki Y, Takeuchi H, Hashizume H, Akitsuki Y, Shigemune Y, et al. Brain training game improves executive functions and processing speed in the elderly: a randomized controlled trial. *PloS one.* 2012;7:e29676.

O'Connor AM. Effects of framing and level of probability on patients' preferences for cancer chemotherapy. *J Clin Epidemiol.* 1989;42:119–126.

O'Connor AM, Fiset V, DeGrasse C, et al. Decision aids for patients considering options affecting cancer outcomes: Evidence of efficacy and policy implications. *J Natl Cancer I Monogr.* 1999;25:67–80.

O'Connor AM, Llewellyn-Thomas HA, Flood AB. Modifying unwarranted variations in health care: shared decision making using patient decision aids. *Health Affairs (Millwood).* 2004;Suppl Variation:VAR63–72.

O'Connor AM, Rostom A, Fiset V, et al.: Decision aids for patients facing health treatment or screening decisions: Systematic review. *BMJ.* 1999;319:731–734.

O'Connor AM, Tugwell P, Wells GA, Elmslie T, Jolly E, Hollingworth G, et al. Randomized trial of a portable, self-administered decision aid for postmenopausal women considering long-term preventive hormone therapy. *Med Decis Making.* 1998;18:295–303.

O'Connor AM, Tugwell P, Wells GA, et al. A decision aid for women considering hormone therapy after menopause: decision support framework and evaluation. *Patient Educ Couns.* 1998;33:267–279.

O'Connor GT, Plume SK, Olmstead EM, Coffin LH, Morton JR, Maloney CT, et al. Multivariate prediction of in-hospital mortality associated with coronary artery bypass graft surgery. Northern New England Cardiovascular Disease Study Group. *Circulation.* 1992;85:2110–2118.

O'Connor AM, Bennett CL, Stacey D, Barry M, Col NF, Eden KB, et al. Decision aids for people facing health treatment or screening decisions. *Cochrane Database Syst Rev.* 2009;(3):CD001431.

O'Loughlin J, Makni H, Tremblay M, et al. Smoking cessation counseling practices of general practitioners in Montreal. *Prev Med.* 2001;33:627–638.

O'Neil J. SMART goals, SMART schools. *Educ Leadership.* 2000;Feb:46–50.

Ockene JK, Zapka JG. Physician-based smoking intervention: a rededication to a five-step strategy to smoking research. *Addict Behav.* 1997;22:835–848.

Office of the National Coordinator for Health IT (ONC). *Meaningful Use Stage II Requirements.* Accessed May 12, 2012, from: http://www.healthit.gov/policy-researchers-implementers/meaningful-use.

Ossip-Klein DJ, McIntosh S, Utman C, Burton K, Spada J, Guido J. Smokers ages 50+: who gets physician advice to quit? *Prev Med.* 2000;31:364–369.

Owen JE, Klapow JC, Hicken B, Tucker DC. Psychosocial interventions for cancer: Review and analysis using a three-tiered outcomes model. *Psycho-Oncology.* 2001;10:218–230.

Pollak KI, Arredondo EM, Yarnall KS, et al. How do residents prioritize smoking cessation for young "high-risk" women? Factors associated with addressing smoking cessation. *Prev Med.* 2001;33: 292–299.

Prochaska JO, Velicer WF. The transtheoretical model of health behavior change. *Am J Health Promot.* 1997; 12(1):38–48.

Project MATCH Research Group. Matching alcoholism treatments to client heterogeneity: Project MATCH posttreatment drinking outcomes. *J Stud Alcohol.* 1997;58:7–29.

Project MATCH Research Group. Matching alcoholism treatments to client heterogeneity: Project MATCH three-year drinking outcomes. *Alcoholism Clin Exp Res.* 1998a; 22:1300–1311.

Project MATCH Research Group. Project MATCH: rationale and methods for a multisite clinical trial matching patients to alcoholism treatment. *Alcoholism Clin Exp Res.* 1993;17:1130–1145.

Project MATCH Research Group. Therapist effects in three treatments for alcohol problems. *Psychother Res.* 1998b;8:455–474.

Rabin BA, Purcell P, Naveed S, Moser RP, Henton MD, Proctor EK et al. Advancing the application, quality and harmonization of implementation science measures. *Implement Sci.* 2012;7(1):119.

Raynor DK, Blenkinsopp A, Knapp P, Grime J, Nicolson DJ, Pollock K, et al. A systematic review of quantitative and qualitative research on the role and effectiveness of written information available to patients about individual medicines. *Health Technol Assess.* 2007;11(5):iii, 1–160.

Raynor DK, Silcock J, Edmondson H. How do patients use medicine information leaflets in the UK? *Int J Pharmacy Practice.* 2007;15:209–218.

Ricciardi L, Mostashart F, Murphy J, Daniel JG, Siminerio EP. A national action plan to support consumer engagement via e-health. *Health Affairs.* 2013; 32 (2): 376–384.

Rice VH. Nursing intervention and smoking cessation: a metaanalysis. *Heart Lung.* 1999;28:438–454.

Rickles NM, Svarstad BL, Stata-Paynter JL, Taylor LV, Kobak KA. Improving patient feedback about and outcomes with antidepressant treatment: a study in eight community pharmacies. Journal of the American Pharmacists Association, 2006;46:25–32.

Ries LAG, Kosary CL, Hankey BF, Miller BA, Edwards BK, eds. *SEER Cancer Statistics Review, 1973–1996.* Bethesda, MD: National Cancer Institute; 1999. Available online from: http://www.seer.ims.nci.nih. gov/.

Rimer BK, Glassman B. Tailoring communications for primary care settings. *Method Inform Med.* 1998;37:171–177.

Rogers LQ, Johnson KC, Young ZM, Graney M. Demographic bias in physician smoking cessation counseling. *Am J Med Sci.* 1997;313:153–158.

Rollnick S, Butler CD, McCambridge J et al. Consultations about changing behavior. *BMJ.* 2005;331(7522):961–963.

Rollnick S, Mason P, Butler C. *Health Behavior Change: A Guide for Practitioners.* New York: Churchill Livingstone; 1999.

Rollnick S, Miller WR. What is motivational interviewing? *Behavioural and Cognitive Psychotherapy.* 1995;23:325–334.

Rorer D, Kinmonth AI. What is the evidence that increasing participation of individuals in self-management improves the processes and outcomes of care? In: Williams R, Kinmonth, A, Warchain N, et al., eds. *The Evidence Base for Diabetes Care.* Hoboken, NJ: John Wiley and Sons, 2002.

Rothman A. Toward a theory-based analysis of behavioral maintenance. *Health Psychol.* 2000;19:64–69.

Sarna LP, Brown JK, Lillington L, Rose M, Wewers ME, Brecht ML. Tobacco interventions by oncology nurses in clinical practice: report from a national survey. *Cancer.* 2000;89:881–889.

Schwartz LM, Woloshin S, Black W, Welch HG. The role of numeracy in understanding the benefit of screening mammography. *Ann Intern Med.* 1997;127:966–972.

Schwartz LM, Woloshin SH, Welch HG. Risk Communication in Clinical Practice: Putting Cancer in Context. *MonogrNatl Cancer I.* 1999;25:124–133.

Secker-Walker RH, Solomon LJ, Flynn BS, Dana GS. Comparisons of the smoking cessation counseling activities of six types of health professionals. *Prev Med.* 1994;23:800–808.

Senathirajah Y, Kukafka R, Guptarak M, Cohall A. Health information seeking and technology use in Harlem—a pilot study using community-based participatory research. *AMIA Annual Symposium Proceedings.* 2006:704–708.

Sepucha KR, Fowler, FJ, Mulley AG Policy support for patient-centered care: the need for measurable improvements In decision quality. *Health Affairs.* 2004. Accessed December 15, 2012, from http://www.dartmouth-hitchcock.org/dhmc-internet upload/file_collection/Policy%20support%20 for%20patient%20centered%20care%20.pdf.

Shaw BR, McTavish F, Hawkins R, Gustafson DH, Pingree S. Experiences of women with breast cancer: exchanging social support over the CHESS computer network. *J Health commun.* 2000;5:135–159.

Sheinfeld Gorin S. Predictors of tobacco control among nursing students. *Patient Educ Couns.* 2001;44:251–262.

Sheinfeld Gorin S, Heck J. Meta-analysis of the efficacy of tobacco counseling by health care providers. *Cancer Epidemiol Biomar Prev.* 2004;13(12):2012–2022.

Sheinfeld Gorin S, Krist A. *Using MOHR for Behavior Change: A Webinar for Clinicians.* Accessed February 29, 2013, from http://healthpolicy.ucla.edu/mohr.

Sheinfeld Gorin S, Wang C, Raich P, Bowen DJ, Hay J. Decision making in cancer primary prevention and chemoprevention. *Ann Behav Med* 2006;32(3):179–187.

Sheridan SL, Harris RP, Woolf SH: Shared decision making about screening and chemoprevention. A suggested approach from the US Preventive Services Task Force. *Am J Prev Med.* 2004;26:56–66.

Skinner CS, Strecher VJ, Hospers H. Physicians' recommendations for mammography: do tailored messages make a difference? *Am J Public Health.* 1994;84:43–49.

Sleath B, Blalock SJ, Bender DE, Murray M, Cerna A, Cohen MG. Latino patients' preferences for medication information and pharmacy services. *J Am Pharm Assoc.* 2009; 49(5), 632–636.

Sleath B, Goldstein M. Chapter 13: Health care professionals. In: Fischhoff B, Brewer NT, Downs JS, eds. *Communicating Risks and Benefits: An Evidence-Based User's Guide,* pp. 121-128. Washington, DC: Food and Drug Administration (FDA), US Department of Health and Human Services, August 2011. Accessed April 13, 2013 from http://www.fda.gov/ downloads/AboutFDA/ReportsManualsForms/ Reports/UCM268069.pdf.

Smith M, Saunders R, Stuckhardt L, McGinnis JM, eds., Committee on the Learning Health Care System in America; Institute of Medicine. *Best Care at Lower Cost: The Path to Continuously Learning Health Care in America,* September 6, 2012. Accessed September 12, 2012, from http://books.nap.edu/openbook. php?record_id=13444.

Smith RA, vonEschenbach AC, Wender R, Levin B, Byers T et al. American Cancer Society Guidelines for the Early Detection of Cancer: update of early detection guidelines for prostate, colorectal, and endometrial cancer. *CA: A Cancer Journal for Clin.* 2001;51:38–75.

Speck BJ, Looney SW. Effects of a minimal intervention to increase physical activity in women: daily activity records. *Nursing Res.* 2001;50(6):374–378.

Speck RM, Hill RK, Pronk NP, Becker MP, Schmitz KH. Assessment and outcomes of HealthPartners 10,000 Steps program in an academic work site. *Health Promot Pract.* 2010;11:741–750.

Stacey D, Bennett CL, Barry MJ, Col NF, Eden KB, Holmes-Rovner M, Llewellyn-Thomas H, Lyddiatt A, Légaré F, Thomson R. Decision aids for people facing health treatment or screening decisions. *Cochrane Database of Systematic Reviews* 5 Oct 2011: doi/10.1002/14651858.CD001431.

Stead LF, Bergson G, Lancaster T. Physician advice for smoking cessation. *Cochrane Database of Systematic Reviews* 2008, Issue 2. Art. No. CD000165. doi: 10.1002/14651858.CD000165.pub3.

Stewart M, Brown J, Weston W, McWhinney I, McWilliam C, Freeman T. *Patient-Centered Medicine: Transforming the Clinical Method.* Thousand Oaks: Sage; 1995.

Stoddard AM, Fox SA. Costanza ME, Lane DS, Andersen MR, Urban N, Lipkus I, Rimer BK. Effectiveness of telephone counseling for mammography: results from 5 randomized trials. *Prev Med.* 2002:90–99.

Strecher VJ. Computer-tailored smoking cessation materials: a review and discussion. *Patient Educ Couns.* 1999;36(2):107–117.

Svarstad BL, Bultman DC, Mount JK. Patient counseling provided in community pharmacies: Effects of state regulation, pharmacist age, and busyness. *Journal Am Pharmacists Assoc.* 2004;44:22–29.

Tilley BC, Vernon SW, Myers RE, Hanz L, et al. The Next Step Trial: impact of a worksite colorectal cancer screening promotion program. *Prev Med.* 1999;28:276–283.

Treasure JL, Katzman M, Schmidt U, Troop N, Todd G, deSilva P. Engagement and outcome in the treatment of bulimia nervosa: first phase of a sequential design comparing motivational enhancement therapy and cognitive behavioural therapy. *Behav Res Ther.* 1998;37:405–418.

Truax CB, Carkhuff RR. *Toward Effective Counseling and Psychotherapy.* Chicago: Aldine; 1967.

Turner-McGrievy GM, Tate D. Weight loss social support in 140 characters or less: use of an online social network in a remotely delivered weight loss intervention. *Transl Behav Med.* 2013 (published online).

Tversky A, Kahneman D. The framing of decisions and the psychology of choice. *Science.* 1981;211:453–458.

UKATT Research Team. Cost effectiveness of treatment for alcohol problems: findings of the randomized UK alcohol treatment trial (UKATT). *BMJ.* 2005a;331:544–548.

US Department of Education, Institute of Education Sciences, National Center for Education Statistics, 1992 National Adult Literacy Survey and and 2003 National Assessment of Adult Literacy. National Cemter for Education Statistics. Acccessed April 13, 2013, from http://nces.ed.gov/naal/kf_demographics.asp.

Vernon SW. Risk perception and risk communication for cancer screening behavior: a review: print communications in cancer risk communication? *JNCI Monogr.* 1999;25:140–148.

Vernon SW, et al. Measures for ascertaining use of colorectal cancer screening in behavioral, health services, and epidemiologic research. *Cancer Epidemiol BiomarPrev.* 2004;13:898–905.

Villanueva M, Tonigan JS, Miller WR. Response of Native American clients to three treatment methods for alcohol dependence. *J Ethnic Subst Abuse.* 2007;6(2):41–48.

Vinson C, Bickmore T, Farrell D, Campbell M, Saunders E, Nowak M, Fowler B, Shaikh A. Adapting research tested computerized tailored interventions for implementation in practice. *Transl Behav Med.* 2011; 1(1), 93–102.

Wagner EH, et al. Quality improvement in chronic illness care: a collaborative approach. *Jt Comm J Qual Im.* 2001;27(2):63–80.

Warsi A, Wang PS, LaValley MP, Avorn J, Solomon DH. Self-management education programs in chronic disease: a systematic review and methodological critique of the literature. *Arch Intern Med.* 2004;164(15):1641–1649.

White MJ, Stark JR, Luckmann R, Rosal MC, Clemow L, Costanza ME. Implementing a computer assisted telephone interview (CATI) system to increase colorectal cancer screening: a process evaluation. *Patient Educ Couns.* 2006;61:419–428.

Whitlock EP, Orleans CT, Pender N, et al. Evaluating primary care behavioral counseling interventions: an evidence:-based approach. *Am J Prev Med.* 2002;22:267–284.

Williams R, Herman W, Kinmouth A-L, Wareham NJ, Goldstein MG. Promoting self management in primary care settings: limitations and opportunities: a commentary. In: Williams R, Herman W, Kinmonth AI, eds. *The Evidence Base for Diabetes Care,* 2nd ed., pp. 701–710. West Sussex, England: John Wiley and Sons; 2002.

Wilson PW, D'Agostino RB, Levy D, Belanger AM, Silbershatz H, Kannel WB, et al. Prediction of coronary heart disease using risk factor categories. *Circulation.* 1998;97:1837–1847.

Winhusen T, Kropp F, Babcock D, Hague D, Erickson SJ, Renz C, Rau L, Lewis D, Leimberger J, Somoza E. Motivational enhancement therapy to improve treatment utilization and outcome in pregnant substance users. *J Subst Abuse Treat.* 2008;35:161–173.

Winterstein AG, Linden S, Lee AE, Fernandez EM, Kimberlin CL. Evaluation of consumer medication information dispensed in retail pharmacies. *Arch Intern Med.* 2010;170:1317–1324.

Woloshin S, Schwartz LM. How can we help people make sense of medical data? *Effective Clin Pract.* 1999;2:176–183.

Yabroff KR, Mandelblatt JS. Interventions targeted toward patients to increase mammography use. *Cancer Epidemiol Biomar Prev.* 1999;8:749–757.

Yabroff KR, Mangan P, Mandelblatt J. Effectiveness of interventions to increase Papanicolaou smear use. *J Am Board Fam Med.* 2003;16:188–203.

Zhu S, Stretch V, Balabanis M, Rosbrook B, Sadler G, Pierce J. Telephone counseling for smoking cessation: effects of single-session and multiple-session interventions. *J Consul Clin Psychol.* 1996;64:202–211.

12

The Future of Prevention in Primary Care

SHERRI N. SHEINFELD GORIN AND YALINI SENATHIRAJAH

Healthcare is in the process of transformation, and prevention is at its core, particularly with the passage of the Affordable Care Act of 2010 (The Patient Protection and Affordable Care Act, P.L. 111-148, March 23, 2010); the wider dissemination of primary care initiatives like the Patient Centered Medical Home with its focus on patient-centeredness, effectiveness, and quality of care; the rising interest in genomics in medicine; the rapid pace of information technology applications in clinical practice; and the pervasive fiscal pressures on the economy. Concurrently, the US population is changing markedly, with the growth in the population of older adults and the increased diversity among its residents overall. These several trends have been well documented in a series of groundbreaking Institute of Medicine (IOM) reports published over the past two decades, including *To Err Is Human: Building a Safer Health System* (2000); *Crossing the Quality Chasm: A New Health System for the 21st century* (2001);*Unequal Treatment: Confronting Racial and Ethnic Disparities in Health Care* (2003); *Best Care at Lower Cost: The Path to Continuously Learning Health Care in America* (2012), and, most recently, *Delivering High Quality Cancer Care: Charting a New Course for a System in Crisis* (2013). This Chapter[1,2] will summarize some of these emerging trends, and offer some suggestions for the near-term future of prevention.

As discussed in Chapter 2, the multi-level perspective—from policy, to provider, and patient—will found the future of prevention, with risk factors, intervention and implementation approaches focused across levels (Sheinfeld Gorin,, Badr, Krebs, & Prabhu Das, 2012).

ADDRESSING THE SHORTER LIVES FOR AMERICANS

Compared to 16 peer countries, lives in the United States are shorter and of poorer health than among those in other high-income democracies in western Europe, as well as Canada, Australia, and Japan. According to the Institute of Medicine's *U.S. Health in International Perspective: Shorter Lives, Poorer Health* (Woolf & Aron, 2013), this disparity in health is strikingly consistent and pervasive over the life course—at birth, during childhood and adolescence, for young and middle-aged adults, and for older adults. Relying on historical trend data beginning in the 1970s through 2008, the Institute of Medicine concluded that, for many years, Americans have been dying at younger ages than people in almost all other high-income countries (see Figures 12-1 and 12-2). This disadvantage has been getting worse for three decades, especially among women. A recent paper by Kindig and Cheng (2013) plumbs the depths of these findings by examining longitudinal trends in 3,140 US counties, reporting that female mortality rates have increased 42.8%, while male mortality rates increased 3.4%. The paper cites a potential causal link in increased smoking and lack of education, with regional differences, notably in the South and the West (Kindig & Cheng, 2013; Dentzer, 2013).

The US health disadvantage spans many types of illness and injury. When compared with the average of peer countries, Americans as a group fare worse in at least nine health areas (Woolf & Aron, 2013). For

---

1 Some of this Chapter is adapted from Sheinfeld Gorin S. Future directions for health promotion. In: Sheinfeld Gorin S, Arnold J. *Health Promotion in Practice,*pp. 543–567. San Francisco, CA: Jossey-Bass, 2006. Evan (Moshe) Gorin contributed technical assistance for the transfer of the figures and tables in this Chapter.

2 We thank Joshua Graff Zivin, Ph.D., Professor of Economics and International Relations, University of California, San Diego for his review of the Chapter.

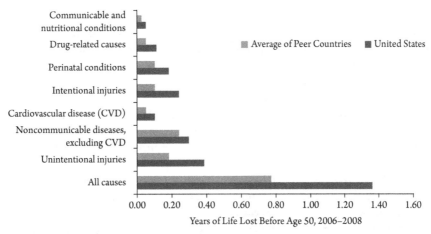

FIGURE 12-1: Causes of Death for US Men Aged 50 and Below, Compared with the Average of Peer Countries, 2006–2008. Reproduced with permission. Woolf SH, Aron L, eds. Panel on Understanding Cross-National Health Differences Among High-Income Countries; Committee on Population; Division of Behavioral and Social Sciences and Education; National Research Council; Board on Population Health and Public Health Practice; Institute of Medicine. *U.S. Health in International Perspective: Shorter Lives, Poorer Health.* Washington, DC : National Academies Press; 2013.

those who reach age 50, these conditions contribute to poorer health and greater illness later in life:

1. Infant mortality and low birth weight;
2. Injuries and homicides;
3. Adolescent pregnancy and sexually transmitted infections;
4. HIV and AIDS;
5. Drug-related deaths;
6. Obesity and diabetes;
7. Heart disease;
8. Chronic lung disease;
9. Disability.

Many of these conditions have a particularly profound effect on young people, reducing the odds that Americans will live to age 50. Within this age group, the single biggest contributor is unintentional injuries, which account for roughly a third of excess US mortality among younger Americans (Ho, 2013). Homicide and suicide contribute to these injuries, fueled by Americans' broad access to guns. In addition, among younger Americans, "accidental poisonings"—literally, deaths from drug overdoses, through abuse of prescription drugs containing hydrocodone and oxycodone, as well as illegal drugs like heroin and cocaine, contribute to

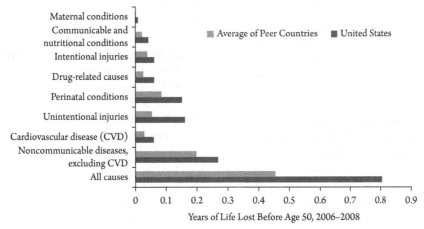

FIGURE 12-2: Causes of Death for US Women Aged 50 and Below, Compared with the Average of Peer Countries, 2006–2008. Reproduced with permission. Woolf SH, Aron L, eds. Panel on Understanding Cross-National Health Differences Among High-Income Countries; Committee on Population; Division of Behavioral and Social Sciences and Education; National Research Council; Board on Population Health and Public Health Practice; Institute of Medicine. *U.S. Health in International Perspective: Shorter Lives, Poorer Health.* Washington, DC : National Academies Press; 2013.

their higher rates of death relative to other groups (Dentzer, 2013).

The United States does enjoy a few health advantages when compared with peer countries, including lower cancer death rates and greater control of blood pressure and cholesterol levels. Americans who reach age 75 can expect to live longer than people in the peer countries. With these exceptions, however, other high-income countries outrank the United States on most measures of health.

The US health disadvantage cannot be fully explained by the health disparities that exist among people who are uninsured or poor, as discussed more fully later in this Chapter. Several studies are now suggesting that even advantaged Americans—those who are white, insured, college-educated, or upper income—are in worse health than similar individuals in other countries.

The Institute of Medicine's report (Woolf & Aron, 2013) found multiple likely explanations for the US health disadvantage:

- *Health systems.* Unlike its peer countries, the United States has a relatively large uninsured population and more limited access to primary care. Americans are more likely to find their health care inaccessible or unaffordable and to report lapses in the quality and safety of care outside hospitals.
- *Health behaviors.* Although Americans are currently less likely to smoke and may drink alcohol less heavily than people in peer countries, they consume the most calories per person, have higher rates of drug abuse, are less likely to use seat belts, are involved in more traffic accidents that involve alcohol, and are more likely to use firearms in acts of violence.
- *Social and economic conditions.* Although the income of Americans is higher on average than in other countries, the United States also has higher levels of poverty (especially child poverty) and income inequality and lower rates of social mobility. Other countries are outpacing the United States in the education of young people, which also affects health. And Americans benefit less from safety net programs that can buffer the negative health effects of poverty and other social disadvantages.
- *Physical environments.* US communities and the built environment are more likely than those in peer countries to be designed around automobiles, and this may discourage physical activity and contribute to obesity.

As cited by the Institute of Medicine (Woolf & Aron, 2013) and as discussed throughout *Prevention Practice in Primary Care*, multilevel prevention (at the policy, provider, and patient levels),across multiple sectors (including health and social services), is key to the US disparity in mortality relative to other peer countries. These findings underscore the need for "increased public and private investment in the social and environmental determinants of health," rather than simply increased health care expenditures. *Most important, however, they point to the primary care practice setting as a critical nexus in the chain of change.*

IMPLICATIONS FOR DIVERSE SUBPOPULATIONS

As discussed previously in Chapters 1 through 3, racial and ethnic minorities (i.e, individuals who do not self-identify as non-Hispanic whites) continue to experience disparities in both health care processes and outcomes compared with majority populations (Edwards, Ward, Kohler, et al., 2010; Ozols, Herbst, Colson, et al., 2007; Institute of Medicine, 2003; Bigby & Holmes, 2005; Biglan & Glasgow, 1991; Sheinfeld Gorin, 2006; Altekruse, Kosary, Krapcho, et al., 2010; Newmann & Garner, 2005; Palmer & Schneider, 2005; Shavers, Fagan, McDonald, 2007; Holmes, Lehman, Hade, et al., 2008; Altekruse, Kosary, Krapcho, et al., 2010). By 2050, 50% of the US population is expected to be racial/ethnic minority, underscoring the significance of disparities in health outcomes (Grieco & Cassidy, 2001). The mechanisms underlying these racial and ethnic disparities are incompletely understood (Institute of Medicine; Smedley, Stith, Nelson, 2003) and may reflect both differences among populations and within them.

For example, Latinos, the fastest growing population in the United States, are a highly diverse racial and ethnic subgroup. According to the US Census (2010), more than half of the growth in the total population of the United States between 2000 and 2010 was due to the increase in the Hispanic population. The US-resident Latino population comprises Mexican Americans (63% of US Latinos), mainland Puerto Ricans (9.2%), Central and South Americans (13.4%), Cubans (3.5%), those from the Dominican Republic (2.8%), Spaniards (1.3%) and "other" Latinos (6.8%), including those who report "Hispanic" or "Latino" (Ennis et al., 2011).

Consequently, Latino subgroups vary in their disease (particularly, cancer) risk factors, including their rates of smoking and drinking alcohol and their patterns of dietary intake and exercise (Winkleby,

Fortmann, & Rockhill, 1993; Loria et al., 1995; Gans et al., 2002; Cervantes, Gilbert, Salgado de Snyder, & Padilla, 1990; Epstein, Botvin, & Diaz, 2001; Gordon-Larsen, Harris, Ward, & Popkin, 2003; Perez-Stable et al., 2001). Their rates of disease (particularly cancer) morbidity and mortality also differ by subgroup (Mallin& Anderson, 1988; Rosenwaike & Shai, 1986; Warshauer, Silverman, Schottenfeld, & Pollack, 1986; Sheinfeld Gorin & Heck, 2005; Sheinfeld Gorin, 2005). Yet, Latinos are less likely overall than whites to obtain recommended cancer screening services, due to economic, educational, cultural, and other structural barriers (Phillips, Morrison, Andersen, & Aday, 1998; National Center for Health Statistics, 2000), Latino subgroups vary in their cancer screening rates (Sheinfeld Gorin & Heck, 2005).

Cancer is now the second leading cause of death among American Indians in the United States, as it is in the US population as a whole, and heart disease is the first (Burhansstipanov, 1998; USDHHS, 2000;NCHS, 2011). The types of cancer experienced within Native communities vary significantly by geographic region(Cobb & Paisano, 1998; USDHHS, 2000; Burhansstipanov, 1998; Burhansstipanov, Hampton,& Wiggins, 1999). Their cancer rates, previously reported to be lower than in other ethnic and racial subgroups, have increased over the past 20 years. These findings suggest the vital importance of tailoring prevention programs to population subgroups that are highly internally diverse.

DEMOGRAPHIC SHIFT TOWARD THE OLDER ADULT

Given the vast differences in mortality between the United States and other peer countries among those aged 50 years and older, these findings are particularly sobering with the aging of the US population (Federal Interagency Forum on Aging-Related Statistics, *Older Americans 2008: Key Indicators of Well-being*, Washington, DC: US Government Printing Office, 2008). Persons aged 65 years and older constitute the fastest growing segment of the population. By 2020, more than 64 million Americans will be aged 65 years or older, constituting nearly 22% of the US population. Women will predominate; minorities, however, will be underrepresented in this age group (Koplan & Livengood, 1994). By the year 2020, the dependency ratio (that is, the proportion of persons not participating in the workforce to those who do participate)

will increase because of the larger numbers of aged persons present (US Senate Special Committee on Aging, 1991).

These projections have obvious implications for changing health services and social support. Chronic diseases are more common among the elderly than the young. For example, the population surge will result in a doubling of cancer diagnoses, from 1.3 million in 2011 to 2.6 million in 2030 (Edwards, Howe, Ries, et al., 2002). As described throughout this book, a considerable number of the major causes of death among persons aged 65 and older—heart disease, cancer, stroke, chronic obstructive pulmonary disease, pneumonia, and influenza—are preventable or can be controlled. As also described throughout *Prevention Practice in Primary Care*, changing certain health behaviors (for example, stopping smoking, eating a balanced diet, reducing sodium, and losing weight) can reduce the risk of disease among older adults (Institute of Medicine [IOM], 1990). Physical activity is a central component of health promotion among the aging (Casperson, 1989).

The 2008 Institute of Medicine (IOM) report on aging underscored that "older persons need to be active partners in their own care" (Institute of Medicine; 2008), a concept emphasized throughout this book. This approach promotes patient preferences and encourages meaningful involvement of older people in their health care interactions, which is central to any successful prevention effort (Sheinfeld Gorin, Gauthier, Hays, Miles, Wardle, 2008; Wagner, Bennett, Austin, Greene, Schaefer, Vonkorff, 2005), as discussed throughout this book. Health promotion among older men and women will include efforts to maintain functional independence and add years of healthy life, rather than simply elongating life.

State and federal programs, such as components of the 2010 federal health care law (Pub. L. No. 111-148, 124 Stat. 119), entitle older people to annual wellness visits, which could offer opportunities to have conversations about a "personalized prevention plan" with an inoculation and cancer screening schedule for the next 5 or 10 years. Clearly, healthy aging is a priority for many public health planners. Assessments of the pros and cons of prevention activities should complement such initiatives. Because of the paucity of randomized cancer screening trials in those aged 76 years and older (US Preventive Services Task Force, 2009), however, questions about the evidence to accompany those intervention choices remain.

From the patient-centered model, the goal is to understand how older persons prioritize disease treatment or prevention and wellness, or how they value extended life years and quality of life (Wagner, Bennett, Austin, Greene, Schaefer, Vonkorff, 2005). Health care decisions for cancer screening could extend beyond age to include health and medical values and preferences, as well as other changes in physical health and life expectancy. As the developmental psychologist Leonard Pearlin remarked, "There is not one process of aging, but many; there is not one life course, but many courses; there is not one sequence of stages, but many" (Haug, Powell, 1981).

With the aging of the US population, and the increased resources that will need to be devoted to the elderly, given a declining workforce, it is not clear from whence the resources will come. As a result, in the United States the issue of reform in the Medicare and Social Security programs has joined the political agenda. For example, increasingly, older Americans will be living alone and may need special assistance to retain their independent functioning. This assistance will involve help with performing activities of daily living (for example, bathing, dressing, and eating) so that individuals may remain residents in the community rather than being placed in long-term nursing care.

Cancer care for older adults, as noted in a recent IOM report, is especially complex. Age is one of the strongest risk factors for cancer. There are many important considerations to understanding the prognoses of older adults with cancer and formulating their care plans. In addition to the factors listed above, these include; altered physiology, functional and cognitive impairment, multiple coexisting morbidities, increased side effects to treatment, distinct goals of care, and the increased importance of social networks for support. Addressing the needs of the aging population will be an integral part of improving the quality of cancer care in the future (IOM, 2013).

Value-based policy decisions to address these challenges will require considerable political will. An ethic of personal and family responsibility for health and the importance of lifestyle changes could again become an ideology to justify resource distributions. By contrast, an ideology that supports a fair, equitable distribution of bargaining power and resources among children, the young, working adults, and the old could be encouraged. A uniform political will, as well as economic munificence— which has been a challenge during the recent worldwide recession—will be required to support the chosen aims.

EVALUATING THE PATIENT-CENTERED MEDICAL HOME

As described in Chapters 2 and 10, primary care providers, health care systems, insurers, state governments, families, and communities are turning to the primary care patient-centered medical home (PCMH) as a solution to many of the troubles of the fragmented US health care system (see Figure 12-3 for an example). What we don't know is whether current models of the medical home achieve these goals and, if so, how to finance them. Rigorous evaluations are critical to determining whether the PCMH model works, and for finding ways to refine, improve, customize, and disseminate the model. Future studies of the PCMH can generate high-quality, reliable evidence about their effectiveness by: (1) focusing evaluations on quality, cost, and experience; (2) including comparison practices; (3) recognizing that the PCMH is a practice-level intervention and account for clustering; (4) including as many intervention practices as possible; (5) being strategic in identifying the right samples of patients to answer each evaluation question; and (6) rethinking the number of patients from whom data are collected to answer key evaluation questions (Peikes, Dale, Lundquist, Genevro, Meyers, 2011).

Patient Activation: Key to the Patient-Centered Medical Home

As discussed in Chapters 2, 3, and 11, "patient activation" refers to a patient's knowledge, skills, ability, and willingness to manage his or her own health. "Patient engagement" is a broader concept that combines patient activation with interventions designed to increase activation and promote positive patient behavior, such as obtaining preventive care or exercising regularly. Patient engagement is one strategy to achieve the "triple aim" of improved health outcomes, better patient care, and lower costs.

Figure 12-4 displays a multilevel model of patient engagement (Carman et al., 2013). The first level is direct patient care, in which patients get information about a condition and answer questions about their preferences for treatment. This form of engagement

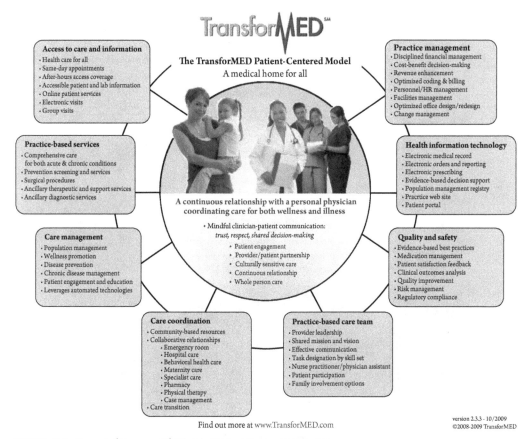

TransforMED℠

The TransforMED Patient-Centered Model
A medical home for all

Access to care and information
- Health care for all
- Same-day appointments
- After-hours access coverage
- Accessible patient and lab information
- Online patient services
- Electronic visits
- Group visits

Practice management
- Disciplined financial management
- Cost-benefit decision-making
- Revenue enhancement
- Optimized coding & billing
- Personnel/HR management
- Facilities management
- Optimized office design/redesign
- Change management

Practice-based services
- Comprehensive care for both acute & chronic conditions
- Prevention screening and services
- Surgical procedures
- Ancillary therapeutic and support services
- Ancillary diagnostic services

Health information technology
- Electronic medical record
- Electronic orders and reporting
- Electronic prescribing
- Evidence-based decision support
- Population management registry
- Practrice web site
- Patient portal

A continuous relationship with a personal physician coordinating care for both wellness and illness

- Mindful clinician-patient communication:
  trust, respect, shared decision-making
  - Patient engagement
  - Provider/patient partnership
  - Culturally sensitive care
  - Continuous relationship
  - Whole person care

Care management
- Population management
- Wellness promotion
- Disease prevention
- Chronic disease management
- Patient engagement and education
- Leverages automated technologies

Quality and safety
- Evidence-based best practices
- Medication management
- Patient satisfaction feedback
- Clinical outcomes analysis
- Quality improvement
- Risk management
- Regulatory compliance

Care coordination
- Community-based resources
- Collaborative relationships
  - Emergency room
  - Hospital care
  - Behavioral health care
  - Maternity care
  - Specialist care
  - Pharmacy
  - Physical therapy
  - Case management
- Care transition

Practice-based care team
- Provider leadership
- Shared mission and vision
- Effective communication
- Task designation by skill set
- Nurse practitioner/physician assistant
- Patient participation
- Family involvement options

Find out more at www.TransforMED.com

version 2.3.3 - 10/2009
©2008-2009 TransforMED

FIGURE 12-3: Example (Commercial) Model of Patient Centered Medical Home.

Source: http://www.transformed.com/

allows patients and providers to join in shared decision making, including assessing the medical evidence, patients' preferences, and using clinical judgment. In the second level of engagement, organizational design and governance, health care organizations reach out for consumer input to ensure that they will be as responsive as possible to patients' needs. In the third level, policy making, consumers are involved in the decisions that communities and society make about policies, laws, and regulations in public health and health care (Carman et al., 2013).

Many studies have shown that patients who are "activated"—that is, have the skills, ability, and willingness to manage their own health and health care—experience better health outcomes at lower costs compared to less activated patients. Using a validated "patient activation measure," Hibbard et al. (2013) studied the relationship between patients' activation scores and their health care costs at Fairview Health Services, a large health care delivery system in Minnesota. In an analysis of more

than 30,000 patients, they found that those with the lowest activation scores, that is, people with the least skills and confidence to actively engage in their own health care, incurred costs that averaged 8–21% higher than patients with the highest activation levels, even after adjusting for health status and other factors. These findings suggest that patient activation could continue to be a significant predictor of health care costs, as patient activation is more widely disseminated throughout the health care system.

CONTINUOUSLY LEARNING HEALTH SYSTEMS

As described in Chapter 1, the US health care system demonstrates pervasive inefficiencies, the health care system offers few rewards and incentives focused on patient needs, and primary care providers—in fact, all health care professionals—experience difficulties managing a rapidly deepening clinical knowledge base; these hinder improvements in the safety and quality of health care. These factors also challenge

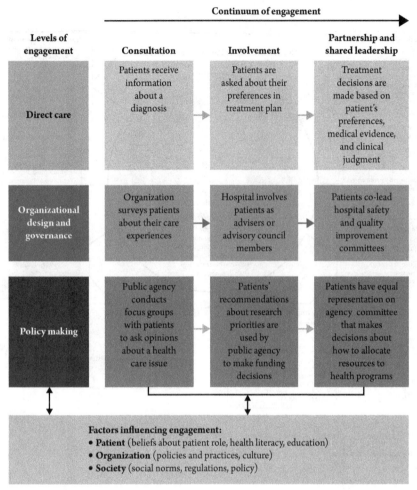

FIGURE 12-4: A Multidimensional Framework for Patient and Family Engagement in Health and Health Care.

US economic stability and global competitiveness (Institute of Medicine, 2012).

The shortcomings of the health care system can be compared to the routine operation of other industries (see Figure 12-5). Builders rely on blueprints to coordinate the work of carpenters, electricians, and plumbers. Banks offer customers financial records that are updated in real time. Automobile manufacturers produce thousands of vehicles that are standardized at their core, while tailored at the margins. While health care must accommodate many competing priorities and human factors unlike those in other industries, the health care system could learn from these industries how to better meet specific needs, expand choices, and shave costs (IOM, 2012). In response, a continuously learning health care system has been proposed, one in which

the lessons from research and each care experience are systematically captured, assessed, and translated into reliable care. To implement this approach, fundamental commitments to changed incentives, culture, and leadership are required, however (Institute of Medicine, 2012).

The continuously learning health care system has several core characteristics that are summarized in Table 12-1, including (1) using information technology more effectively with clinicians and patients having real-time access to medical records and using technology to streamline administrative tasks; (2) creating systems to manage complexity with prompts, technologies, and delivery systems that help clinicians the growing complexity of medical knowledge and care required; (3) making health care safer with hospitals and providers constantly

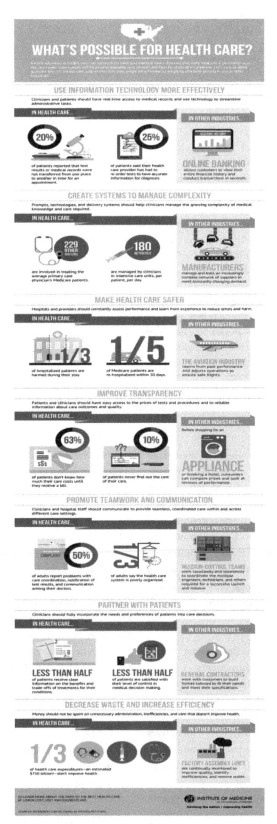

FIGURE 12-5: Infographic Comparing Health Care to Other Industries.

Source: Institute of Medicine. http://www.iom.edu/Reports/2012/Best-Care-at-Lower-Cost-The-Path-to-Continuously-Learning-Health-Care-in-America/Infographic.aspx. Reproduced with permission

---

TABLE 12-1. CHARACTERISTICS OF A CONTINUOUSLY LEARNING HEALTH
CARE SYSTEM

Science and Informatics

Real-time access to knowledge—A learning health care system continuously and reliably captures, curates, and delivers the best available evidence to guide, support, tailor, and improve clinical decision making and care safety and quality.

*Digital capture of the care experience—A learning health care system captures the care experience on digital platforms for real-time generation and application of knowledge for care improvement.

Patient-Clinician Relationships

*Engaged, empowered patients—A learning health care system is anchored on patient needs and perspectives and promotes the inclusion of patients, families, and other caregivers as vital members of the continuously learning care team.

Incentives

*Incentives aligned for value—In a learning health care system, incentives areactively aligned to encouragecontinuous improvement, identify and reduce waste, and reward high-value care.

*Full transparency—A learning health care system systematically monitors the safety, quality, processes,prices, costs, and outcomes of care, and makes information available for care improvement and informed choices and decision making by clinicians, patients, and their families.

Culture

Leadership-instilled culture of learning—A learning health care system is stewarded by leadership committed to a culture of teamwork, collaboration, and adaptability in support of continuous learning as a core aim.

*Supportive system competencies—In a learning health care system, complex care operations and processes are constantly refined through ongoing team training and skill building, systems analysis and information development, and creation of the feedback loops for continuous learning and system improvement.

---

*From: Smith M, Saunders R, Stuckhardt L, McGinnis JM, eds.; Committee on the Learning Health Care System in America; Institute of Medicine. Best Care at Lower Cost: The Path to Continuously Learning Health Care in America, September 6, 2012; Accessed September 12, 2012, from http://books.nap.edu/openbook.php?record_id=13444. Reproduced with permission

---

assessing performance and learning from their experiences to reduce errors and harm; (4) improving transparency with patients and clinicians having easy access to the prices of tests and procedures and to reliable information about care outcomes and quality; (5) promoting teamwork and communication with clinicians and hospital staff communicating to provide seamless, coordinated care within and across different care settings; and (6) partnering with patients to fully incorporate the needs and preferences of patients into all care decisions (Institute of Medicine, 2012).

At its core, the continuously learning health care system involves four components: (1) science and informatics with real-time access to knowledge and digital capture of the care experience; (2) patient-clinician relationships with engaged, empowered patients; (3) incentives aligned for value and full transparency; and (4) a leadership-instilled culture of learning with supportive system competencies.

In practice, the continuously learning system converts data about care and operations into knowledge for evidence-based clinical practice and health system change. In so doing, the continuously learning system incorporates health information technology, databases, the electronic health care record, and, importantly, a research infrastructure. In addition, new research criteria, including comparative effectiveness, and research methods will be required to fully implement the continuously learning health care system in practice.

Comparative Effectiveness Research

One of the research approaches integral to the continuously learning health care system is comparative effectiveness research (CER). The US Federal Coordinating Council for CER defines it as:

the conduct and synthesis of research comparing the benefits and harms of different interventions and strategies to prevent, diagnose, treat and monitor health conditions in "real world" settings. The purpose of this research is to improve health outcomes by developing and disseminating evidence-based information to patients, clinicians, and other decision-makers, responding to their expressed needs, about which interventions are most effective for which patients under specific circumstances.

CER involves the comparison of strategies for prevention, diagnosis, treatment, or delivery system designs that are feasible in the day-to-day practice of clinical medicine or public health. Conventional biomedical research has long been dominated by the paradigm of the "phase III" randomized clinical trial, in which two therapeutic options—usually medications—are compared in highly selected patients and a carefully controlled research environment (Rothwell, 2006; Kessler& Glasgow, 2011). The phase III randomized clinical trial (RCT) provides the best data, but by its very nature, is separate from the workings of clinical care in a given health care system. The RCT is both costly and time-consuming, and its rather narrow entry criteria may diminish its ability to be generalized to routine patients (e.g., those with comorbidities, or those outside the entry criteria of age and severity). Further, the translation of findings into practice

is often slow and cumbersome, with many years passing before research findings find their way into patient care (Balas& Boren, 2000).

In CER, a wide array of research designs may be used in addition to the RCT, including; novel randomized trials, quasi-experimental evaluations, observational studies using existing databases, and modeling or simulation studies. The pragmatic trial has been proposed as an alternative to the RCT, to more rapidly test hypotheses and translate scientific findings into practice. Table 12-2 summarizes the key characteristics of pragmatic trials compared to traditional efficacy trials in terms of measures, costs, focus, and other dimensions. As shown in Table 12-2, there are major differences in the formulation of study questions, methods, issues receiving the greatest priority, outcomes and analyses, and level of stakeholder involvement (Krist, Glenn, Glasgow, Balasubramanian, Chambers et al., 2013).

Because the outcomes are varied in CER, multiple data sources may be required to conduct these studies. Primary data collected for a CER study

---

TABLE 12-2. DISTINGUISHING BETWEEN PRAGMATIC AND TRADITIONAL CLINICAL EFFICACY TRIALS

	Pragmatic Study	Traditional Clinical Efficacy
Stakeholder Involvement	Engaged in all study phases including study design, conducting the study, collecting data, interpreting results, disseminating findings	Limited engagement, often in response to investigator ideas or study subjects
Research Design	Includes internal and external validity, design fidelity and local adaptation, real-life settings and populations, contextual assessments	Focus on limiting threats to internal validity, typically uses randomized controlled trial, participants and settings typically homogenous
Outcomes	Reach, effectiveness, adoption, implementation, comparative effectiveness, sustainability	Efficacy, mechanism identification, component analysis
Measures	Brief, valid, actionable with rapid clinical utility, feasible in real-world and low-resource settings	Validated measures that minimize bias, focus on internal consistency and theory rather than clinical relevance
Costs	Assessments include intervention costs and replication costs in relation to outcomes	Often not collected or reported
Data Sources	May include existing data (electronic health records, administrative data) and brief patient reports.	Data generation and collection part of clinical trial
Analyses	Process and outcome analyses relevant to stakeholders and from different perspectives	Specified *a priori* and typically restricted to investigator hypotheses
Availability of findings	Rapid learning and implementation	Delay between trial completion and analytic availability

From: Krist AH, Glenn BA, Glasgow RE, Balasubramanian B, Chambers DA, Fernandez M, Heurtin-Roberts S, Kessler R, Ory MG, Phillips SM, Ritzwoller DP, Roby DH, Rodriguez H, Sheinfeld Gorin S, Stange K, The MOHR Study Group. Designing a Flexible, Pragmatic Primary Care Implementation Trial: The My Own Health Report (MOHR) Project. Implementation Science, http://www.implementationscience.com/content/8/1/73.

can be augmented by data from electronic medical records, administrative claims, patient reports, and other sources. The outcomes assessed in CER should be those that patients and practitioners value and can readily use to assess the effectiveness of the strategy. As a result, a wide array of outcomes generally must be measured. For example, for cancer prevention, rather than only pathologist confirmed breast cancer, mammographic density is increasingly used both as a surrogate end point biomarker of drug effect and as a predictive biomarker of clinical drug efficacy when evaluated with tamoxifen and aromatase inhibitors in women with high breast density at baseline (Cuzick et al., 2011; Kim et al., 2012; Umar, Dunn, & Greenwald, 2012).

CER dramatically expands the range of research possibilities. Although it is likely that, in practice, the bulk of CER research will focus on pharmacological therapies, medical devices, or clinical procedures, all definitions emphasize that CER include behavioral interventions, evaluation of alternative systems of care for delivery of public health services, clinical preventive services, or treatments, and new strategies for early diagnosis or individualization of treatment, such as genomic testing. Though rarely stated, these definitions also imply that CER can expand to examine and compare the effectiveness of environmental and policy interventions(Glasgow & Steiner, 2011). Importantly, the aims of CER are focused on applications in ongoing care, and thus could greatly advance the *usability* of the evidence that is developed for prevention in primary care.

DISSEMINATING EVIDENCE TO PRIMARY CARE PROVIDERS: ACADEMIC DETAILING

As described in Chapter 10, one promising strategy to increase physician compliance with *evidence-based* guidelines and to overcome primary care physician barriers to prevention practice is academic detailing. Academic detailing applies to physician involvement in health promotion, using a similar approach to that used by pharmaceutical salespeople (Ashford, Gemson, Sheinfeld Gorin, Bloch, Lantigua, Ahsan & Neugut, 2000). These salespeople employ a brief, focused intervention repeated at periodic intervals with the physician. Academic detailers do the same, sharing with the physician materials and approaches that are tailored to the physician's barriers to, for example, preventive screening. In the future, emerging new systems of care will consider their clinicians to be responsible for the quality and appropriateness of the tests and procedures that they order or the medications that they prescribe, and will be able to encourage, mandate, and even pay for participation in educational outreach activities such as academic detailing. The mergers or alignments of payers that often accompany the integration of systems will also encourage joint funding of academic detailing programs, helping to overcome the fear of "free-riding" by competitors that often chills the enthusiasm of private health insurers for sponsoring such programs (Avorn, 2012).

MEDICAL INFORMATICS AND A CONTINUOUSLY LEARNING HEALTH CARE SYSTEM

In 1990, Shortliffe and Perrault wrote that for health professionals "it is increasingly difficult to practice modern medicine without information technologies," a statement that is even more accurate today (Shortliffe & Perrault, 1990; Eysenbach, 2000). The focus of medical informatics has been the development of applications for health professionals: medical informaticians have looked at medical practice mainly through the eyes of health professionals rather than through the eyes of patients (Eysenbach, 2000). In the future (as in the present), this will continue to change. It is increasingly unlikely that health professionals will encounter patients who have not used information technology to influence their health knowledge, attitudes and beliefs toward change, and perception of symptoms. Health professionals should, therefore, not only understand consumer health applications but also ensure that these applications are developed, applied, and evaluated properly (Eysenbach, 2000; see Figure 12-6).

Further, as incentives for minimal use (see Chapter 10), pay for performance (see Chapter 9) and other similar approaches enhancing both efficiency and quality across systems of care become more widespread, those offices that have adopted medical informatics, including computerized information technologies (IT), to improve care management will be rewarded (Medpac, 2011). Minimal use criteria, in particular, promise to remain highly influential on the use of information technologies in primary care in the future. Stage 3 criteria, proposed for implementation in 2016 (and still in formation), are designed to improve clinical outcomes.

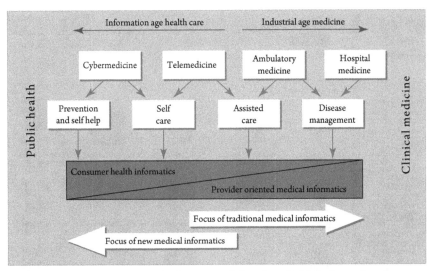

FIGURE 12-6: The Focus of Traditional Medical Informatics Is Shifting from Health Professionals to Consumers.

Source: Eysenbach G. Consumer health informatics. *BMJ.* 2000 June 24; 320(7251):1713–1716.

Stage 3 will build on the infrastructure and quality data that are collected and incorporated in clinical processes through stages 1 and 2 (http://www.cdc.gov/ehrmeaningfuluse/). These approaches begin with the use of the electronic medical record to track the numerous patient interactions over multiple settings of care, pharmaceutical use, test results, and continually evolving clinical guidelines, as described in Chapter 11. Implementation of electronic medical record varies, and may still be daunting to many clinicians as the rigor of the CMS criteria increase, however.

Despite these drawbacks, and amidst the rapid change in the field, some forward-looking approaches to medical informatics are described briefly in Figures 12-7 through 12-10.

Mobile Health

Mobile health (*mHealth*) interventions are one of the fastest growing areas of activity in prevention-focused medical informatics. *mHealth* uses mobile devices, including any wireless device carried by a person, that transmits or accepts health information. The growth in cell phones that are carried by a majority of the US adult population, with their rapidly increasing capabilities, screen resolutions, add-ons such as sensors, video chat, and increased storage, has resulted in an explosion in new ways to foster health management and preventive services. As of June 2013, 40,000 health-related applications ("apps") were available for download

on smartphones and tablets(http://medcitynews.com/2013/06/40000-health-related-apps-and-no-easy-way-to-know-which-ones-work/). Testing of these apps is rare, however, with resultant fraud, abuse, or even patient harm. For example, in a recent case-control study, the performance of smartphone applications in assessing melanoma risk from photographs of skin lesions was evaluated; diagnostic accuracy of the apps varied considerably. Three of four smartphone applications incorrectly classified 30% or more of melanomas as unconcerning. Reliance on these applications, which are not subject to regulatory oversight, in lieu of medical consultation can delay the diagnosis of melanoma (and other diseases) and harm users, however (Wolf et al., 2013).

A promising use of *mhealth* on the cell phone is ecological momentary assessment, which has been used to monitor smoking cessation or food choices. Unlike self-report that can be biased and intermittent, the phone—which is carried throughout each day—can monitor behavior using sensors and/or self-reports. This monitoring can be timed appropriately (for example, near lunch to querie food choices) and can ask the patient specific questions in an easy-to-respond format. Data can be uploaded to centralized databases with online or mobile tracking tools; visualizations can be viewed by the health care team and the patient, decisions made, and programs of treatment adjusted. Monitoring between visits is also possible with mobile health technologies. For example, sleep disorders or smoking lapses

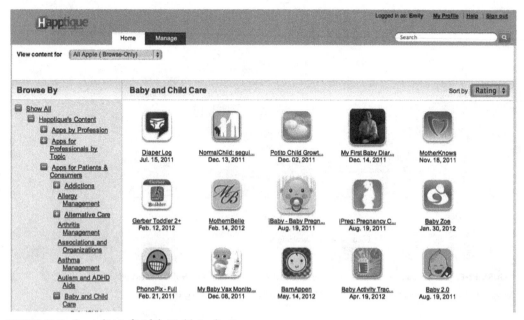

FIGURE 12-7: Curated List of Mobile Health Applications.

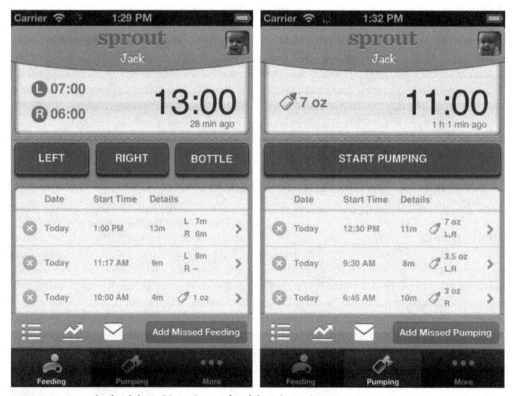

FIGURE 12-8: Example of Mobile Health Application (App) for Baby Feeding Times.

Source: http://www.happtique.com.

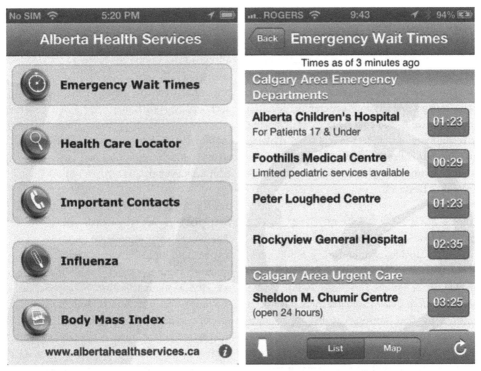

FIGURE 12-9: Example of Mobile Health Application (App) for Emergency Wait Times.

Source: http://www.happtique.com

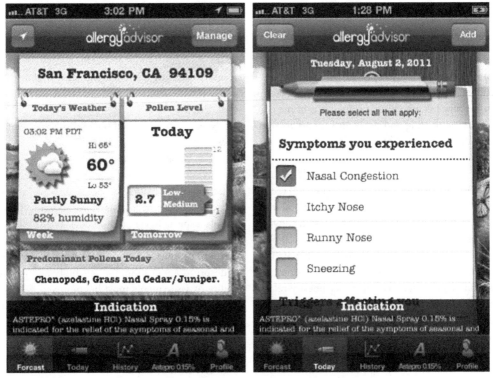

FIGURE 12-10: Example of Mobile Health Application (App) for Health Self-Report.

Source: http://www.happtique.com

may be recorded in real time by monitoring breathing patterns or movements.

Mobile health applications have the advantage of potential scalability to a large population, as devices are cheap and often already owned by the patient. They can be attached to specialized sensors, contain accelerometers and geographic location detection functions; can collect, store, and transmit massive amounts of rich data in real time, allowing continuous data collection at many geographic locations; and can accommodate applications that provide real-time feedback.

Sensors

A number of sites (and apps) provide small wearable sensors capable of monitoring blood pressure, glucose, and walking (e.g., *Bodymedia; Fit Armband BW 2; Philips DirectLife; FitBit; Gruve; Zeo Personal Sleep Coach*); of late, these have been augmented by new sensors capable of accurate physiological measures (such as cortisol to track stress levels). Sensor data can allow rapid reactions to events or environments, and different interfaces for health care providers and patients or their families to facilitate comprehension. These approaches, called sensor-enhanced health information systems (*seHIS*), have already been used for cardiac monitoring. Continuous monitoring, for example of gait abnormalities (Marschollek et al., 2012), can assist with the diagnosis and treatment of musculoskeletal conditions such as knee arthritis, using data from the patient's experiences with the activities of daily living. With the aging of the population, sensors may become more useful for at-home continuous monitoring and decision support to allow patients to remain at home with remote provider support.

As one example of the promise of *seHIS*, theK-NOWME Network, which is designed to reduce obesity among minority youth, is a suite of wearable, wireless sensors (a wireless body area network, or WBAN) that sends streaming data to a mobile phone for non-intrusive monitoring of metabolic health, vital signs such as heart rate and stress levels, and physical activity and other obesity-related behaviors. The mobile phone collects, stores, and transmits data to a secure web server where data are analyzed and translated in real time. A record of behavior and health data that is time-stamped, synchronized, and geographically localized can be made available via secure Internet to interventionists or health care professionals.The phone allows for immediate, real-time feedback through the phone display and through text messaging, image, and voice tags. Some data will be immediately visualized on the phone for participants (for instance, a running tally of minutes of moderate to vigorous physical activity per day). In the future, networks such as *KNOWME* may yield a new generation of adaptive, personalized interventions for real-time monitoring, immediate data delivery, and rapid adaptive intervention response (www.knowme.usc.edu; Emken et al., 2012).

seHIS and Personalized Decision Support

The successful implementation of *seHIS* that involves multiple providers, using multiple data sources, requires strict requirements for data security, a standardization of approaches across providers and institutions, and the use of methods of multimodal (e.g., multimedia data such as images and videos) mass data analysis (Wu, Chang, Chang, & Smith, 2004; Marschollek et al., 2012). Given this complexity, decision support programs based on these data must allow rapid response, prioritization, customizability, and explanations of decisions (Marschollek et al., 2012). For example, Ali et al. (2012) and Goodwin et al. (2012) used machine learning to model data from 13 features of the ECG (electrocardiogram) from cell phones, and were able to distinguish between smoking, stress, running, and conversation. In the future, machine learning from cell phones would facilitate development of feedback programs in real time (Ali et al., 2012).

Newer applications of this approach use gaming sites to engage patients and encourage the logging of health behaviors. These applications have *crowdsourced* support. (Crowdsourcing is the practice of obtaining participants, services, ideas, or content by soliciting contributions from a large group of people, especially via the Internet). While this field is in its infancy, for *seHIS*-informed personalized decision support to be safe, useful, effective, and of widespread application, the reliability and predictability of assessments must be improved. Methods for making the large amounts of data interpretable by clinicians are key.

Crowdsourced Health Research Studies

Crowdsourced health research studies have arisen as a natural extension of the activities of online health interest communities, as described previously in this Chapter, and can be researcher-organized or participant-organized. In the last few years, professional researchers have been crowdsourcing cohorts from health social networks for the conduct of traditional studies. Participants have also begun to organize their own research studies through health social networks and health collaboration communities created especially for the purpose of self-experimentation and the investigation of health-related concerns (Wicks, Pickard, Francke, & Swan, 2012).

For example, the *HealthTracking Network* (http://www.healthtracking.net) uses crowdsourcing to monitor common illnesses worldwide; it also enables individuals to monitor their own health online.

Short Message Service (SMS) Text Reminders

Reminders are effective in engaging patients and prompting desired behaviors in a just-in-time manner. Two-way SMS text reminders can provide psychological support, triage, and verification of reported behaviors.

Text4baby (https://text4baby.org) is a widely disseminated application that provides advising prompts on healthy behaviors for pregnant women, as well as mothers, for example, prenatal care, safe sleep, immunizations, breastfeeding, and oral health, based on the stage of pregnancy. Other applications include SMS text reminders for AIDS medication adherence, both in the United States and abroad.

A recent comprehensive meta-analysis of mobile health interventions found modest but significant effectiveness of SMS for improving appointment adherence relative to no reminders. SMS reminders were no more effective than postal or phone call reminders, and texting reminders to patients who persistently missed appointments did not significantly change the number of cancelled appointments, however (Free, Phillips, Watson, Galli, Felix, et al., 2013). A study conducted after the meta-analysis, however, found that text message reminders improved adherence to malaria treatment guidelines by 23% (Zurovac, Sudoi, Akhwale, Hamer, Rowe, & Snow, 2011). Militello's (2012) systematic review showed that SMS messages may be more effective as reminders supporting disease management behavior change in children and teens than in adults. The authors note that many studies

were not of high quality, and more rigorous studies are needed to establish the benefits of mobile intervention for various modalities, however. Particularly as cell phone capabilities expand rapidly to include video and photo transmission, more rigorous trials of these interventions will be warranted.

It is important to note that mobile health technologies, their financial models, and health interventions are growing rapidly in developing countries. Because of cheap cell phone plans and phones, they may be the most widely owned computing devices. Developing countries have often been able to rapidly "leapfrog" toward widespread implementation of mobile phone systems. Thus developers of health interventions in wealthy countries are likely to find innovation transmission moving from developing countries to the developed.

Medical Informatics and Behavioral Health

Medical Informatics is particularly important for behavioral health providers, but the incentives that have been offered to other health care providers have not yet been extended to this group. Further, few behavioral health providers have fully implemented electronic records (Major & Turner, 2003). Privacy and confidentiality of recorded substance abuse is of particular concern with shared electronic medical records, due to the stigma attached to the disease, and concerns about the applications of the federal substance abuse confidentiality regulations (42 CFR).

EMERGING THEORETICAL MODELS

As discussed in Chapter 3, there are a number of explanatory models for prevention in primary care. New models that better describe the phenomena under observation—particularly the primary care consultation (Love & Burton, 2005)—continue to emerge. One of the most promising of these is the model of complex adaptive systems (CAS). Constructs from complexity theory undergird models of CAS.

In short, complex adaptive systems are networks of elements that exchange information such that change in the context of one element changes the context of all others. Complexity is the pattern of behavior that emerges from the interaction of elements that respond to the limited information with which they are presented (Cilliers, 1998; Kernick, 2006; Waldrop, 1992; Lewin, 1993).

As these concepts are discussed in Chapter 3, some examples of the applications of the study of complex adaptive systems that may inform future understandings of prevention in practice follow. Due to non-linear characteristics, small changes in one area can occasionally have large effects across the whole system. This has been called the "butterfly effect." (A butterfly in New York can flap its wings and cause a hurricane in Tokyo.) For example, the televised colorectal cancer screening of Katie Couric, a celebrity, had a large effect on colorectal cancer screening among the US population (Cram et al., 2003); the riding accident of actor Christopher Reeves had a large but probably inappropriate impact on the redistribution of research funding into spinal injuries in the United States (Greenberg, 1997).

A system is different from the sum of the parts. Therefore, no one can stand outside the system and hope to understand and engineer it to a predetermined future, as approaches to organizational change in the NHS in England have repeatedly demonstrated (Kernick, 1993). Further, system boundaries are often based on the observer's needs and prejudices rather than any intrinsic property of the system itself. For example, primary care practitioners find it difficult to define the boundaries between health and social care in their work, but these organizational demarcations have historically been rigorously enforced (Kernick, 2006).

In the future, research founded in complexity theory and models of complex adaptive systems may continue to offer understandings of the primary care context, and the changing provider/patient interchange. With its focus on the characteristics of complex, non-linear systems, complexity theory could guide research toward richer, more nuanced understandings of primary care as it evolves (Kernick, 2006; Miller, Crabtree, McDaniel, Stange, 1998).

PAYMENT REFORM

As discussed in Chapter 1, and implicit throughout this book, better targeting health spending and concomitantly improving the quality of health care rests on a fundamental change in the way physicians are paid. As displayed in Figures 12-11 and 12-12, the growth in health care spending over time has been considerable, particularly by comparison to other peer countries. As discussed previously in this

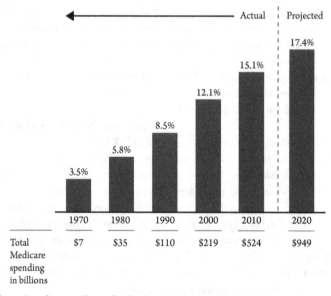

FIGURE 12-11: Medicare Spending as a Share of Federal Budget Outlays, 1970–2020.

* Estimates for 1970–2010 represent total Medicare outlays; estimate for 2020 represents projection of mandatory Medicare outlays. CBO (August 2010) projects that discretionary Medicare outlays will be $9 billion in 2020.

Source: Henry J. Kaiser Family Foundation and Congressional Budget Office, Budget and Economic Outlook, January 2010 (for 1970 data) and January 2011 (for 1980–2020 data, except 2010, which comes from CBO August 2010 Baseline: Medicare). Historical total spending for 1970–2000 from 2010 Annual Report of the Boards of Trustees of the Federal Hospital Insurance and Federal Supplementary Medical Insurance Trust Funds. The National Commission on Physician Payment Reform, http://physicianpaymentcommission.org/wp-content/uploads/2013/03/physician_payment_report.pdf.

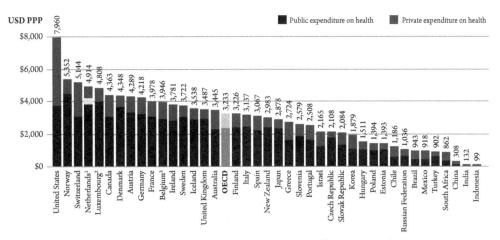

FIGURE 12-12: Total Health Expenditure per Capita, Public and Private, 2009 (or Nearest Year).

[1] In the Netherlands, it is not possible to clearly distinguish the public and private share related to investments.

[2] Health expenditure is for the insured population rather than the resident population.

[3] Total expenditure excluding investments.

Source: OECD Health Data 2011; WHO Global Health Expenditure Database. The National Commission on Physician Payment Reform, http://physicianpaymentcommission.org/wp-content/uploads/2013/03/physician_payment_report.pdf.

Chapter, any growth in health care spending should be accompanied by concomitant increases in health-care quality and public health.

Concentrated Health Care Markets

The question of payment reform is a large one, fraught with both political and economic tensions. While these debates will not be reviewed here, most economists agree that US health care markets are highly concentrated, offering limited competition. Highly concentrated hospital and private insurer markets tend to lead to inefficient (and highly varied) pricing, and for individuals, increased monies spent on their own health care (Hartman et al., 2013), including higher premium costs, alongside less coverage.

The picture is more nuanced within concentrated health plan markets, however, as these environments tend to benefit consumers through lower hospital prices as long as health plan markets remain competitive (Melnick, Shen, & Wu, 2011). According to a recent study (Melnick, Shen, & Wu, 2011), 64% of hospitals operate in markets where health plans are not very concentrated, and only 7% are in markets that are dominated by a few health plans. Further, in most markets, hospital market concentration exceeds health plan concentration. Generally, greater hospital market concentration leads to higher hospital prices, with hospital prices in

the most concentrated health plan markets approximately 12% lower than in more competitive health plan markets. As a result, concentrated health plan markets can counteract the price-increasing effects of concentrated hospital markets, so—contrary to conventional wisdom—increased health plan concentration benefits consumers through lower hospital prices as long as health plan markets remain competitive.

Rather than being influenced by competition, health care prices are largely set by insurers and providers with monopoly power to maximize profits. According to a paper in the *Harvard Business Review* (Porter & Teisberg, 2004) the kind of competition now prevalent in the health care system tends to drive up costs, and the kinds of competition that might push costs down are limited. Similarly, scholars from another political perspective than Porter and Teisberg (2004) have illustrated that Medicare controls costs much more effectively than private insurers:

Within the private sector, patients enrolled in large health plans are perversely subsidized by members of smaller groups, the uninsured and out-of-network patients. This administrative complexity of dealing with multiple prices adds costs with no benefit. The dysfunctional competition that has been created by price discrimination far outweighs any short-term advantages individual system participants gain from it, even for those participants who currently enjoy the biggest discounts. The lesson is simple: skewed incentives motivate activities that push costs higher. All these incentives and distortions reinforce zero-sum competition and work against value creation. (Porter & Teisberg, 2006, p. 66)

Big hospital chains and provider groups dominate many local markets (Federal Trade Commission & Department of Justice, 2004), obtaining higher rates from dominant insurers, who are motivated by fear of losing market share if they fail to attract these providers to their networks. Research indicates that hospitals can change their business practices and control their costs effectively when faced with competitive pressure (Robinson, 2004; Archer, 2013), but health care markets have concentrated in the last few decades. Other than health plans, many providers have not had to compete to offer high-value care.

Commercial health plans have little bargaining power when they negotiate prices with monopolistic providers, so they tend to adapt to this non-competitive environment. At the extreme, this may result in collusion (Boston Globe, 2009); big insurers may negotiate "most-favored nation" clauses with providers (Crinicker, 1990–1991; Archer, 2013); the subsequent limited competition offers less pressure to push rates downward.

Cost Shifting

The debates about health care policy have similarly addressed "price discrimination" (Reinhardt, 2006) or hospital cost shifting—that private payers are charged more in response to shortfalls in public payments. It is well-known that hospitals charge different payers (health plans and government programs) different amounts for the same service *even at the same point in time*, a phenomenon known to economists as "price discrimination" (Reinhardt, 2006). Price discrimination is not unusual for airlines (charging passengers on the same flight different ticket prices depending on purchase date), hotels (different room rates by date of purchase), colleges (via financial aid), and movie theaters (senior and child discounts; Frakt, 2011; http://theincidentaleconomist.com/wordpress/tag/simply-put). Further, price discrimination does not necessarily mean that someone pays more *because* someone else paid less. Nonetheless, it is widely

believed that private insurers have to pay more *because* public programs pay less (Morrisey 1993, 1994, 1996; Ginsburg 2003).

The evidence suggests, however, that there is likely only a small cost shifting effect for hospital services today, though not for physician services or pharmaceuticals. The greater an organization maximizes profits, or the greater the competition it faces for customers (patients), the less scope there is for cost shifting (Frakt, 2011; http://theincidentaleconomist.com/wordpress/tag/simply-put).

Many hospitals do not maximize profits and do not face stiff price competition, so can cost shift. Over all, hospitals probably cost shift about 20 cents of each dollar shortfall in Medicare payments. In other words, if Medicare cut its payments to hospitals (for a particular service) by one dollar, private insurers would pay 20 cents more for that service. The remaining 80 cents would be made up by decreases in the costs of providing that service (e.g., changes in staffing or reductions in quality). In the past, the cost shifting varied from dollar-for-dollar, to zero, depending upon how much hospitals had to compete for privately insured patients (Frakt, 2011; http://theincidentaleconomist.com/wordpress/tag/simply-put).

Declining Utilization

Declining utilization is not a new trend, but one that has been developing for the past 5 to 10 years. The cumulative inpatient discharges per fee-for-service (FFS) Medicare beneficiary declined 6.0% from 2004 to 2010 (Grube, Kaufman, York, 2013). These data may reflect the effect of federal efforts to shift the care of Medicare beneficiaries to outpatient settings, clinical observation, or decision units (see Chapter 5). The trend toward declining inpatient hospital use are expected to continue until 2021. Use is expected to be lowest in well-managed hospitals with low patient admissions (see Figure 12-13).

Some Proposals for the Future of Payment Reform

There are numerous proposals for change in the future, some of which (for example, guaranteeing access to coverage for all Americans) have already been incorporated in the Affordable Care Act. Others remain to be considered by policy makers and legislators in the future.

As the health care exchanges that are within the Act have not yet become fully functional, with

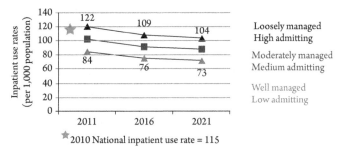

FIGURE 12-13: Projections for Inpatient Use Rates for Total Population (2011–2021).

Source: Private study conducted in 2011 by Milliman for Kaufman, Hall & Associates, Inc. Grube M, Kaufman K, York R. Decline in utilization rates signals a change in the inpatient business model. *Health Affairs* blog, March 8, 2013.

October 1, 2013 (without additional website problems, Congressional defunding or delay) signaling the first enrollee, and rate assessment in 2014 (March 1, 2013, "Letter to Issuers on Federally-facilitated and State Partnership Exchanges"; http://cciio.cms.gov/resources/files/issuer-letter-3-1-2013.pdf), there is no evidence yet that the newly created exchanges will exert any downward pressure on prices, given the experience of private plans to date. Thus, federal legislators and policy makers would have four other options to increase the incentives to reduce costs: They can use Medicare-style techniques to set rates or rate ceilings in the commercial marketplace (Reinhardt, 2009; Archer, 2013), including in the new health insurance exchanges, just as every other developed nation does. They can give people under 65 the choice of a public health insurance plan (Holahan et al., 2013) that works like Medicare (Congressional Budget Office, 2010), competes against the private health plans, and brings down costs. Or they can do both. To increase competition in concentrated markets, stricter enforcement of antitrust laws could be used to break up monopolies in health care markets, although even heavily regulated insurance markets—such as Medicare Advantage or the exchange system in Massachusetts—have not been particularly successful at controlling costs. Nonetheless, health care consumers tend to benefit from policies that maintain competition in hospital markets or that restore competition to hospital markets that are uncompetitive (Melnick, Shen, & Wu, 2011),

Economist Uwe Reinhardt has addressed the limited competition and burdensome administrative costs endemic to the current fee-for-service healthcare system by adopting a common relative value platform, at least for physicians and hospitals, to be used as a basis for charging all patients. These include the diagnosis-related groups (DRGs) and

resource-based relative value scale (RBRVS), which could be refined over time on the basis of either cost or imputed value (2009).

If price competition among providers were desired, providers could set their own monetary conversion factors for their relative value scales and compete on a simple, one-dimensional price indicator. Employers, insurers, and patients all would be able to understand this price indicator. It would replace the 20,000 or so itemized "charges" (list prices) now in each hospital's charge master, and the 9,000 or so prices in the physicians' fee schedule (Reinhardt, 2009).

One could also, however, have these conversion factors negotiated between associations of providers and associations of insurers with a region (e.g., a state) and make them binding on all providers and insurers in the region, as is now done in some European countries—notably Germany—which operate all-payer systems within regions. Under these conditions, a physician or a hospital would charge all insurance carriers or patients the same price for identical procedures. The system would work best if there were not a large number of uninsured people and if the public insurance programs—Medicare, Medicaid, and the Children's Health Insurance Program (CHIP)—were part of the arrangement (Reinhardt, 2009).

Longer term, Reinhardt has suggested incremental moves toward "bundled payments," as most hospital episodes are already bundled substantially though the DRG (Diagnosis-Related Group) system. Convalescent care or the mainly hospital-based services of radiologists, anesthesiologists, and pathologists could be added. Bundled payments may, however, disadvantage small private physicians' offices through the costs of payment administration.

As discussed previously in this Chapter, Medicare, in line with overall health spending, continues to represent a growing share of gross domestic product (GDP) each year, a trend (Congressional Budget Office, 2012) that is expected to continue in the years ahead. Spending on Medicare and Medicaid currently represents 21% (Center on Budget and Policy Priorities, 2012) of all federal expenditures. As discussed previously in this Chapter and Chapters 1 and 2, these figures are daunting, and for a government facing extraordinary pressure to reduce expenditures, real reforms are needed to achieve financial solvency for Medicare and maintain the integrity of the program (Holtz-Eakin & Thorpe, February 12th, 2013; http://www.futureofmedicare.org. Similarly, Medicaid has expanded in states that have accepted this provision of the ACA, furthering both federal and future state budgetary pressures from this program as well.

The bipartisan Partnership for the Future of Medicare ("Partnership") has devised a set of principles to serve as "guard rails" to help policy makers chart a productive course for Medicare that will guide future changes in the program, including, at its core, replacing the antiquated fee-for-service (FFS) payment model with a more modern delivery model that changes economic incentives from volume to value and introduces accountability. In addition, the Partnership recommends that Medicare support vulnerable populations and address the increasing prevalence of chronic diseases. For example, the Partnership recommends improving efforts to serve vulnerable populations like those dually eligible for Medicare and Medicaid and those who have special needs. Coordinated care efforts that increase quality and accountability of care for these populations will improve outcomes and lower costs. Medicare needs to insure that it includes better efforts to avert the rise in preventable chronic diseases such as diabetes.

Like the Partnership for the Future of Medicare, the National Commission on Physician Payment Reform ("National Commission") on March 4, 2013, recommended the elimination of fee-for-service payments to health care providers. The National Commission, formed by the Society of General Internal Medicine, recently issued 12 recommendations to provide a 5-year blueprint for transitioning to a blended payment system. The National Commission contends that the following recommendations will lead to better results for both public and private payers, as well as patients:

1. Over time, payers should largely eliminate stand-alone fee-for-service payment to medical practices because of its inherent inefficiencies and problematic financial incentives.

2. The transition to an approach based on quality and value should start with the testing of new models of care over a 5-year time period, incorporating them into increasing numbers of practices, with the goal of broad adoption by the end of the decade.

3. Because fee-for-service will remain an important mode of payment into the future, even as the nation shifts toward fixed-payment models, it will be necessary to continue recalibrating fee-for-service payments to encourage behavior that improves quality and cost-effectiveness and to penalize behavior that misuses or overuses care.

4. For both Medicare and private insurers, annual updates should be increased for evaluation and management codes, which are currently undervalued. Updates for procedural diagnosis codes should be frozen for a period of three years, except for those that are demonstrated to be currently undervalued.

5. Higher payment for facility-based services that can be performed in a lower-cost setting should be eliminated.

6. Fee-for-service contracts should always incorporate quality metrics into the negotiated reimbursement rates.

7. Fee-for-service reimbursement should encourage small practices (those having fewer than five providers) to form virtual relationships and thereby share resources to achieve higher quality care.

8. Fixed payments should initially focus on areas where significant potential exists for cost savings and higher quality, such as care for people with multiple chronic conditions and in-hospital procedures and their follow-up.

9. Measures to safeguard access to high-quality care, assess the adequacy of risk-adjustment indicators, and promote strong physician commitment to patients should be put into place for fixed payment models.

10. The sustainable growth rate (SGR; the Medicare sustainable growth rate formula that helps determine physician pay) should be eliminated.

11. Repeal of the SGR should be paid for with cost savings from the Medicare program as a whole, including both cuts to physician payments and reductions in inappropriate utilization of Medicare services.

12. The Relative Value Scale Update Committee (RUC) should make decision making more transparent and diversify its membership so that it is more representative of the medical profession as a whole. At the same time, the Centers for Medicare and Medicaid Services (CMS) should develop alternative open, evidence-based, and expert processes to validate the data and methods it uses to establish and update relative values.[3]

As discussed in Chapter 9, pay for performance (P4P), a recent policy initiative in which explicit

---

3 In 1992, Medicare significantly changed the way it pays for physicians' services. Instead of basing payments on charges, the federal government established a standardized physician payment schedule based on a resource-based relative value scale (RBRVS). In the RBRVS system, payments for services are determined by the resource costs needed to provide them. The cost of providing each service is divided into three components: physician work, practice expense, and professional liability insurance. Payments are calculated by multiplying the combined costs of a service by a conversion factor (a monetary amount that is determined by the Centers for Medicare and Medicaid Services). Payments are also adjusted for geographical differences in resource costs. The physician work component accounts, on average, for 48% of the total relative value for each service (http://www.ama-assn.org/ama/pub/physician-resources/solutions-managing-your-practice/coding-billing-insurance/medicare/the-resource-based-relative-value-scale/overview-of-rbrvs.page?). To ensure that physician services across all specialties are well-represented, the AMA established the AMA/Specialty Society Relative Value Scale Update Committee (RUC). The RUC makes annual recommendations regarding new and revised physician services to the Centers for Medicare and Medicaid Services (CMS) and performs broad reviews of the RBRVS every 5 years (http://www.ama-assn.org/ama/pub/physician-resources/solutions-managing-your-practice/coding-billing-insurance/medicare/the-resource-based-relative-value-scale.page?).

financial incentives are offered by purchasers and health plans to primary care physicians, specialists, and hospital providers for achieving predefined quality targets, may also influence provider payment approaches (including fee-for-service, capitation, and salary). As described in Chapter 9, pay-for-performance systems are intended to improve the quality of care for beneficiaries, and could result in higher or lower payments for individual health care providers, depending on the quality of their care.

A recent study examining P4P policies analyzed Medicare claims from 2000 through 2002 for 1.79 million fee-for-service beneficiaries treated by 8,604 respondents to the Community Tracking Study Physician Survey in 2000 and 2001. They assigned each patient to the physician with whom the patient had had the most visits, and assessed the amount of care received (Pham et al., 2007). Their findings revealed that in fee-for-service Medicare, the dispersion of patients' care among multiple physicians will limit the effectiveness of pay-for-performance initiatives that rely on a single retrospective method of assigning responsibility for patient care (Pham et al., 2007). There is also some evidence that performance incentives work best in combination with reminder systems and standing orders (Christianson, Leatherman, & Sutherland, 2008).The effectiveness of P4P programs will continue to depend on the coordination of patient care over time, the soundness of measures of health care quality to be used, the appropriate monitoring, and follow-up. In addition to the Affordable Care Act, some of these (often contradictory) proposals will guide the US health care system through the fiscal challenges that it will face over the next 10 years.

ADDRESSING THE PRIMARY CARE WORKFORCE

The primary care workforce is key to health care reforms in prevention, as reflected in part in the Affordable Care Act. As discussed in Chapter 2, the act will have a major impact on the practice of primary care, particularly in the legislative and financial support for prevention. To prevent disease and promote health and wellness, the Act breaks new ground. A paper by Koh and Sibelius (2010) states that the law reaffirms the principle that "the health of the individual is almost inseparable from the health of the larger community. And the health of each community and territory determines the overall health status of the Nation."Moving prevention toward the mainstream of health may well be one of the most lasting legacies of this landmark legislation (Koh & Sibelius, 2010).

Figure 12-14 summarizes the major components of the act and their likely impact on the provider shortages in primary care that were discussed in Chapter 1. Many of the 10 major titles in the law, especially Title IV, Prevention of Chronic Diseases and Improving Public Health, advance a prevention theme through a wide array of new initiatives and funding that could enrich the supply of primary care providers. In the future, the Act will reinvigorate public health on behalf of individuals, worksites, communities, and the nation at large and could usher in a revitalized era for prevention at every level of society (Koh & Sibelius, 2010).

Team-Based Care

The implementation of some increasingly popular operational changes in the ways clinicians deliver care—including the use of teams or "pods," better information technology and sharing of data, and the use of non-physicians (described further forthwith)—have the potential to offset completely the increase in demand for physician services while improving access to care, thereby averting the looming primary care physician shortage that is discussed in Chapter 1 (Green, Savin, & Lu, 2013).

One of these approaches, team-based health care, has particular resonance in primary care prevention. It has been touted by policy leaders as a means to encourage greater efficiency, more shared responsibility, and a means for implementing outcomes-driven health care (Daschle, 2013). Team-based care has often formed the basis of coordinated care, as discussed more fully in Chapter 10.

PPACA Section	Focus	Impact on Physicians
1001, 1201	Immediate insurance industry reforms-require coverage without pre-existing conditions, expansion of dependent coverage, elimination of annual and lifetime limits, etc.	Increases access to commercially insured patients; Increases practice revenue, especially for primary care physicians (PCPs)
1104	Required implementation of administrative simplification	Reduces costs of billing, credit and collections with insurance plans; reduced costs for answering patients questions about insurance coverage
1416	Authorizes study of geographic vacation in coverage; care provided	Possible spotlight on overuse of services (diagnostics, surgery, prescribing patterns) might prompt increased attention to variability and non-evidence-based practice patterns of physicians
1501	Individual mandate expected to expand commercial insurance coverage for 16 million who are currently uninsured	Increases commercial market for physicians, but rate might be closer to Medicare than commercial
2001-2004, 2301-2303, 2401-2403, 10202, 2601-2602	Expansion and federal funding for Medical and Children's Health insurance programs (CHIP); expanded coverage for community-based care, hospice care; expansion of plots for dual eligibles	Expanded funding opportunities for primary care providers (physicians, nurses); additional funding via pilots for dual eligibles
2702-2706	Pilot funding for accountable care organizations (ACOs) medical homes and avoidable readmissions programs	Encourages alignment of physicians and hospitals and clinical integration across specialties (accountable care models do not require hospital affiliation)
2951-2954, 4101-4108	Funding for maternal child health; patient education; preventive health; expansion of preventive health services under oversight of the U.S. Department of Health and Human Services (HHS)via school based clinics, annual wellness visits for Medicare enrollees, etc.	Additional funding for primary care services targeted to underserved populations, especially services for women and children
3002, 3003-3007, 10327, 10331	Increased transparency of physician performance	More visibility about physician performance: Safety, outcomes, efficiency, patient satisfaction

FIGURE 12-14: Components of the Affordable Care Act That Address the Primary Care Workforce.

Source: The Patient Protection and Affordable Care Act, P.L. 111-148, 23 March 2010;

Deloitte Center for Health Solutions. The Physician Workforce: Opportunities and Challenges Post-Health Care Reform, 2010. Retrieved December 3, 2012, from http://www.deloitte.com/view/en_US/us/Insights/Browse-by-Content-Type/Newsletters/health-care-reform-memo/a4edfe-ab5ffbb210VgnVCM3000001c56f00aRCRD.htm?id=us_furl_physicianworkforce_030512.

"Team-based health care is the provision of health services to individuals, families, and/or their communities by at least two health providers who work collaboratively with patients and their caregivers—to the extent preferred by each patient—to accomplish shared goals within and across settings to achieve coordinated, high-quality care" (Naylor, Coburn, Kurtzman, et al., 2010). The principles of team-based health care are summarized below.

- *Shared goals*: The team—including the patient and, where appropriate, family members or others in the social network—works to establish shared goals that reflect patient and family priorities, and can be clearly articulated, understood, and supported by all team members.
- *Clear roles*: There are clear expectations for each team member's functions, responsibilities, and accountabilities, which optimize the team's efficiency and often make it possible for the team to take advantage of a division of labor, thereby accomplishing more than the sum of its parts.
- *Mutual trust*: Team members earn each others' trust, creating strong norms of reciprocity and greater opportunities for shared achievement.
- *Effective communication*: The team prioritizes and continuously refines its communication skills. It has consistent channels for candid and complete communication, which are used by all team members across all settings.
- *Measurable processes and outcomes*: The team agrees on and implements reliable and timely feedback on successes and failures in both the functioning of the team and achievement of the team's goals. These are used to track and improve performance immediately and over time (Mitchell, Wynia, Golden, McNellis, Okun, et al., 2012).

Expanding the Health Care Team in Primary Care

With the Affordable Care Act of 2010, policy leaders have supported the importance of incentives to encourage even higher numbers of primary care providers in all health-related schools: doctors, nurses, physician assistants, and pharmacists.

Changed "scope of practice" laws have been proposed to allow all primary care practitioners to practice to the fullest extent of their training (Daschle, 2013). Some of these approaches have been discussed previously in this Chapter, as well as in Chapters 1 and 2.

A promising addition to the primary care team is the community health worker (CHW), including lay health advisors and navigators who are members of both the racial/ethnic target community and a part of the organization or intervention, and thus "span boundaries." These individuals communicate health information to the target group through their existing social networks, tailor messages to the cultural contexts of their communities, and broker resources for the individual (Sheinfeld Gorin, Badr, Krebs, Prabhu Das, 2012; Bartel, 2001; Eng, 1992; Zaheer, McEvily, Perrone, 1998). A recent review article reported that CHWs are effective in improving chronic disease care and health outcomes. CHWs have contributed to significant improvements in community members' access to and continuity of care and adherence to treatment for the control of hypertension (Brownstein, 2007). They assume multiple roles, including patient and community education, patient counseling, monitoring patient health status, linking people with health and human services, and enhancing provider-patient communication and adherence to care. Adequate translation of research into clinical practice remains a major challenge, however. Addressing this issue, which has national implications, will require sustainable funding; appropriate reimbursement; enhanced efforts to incorporate CHWs into health care teams; better utilization of their skills; improved CHW supervision, training, and career development; policy changes; and ongoing evaluation, including a reporting of costs (Brownstein, Bone, Dennison, Hill, Kim & Levine, 2005).

Viewed from the perspective of disruptive innovations (cheaper, simpler, more convenient products or services that start by meeting the needs of less-demanding customers; Christensen, Bohmer, & Kenagy, 2000), expansion of the primary care team to include more types of providers, including CHWs, team-based care, and changes in "scope of practice" laws, could better match the clinician's skill level to the difficulty of the medical problem. In the future, these changes could allow primary care physicians to move "upmarket," using advances in diagnostic and therapeutic technologies, alongside additional training, to perform many of the services they now refer to costly hospitals and specialists.

PERSONALIZED MEDICINE

As described in Chapter 8, the basis of prevention has been enlarged by the findings from the Human Genome Project, and the publication of *The Cancer Genome Atlas* (TCGA), which catalogues genetic mutations that are found in cancers. A recent IOM report defined personalized medicine as"...medical care based on the particular biological characteristics of the disease process in individual patients. By using genomics and proteomics, individuals can be classified into subpopulations based on their susceptibility to a particular disease or response to a specific treatment. They may then be given preventive or therapeutic interventions that will be most effective given their particular characteristics" (IOM, 2010). In addition to the examples given in Chapter 8, the application of these emerging approaches to future cancer prevention follow.

Example: Cancer Prevention

In addition to genomics, cancer prevention strategies in the future will incorporate a variety of new modalities, including imaging, proteomic, metabolomic, glycomic, and epigenetic, to identify and validate surrogate biomarkers for use in phase I and II prevention trials.[4] Phase I trials involve a small number of patients to test safety in humans and determine the correct dose of a drug. These trials also help determine the best way to give the drug, whether oral or intravenously. After determining that a treatment is reasonably safe in people, it enters phase II trials. Phase II trials are done to test for effectiveness, asking if the treatment works. Since a larger number of people are studied, further information is gained on safety during phase II trials (http://lungcancer.about.com/od/treatmentoflungcancer/a/phase-trial.htm).

Overdiagnosis, Underdiagnosis, and Risk Stratification

Overdiagnosis of cancerous lesions, the clinical significance of which is undetermined, provides a great challenge for the screening and cancer prevention community (Welch & Black, 2010).

In addition, screening can identify pre-cancers, the clinical relevance of which is also unknown. The problem is further complicated by the fact that pre-cancers of undetermined significance are being identified at an alarmingly high rate, partly due to the improvement in detection technologies. By contrast, underdiagnosis occurs when lesions that are destined to progress to cancer are either not diagnosed or are hidden in pre-cancers. For example, although individuals with Barrett's esophagus are at a high risk of developing esophageal adenocarcinoma, 95% of patients with Barrett's esophagus never develop cancer. Conversely, most esophageal adenocarcinoma cases are missed, as they are diagnosed as Barrett's esophagus (Reid, Li, Galipeau, & Vaughan, 2010). In the future, genomic analyses akin to the *The Cancer Genome Atlas* (TCGA) projects could discern which of the screen-diagnosed pre-cancerous and small invasive lesions pose actual threats to the health of individuals and which do not. These analyses could avoid morbid and costly follow-up medical intervention in individuals whose newly revealed lesions are predicted never to progress to cancer (Umar, Dunn, & Greenwald, 2012).

Immunoprevention modalities

Cancer prevention is ideal for interventions involving the modulation of the immune response. The small size of pre-invasive lesions that confer high cancer risk, combined with the robust nature of the immune system, promises success with immune modalities in prevention. Vaccines, already well-established tools for preventing a variety of infectious diseases, have been applied to the prevention of some of the 20% of cancers that are known to have infectious aetiologies. Building on past successes with prophylactic HBV (Hepatitis B) and HPV (human papillomavirus) vaccines, as described in Chapter 4, research is beginning to address the cancer-preventive effects of therapeutic vaccines in individuals who are already infected with oncogenic viruses. The immune evasiveness of highly mutable cancer-causing viruses poses a special challenge to vaccine development, but, in the future, improved understanding of the immune system should allow this obstacle to be overcome. In the near future, an important challenge for successful vaccines, such as those for HPV (human papillomavirus) and HBV (hepatitis B), will be to increase uptake in the United States (Sheinfeld Gorin, Glenn, & Perkins, 2011), as well as in developing countries, which lack

---

4 This section is adapted from Umar, Dunn, & Greenwald, 2012.

the resources for the treatment of infection-associated (and other) cancers.

Dissemination of Personalized Prevention

As discussed previously in this Chapter and in Chapter 11, the real challenge to personalized prevention of the future is "How do we integrate new evidence [from personalized medicine about prevention] into existing clinical practice?" (IOM, 2010). A telling example is found not in the dissemination of emerging genomics and proteomics findings, but in the adoption in clinical practice of the SERMs (selective estrogen receptor modulators), tamoxifen and raloxifene. There is strong evidence from well-designed phase III trials (RCTs) over more than a decade that the SERMs tamoxifen and raloxifene are effective risk-reducing agents for breast cancer; both tamoxifen and raloxifene have FDA approval and endorsement by respected professional organizations for this indication (Nelson et al., 2009; Visvanathan et al., 2009; see Chapter 4). The use of preventive tamoxifen and raloxifene by high-risk women has been limited, however, primarily because of concerns over perceived unacceptable toxicity (Decensi et al., 2010; Waters et al., 2010).

The relatively limited uptake of these SERMs, despite a strong benefit to risk profile among high risk women diagnosed with breast cancer, is due to a number of factors, including limited dissemination of the evidence into primary care practices. Methods to improve the communication of evidence to and by providers through approaches such as academic detailing (as described previously in this Chapter and in Chapters 10 and 11) must be more widely disseminated (Dreyfuss, 2010). Approaches directed toward the clinician must be coupled with both office-based approaches and best practices for patient risk education to reduce the barriers to patient understanding (see Chapter 11). If physicians and other health care professionals are to increase the use of evidence-based cancer-preventive agents, whether drugs, nutrients, vaccines, or gene therapies, a clear message must be given that the benefits far outweigh the identified side effects, especially if clinicians are to be successful in recommending these interventions to otherwise healthy individuals.

The importance of effective communication with patients about prevention will become even more critical as the complex findings from genetics, genomics, and proteomics that are most often associated with "personalized medicine" move further into clinical practice (see Chapter 8). As discussed throughout *Prevention Practice in Primary Care* and particularly in Chapter 11, the way primary care providers communicate these findings to patients is a powerful influence on how patients process the information. Over time, even legal pressures to disclose findings about the implications of strong family histories of cancer on individual genetic risk profiles will increase the importance of this communication (Penson et al., 2000).

Effective communication about "personalized prevention" must be equally accessible to varied population subgroups, by race and ethnicity, income and education, level of acculturation, and psychologic profiles. For example, while awareness of current genetic risk assessment and testing (in cancer) has increased over time, with about one-half of the US population aware in 2000 (Wideroff et al., 2003), it has been uneven across subpopulations (Heck et al., 2008; Wideroff et al., 2003). Uptake of genetic testing, too, varies, with African American women less likely than others to engage in BRCA1 or BRCA2 testing for breast cancer, for example (Sherman et al., 2013). Even when the possible confounding effects of access to care (location and number of testing sites and cost) are minimized, rates of genetic testing uptake among African American women lag behind those of Caucasian American women (Susswein et al., 2008). This suggests the importance of further study of the underlying psychological and/or social factors to the uptake of current genetic risk services among African American women (Sherman et al., 2013). These findings also suggest that the uptake of future genomic and proteomic testing may be similarly uneven across the US population, potentially leading to inequities and poorer health outcomes.

Increased Participation of Primary Care in Clinical Trials for Prevention

Clinical trials are the primary mechanism by which new approaches to cancer treatment can be evaluated, yet only a small proportion of eligible cancer patients are offered the opportunity to participate, and fewer are actually enrolled. Estimates of trial accrual range from as few as 2–3% of adult cancer patients to as many as 20% of eligible patients.

Ethnic and racial minorities, as well as older adults, are under-represented in clinical trials. American Indians, in particular, are under-represented in this research. Challenges that researchers and providers may face in clinical trial recruitment among American Indian communities include a complex mixture of cultural, physical, and societal factors (Hodge et al., 2000; Buchwald et al., 2006; LaVallie, Wolf, Jacobsen, Buchwald, 2008; Petereit & Burhansstipanov, 2008), including the huge cultural distance between traditional American Indian cultures and the clinical/medical culture of the Western medical establishment. For example, to the Navajo, cancer etiology involves powers and influences such as wind and lightning, other animate beings such as bears and snakes, prenatal influences, and the intentional actions of other persons (Justice, 1990).

Four types of barriers have been shown to inhibit participation in clinical trials: (1) physician barriers, including time constraints imposed by enrolling and educating patients, treatment preferences/ biases, concern about the doctor-patient relationship, lack of experience with clinical trials, lack of interest in research in general or the particular study, and economic disincentives; (2) patient barriers, including a lack of awareness about the availability of trials, unwillingness to be randomized, mistrust of medical experimentation, confusion over informed consent, language, cultural and sociodemographic factors; (3) barriers at the organizational level, including the lack of research infrastructure, an organizational culture that may be unfriendly to research, and fear of the increased cost of medical care; and (4) trial-related barriers to participation, including strict eligibility criteria, lack of equipoise/uncertainty, trial-recommended therapy that is not appropriate for the full cohort of patients because of age, comorbidity, or performance status, as well as the timing of the trial, whether offered at diagnosis, during active treatment, or post-curative treatment (Ellis, 2000; Ross et al., 1999; Cornis et al., 2003; Kornblith et al., 2002; Mannel et al., 2003; Siminoff et al., 2000; Shavers, Lynch, Burmeister, 2002; Murthy, Krumholz, Gross, 2004; Somkin et al., 2005; Langley et al., 2000; Gross et al., 2005; Cassileth, 2003).

Prevention trials, in particular, pose particular challenges. Whereas past definitive phase III prevention trials have served us well in documenting or rejecting the efficacy of promising preventive interventions for high-risk individuals on the risk of developing invasive breast cancer and other disease outcomes (Lippman et al., 2009; Klein et al., 2011; e.g., the NSABP Study of Tamoxifen and Raloxifene [STAR] P-2 trial, 2006;

Vogel et al., 2010; Thompson et al., 2003; Fisher et al.,1998; Fisher et al., 2005), the necessarily large size of such trials requires substantial investment of both monetary and human resources. For these reasons, alternative designs for definitive clinical prevention trials, aiming for shorter intervention durations and smaller participant cohorts, are beginning to be investigated. In addition to the suggestions made earlier in this Chapter regarding research methods, future large prevention trials should be prospectively designed to cut across multiple disease entities in a manner resembling the Women's Health Initiative (The Women's Health Initiative Study Group, 1998). In addition, in cancer, more efficient approaches for the development of preventive agents from *in vitro* testing, though *in vivo* animal model evaluation to clinical trials are currently being explored (Steele & Lubet, 2010; Umar, Dunn, & Greenwald, 2012).

Returning Research Results to Participants in Clinical Trials for Prevention

According to recent surveys, nearly all research participants expect researchers to return clinically useful information from studies, particularly genetic findings (Meulenkamp et al., 2010; Kaufman et al., 2008; Ceballos et al., 2008). There are some agreed-upon ethical principles for the return of genetic results in epidemiological research studies (Bookman et al., 2006; Roberts et al., 2010; Dressler, 2009). And, Kollek and Petersen (2011) have suggested a set of key questions to be addressed to return genetic findings, including: What feedback to return? To whom? By whom? How? The National Health, Lung, and Blood Institute 28-member multidisciplinary working group recently proposed a 5-recommendation guideline on ethical and practical considerations when research genetic test results are provided to study participants (Fabsitz et al., 2010). There is increasing discussion about whether incidental findings as well as expected genetic findings should be returned from participation in research, however (Wolf et al., 2012; Green et al., 2012).

Findings from a recent study among 107 patients participating in the Colon Cancer Family Registry revealed that a telephone disclosure process for the return of research-based genetic results (of the DNA mismatch repair gene; MMR) led to high rates of result uptake (Graves et al., 2013). The Lynch syndrome families who received the telephone disclosure were more likely to communicate the results to providers and family members than others. Additional practical guidance is necessary for the primary care provider to apply these research standards and intervention approaches in clinical practice (Keogh et al., 2013).

Genomic databases hold great promise for improving the health of all and will revolutionize medical research and practice. Patients, as well as the larger public, should understand both the benefits of *big data* and its potential perils to individual privacy, however. In addition to anonymization of data, database security and a number of protective laws that have been passed over the past 40 years have been the primary safeguards against security lapses in genomic data made partially or largely available to the public. The Presidential Commission for the Study of Bioethical Issues' recent report, "Privacy and Progress in Whole Genome Sequencing," among other initiatives, has also addressed genomic data privacy (2012). Yet, under the right circumstances, a persistent individual can overcome barriers to identification and "re-identify" an individual in an anonymized database. Various factors, including formation of very large databases, data sharing, and access by large numbers of individuals have put new strains on genomic security for those altruistic enough to volunteer their tissue and health information (Kupersmith, 2013). The addition of additional oversight by bodies of experts and legislation are warranted in the future to balance the values of scientific discovery and patient privacy.

DEFINITIONS OF HEALTH

It has been suggested that the focus of prevention in the twenty-first century is finding the answer to the question, What makes people healthy? Policies and programs designed to build healthy communities and workplaces, strengthen social networks for health, and increase people's abilities to lead healthy lives are considered key to health promotion. The effects of health on wealth creation are yet to be fully measured.

A central question at the heart of these efforts, however, concerns obtaining a clear and consistent measurement of health (Sheinfeld Gorin, 2006). Health is a multifaceted concept. Measures of mortality, morbidity, and the use of health services are insensitive to short-term and small effects. Measures of health at the population level, such as the population attributable fraction or quality-adjusted life-years (that is, measures of the benefit of a health intervention in terms of a person's time spent in a series of quality-weighted health states) are imperfect. Measures and analyses of the impact of important lifestyle factors such as diet, physical activity, and obesity are increasingly rigorous (e.g., Harvard Food Frequency Questionnaire, Block Food Frequency Questionnaire, and the Diet History Questionnaire; Block, Thompson, Hartman, Larkin, Guire, 1992; Block, Woods, Potosky, Clifford, 1990; Block, Patterson, Subar, 1992; Field, Byers, Hunter, et al., 1999; Oh, Hu, Cho, et al., 2005; Subar, Thompson, Kipnis, et al., 2001; Thompson, Subar, Brown, et al., 2002; Willett, Stampfer, Underwood, Speizer, Rosner, Hennekens, 1983). It is often difficult to select control populations against which to measure changes in programs and policies, however, as with the PCMH. In addition to the challenges of defining, choosing, and evaluating evidence, numerous methodological and political difficulties arise in consulting with patients (e.g., see Chapter 11, regarding patient-reported measures), and community-based groups that are stakeholders in prevention so that the findings from their participation are balanced and reliable.

Mental Health Promotion

The definition of health includes mental health. Depression will be one of the largest health problems worldwide by the year 2020 (Herrman, 2001). According to the USPSTF, depressive disorders include major depressive disorder (MDD), dysthymia, and minor depression. Other conditions that include depressive features (for example, bipolar disorder) are not considered depressive disorders. Depressive symptoms are associated with the development of ischemic disease as well as with poorer outcomes among patients who have preexisting cardiovascular disease (as described in Chapter 5; Glassman & Shapiro, 1998). In addition to cardiovascular risks, depressive symptoms are linked to higher morbidity and mortality in a number of other diseases, such as risk for cancer in older persons (Penninx et al., 1998); all-cause mortality in medical inpatients (Herrman et al., 1998); risk for osteoporosis (Michelson et al., 1996); lessened physical, social, and role function; worse perceived current health; and greater bodily pain (Wells et al., 1989; IOM, 2000). It is a major risk factor for suicide.

As one example of the prevalence of depression, postpartum depression may affect as many as 1 in every 7 women (Wisner et al., 2013). The largest study to date with a cohort of 10,000 women who delivered infants at one obstetrical hospital in Pittsburgh were asked to take part in a short telephone interview 4 to 6 weeks after they had their babies. Among women followed for a year after delivery, some 22% had been depressed. The study recommends that all pregnant women and new mothers be screened for depression (Wisner et al., 2013).

According to the USPSTF, in primary care settings, the prevalence of major depressive disorder (MDD) ranges from 5% to 13% in adults and from 6% to 9% in older adults. The prevalence of dysthymia in adults in primary care settings is estimated to range from 2% to 4%. One-third to one-half of adults and nearly two-thirds of older adults who receive treatment for depression receive it in a primary care setting (http://www.uspreventiveservicestaskforce.org/uspstf/uspsdepr.htm; O'Connor, Whitlock, Gaynes, Beil, 2009). Large-scale studies of patients initiating treatment of depression show that approximately two-thirds achieve remission within 1 year. Older patients have similar or slightly lower recovery rates than other adults, possibly because of a higher rate of comorbid medical conditions. Despite fairly high rates of recovery from particular episodes, depression is highly recurrent. A large scale community care–based study of depression treatment found that about half of patients who achieved remission had relapse during the subsequent year (http://www.uspreventiveservicestaskforce.org/uspstf/uspsdepr.htm; O'Connor, Whitlock, Gaynes, Beil, 2009).

In clinical practice, the USPSTF recommends screening adults for depression when staff-assisted depression care supports are in place to assure accurate diagnosis, effective treatment, and follow-up. "Staff-assisted depression care supports" refer to clinical staff that assist the primary care clinician by providing some direct depression care, such as care support or coordination, case management, or mental health treatment. Screening approaches for depression are described further in Chapter 11, and will continue to expand across primary care settings in the future, primarily by using electronic health records.

The USPSTF has not yet recommended routine screening for illicit drug use, as current evidence is insufficient to assess the balance of benefits and harms of screening adolescents, adults, and pregnant women (http://www.uspreventiveservicestaskforce.org/uspstf/uspsdrug.htm; Pollen et al., 2008). Nonetheless, illicit drug use and abuse are serious problems among adolescents, adults, and pregnant women in the United States. Approximately 3.2% of the population age 12 and over meet criteria for a drug use disorder. Many individuals with drug use disorders have coexisting mental and physical health conditions. A recent literature review compared the diagnoses, heritability, etiology (genetic and environmental factors), pathophysiology, and response to treatments (adherence and relapse) of drug dependence versus type 2 diabetes mellitus, hypertension, and asthma, all chronic illnesses.. The findings of this study—that long-term care strategies of medication management and continued monitoring produce lasting benefits—suggest that drug dependence should be insured, treated, and evaluated like other chronic illnesses, including within the primary care environment, generally by referral(McLellan, Lewis, O'Brien, &Kleber, 2000).

The integration of services for individuals with serious mental illness or individuals that have co-occurring serious mental illness and substance use disorder is important to reducing the stigma of mental illness, health care cost reduction, and reducing morbidity and mortality among a large swath of the US population. The Substance Abuse and Mental Health Services Administration (SAMHSA) and the Health Resources and Services Administration (HRSA) Primary Care Behavioral Health Integration Initiative program seek to provide some primary care capacity in community mental health centers. These efforts must be expanded, alongside an increased workforce and increased resources. The reduction of stigma associated with mental illness and substance abuse is of particular importance with this integration (Shim & Rust, 2013).

Mental health promotion involves an orientation toward health and not just mere treatment of illness. In the future, mental health promotion will involve a better understanding of the nature of mental health and mental illness, as well as the development of policies and programs across multiple sectors, including law, social services, housing, and health, to alter the conditions that are conducive to health in its entirety. Similarly, in the future, mental health may be viewed more broadly, as happiness, well-being, and resilience.

CONCERN FOR SOCIAL JUSTICE: EQUITY IN PREVENTION

America's citizens who are poor—particularly poor children, the unemployed, and the economically marginal or exploited among racial and ethnic minorities—face social situations that place them at high risk for disease and premature death. In fact, poverty—partly because it is often associated with comparatively low levels of education—leads to poorer health prospects overall (Marmot et al., 1991; Tyroler, 1989; Salonen, 1982; Dayal, Power, & Chiu, 1982; Haan, Kaplan, & Camacho, 1987; Baquet, Horm, Gibbs, & Greenwald, 1991; Winkleby, Jatulis, Frank, & Fortmann, 1992; Guralink, Land, Blszer, Fillenbaum, & Branch, 1993; Charlton & White, 1995; Pappas, Queen, Hadden, & Fisher, 1993). At present, many Americans have not even received the clinical preventive services they need, in part due to financial barriers, thus contributing to the high levels of preventable morbidity and mortality in the population. In particular, African Americans have shown less movement toward health and are less likely to continue to move forward. For example, although white women have the highest incidence of breast cancer, black women have higher death rates from this disease. This finding is of particular concern for those committed to equitable health care.

In addition, the number of individuals who are uninsured remains a problem, one that the Affordable Care Act seeks to address. Uninsured children are more likely than the insured to lack a usual source of health care, to go without needed care, and to experience worse health outcomes (Institute of Medicine, 2002). Despite the availability of Medicaid coverage, more than one in five poor children are uninsured. While near-poor children are more likely to have private insurance, 17% remain uninsured. Almost all of these children (96%) are eligible for Medicaid or State Children's Health Insurance Program (SCHIP), but either their parents never enrolled them in one of these programs or they were previously covered and were not re-enrolled (Kaiser Family Foundation, 2007). Of course, access to preventive services depends on more than insurance coverage. Access also depends on the provision of enabling services, such as transportation services and the means to reduce language barriers. National health policies could encourage equity in access to health services. These policies could be implemented by local coordinating bodies, such as the public health department, and overseen by a federal agency, such as the Centers for Disease Control and Prevention (CDC) or the Centers for Medicare and Medicaid Services (CMS). Continued advocacy by primary care providers, coupled with federal legislation and strong federal public health leadership, will be necessary to promote health among society's most vulnerable members.

Values for the Practice of Prevention

Because of major changes in the sociodemographics of the American populace and in the delivery of health care, in accountability, in technology, and in health promotion, ethical issues will emerge as critical to future practice. Some of the ethical questions to be answered in the near future are being posed now: for example, Should decisions about the allocations of monies from federal and foundation sources be made on the basis of the health of a community? Should health promotion interventions be targeted to those most in need or those in largest number? Is it morally acceptable to smoke, or to remain overweight? What genetic testing should individuals undertake? What feedback should be returned? To whom? By whom? How? Who should see the results? How should the results be protected? What kinds of decisions about insurance, work, and family life should be made on the basis of these results?

Core Values

Given the challenges that primary care providers face now and will face in the future, they must articulate their personal and collective vision of the good life, health, and the good society. They should make clear the values, models, and ideals they wish for individuals and for societies, as they are encouraging patients to do the same, particularly to clarify their preferences in shared decision making. For example, do they hold an individualist or a collectivist vision of society? They need "to explore and define what, very specifically, would be right. Toward what, stated as clearly as may be possible, should we aim?" (Galbraith, 1996, p. 1).

In the United States, liberal philosophies of self-determination and rugged individualism generate fears of moralizing others' actions or intruding into someone else's moral space (Etzioni, 1993; Sandel, 1996). Yet without moral direction, primary care providers' assumptions and practices may lead to abuses of power through their presuming to know best what patients need, stigmatizing them with labels that imply deficits, or neglecting to consider social injustices (Prilleltensky, 1997).

Commitment to Change

The ethical decisions that primary care providers make on a daily basis emerge within a particular political context. Although the Affordable Care Act of 2010 includes some landmark provisions to support prevention, at present, health care policy is fragmented and fails to make use of the variety of strategies available to influence health-promoting behaviors of individuals and institutions, as has been discussed throughout *Prevention Practice in Primary Care*.

The political environment, increasingly conservative and polarized, reflects a move away from "comprehensive" governmental solutions and toward incremental approaches in which a few problems are tackled at a time as an increasingly difficult bipartisan consensus is built. At present, Congress tends to model this practice.

Thus the leadership for comprehensive health promotion must arise from among those most interested in it. A comprehensive national health policy that is fully implemented and funded is needed to achieve equity in access to clinical prevention services. Even more critical is an equitable sharing of society's basic health determinants: nutritious food, basic education, safe water, decent housing, secure employment, adequate income, and peace (McBeath, 1991). Leadership from all sectors—government, insurers, health care organizations, academic researchers, communities, and primary care providers in partnership with patients and their families—is vital to ensuring fair allocation of these resources. The focus of health care professionals concerned with prevention—and health promotion *writ large*—must continue to move society toward the broadest aims of social justice so that all may be healthy.

CONCLUSIONS

In this final Chapter, the profound sociodemographic changes resulting from the aging of the population have been outlined. In addition, accountability for performance in the provision of services and applying evidence-based interventions will remain strong themes for future practice, as health care costs continue to rise. Payment reform is thus key to future change in primary care prevention. Personalizing prevention, based on an increasing knowledge of a patient's genome will pose profound ethical questions in daily practice. Social justice—ensuring accessible and equitable care for society's most vulnerable—should remain a core value for primary care providers, even as the challenge of promoting health in partnership with their patients remains a daunting one.

REFERENCES

Ali A, Hossain M, Hovsepian K, Rahman M, Kumar S. SmokeTrack: automated detection of cigarette smoking in the Mobile Environment from Respiration. Proceedings of the 11th International Conference on Information Processing in Sensor Networks. Beijing, China: ACM; 2012, pp. 269–280.

Altekruse SF, Kosary CL, Krapcho M, et al., eds. *SEER Cancer Statistics Review, 1975–2007*. National Cancer Institute. Published 2010. Accessed August 3, 2011, from http://seer.cancer.gov/csr/1975_2007/.

American Medical Informatics Association. *Frequently Asked Questions*. Accessed May 13, 2012, from http://www.amia.org/about/faqs/f7.html.

Archer D. No competition: the price of a highly concentrated health care market. *Health Affairs* blog posting, March 6, 2013. Accessed January 13, 2013, from 2013/03/06/no-competition-the-price-of-a-highly-concentrated-health-care-market/

Ashford A, Gemson D, Sheinfeld Gorin S, Bloch S, Lantigua R, Ahsan H, Neugut AI. Cancer screening and prevention practices of inner city physicians. *Am J Prev Med*. 2000;19:59–62.

Avorn J. AD History Part III: the future of academic detailing. *Academic Detailing Today* newsletter, Fall/Winter 2012.

Balas EA, Boren SA. Managing clinical knowledge for health care improvement. In: *Yearbook of Medical Informatics*, pp. 65–70. Bethesda, MD: National Library of Medicine; 2000.

Baquet CR, Horm JW, Gibbs T, Greenwald P. Socioeconomic factors and cancer incidence among blacks and whites. *J Am Cancer Inst*. 1991;83:553–557.

Bartel CA. Social comparisons in boundary-spanning work: effects of community outreach on members' organizational identity and identification. *Admin Sci Q*. 2001;46:379–413.

Bigby J, Holmes MD. Disparities across the breast cancer continuum. *Cancer Causes Control*. 2005;16(1):35–44

Biglan A, Glasgow RE. The social unit: an important facet in the design of cancer control research. *Prev Med*. 1991;20(2):292–305.

Block G, Patterson B, Subar A. Fruit, vegetables, and cancer prevention: a review of the epidemiologic evidence. *Nutr Cancer*. 1992;18:1–29.

Block G, Thompson FE, Hartman AM, Larkin FA, Guire KE: Comparison of two dietary questionnaires validated against multiple dietary records collected during a 1-year period. *J Am Diet Assoc*. 1992;92:686–693.

Block G, Woods M, Potosky A, Clifford C: Validation of a self-administered diet history questionnaire using multiple diet records. *J Clin Epidemiol* 1990;43:1327–1335.

Bookman E, Langehorne A, Eckfeldt J, Glass K, Jarvik G, Klag M, Koski G, Motulsky A, Wilfond B, Manolio T, Fabsitz R, Luepker R. Reporting genetic results in research studies: summary and recommendations of an NHLBI working group. *Am J Med Genet A* 2006;140A:1033–1040.

Brown LS. *Subversive Dialogues: Theory in Feminist Therapy*. New York: Basic Books; 1994.

Brownstein JN, Bone LR, Dennison CR, Hill MN, Kim MT, Levine DM. Community health workers as interventionists in the prevention and control of heart disease and stroke: review article. *Am J Prev Med*. 2005;29(5)Suppl 1:128–133.

Buchwald D, et al. Attitudes of urban american indians and alaska natives regarding participation in research. *J Gen Intern Med*. 2006;21:648–651.

Burhansstipanov L, Hampton J, Higgins C. Issues in cancer data and surveillance for American Indian and Alaska Native populations. *J Registry Management*. 1999;26(4):153–157.

Burhansstipanov L. Cancer mortality among Native Americans. *Cancer*. 1998;83(11):2247–2250.

Car J, Gurol-Urganci I, de Jongh T, Vodopivec-Jamsek V, Atun R. Mobile phone messaging reminders for attendance at healthcare appointments. *Cochrane Database of Systematic Reviews*. 2012;7:CD007458.

Casperson CJ. Physical activity epidemiology: concepts, methods and applications to exercise science. *Exercise Sports Sci Rev*. 1989;17:423–473.

Cassileth BR. Clinical trials: time for action. *J Clin Oncol*. 2003;21:765–766.

Ceballos R, Newcomb P, Beasley J, Petersen S, Templeton A, Hunt J. Willingness to disclose genetic status to family members: acomparison of colon cancer cases and relatives. *Genet Test Mol Biomark*. 2008;12(3):415–420.

Center on Budget and Policy Priorities. *Policy Basics: Where Do Our Federal Tax Dollars Go?* Revised August 13, 2012. Accessed January 13, 2013, from http://www.cbpp.org/cms/index.cfm?fa=view&id=1258.

Centers for Disease Control and Prevention. *Inventory of Managed Care Projects for FY 1995–1996*. Atlanta, GA: Author; 1996.

Centers for Disease Control and Prevention. Prevention and managed care: Opportunities for managed care organizations, purchasers of health care, and public health agencies. *MMWR*. 1995;44(RR-14):1–12.

Cervantes RC, Gilbert MJ, Salgado de Snyder N, Padilla AM. Psychosocial and cognitive correlates of alcohol use in younger adult immigrant and U.S.-born Hispanics. *Int J Addict*. 1990;25:687–708.

Charlton BG, White M. Living on the margin: a salutogenic model for socio-economic differentials in health. *Public Health*. 1995;109:235–243.

Christianson JB, Leatherman S, Sutherland K. Lessons from evaluations of purchaser pay-for-performance programs. a review of the evidence. *Med Care Res Rev*. December 2008;65(6):suppl.5S–35S.

Christensen CM, Bohmer R, Kenagy J. Will disruptive innovations cure health care? *Harvard Business Review*, 2000.

Cobb N, Paisano R. Patterns of cancer mortality among Native Americans. *Cancer*. 1998;83(11):2377–2383.

Congressional Budget Office. *Analysis of a Proposal to Offer a Public Plan Through the New Health Insurance Exchanges*. 2010. Accessed January 13, 2013, from http://www.cbo.gov/publication/21654.

Congressional Budget Office. *The 2012 Long-Term Budget Outlook*. June 2012. Accessed January 13, 2013, from http://www.cbo.gov/sites/default/files/cbofiles/attachments/06-05-Long-Term_Budget_Outlook_2.pdf

Cram P, Fendrick AM, Inadomi J, Cowen ME, Carpenter D, Vijan S. The impact of a celebrity promotional campaign on the use of colon cancer screening: the Katie Couric effect. *Arch Intern Med*. 2003 Jul 14;163(13):1601–1605.

Crinicker A. A competitive analysis of most favored nations clause in contracts between health care providers and insurers. *NCL Review*. 1990–1991;69:863.

Cuzick J, et al. Tamoxifen-induced reduction in mammographic density and breast cancer risk reduction: a nested case-control study. *J. Natl Cancer Inst*. 2011;103:744–752.

Daschle T. Creating a workforce for the new health care world. *Health Affairs blog*, March 7, 2013.

Dayal HH, Power RN, Chiu C. Race and socioeconomic status in survival from breast cancer. *J Chron Dis*. 1982;35:675–683.

Decensi A, et al. Metformin and cancer risk in diabetic patients: a systematic review and meta-analysis. *Cancer Prev. Res*. 2010;3:1451–1461.

Dentzer S. America's health deficit: dying from policy neglect. *Health Affairs*. March 2013;32(3):446.

Dressler LG. Disclosure of research results from cancer genomic studies: state of the science. *Clin Cancer Res*. 2009;15(13):4270–4276. doi:10.1158/1078-0432. ccr-08-3067.

Dreyfuss JH. Tamoxifen infrequently used by women at risk for breast cancer. *CA Cancer J Clinic*. 2010;60: 204–206.

Edwards BK, Ward E, Kohler BA, et al. Annual report to the nation on the status of cancer, 1975–2006, featuring colorectal cancer trends and impact of interventions (risk factors, screening, and treatment) to reduce future rates. *Cancer*. 2010;116(3):544–573.

Ellis PM. Attitudes towards and participation in randomised clinical trials in oncology: a review of the literature. *Ann Oncol*. 2000;11:939–945.

Emken BA, Li M, Thatte G, Lee S, Annavaram M, Mitra U, et al. Recognition of physical activities in overweight

Hispanic youth using KNOWME Networks. *J Phys Activ Health.* 2012;9:432–441.

Eng E, Young R. Lay health advisors as community change agents. *J Fam Comm Health.* 1992;15:24–40.

Ennis SR, Ríos-Vargas M, & Albert NG. *The Hispanic Population: 2010: 2010 Census Brief.* May 2011. Accessed January 15, 2013, from: http://www.census.gov/prod/cen2010/briefs/c2010br-04.pdf.

Epstein JA, Botvin GJ, Diaz T. Alcohol use among Dominican and Puerto Rican adolescents residing in New York City: role of Hispanic group and gender. *J Dev Behav Pediatr.* 2001;22:113–118.

Etzioni A. *The Spirit of Community.* New York: Touchstone; 1993.

Eysenbach G. Consumer health informatics. *BMJ.* 2000 June 24;320(7251):1713–1716.

Fabsitz R, McGuire A, Sharp R, Puggal M, Beskow L, Biesecker L, Bookman E, Burke W, Burchard E, Church G, Clayton E, Eckfeldt J, Fernandez C, Fisher R, Fullerton S, Gabriel S, Gachupin F, James C, Jarvik G, Kittles R, Leib J, O'Donnell C, O'Rourke P, Rodriguez L, Schully S, Shuldiner A, Sze R, Thakuria J, Wolf S, Burke G. Ethical and practical guidelines for reporting genetic research results to study participants. Updated guidelines from a National Heart, Lung, and Blood Institute Working Group. *Circ Cardiovasc Genet.* 2010;3:574–580.

Federal Trade Commission and Department of Justice. *Improving Health Care: A Dose of Competition.* 2004. Accessed January 13, 2013, from http://www.justice.gov/atr/public/health_care/204694.htm.

Field AE, Byers T, Hunter DJ, Laird NM, Manson JE, Williamson DF, Willett WC, Colditz GA. Weight cycling, weight gain, and risk of hypertension in women. *Am J Epidemiol.* 1999;150:573–579.

Fisher B, et al. Tamoxifen for prevention of breast cancer: report of the National Surgical Adjuvant Breast and Bowel Project P-1 Study. *J. Natl Cancer Inst.* 1998;90:1371–1388.

Fisher B, et al. Tamoxifen for the prevention of breast cancer: current status of the National Surgical Adjuvant Breast and Bowel Project P-1 study. *J. Natl Cancer Inst.* 2005; 97, 1652–1662.

Frakt A. How much do hospitals cost shift? a review of the evidence. *Milbank Q.* 2011 March;89(1).

Free C, Phillips G, Felix L, Galli L, Patel V, Edwards P. The effectiveness of M-health technologies for improving health and health services: a systematic review protocol. *BMC Research Notes.* 2010:3:25.

Free C, Phillips G, Watson L, Galli L, Felix L, et al. The effectiveness of mobile-health technologies to improve health care service delivery processes: a systematic review and meta-analysis. *PLoS Med* 2013;10(1): e1001363.

Galbraith JK. *The Good Society.* Boston: Houghton Mifflin; 1996.

Gans KM, Burkholder GJ, Upegui DI, Risica PM, Lasater TM, Fortunet R. Comparison of baseline fat-related eating behaviors of Puerto Rican, Dominican, Colombian, and Guatemalan participants who joined a cholesterol education project. *J Nutr Educ Behav.* 2002;34:202–210.

Ginsburg P. Can hospitals and physicians shift the effects of cuts in Medicare reimbursement to private payers? *HealthAffairs* 2003; Suppl Web Exclusives:W3-472-9.

Glasgow RE, Steiner JF. Comparative effectiveness research to accelerate translation: recommendations for an emerging field of science; In: Brownson RC, Colditz GA, Proctor EK, eds. *Dissemination and Implementation Research in Health: Translating Science to Practice.* Oxford Scholarship Online, 2012.

Glassman AH, Shapiro PA. Depression in the course of coronary artery disease. *Am J Psychiat.* 1998;155: 4–11.

Goodwin et al. Why mHealth? Presentation at mHealth Summer Institute 7/30/2012, http://obssr.od.nih.gov/mHealth_Summer_2012/Presentations/7_31_2012_Principles_of_mHealth_Desigh_III.pdf.

Gordon-Larsen P, Harris KM, Ward DS, Popkin BM. Acculturation and overweight-related behaviors among Hispanic immigrants to the US: The National Longitudinal Study of Adolescent Health. *Soc Sci Med.* 2003;57:2023–2034.

Graves KD, Sinicrope PS, Esplen MJ, Peterson SK, Patten CA, Lowery J, Sinicrope FA, Nigon SK, Borgen J, Sheinfeld Gorin, S, Keogh L, Lindor NM. Communication of genetic test results to family and health care providers following disclosure of research results. *Genetics in Medicine* epub October 3, 2013. Accessed October 3, 2013 from: http://www.nature.com/gim/journal/vaop/ncurrent/abs/gim2013137a.html.

Green LV, Savin S, Lu Y. Primary care physician shortages could be eliminated through use of teams, nonphysicians, and electronic communication. *Health Aff.* January 2013;32(1):11–19.

Green RC, Berg JS, Berry GT, Biesecker LG, Dimmock DP, Evans JP, Grody WW, Hegde MR, Kalia S, Korf BR, Krantz I, McGuire AL, Miller DT, Murray MF, Nussbaum RL, Plon SE, Rehm HL, Jacob HJ. Exploring concordance and discordance for return of incidental findings from clinical sequencing. *Genet Med.* 2102;14(4):405–410.

Greenberg D. NIH resists research funding linked to patient load. *Lancet.* 1997; 349: 1229.

Grieco E, Cassidy R. *Overview of Race and Hispanic Origin: Census 2000 Brief.* Washington, DC: US Department of Commerce, Economics and Statistics Administration, US Bureau of the Census; 2001.

Gross CP, Herrin J, Wong N, Krumholz HM. Enrolling older people in cancer trials: the effect of sociodemographic, protocol, and recruitment center characteristics. *J Clin Oncol.* 2005;23:4755–4763.

Grube M, Kaufman K, York R. Decline in utilization rates signals a change in the inpatient business model. *Health Affairs blog*, March 8, 2013.

Guralink JM, Land KC, Blszer D, Fillenbaum GG, Branch LG. Educational status and active life expectancy among older blacks and whites. *New Engl J Med*. 1993;329:110–116.

Haan M, Kaplan GA, Camacho T. Poverty and health: prospective evidence from the Alameda County study. *Am J Epidemiol*. 1987;125:989–999.

Harris JM, Salasche SJ, Harris RB. Can Internet-based continuing medical education improve physicians' skin cancer knowledge and skills? *J Gen Intern Med*. 2001;16:50–56.

Hartman M, Martin AB, Benson J, Catlin A. National health expenditure accounts team. national health spending in 2011: overall growth remains low, but some payers and services show signs of acceleration. *Health Affairs*. 2013;32(1):87–99.

Health Insurance for the Aged Act (Medicare Act), 42 U.S.C. §§ 301 et seq. (1994).

Health Resources and Services Administration. http://www.integration.samhsa.gov/about-us.

Heck JE, Franco R, Jurkowski JM, Sheinfeld Gorin S. Awareness of genetic testing for canceramong United States Hispanics: the role of acculturation. *Community Genetics*. 2008;11:36-42.

Herrman H. The need for mental health promotion. *Aust NZ J Psychiat*. 2001;35:709–715.

Hodge F, Weinmann S, Roubideaux Y. Recruitment of American Indians and Alaska Natives into clinical trials. *Ann Epid*. 2000;10:S41–S48.

Holahan J, Blumberg LJ, McMorrow S, Zuckerman S, Waidmann T, Stockley K. *Containing the Growth of Spending in the US Health System*. The Urban Institute Health Policy Center. October 2011. Accessed January 13, 2013, from http://www.urban.org/uploadedpdf/412419-Containing-the-Growth-of-Spending-in-the-US-Health-System.pdf.

Holmes JH, Lehman A, Hade E, et al. Challenges for multilevel health disparities research in a transdisciplinary environment. *Am J Prev Med*. 2008;35(2 suppl):S182–S192.

Innes A, Campion P, Griffiths F. Complex consultations and the edge of chaos. *Br J Gen Pract*. 2005;55:47–52.

Institute of Medicine; Smedley BD, Stith AY, Nelson AR, eds. *Unequal Treatment: Confronting Racial and Ethnic Disparities in Health Care*. Washington, DC: National Academies Press; 2003.

Institute of Medicine. *Crossing the Quality Chasm: A New Health System for the 21st century*. Washington: National Academies Press; 2001.

Institute of Medicine. *Delivering High-Quality Cancer Care: Charting a New Course for a System in Crisis*. Washington, DC: The National Academies Press; 2013.

Institute of Medicine. *Health Insurance Is a Family Matter*. Washington, DC: National Academies Press; 2002.

Institute of Medicine. *Policy Issues in the Development of Personalized Medicine in Oncology: Workshop Summary*. 2010. Accessed January 2013 from http://www.nap.edu/catalog.php?record_id=12779

Institute of Medicine. *Promoting Health: Intervention Strategies from Social and Behavioral Research*. Washington, DC: National Academies Press; 2000.

Institute of Medicine. *Retooling for an Aging America: Building the Health Care Workforce*. Washington: National Academies Press; 2008.

Institute of Medicine. *The Second Fifty Years: Promoting Health and Preventing Disability*. Washington, DC: National Academies Press; 1990.

Brownstein JN, Chowdhury FM, Norris SL, Horsley T, Jack L Jr, Zhang X, Satterfield D. Effectiveness of community health workers in the care of people with hypertension. *Am J Prev Med*. 2007;32(5):435–447.

Justice J. *Cancer in American Indians and Alaska Natives*. Tucson, AZ; Native American Research and Training Center; 1990.

Kaiser Family Foundation. *Health Coverage for Low-Income Children*. 2007. Accessed January 13, 2013, from http://www.allhealth.org/briefingmaterials/HealthCoverageForLow-IncomeChildren-530.pdf.

Kaufman D, Murphy J, Scott J, Hudson K. Subjects matter: asurvey of public opinions about a large genetic cohort study. *Genet Med*. 2008;10(11):813–839.

Keogh LA, Fisher D, Sheinfeld Gorin S, Schully SD, Lowery JT, Ahnen DJ, Maskiell JA, Lindor NM, Hopper JL, Burnett T, Holter S, Arnold JL, Gallinger S, Laurino M, Esplen MJ, Sinicrope PS, Colon Cancer Family Registry. How do researchers manage genetic results in practice? The experience of the multinational Colon Cancer Family Registry. *J Community Genetics* May 24, 2013 (published online). Accessed May 24, 2013 from: http://www.ncbi.nlm.nih.gov/pubmed/23703702.

Kernick D. Wanted—new methodologies for health service research. Is complexity theory the answer? *Family Practice*. 2006; 23: 385–390.

Kessler R, Glasgow RE. A proposal to speed translation of healthcare intervention research into practice: Dramatic change is needed. *Am J Prev Med*. 2011;40(6):637–644.

Kim J, et al. Breast density change as a predictive surrogate for response to adjuvant endocrine therapy in hormone receptor positive breast cancer. *Breast Cancer Res*. 2012;14, R102.

Klein EA, et al. Vitamin E and the risk of prostate cancer: the Selenium and Vitamin E Cancer Prevention Trial (SELECT). *JAMA*. 2011;306:1549–1556.

Koh HK, Sebelius KG. Promoting prevention through the Affordable Care Act. *New Engl J Medicine*. 2010;363:1296–1299.

Kollek R, Petersen I. Disclosure of individual research results inclinico-genomic trials: challenges, classification and criteria for decision-making. *J Med Ethics.* 2011;37:271–275.

Koplan JP, Livengood JR. The influence of changing demographic patterns on our health promotion priorities. *Am J Prev Med.* 1994;10(Suppl 1):42–44.

Kornblith AB, Kemeny M, Peterson BL, et al. Survey of oncologists' perceptions of barriers to accrual of older patients with breast carcinoma to clinical trials. *Cancer.* 2002;95:989–996.

Krist AH, Glenn AB, Glasgow RE, Balasubramanian B, Chambers DA, Fernandez M, Heurtin-Roberts S, Kessler R, Ory MG, Phillips SM, Ritzwoller DP, Roby DH, Rodriguez HP, Sabo RT, Sheinfeld Gorin S, Stange KC. Designing a valid randomized pragmatic primary care implementation trial: the my own health report (MOHR) project. *Implementation Science.* 2013;8:73.   http://www.implementationscience. com/content/8/1/73.

Kupersmith J. The privacy conundrum and genomic research: re-identification and other concerns. *Health Affairs.* September 11, 2013. Accessed September 11, 2013, from http://healthaffairs. org/blog/ 2013/09/ 11/the-privacy-conundrum-and-genomic-research-re-identification-and- other-concerns/.

LaVallie DL, Wolf FM, Jacobsen C, Buchwald D. Barriers to cancer clinical trial participation among Native elders. *Ethnicity Dis.* 2008;18(2):210–217.

Lewin R. *Complexity: Life on the Edge of Chaos.* London: Phoenix; 1993.

Lippman SM, et al. Effect of selenium and vitamin E on risk of prostate cancer and other cancers: the Selenium and Vitamin E Cancer Prevention Trial (SELECT). *JAMA.* 2009;301: 39–51.

Loria CM, Bush TL, Carroll MD, Looker AC, McDowell MA, Johnson CL, et al. Macronutrient intakes among adult Hispanics: a comparison of Mexican Americans, Cuban Americans, and mainland Puerto Ricans. *Am J Public Health.* 1995;85:684–689.

Love T, Burton C. General practice as a complex system: novel analysis of consultation data. *Fam Pract.* 2005;22:347–352.

Major LF, Turner MG. Assessing the information management requirements for behavioral health providers. *Journal of Healthcare Management / American College of Healthcare Executives.* 2003;48(5):323–333.

Mallin K, Anderson K. Cancer mortality in Illinois Mexican and Puerto Rican immigrants, 1979–1984. *Int J Cancer.* 1988;41:670–676.

Mannel RS, Walker JL, Gould N, et al. Impact of individual physicians on enrollment of patients into clinical trials. *Am J Clin Oncol.* 2003;26:171–173.

Marmot MG, Smith GD, Stansfeld S, Patel C, North F, Head J, et al. Health inequalities among British civil servants: the Whitehall II study. *Lancet.* 1991;337:1387–1393.

Marschollek M, Gietzelt M, Schulze M, Kohlmann M, Song B, Wolf KH. Wearable sensors in healthcare and sensor-enhanced health information systems: all our tomorrows? *Healthcare Informatics Res.* 2012;18:97–104.

McLellan AT, Lewis DC, O'Brien CP, Kleber HD. Drug dependence, a chronic medical illness: implications for treatment, insurance, and outcomes evaluation. *JAMA.* 2000 Oct 4;284(13):1689–1695.

Medicaid Act, 42 U.S.C. §§ 1396 et seq. (1994).

Medicare Payment Advisory Commission. *Report to the Congress: Medicare Payment Policy.* Washington, DC: Author; 2011.

Melnick GA, Shen YC, Wu VY. The increased concentration of health plan markets can benefit consumers through lower hospital prices. *Health Affairs.* 2011;30(9):1728–1733.

Meulenkamp T, Gevers S, Bovenberg J, Koppelman G, van Hylckama VA, Smets E. Communication of biobanks' research results: what do (potential) participants want? *Am J Med Genet.* 2010;152A(10):2482–2492.

Militello LK, Kelly SA, Melnyk BM. Systematic review of text-messaging interventions to promote healthy behaviors in pediatric and adolescent populations: implications for clinical practice and research. *Worldviews on Evidence-Based Nursing/Sigma Theta Tau International, Honor Society of Nursing.* 2012;9: 66–77.

Miller W, Crabtree B, McDaniel R, Strange K. Understanding change in primary care practice using complexity theory. *J Fam Pract.* 1998;46:369–376.

Mitchell P, Wynia M, Golden R, McNellis B, Okun S, Webb CE, Rohrbach V, Von Kohorn I. *Core Principles & Values of Effective Team-Based Health Care.* The Institute of Medicine: National Academies Press, October 2012. Accessed February 28, 2013, from http://www.iom.edu/~/media/Files/Perspectives-Files/2012/Discussion-Papers/VSRT-Team-Based-Care-Principles-Values.pdf.

Morrisey M. Competition in hospital and health insurance markets: a review and research agenda. *Health Services Res.* 2001;36(1, part 2):191–221.

Morrisey M. *Cost Shifting in Health Care: Separating Evidence from Rhetoric.* Washington, DC: AEI Press; 1994.

Morrisey M. *Hospital Cost Shifting: A Continuing Debate.* EBRI Issue Brief. December 1996; (180). Accessed January 2013 from: http://www.ebri.org/pdf/briefspdf/1296ib.pdf

Morrisey M. *Hospital Pricing: Cost Shifting and Competition.* EBRI Issue Brief. 1993;(137):1-17.

Morrisey M, Cawley J. Health economists' views of health policy. *J Health Polit Polic.* 2008;33:4.

Murthy VH, Krumholz HM, Gross CP. Participation in cancer clinical trials: race-, sex-, and age-based disparities. *JAMA.* 2004 Jun 9;291:2720–2726.

National Center for Health Statistics, NVSS, V60, N3, Dec. 29, 2011, Deaths, Final Data for 2009. Accessed

January 2013 from http://www.cdc.gov/nchs/data/nvsr/nvsr60/nvsr60_03.pdf.

National Center for Health Statistics. *2000 National Health Interview Survey Cancer Screening Public Use.* Hyattsville, MD: Author; 2000.

National Commission on Physician Payment Reform. Accessed March 4, 2013, from http://physicianpaymentcommission.org/wp-content/uploads/2013/03/physician_payment_report.pdf.

Naylor MD, Coburn KD, Kurtzman ET, et al. *Inter-Professional Team-Based Primary Care for Chronically Ill Adults: State of the Science.* Unpublished white paper presented at the ABIM Foundation meeting to Advance Team-Based Care for the Chronically Ill in Ambulatory Settings. Philadelphia, PA; March 24–25, 2010.

Nelson HD, et al. Systematic review: comparative effectiveness of medications to reduce risk for primary breast cancer. *Ann. Intern. Med.* 2009;151:703–715.

Newmann SJ, Garner EO. Social inequities along the cervical cancer continuum: a structured review. *Cancer Causes Control.* 2005;16(1):63–70.

O'Connor EA, Whitlock EP, Gaynes BN, Beil TL. *Screening for Depression in Adults and Older Adults in Primary Care: An Updated Systematic Review.* Evidence Synthesis No. 75. AHRQ Publication No. 10-05143-EF-1. Rockville, MD: Agency for Health Care Research and Quality; 2009.

Oh K, Hu FB, Cho E, Rexrode KM, Stampfer MJ, Manson JE, Liu S, Willett WC: Carbohydrate intake, glycemic index, glycemic load, and dietary fiber in relation to risk of stroke in women. *Am J Epidemiol.* 2005;161:161–169.

Organizacion Pan Americana de la Salud. *Pronunciamiento de consenso sobre politicas de atencion a los ancianos en America Latina* [Consensus statements about the policies regarding the elderly in Latin America]. Santiago: Centro Latinoamericano de Demografia, Central Internacional del Envejecimiento; 1992.

Ozols RF, Herbst RS, Colson YL, et al. Clinical cancer advances 2006: major research advances in cancer treatment, prevention, and screening—a report from the American Society of Clinical Oncology. *J Clin Oncol.* 2007;25(1):146–162.

Palmer RC, Schneider EC. Social disparities across the continuum of colorectal cancer: a systematic review. *Cancer Causes Control.* 2005;16(1):55–61.

Pappas G, Queen S, Hadden W, Fisher G. The increasing disparity in mortality between socioeconomic groups in the United States, 1960 to 1986. *New Engl J Med.* 1993;329:103–109.

Peikes D, Dale S, Lundquist E, Genevro J, Meyers D. *Building the Evidence Base for the Medical Home: What Sample and Sample Size Do Studies Need?* AHRQ Publication No. 11-0090-EF. Rockville, MD: Agency for Healthcare Research and Quality; September 2011.

Penninx BWJH, Guralnik JM, Paho, M, Ferrucci L, Cehan JR, Wallace RB, et al. Chronically depressed mood and cancer risk in older persons. *J Natl Cancer I.* 1998;90:1888–1893.

Penson RT, Seiden MV, Shannon KM, Lubratovich ML, Roche M, Chabner BA, Lynch TJ Jr. Communicating genetic risk: pros, cons, and counsel. *Oncologist* 2000;5:152–161.

Perez-Stable EJ, Ramirez A, Villareal R, Talavera GA, Trapido E, Suarez L, et al. Cigarette smoking behavior among US Latino men and women from different countries of origin. *Am J Public Health.* 2001;91:1424–1430.

Petereit DG, Burhansstipanov L. Establishing trusting partnerships for successful recruitment of American Indians to clinical trials. *Cancer Control.* 2008;15(3):260–268.

Pham HH, Schrag D, O'Malley AS, Wu B, Bach PB. Care patterns in Medicare and their implications for pay for performance. *New Eng J Med.* 2007; 356 (11):1130–1139.

Phillips KA, Morrison KR, Andersen R, Aday LA. Understanding the context of healthcare utilization: Assessing environmental and provider-related variables in the behavioral model of utilization. *Health Serv Res.* 1998;33:571–596.

Polen MR, Whitlock EP, Wisdom JP, Nygren P, Bougatsos C. *Screening in Primary Care Settings for Illicit Drug Use: Staged Systematic Review for the U.S. Preventive Services Task Force.* Evidence Synthesis No. 58, Part 1. (Prepared by the Oregon Evidence-based Practice Center under Contract No. 290-02-0024.) AHRQ Publication No. 08-05108-EF-s. Rockville, MD, Agency for Healthcare Research and Quality; January 2008.

Porter ME, Teisberg EO. Redefining competition in healthcare. *Harvard Business Review*, 2004. Accessed January 13, 2013, from http://hbr.org/web/extras/insight-center/health-care/redefining-competition-in-health-care.

Porter ME, Teisberg EO. *Redefining Health Care.* Boston, MA: Harvard Business Review Press; 2006.

Presidential Commissionfor the Study of Bioethical Issues. PRIVACY and PROGRESSin Whole Genome Sequencing. October 2012. Accessed February 2013 from http://bioethics.gov/sites/default/files/PrivacyProgress508_1.pdf.

Prilleltensky I. Values, assumptions, and practices: assessing the moral implications of psychological discourse and action. *Am Psychol.* 1997;52(5):517–535.

Reid BJ, Li X, Galipeau PC, Vaughan TL. Barrett's oesophagus and oesophageal adenocarcinoma: time for a new synthesis. *Nature Rev. Cancer.* 2010;10:87–101.

Reinhardt U. The pricing of US healthcare services: chaos behind a veil of secrecy. *Health Affairs* 2006;25(1):57–69. Accessed January 13, 2013, from http://healthaffairs.org/blog/2009/07/24/a-modest-proposal-on-payment-reform/.

Roberts J, Shalowitz D, Christnesen K, Everett J, Kim S, Raskin L, Gruber S. Returning individual results: development of a cancer genetics education and risk communication protocol. *J Empir Res Hum Res Ethics*. 2010;15(3):17–30.

Robinson JC. Consolidation and the transformation of competition in health insurance. *Health Affairs*. 2004;23(6):11–24.

Rosenwaike I, Shai D. Trends in cancer mortality among Puerto Rican-born migrants to New York City. *Int J Epidemiol*. 1986;15:30–35.

Ross S, Grant A, Counsell C, Gillespie W, Russell I, Prescott R. Barriers to participation in randomised controlled trials: a systematic review. *J Clin Epidemiol*. 1999;52:1143–1156.

Rothwell PM. Factors that can affect the external validity of randomised controlled trials. *PLoS Clin Trials*. 2006;1:e9.

Salonen JT. Socioeconomic status and risk of cancer, cerebral stroke, and death due to coronary heart disease and any disease: a longitudinal study in eastern Finland. *J Epidemiol Commun Health*. 1982;26:294–297.

Sandel MJ. *Democracy's Discontent: America in Search of a Public Philosophy*. Cambridge, MA: Harvard University Press; 1996.

Shapiro AK, Morris LA. The placebo effect in medical and psychological therapies. In: Bergin A, Garfield, S, eds. *Handbook of Psychology and Behavior Change*, pp. 369–410. New York: Wiley; 1978.

Shavers VL, Fagan P, McDonald P. Health disparities across the cancer continuum. *J Health Care Poor Underserved*. 2007;18(4 suppl):1–5.

Shavers VL, Lynch CF, Burmeister LF. Racial differences in factors that influence the willingness to participate in medical research studies. *Ann Epidemiol*. 2002;12:248–256.

Sheinfeld Gorin S. Colorectal cancer screening compliance among urban Hispanics. *J Behav Med*. 2005;28:125–137.

Sheinfeld Gorin S. Future directions for health promotion. In: Sheinfeld Gorin S, Arnold J, eds. *Health Promotion in Practice*, pp. 543–567. San Francisco, CA: Jossey-Bass, 2006.

Sheinfeld Gorin S. Models of health promotion. In: Sheinfeld Gorin S, Arnold J, eds. *Health Promotion in Practice*, pp. 21–66. San Francisco, CA: Jossey-Bass; 2006.

Sheinfeld Gorin S, Badr H, Krebs P, Prabhu Das I. Multilevel interventions and racial/ethnic health disparities. *J Natl Cancer I Monogr*. 2012;44:100–111.

Sheinfeld Gorin S, Gauthier J, Hays J, Miles A, Wardle J. Cancer screening and ageing: a research agenda. *Cancer*. 2008;113:3493–3504.

Sheinfeld Gorin S, Glenn B, Perkins RB. The human papillomavirus (HPV) vaccine and cervical cancer: uptake and next steps. *Advances in Therapy*. 2011;(28)8:615–639.

Sheinfeld Gorin S, Heck J. Cancer screening among Latino subgroups in the United States. *Prev Med*. 2005;40:515–526.

Sheinfeld Gorin S, Wang C, Raich P, Bowen DJ, Hay J. Decision making in cancer primary prevention and chemoprevention. *Ann Behav Med*. 2006;32(3):179–187.

Sherman KA, Miller SM, Shaw L, Cavanagh K, Sheinfeld Gorin S. Psychosocial approaches to participation in BRCA1/2 genetic risk assessment among African American women: a systematic review. *J Community Genetics* August 10, 2013 (published online). Accessed August 10, 2013 from: http://link.springer.com/article/10.1007/s12687-013-0164-y/fulltext.html.

Shim R, Rust G. Primary care, behavioral health, and public health: partners in reducing mental health stigma. *Am J Public Health*. 2013;103(5):774–776. doi: 10.2105/AJPH.2013.301214.

Shortliffe EH, Perrault L. *Medical Informatics: Computer Applications in Health Care*. Reading, MA: Addison-Wesley; 1990.

Siminoff LA, Zhang A, Colabianchi N, Sturm CM, Shen Q. Factors that predict the referral of breast cancer patients onto clinical trials by their surgeons and medical oncologists. *J Clin Oncol*. 2000;18:1203–1211.

Smith M, Saunders R, Stuckhardt L, McGinnis JM, eds. Committee on the Learning Health Care System in America, Institute of Medicine. *Best Care at Lower Cost: The Path to Continuously Learning Health Care in America*. Washington, DC: National Academies Press; 2012.

Somkin CP, Altschuler A, Ackerson L et al. Organizational barriers to physician participation in cancer clinical trials. *Am J Manag Care*. 2005;11:413–421.

Speck RM, Hill RK, Pronk NP, Becker MP, Schmitz KH. Assessment and outcomes of HealthPartners 10,000 Steps program in an academic work site. *Health Promot Pract*. 2010;11:741–750.

Steele VE, Lubet RA. The use of animal models for cancer chemoprevention drug development. *Semin. Oncol.* 2010;37:327–338.

Subar AF, Thompson FE, Kipnis V, Midthune D, Hurwitz P, McNutt S, McIntosh A, Rosenfeld S. Comparative validation of the Block, Willett, and National Cancer Institute Food Frequency Questionnaires: The Eating at America's Table Study. *Am J Epidemiol* 2001;154:1089–1099.

Susswein LR, Skrzynia C, Lange LA, Booker JK, Graham ML, 3rd, Evans JP. Increased uptake of BRCA1/2 genetic testing among African American women with a recent diagnosis of breast cancer. *J Clin Oncol*. 2008;26 (1):32-36. doi: 26/1/32[pii]10.1200/JCO.2007.10.6377.

The NSABP Study of Tamoxifen and Raloxifene (STAR) P-2 trial. *JAMA*. 2006;295:2727–2741.

The Office of the National Coordinator for Health IT (ONC) Meaningful Use Stage II requirements. Accessed May 12, 2012, from: http://www.healthit.gov/policy-researchers-implementers/meaningful-use.

The Patient Protection and Affordable Care Act, P.L. 111–148, March 23, 2010.

The Women's Health Initiative Study Group. Design of the Women's Health Initiative clinical trial and observational study. *Control Clin Trials.* 1998;19: 61–109.

Thompson FE, Subar AF, Brown CC, Smith AF, Sharbaugh CO, Jobe JB, Mittl B, Gibson JT, Ziegler RG. Cognitive research enhances accuracy of food frequency questionnaire reports: results of an experimental validation study. *J Am Diet Assoc.* 2002;102: 212–225.

Thompson IM, et al. The influence of finasteride on the development of prostate cancer. *N. Engl. J. Med.* 2003;349:215–224.

Tyroler HA. Socioeconomic status in the epidemiology and treatment of hypertension. *Hypertension.* 1989;13(Suppl. 1):194–197.

Umar A, Dunn K, Greenwald P. Future directions in cancer prevention. *Nature Reviews: Cancer.* 2012;12:835–848.

US Bureau of the Census. Health Insurance Statistics: Low Income Uninsured by State. 2004. Retrieved December 3, 2012, from http://www.census.gov/hhes/hlthins/liuc03.html.

US Bureau of the Census. *The Hispanic Population of the United States: Population Characteristics.* Washington, DC: Author; 2000.

US Department of Health and Human Services, IHS. *Regional Differences in Indian Health 1998–99.* Rockville, MD: Department of Health and Human Services, Indian Health Service; 2000.

US Department of Health and Human Services, Public Health Service. *Healthy People 2000: Midcourse Review and 1995 Revisions.* Washington, DC: US Government Printing Office; 1995.

US Preventive Services Task Force. *Guide to Clinical Preventive Services.* 2nd ed. Alexandria, VA: International Medical Publishing; 2009.

US Senate Special Committee on Aging, American Association of Retired Persons, Federal Council on the Aging, and US Administration on Aging. *Aging America: Trends and Projections.* Washington, DC: US Government Printing Office; 1991.

Visvanathan K, et al. American society of clinical oncology clinical practice guideline update on the use of pharmacologic interventions including tamoxifen, raloxifene, and aromatase inhibition for breast cancer risk reduction. *J. Clin. Oncol.* 2009;27: 3235–3258.

Vogel VG, et al. Update of the National Surgical Adjuvant Breast and Bowel Project Study of Tamoxifen and Raloxifene (STAR) P-2 Trial: preventing breast cancer. *Cancer Prev. Res.* 2010;3:696–706.

Wagner EH, Bennett SM, Austin BT, Greene SM, Schaefer JK, Vonkorff M. Finding common ground: patient-centeredness and evidence-based chronic illness care. *J Altern Complem Med.* 2005;11: S7–S15.

Waldrop M. *Complexity: The Emerging Science at the Edge of Order and Chaos.* London: Penguin; 1992.

Warshauer ME, Silverman DT, Schottenfeld D, Pollack ES. Stomach and colorectal cancers in Puerto Rican–born residents of New York City. *J Natl Cancer I.* 1986;76, 591–595.

Waters EA, McNeel TS, Stevens WM, Freedman AN. Use of tamoxifen and raloxifene for breast cancer chemoprevention in 2010. *Breast Cancer Res Treat.* 2012 Jul;134(2):875–880.

Welch HG, Black WC. Overdiagnosis in cancer. *J. Natl Cancer Inst* 2010;102:605–613.

Wells KB, Stewart A, Hays RD, Burnam A, Rogers, W, Daniels M, et al. The functioning and well-being of depressed patients. *JAMA.* 1989;262:914–919.

Wicks P, Pickard T, Francke U, Swan M. Crowdsourced health research studies: an important emerging complement to clinical trials in the public health research ecosystem. *J Med Internet Res.* 2012;14(2):e46.

Wideroff L, Vadaparampil TS, Breen N, Croyle RT, Freedman AN. Awareness of genetic testing for increased cancer risk in the year 2000 National Health Interview Survey. *Community Genet.* 2003;6:147–156.

Willett WC, Stampfer MJ, Underwood BA, Speizer FE, Rosner B, Hennekens CH. Validation of a dietary questionnaire with plasma carotenoid and alpha-tocopherol levels. *Am J Clin Nutr.* 1983;38:631–639.

Winkleby MA, Fortmann SP, Rockhill B. Health-related risk factors in a sample of Hispanics and whites matched on sociodemographic characteristics: The Stanford Five-City Project. *Am J Epidemiol.* 1993;137: 1365–1375.

Winkleby MA, Jatulis DE, Frank E, Fortmann SP. Socioeconomic status and health: How education, income, and occupation contribute to risk factors for cardiovascular disease. *Am J Public Health.* 1992;82: 816–820.

Wisner KL, Sit DKY, McShea MC, Rizzo DM, Zoretich RA, Hughes CL, Eng HF, Luther JF, Wisniewski SR, Costantino ML, Confer AL, Moses-Kolko EL, Famy CS, Hanusa BH. Onset timing, thoughts of self-harm, and diagnoses in postpartum women with screen-positive depression findings. *JAMA Psychiatry.* 2013;70:490–498. doi: 10.1001/jamapsychiatry.2013.87.

Wolf JA, Moreau JF, Akilov O, Patton T, English JC, Ho J, Ferris LK. Diagnostic inaccuracy of smartphone applications for melanoma detection. *JAMA Dermatol.* 2013;149(4):422–426.

Wolf SM, Crock BN, Van Ness B, Lawrenz F, Kahn JP, Beskow LM, Cho MK, Christman MF, Green RC, Hall R, Illes J, Keane M, Knoppers BM, Koenig BA, Kohane IS, LeRoy B, Maschke KJ, McGeveran W, Ossorio P, Parker LS, Petersen GM, Richardson HS,

Scott JA, Terry SF, Wilfond BS, Wolf WA. Managing incidental findings and research results in genomic research involving biobanks and archived datasets. *Genet Med.* 2012;14(4):361–384.

Woolf SH, Aron L, eds. Panel on Understanding Cross-National Health Differences Among High-Income Countries; Committee on Population; Division of Behavioral and Social Sciences and Education; National Research Council; Board on Population Health and Public Health Practice; Institute of Medicine. *U.S. Health in International Perspective: Shorter Lives, Poorer Health.* Washington, DC: National Academies Press; 2013.

Wu Y, Chang EY, Chang KCC, & Smith JR. Kevin Chen-Chuan Chang. Optimal multimodal fusion for multimedia data analysis. *ACM.* 2004;572–579.

Zaheer A, McEvily B, Perrone V. Does trust matter? Exploring the effects of interorganizational and interpersonal trust on performance. *Org Sci.* 1998;9(2):141–159.

Zurovac D, Sudoi RK, Akhwale WS, Ndiritu M, Hamer DH, Rowe AK, Snow RW. The effect of mobile phone text-message reminders on Kenyan health workers' adherence to malaria treatment guidelines: a cluster randomised trial. *Lancet.* 2011;378(9793):795–803.

INDEX